Sterile Processing Technical Manual

Ninth Edition

Disclaimer

This publication is designed to provide accurate and authoritative information in regard to the subject matter covered. It is sold with the understanding that the publisher is not engaged in rendering legal, accounting or other professional services. The authors are solely responsible for the contents of this publication. All views expressed herein are solely those of the authors and do not necessarily reflect the views of the Healthcare Sterile Processing Association (HSPA). Nothing contained in this publication shall constitute a standard or recommendation from HSPA. HSPA also disclaims any liability with respect to the use of any information, procedure or product, or reliance thereon by any member of the healthcare industry.

By the Healthcare Sterile Processing Association
55 West Wacker Drive, Suite 501
Chicago, IL 60601

The Healthcare Sterile Processing Association is a not-for-profit corporation that provides educational and certification programs and support for healthcare Sterile Processing professionals. For more information about HSPA, visit www.myhspa.org.

Printed in the United States of America

ISBN: 979-8-3507-0521-8

Contents

Sterile Processing Technical Manual

Ninth Edition

Chapter 1

Introduction to Sterile Processing

Learning Objectives

As a result of successfully completing this chapter, the reader will be able to:

1. Explain the importance of the Sterile Processing department, with an emphasis on the service provided and the role of Sterile Processing in quality patient care
2. Review the workflow process in an organized Sterile Processing department
3. Identify basic knowledge and skills required for Sterile Processing technicians
4. Define job responsibilities of Sterile Processing technicians
5. Discuss the roles of education and training in the field of Sterile Processing profession

INTRODUCTION

The majority of medical procedures require the use of supplies, instruments and/or equipment. Some items are used once and then discarded, while others are reused multiple times. Reusable items must be thoroughly cleaned, inspected, disinfected and/or sterilized before they can be used to treat other patients. The Sterile Processing department (SPD) in a healthcare facility performs these important reprocessing activities.

Advancing Technologies

Medical technology is rapidly advancing. The medical devices used in the Operating Room (OR) and throughout the healthcare facility have changed dramatically over the years. (See **Figure 1.1**) As these devices become more complex, the same can be said of the methods required to reprocess them. (See **Figure 1.2**)

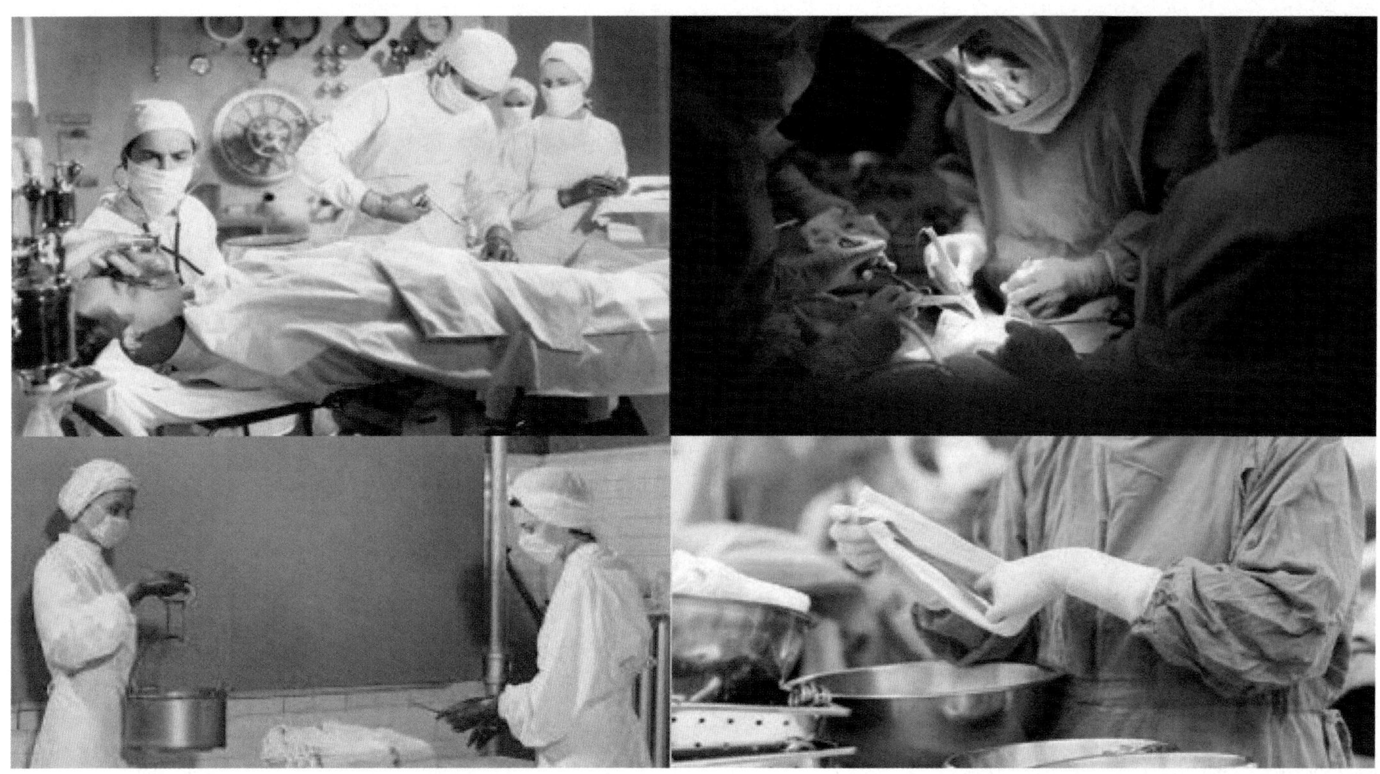

Figure 1.1 Operating Room advancements

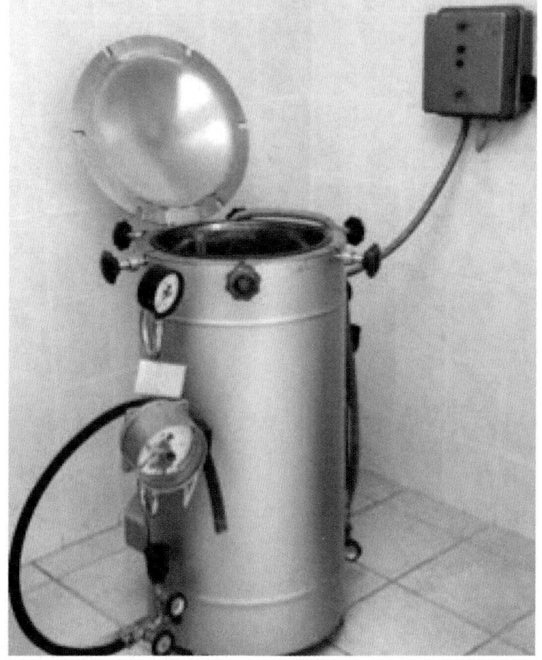

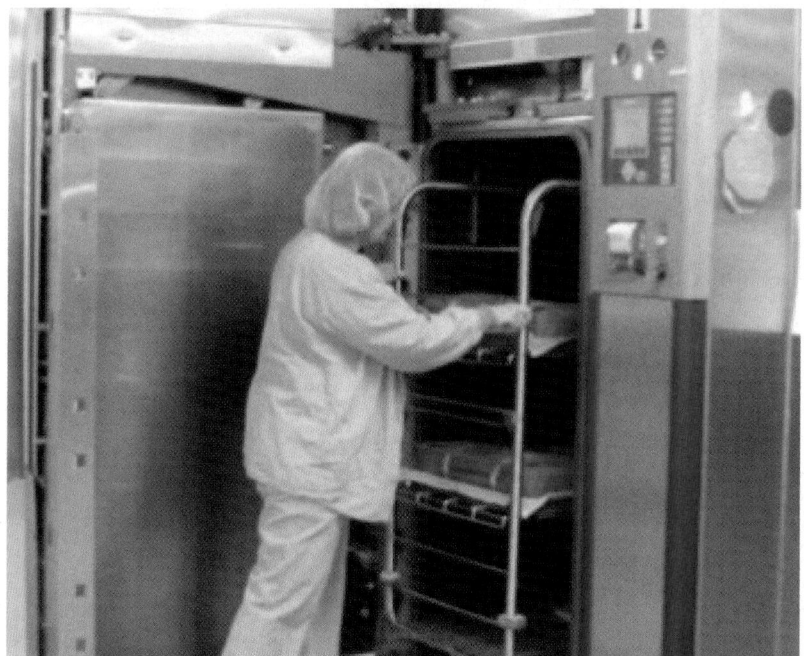

Figure 1.2 Sterile Processing advancements

Like the entire medical field, the Sterile Processing (SP) profession has evolved significantly. The advances experienced in patient treatment and care have come with advances in the medical devices used to provide those services. Today's increasingly sophisticated medical devices require more complex handling and processing, which has resulted in many changes for SP technicians. These changes have not happened overnight but have been introduced steadily throughout the past years. For example, one need only to look back a short time to identify changes that have enabled increases in **minimally invasive surgery (MIS)**. (See **Figure 1.3**) These procedures provide many benefits to patients, including shortened hospital stays, smaller incisions, reduced trauma and shorter recovery times. These procedures require complex instrumentation, which requires complex processing protocols.

Medical technologies will continue to advance, devices will become more complex and SP technicians will be required to keep up with advances. This chapter will introduce the field of SP and provide an overview of the knowledge and skills required to meet the demand for timely, safe and functional medical devices.

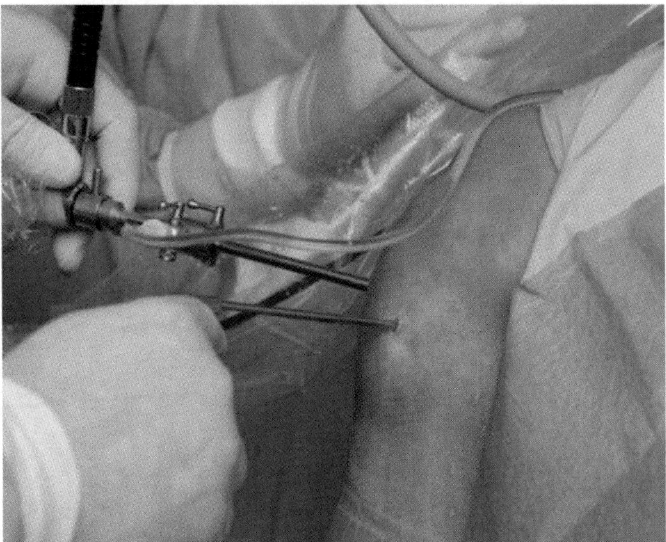

Figure 1.3 Example of a minimally invasive procedure (arthroscopy)

Minimally invasive surgery (MIS) A surgical procedure performed in a manner that causes little or no trauma or injury to the patient; it is often performed through a cannula using lasers, endoscopes or laparoscopes. Compared with other procedures, minimally invasive procedures involve smaller incisions, less tissue damage and bleeding, smaller amounts of anesthesia, less pain and minimal scarring.

What's in a Name? Central Processing, Sterile Processing, Surgical Supply and Processing

SPD goes by many names. No matter the name, the department supports caregiver departments by processing reusable medical devices. Many SPDs dispense sterile supplies for performing patient procedures and some departments also provide medical equipment for patient use.

This vital department is an important part of the facility's infection prevention and quality processes throughout many patient care areas.

STERILE PROCESSING WORKFLOW

The SPD is the central location for the delivery of soiled (used) medical devices and the distribution of clean and sterile items. In order to provide a safe working environment, facilities should implement processes and procedures with specific workflows for medical devices to help ensure safety. Soiled materials must be isolated from their clean counterparts to ensure acceptable processing conditions. A one-way flow of materials from the soiled area to the clean processing area and on to the sterile storage area is required. (See **Figure 1.4**)

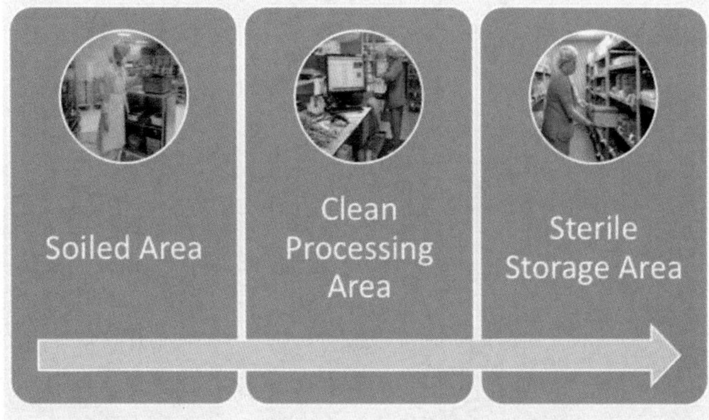

Figure 1.4 One-way flow

To facilitate one-way flow of goods and maintain distinction between soiled and clean work areas, physical barriers or walls are used to separate the functional areas of the SPD. These areas include decontamination, preparation and packaging (prep and pack), sterilization and sterile storage/distribution.

Decontamination

Decontamination is the physical or chemical process that renders an inanimate object—such as a medical device that may be contaminated with harmful microbes—safe for further handling. The decontamination area is where all soiled instruments from the OR are received, along with other items such as medical equipment. Instrumentation and medical equipment can be collected from different places within the healthcare facility [e.g., Labor and Delivery (L&D), the Emergency Department (ED) and patient care units like the Intensive Care Unit (ICU)]. When medical devices are received, they must be properly sorted, disassembled and **cleaned** using established protocols. (See **Figure 1.5**) All items returned to the decontamination area are considered contaminated and potentially infectious. Decontamination is an important process because items cannot be considered sterile or high-level disinfected if they are not effectively cleaned; therefore, cleaning is the first step in the sterilization process. An effective cleaning process may be accomplished with manual and/or mechanical cleaning techniques. SP technicians must have an in-depth knowledge of the items to be cleaned in this area and must select the appropriate method of decontamination as recommended by the device manufacturer. After thorough cleaning, many items in the decontamination area will be sent to the preparation and packaging area for further processing.

> **Decontamination** To make safe by removing or reducing contamination by infectious organisms or other harmful substances to an acceptable level.
>
> **Cleaning** The removal of all visible and non-visible soil and any other foreign material from medical devices being processed.

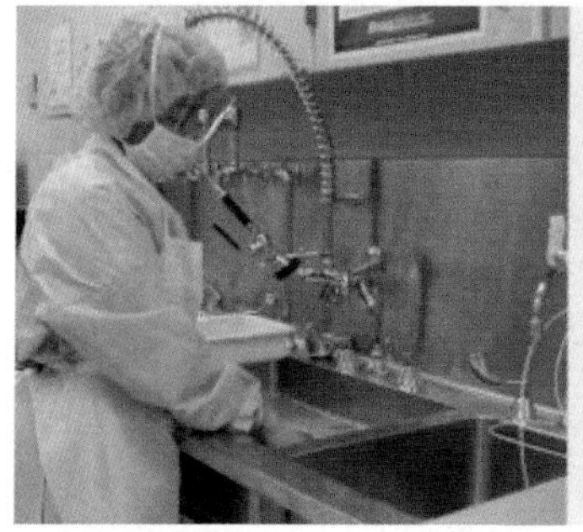
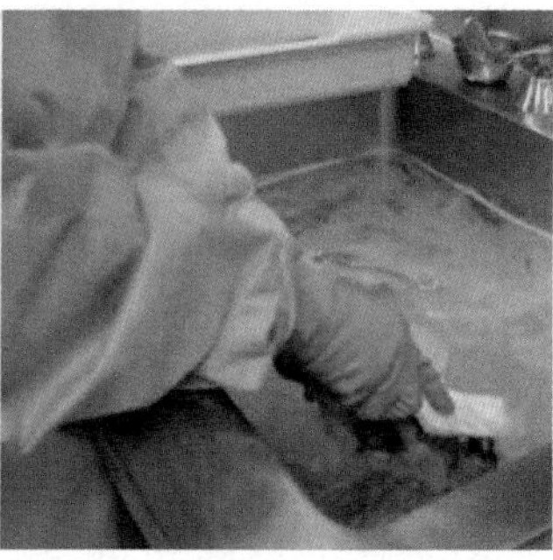

Figure 1.5 Manual cleaning in the decontamination area

Working in the decontamination area requires a thorough knowledge and understanding of microbiology and the decontamination process. SP staff must be able to identify and clean a wide variety of medical devices. Knowledge about cleaning and disinfecting agents and their use is critical. Protocols for waste disposal, transportation of contaminated items and operation of equipment used in the cleaning process, including washer-disinfectors, ultrasonic cleaners, cart washers, steam guns and specialty washers, is required. (See **Figure 1.6**)

SP technicians working in the decontamination area must be protected from the environment. The physical layout of this area, as well as cleaning equipment used in it, must meet the appropriate standards of governmental agencies and the recommendations of professional organizations. Policies and procedures must be developed and followed to ensure that work practices minimize employee injury and exposure to pathogens. To meet the facility's and the Occupational Safety and Health

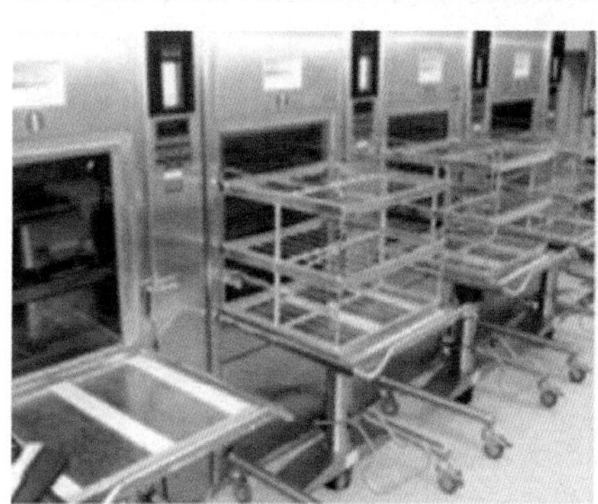
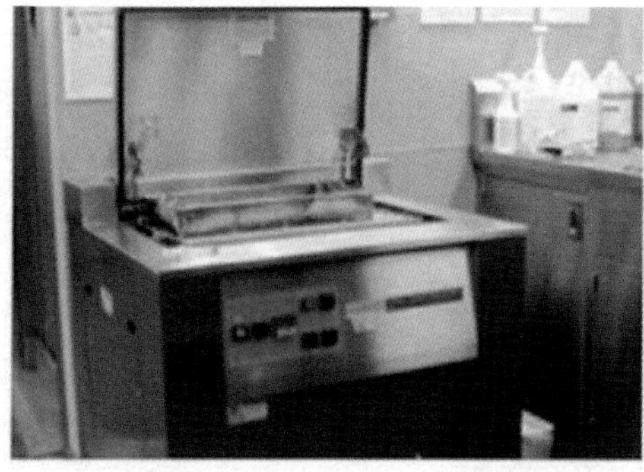
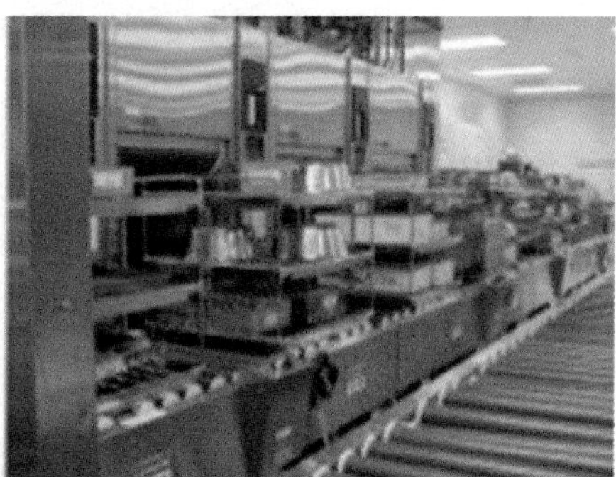
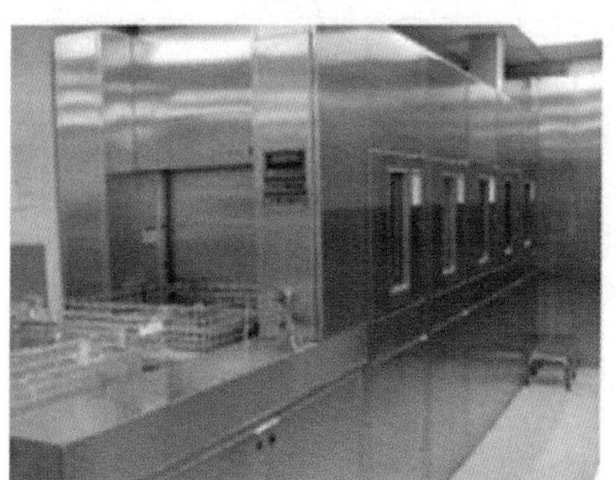
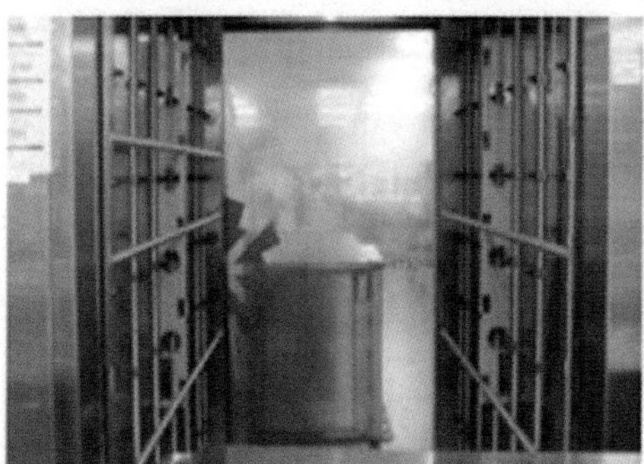
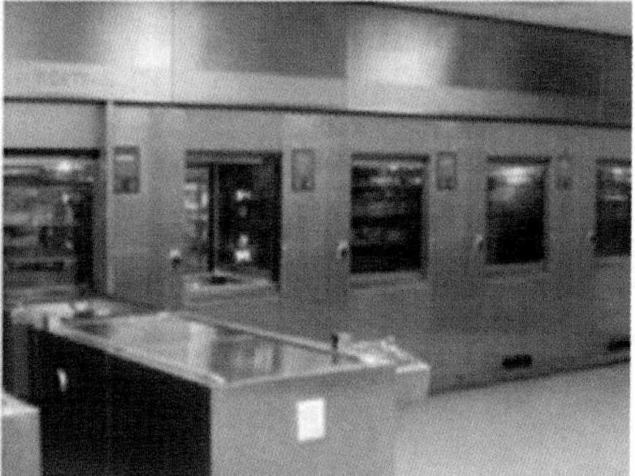

Figure 1.6 Examples of mechanical cleaners in the decontamination area

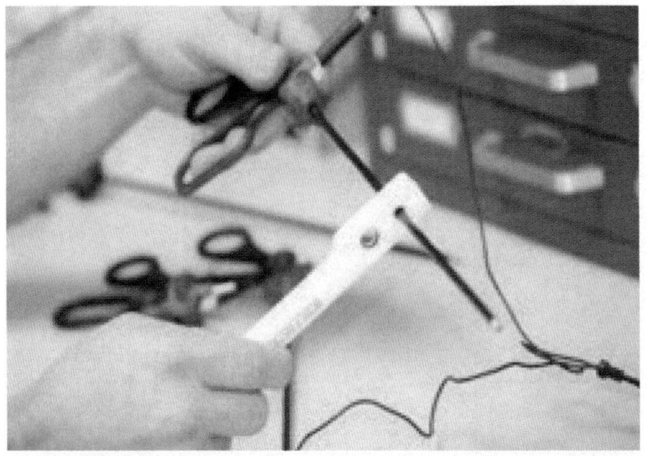

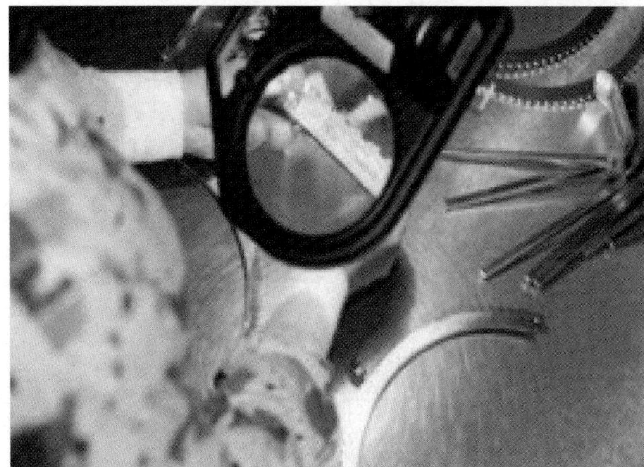

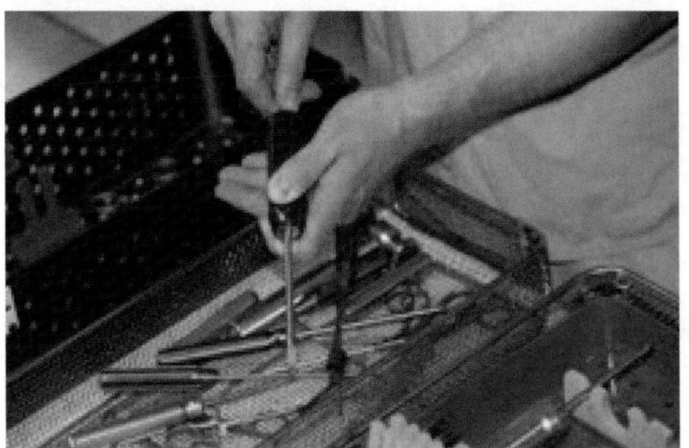

Figure 1.7 Instrument inspection processes

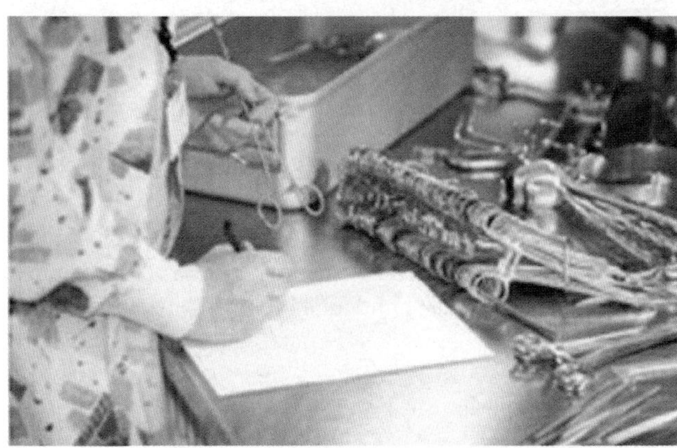

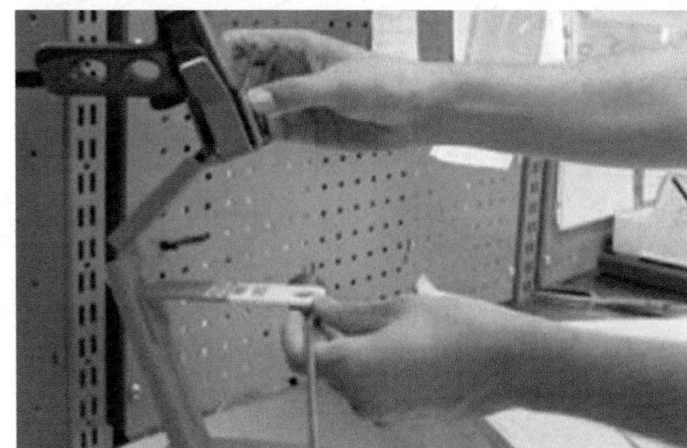

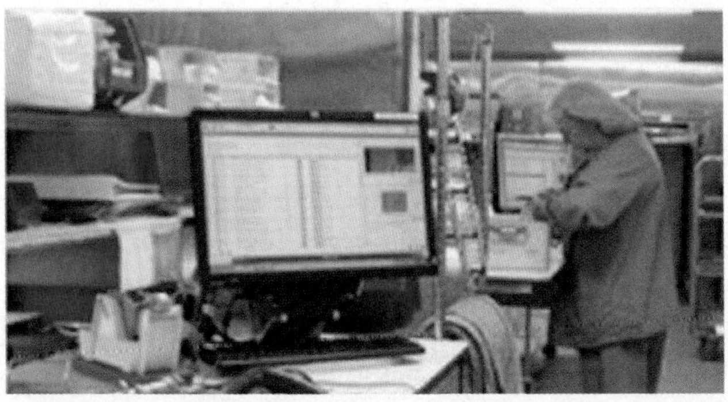

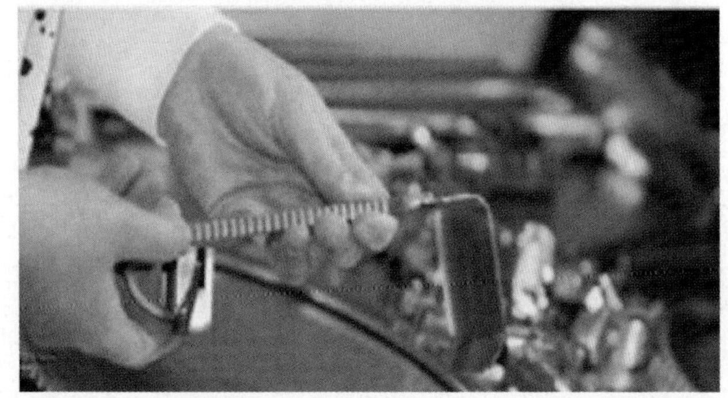

Figure 1.8 Instrument assembly processes

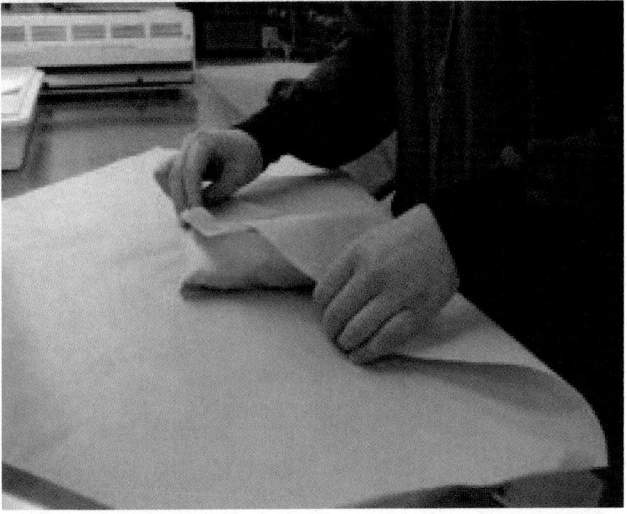

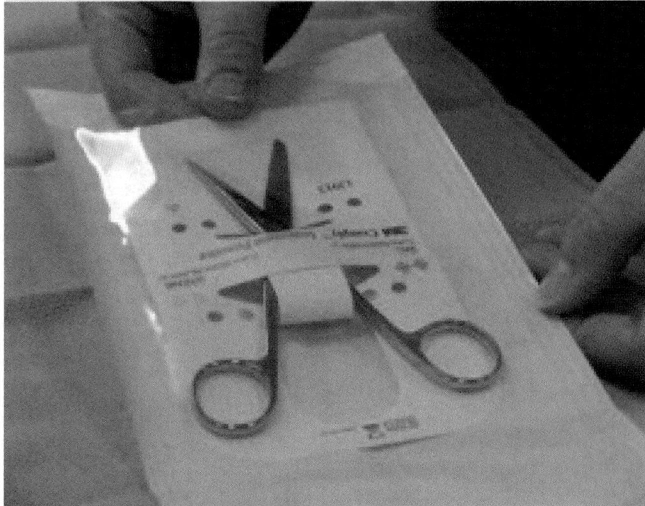

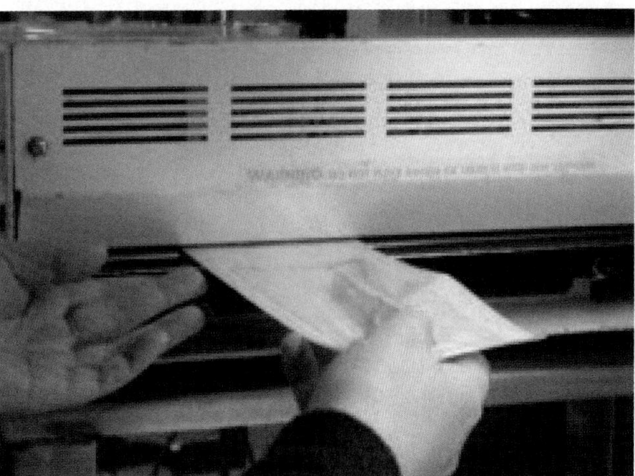

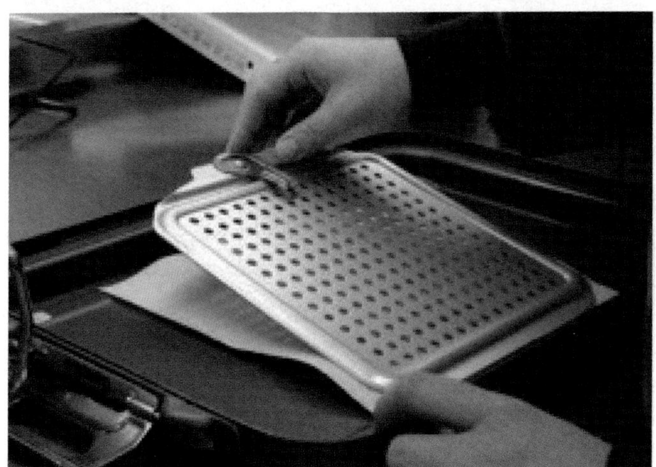

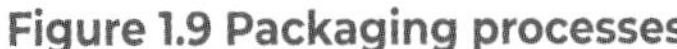

Figure 1.9 Packaging processes

Administration's (OSHA's) safety requirements, SP technicians must wear special attire, called **personal protective equipment (PPE).** PPE minimizes exposure to bloodborne pathogens and other contaminants. PPE includes a fluid-resistant facemask, eye protection, a fluid-resistant cover gown, general purpose utility gloves and fluid-resistant shoe covers.

> **Personal protective equipment (PPE)** A part of Standard Precautions for all healthcare workers to prevent skin and mucous membrane exposure when in contact with blood and body fluids of any patient. PPE includes fluid-resistant protective clothing, disposable gloves, eye protection, face masks and shoe covers.

Preparation and Packaging

After items are safe for handling, they are delivered to the prep and pack area of the SPD. Each item should be carefully inspected for cleanliness, proper function and possible defects. Instruments and other devices should be inspected, packaged and labeled in preparation for sterilization.

SP technicians must be able to identify thousands of surgical instruments. They must understand how instruments are manufactured, how they are constructed, how to test them and how to best maintain them. It is essential that SP professionals have the knowledge and training to maintain instruments properly, consistently and safely. (**Figures 1.7** and **1.8** provide examples of inspection and assembly activities.)

Surgical specialty instruments, equipment and implants also require special knowledge and expertise. SP technicians must be able to select the proper packaging system and use proper techniques for packaging items for sterilization. (See **Figure 1.9**)

Sterilization

Items to be sterilized must be properly identified and the correct methods and parameters for **sterilization** must be followed according to the manufacturer's **instructions for use (IFU)**. The

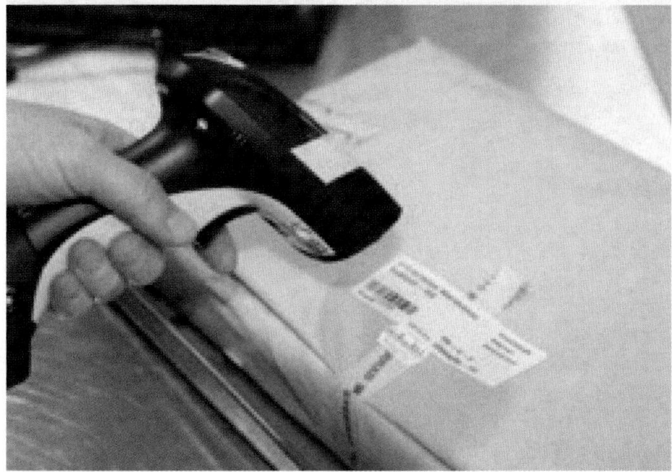

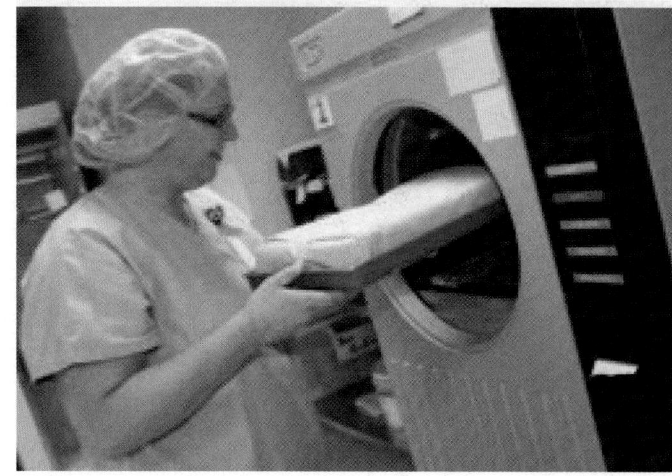

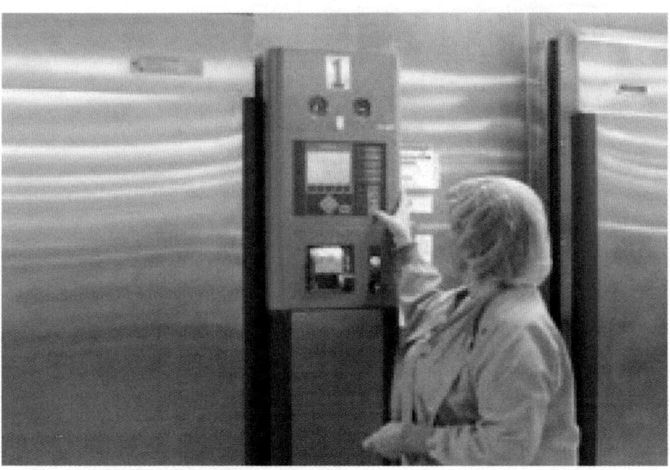

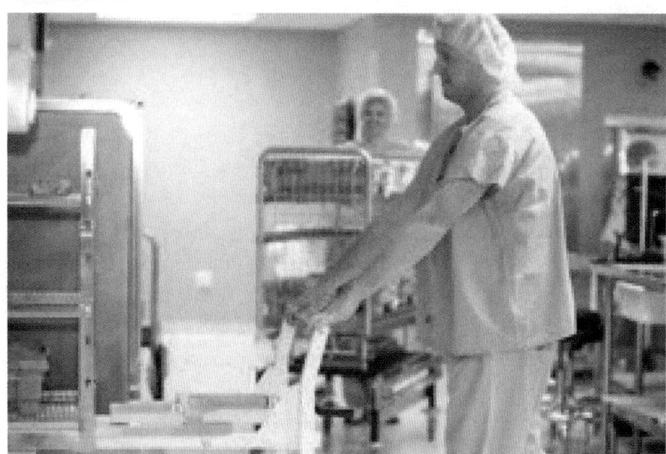

Figure 1.10 Examples of sterilization activities

principles necessary to achieve sterilization must be understood and applied. Sterilizers must be loaded and operated properly, and sterilization quality assurance measures must be followed to help ensure that sterilization parameters have been met. Records must be maintained, and SP technicians must be aware of factors that can compromise sterile packaging. (See **Figure 1.10**)

Sterilization Process by which all forms of microbial life, including bacteria, viruses, spores and fungi, are completely destroyed.

Instructions for use (IFU) Information provided by a device manufacturer that provides detailed instructions on how to properly use and/or process the device.

Personnel working in the preparation, packaging and sterilization areas of SP must wear facility-required attire such as a scrub suit and hair coverings. It is essential that SP technicians diligently adhere to dress codes and safe work practices to protect the environment from contamination.

Sterile Storage and Distribution

The supply area of SP is dedicated to the storage of sterile instruments and clean or sterile supplies. A separate area for removing supplies from shipping cartons and containers should be provided. The major portion of the work in this area involves receiving, storing and dispensing supplies and sterile instruments. (See **Figure 1.11**)

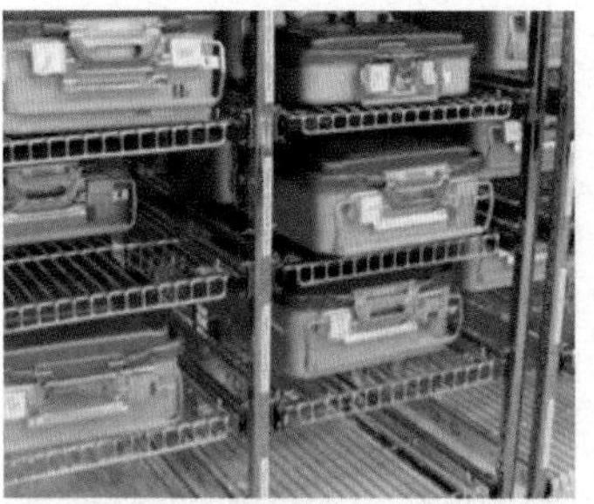

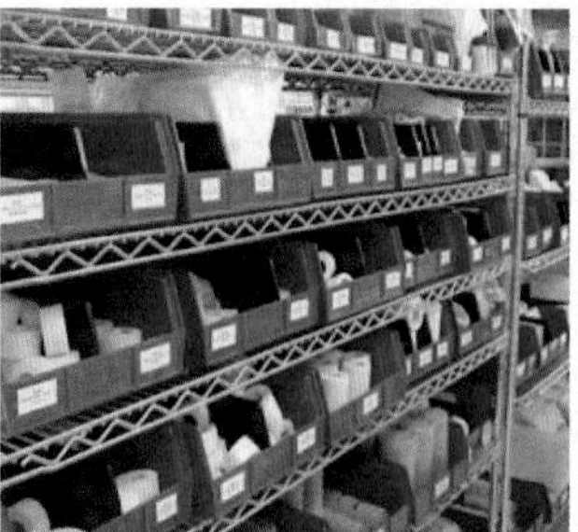

Figure 1.11 Sterile storage areas

While items may be dispensed to almost all departments within a healthcare facility, the major focus of this area is servicing the

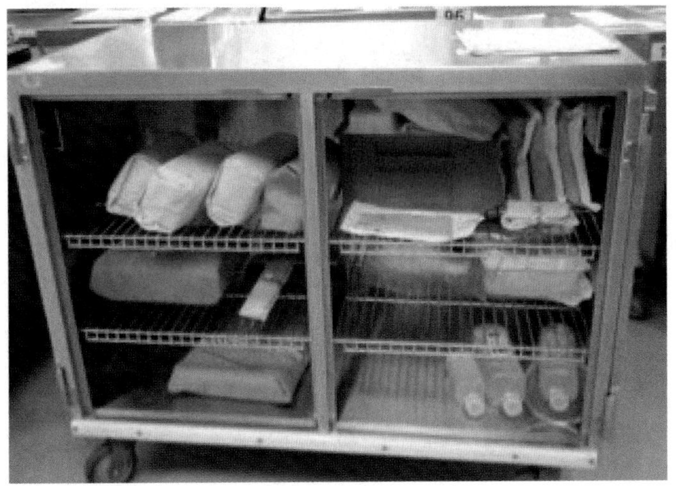

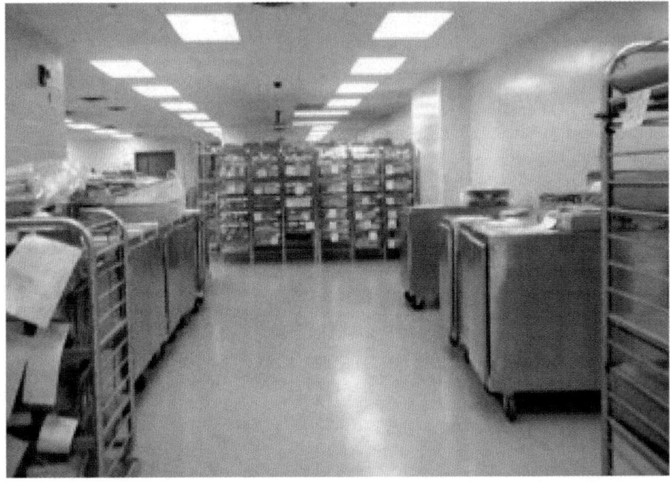

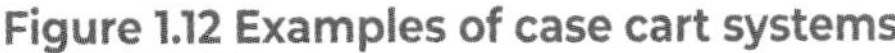

Figure 1.12 Examples of case cart systems

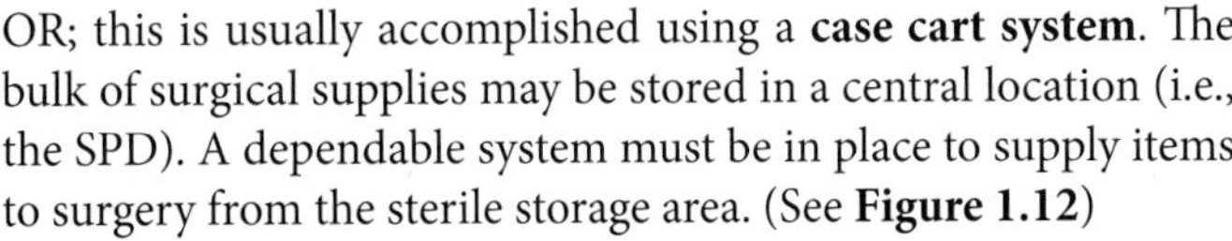

OR; this is usually accomplished using a **case cart system**. The bulk of surgical supplies may be stored in a central location (i.e., the SPD). A dependable system must be in place to supply items to surgery from the sterile storage area. (See **Figure 1.12**)

Surgical procedures are usually scheduled through a surgery scheduling office using a special computer program. When surgical procedures are scheduled, authorized personnel assign a **case cart** or **doctor's (physician's) preference card** to each procedure. This generates a **case cart pull sheet (pick list)** that identifies items specific to the doctor and procedure. SP technicians use this sheet to place supplies from the sterile storage area onto the case carts that transport these items to the appropriate OR/surgical suite. Personnel working in this area usually gather instruments and supplies needed for all scheduled surgical procedures during the day or evening before they will be used.

Other areas within the healthcare facility may be supplied from the sterile storage area. Also, facility personnel from different departments frequently require items that are only available from SP. Those working in the sterile storage area must be familiar with all supplies within the location in order to provide fast and accurate customer service.

Open lines of communication must be maintained between those in SP and sterile storage areas to help ensure that an adequate stock of sterile items is always available. Also, the **Supply Chain Management** department, also known as the Materials Management department, is an important link in the supply process; therefore, effective communication and problem-solving skills must be fostered between personnel in these two important departments.

Case cart system An inventory control system for products/equipment typically used in an OR that involves use of an enclosed or covered cart (generally prepared for one surgical case and not used for general supply replenishment).

Case cart A cart prepared for an individual procedure. Case carts usually contain all instruments, supplies and utensils needed for a specific procedure.

Doctor's (physician's) preference card A document that identifies a physician's needs (requests and preferences) for a specific medical procedure. Preference cards usually contain information regarding the instruments, equipment, supplies and utensils used by a specific physician. They may also include reminders for the staff of the physician's preferences regarding patient draping, instruments and supplies.

Case cart pull sheet (pick list) A list of specific supplies, utensils and instruments for a specific procedure. SP technicians use these lists to assemble the items needed for individual procedures.

Supply Chain Management Department that procures and distributes resources and manages supplies, goods and services to providers and patients.

Personnel working in the sterile storage area must have thorough knowledge of every item, how it is used, where it is located, and the process for obtaining it. Other knowledge and skills include those needed for:

- Inventory control and supply distribution
- Surgical specialties and procedures
- Sterile storage and handling requirements

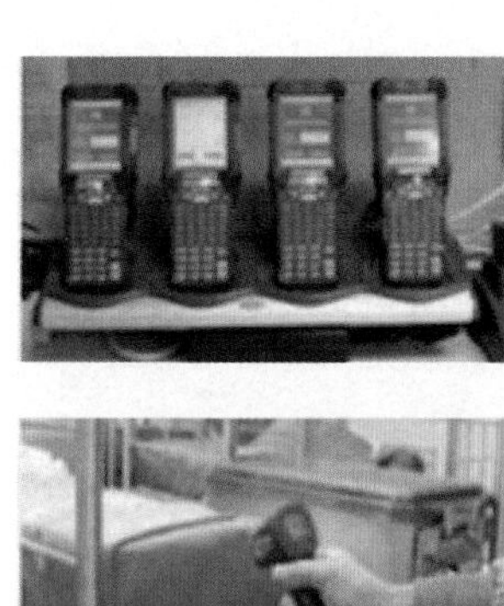
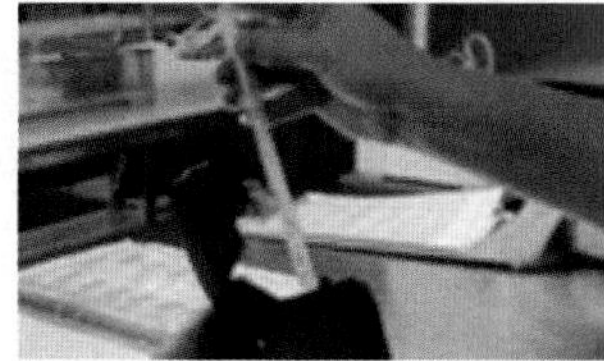
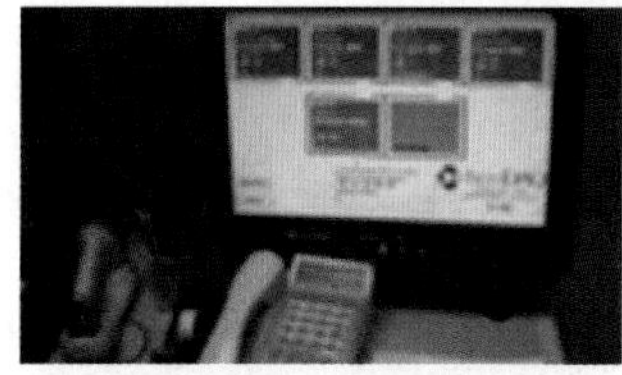
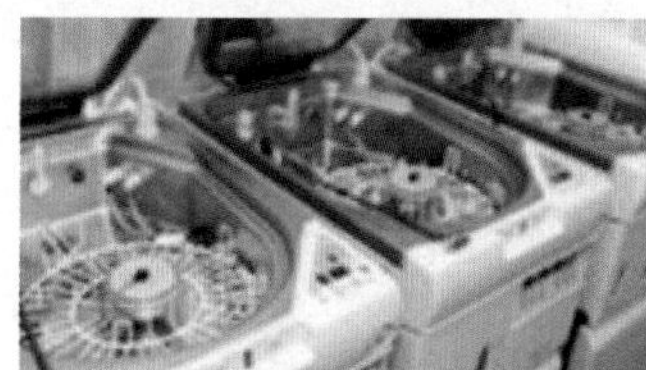
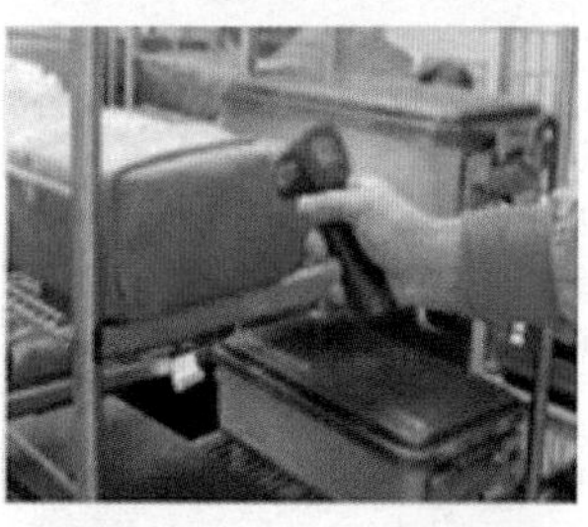
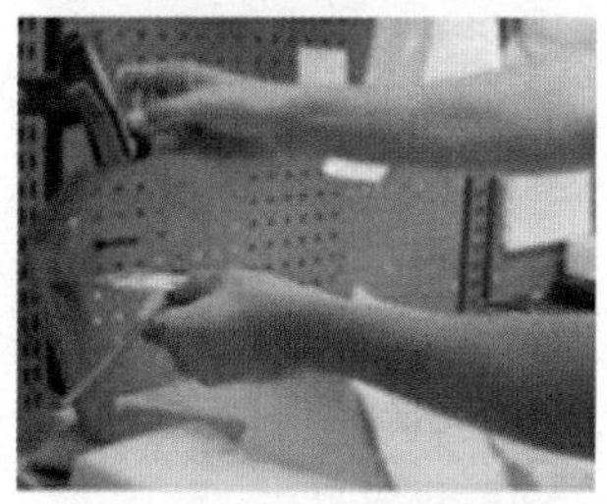
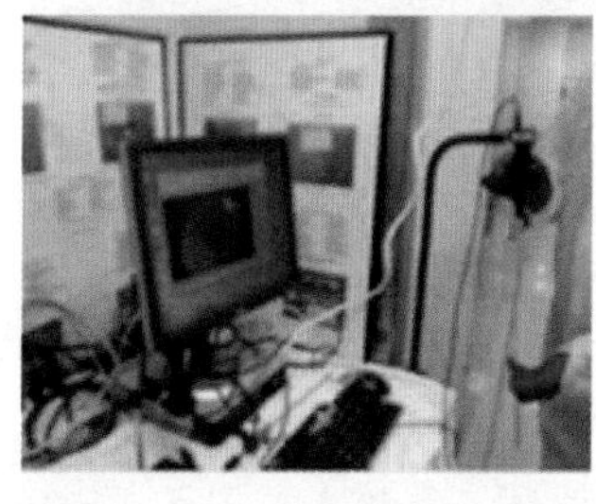
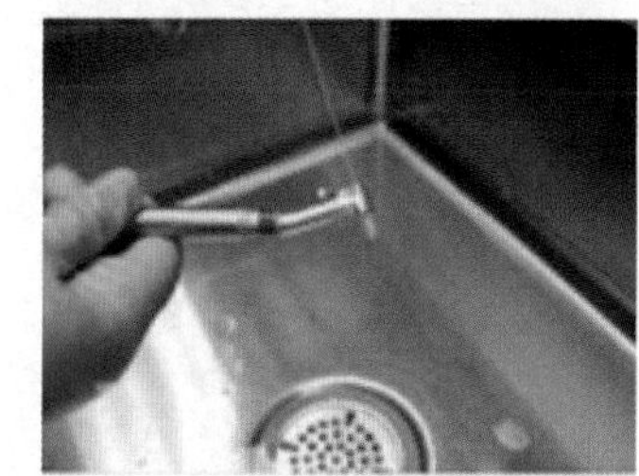
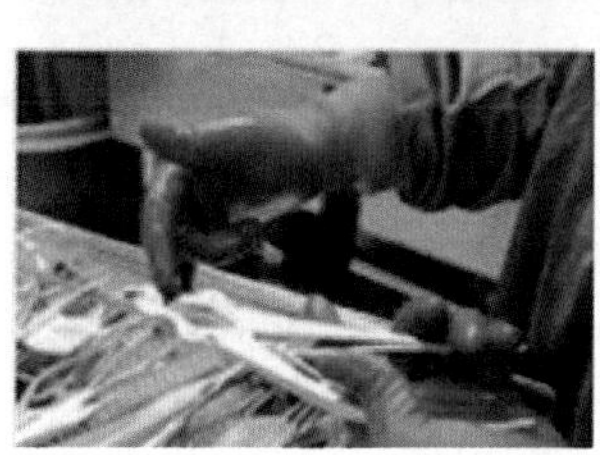
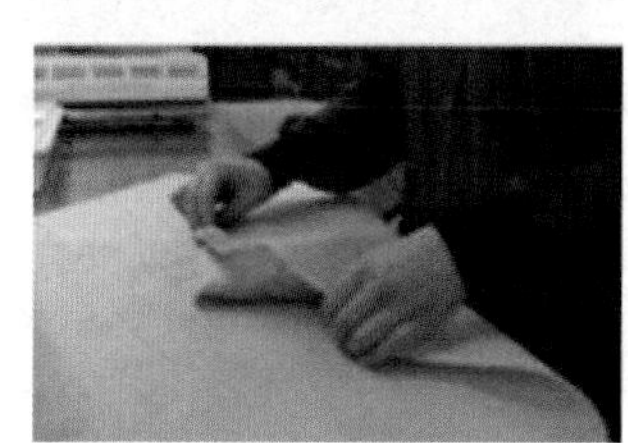
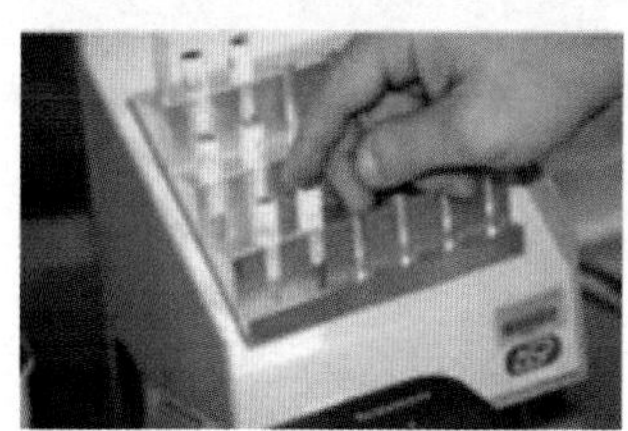
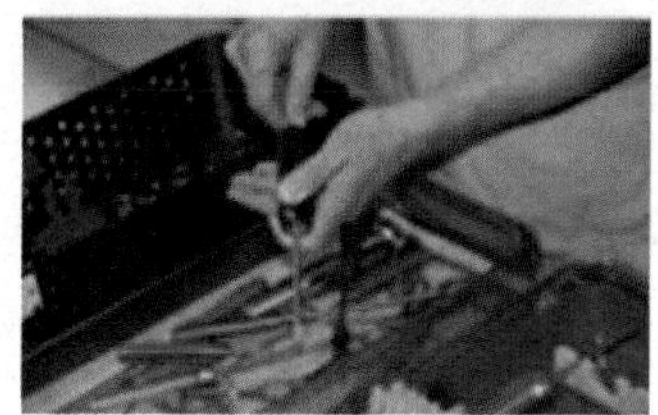

Figure 1.14 The tasks performed by Sterile Processing technicians require specialized skills.

- Computer systems relating to inventory and case carts
- Acquisition and disposition of supplies
- Resolution of supply problems

All SP areas must exercise careful environmental control conditions. Each work area should be restricted to assigned and authorized personnel who consistently follow the facility's dress code policies. Strict traffic control patterns must control the movement of people and goods through the department. Air pressure levels must be maintained to control air movements. Proper air pressure control helps to prevent the flow of bacteria-laden particulates and dust from soiled to clean areas.

Ancillary Areas and Equipment

The SPD performs the primary medical device processing for the healthcare facility. Specialty procedure carts, such as isolation, urology and emergency carts, can be processed by the SPD. These specialty carts are cleaned, inventoried and restocked between patient use and may be stored in the SP area until needed. Other patient care equipment, such as IV pumps, can also be processed and stored in the department.

Loaned Instruments

Loaned instruments are brought in for a specific patient procedure, for evaluation of new technology or to use while existing devices are being repaired. There should be a designated location and processes for receiving, processing, distribution, cleaning, and return.

THE PROCESSING CYCLE

Work performed in the SPD usually follows a processing cycle. (See **Figure 1.13**) After use, items that can be reprocessed are returned to the decontamination area to start the process all over again. It is important to note that at each step in the process, items are inspected to ensure that they are clean, in good repair, assembled, and processed correctly.

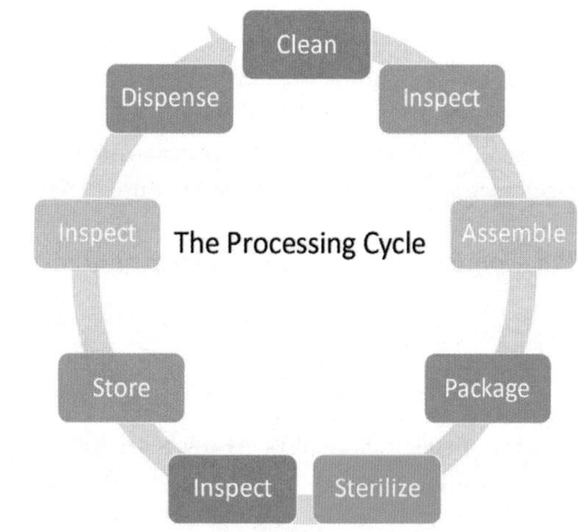

Figure 1.13 Tasks in the processing cycle follow a specific order and must not be rushed or skipped.

SP technicians must not only master specific skills in each work area, but they must also learn new ones as technologies, regulations, standards and best practices evolve. **Figure 1.14** provides some examples of skills SP technicians may routinely perform.

A Basic Educational Foundation Is Needed

Numerous dimensions of knowledge and skills are required for SP technicians to be successful in their jobs. A basic educational foundation is necessary to form the base for more specialized knowledge and skills. Examples of these skills include the ability to:

- Read and write, including the use of reports, manuals and IFU.
- Communicate clearly with inter- and intra-departmental team members.
- Interpret technical materials used for SP practices and procedures.
- Understand concepts of microbial transmission and infection prevention.
- Understand and use surgical and medical terminology.

BASIC JOB KNOWLEDGE AND SKILLS

SP professionals require significant knowledge and skill sets to perform effectively on the job. Knowledge and skill sets should include the following:

Communication Skills

SP technicians must know alternative methods of providing and obtaining information. They must be effective verbal and written communicators. To do so, they must be able to:

- Assess the ability of other people to understand what is being communicated
- Adapt the communication style to individual needs
- Apply active listening skills using reflection, restatement and clarification techniques
- Interact appropriately and respectfully with diverse groups in numerous situations
- Communicate in a manner that is straightforward, understandable, accurate and timely
- Use facility-specific guidelines and methods to send and receive information
- Access and use electronically produced information

Facility Systems

SP technicians must understand how their role fits into their department, their organization and the overall healthcare environment. They must be able to identify how key systems affect the services they perform and the quality of care they provide. To do so requires that they:

- Are aware of the range of services offered to customers
- Prevent unnecessary waste and duplication
- Participate in quality improvement activities
- Use resources, including other staff members and training opportunities

Employability Skills

Successful SP technicians use employability skills to enhance their employment opportunities and job satisfaction, and they maintain and upgrade those skills as required. Examples include:

- Maintaining appropriate personal skills, such as attendance and time management, and assume individual responsibility for their actions
- Maintaining professional conduct standards
- Using analytical skills to solve problems and make decisions
- Formulating solutions to problems using critical thinking skills, independently and in teams
- Adapting to changing situations
- Practicing personal integrity and honesty
- Engaging in ongoing self-assessment and goal modification for their personal and professional improvement
- Exhibiting respectful and empathetic behavior as they interact with peers, superiors, subordinates and customers
- Listening attentively to verbal instructions, requests and other information

Legal Responsibilities

SP technicians must understand and maintain an awareness of the legal responsibilities and limitations and the implications of their actions within the healthcare delivery setting. To do so, they must:

- Comply with established risk management factors and procedures

- Determine when an incident must be reported
- Maintain confidentiality
- Operate within the required scope of practice
- Follow mandated standards for workplace safety
- Comply with legal requirements for documentation

Ethics

Ethics relates to knowing the difference between "right" and "wrong." In the healthcare environment, it means conforming to accepted and professional standards of conduct. Ethical behavior is "doing the right thing in the right way." Ethics should govern and guide the way SP technicians act and make decisions. They must always:

- Respect patient rights
- Promote justice and the equal treatment of all individuals
- Recognize the importance of the patient's needs over other considerations
- Report any activity that adversely affects the health, safety or welfare of patients, visitors or fellow workers
- Comply with regulatory guidelines, facility policies, and departmental policies and procedures
- Respect differences among team members
- Demonstrate professionalism when interacting with customers and co-workers

Safety Practices

Successful SP technicians understand existing and potential hazards to patients, co-workers and themselves. They prevent injury or illness through safe work practices, and they consistently follow health and safety policies and procedures. They do so as they:

- Practice infection prevention procedures
- Use **Standard Precautions** to control the spread of infection
- Practice appropriate cleaning, disinfecting and sterilizing protocols
- Apply principles of body mechanics
- Identify and report fire and electrical hazards
- Use equipment properly
- Follow emergency procedures and protocols
- Comply with regulatory guidelines

Standard Precautions Method of using appropriate barriers to reduce the risk of transmission of bloodborne and other pathogens. This standard applies to all patients, regardless of diagnosis or presumed infectious status.

Resource Management

SP technicians must understand the roles and responsibilities of individual members as part of the healthcare team. Examples include:

- Controlling costs and reducing waste
- Providing quality service
- Practicing time management skills
- Identifying and solving potential problems
- Using inventory appropriately

Other skills are also required of SP technicians. For example, they must:

- Practice established policies and procedures to prevent **healthcare-associated infections (HAIs)**
- Keep their work environment clean and organized

New healthcare roles demand higher levels of skill than ever before for those working in SP. The complexities created by technology continue to grow and a new generation of healthcare professionals is emerging.

Healthcare-associated infection (HAI) An infection that is not present when a patient is admitted to a healthcare facility. If the infection develops in a patient on or after day three of admission to the healthcare facility, the infection is referred to as a HAI.

BASIC JOB RESPONSIBILITIES

SP technicians are accountable for many tasks. **Job descriptions** are used to define and communicate job duties and requirements to employees within an organization. They are intended to be overviews that capture the general purpose and major accountabilities of a job, and they are used for the following reasons:

- To evaluate positions and determine compensation. They can be used in conjunction with other resources to establish a pay range for a given position.
- To clarify expectations. Job descriptions outline key job duties, which can be reviewed at the time of hire to clarify performance standards and expectations. They should be reviewed regularly (typically annually) by both the supervisor and those who occupy the position.
- To review performance. Job descriptions can be used during annual performance reviews.

Because SPDs vary in size and scope of service and because jobs within the SPD vary, there is no single job description that applies to all situations.

Job description A Human Resources tool that identifies the major tasks performed by individuals in specific positions.

CONCLUSION

The SP environment is dynamic and fast paced. The work is challenging, highly technical and complex. The performance of this vital department has a major impact on the successful operation of many departments.

Inefficiencies in productivity, errors that create the need for rework, and poor-quality performance are costly to hospitals. With the ever-increasing costs of healthcare, SP professionals must conserve resources and minimize expenses.

SP is an evolving occupational discipline. Over the years, there have been dramatic changes and changes continue at a rapid pace. Conscientious SP professionals will find great satisfaction in knowing their efforts, service, special skills and due diligence are a part of every surgical procedure, every patient's recovery and every positive outcome.

RESOURCES

U.S. Department of Labor. Medical Equipment Preparers. https://www.bls.gov/oes/current/oes319093.htm.

Colbert BJ. *Workplace Readiness for Health Occupations.* Second Edition. Thomson Delmar Learning. 2006.

Booth KA. *Health Care Science Technology: Career Foundations.* McGraw-Hill Companies Inc. 2004.

U.S. Department of Education. *National Health Care Skill Standards.* The National Consortium on Health Science & Technology Education.

STERILE PROCESSING TERMS

Minimally invasive surgery (MIS)

Decontamination

Cleaning

Personal protective equipment (PPE)

Sterilization

Instructions for use (IFU)

Case cart system

Case cart

Doctor's (physician's) preference card

Case cart pull sheet (pick list)

Supply Chain Management

Standard Precautions

Healthcare-associated infection (HAI)

Job description

Chapter 2

Medical Terminology for Sterile Processing Technicians

Learning Objectives

As a result of successfully completing this chapter, the reader will be able to:

1. Explain the importance of medical terminology for Sterile Processing technicians
2. Identify the various elements used in medical terminology, including prefixes, roots and suffixes
3. Discuss how medical terminology can refer to human anatomy, disease processes, surgical instruments and surgical procedures
4. Understand medical terminology used in reference to surgical procedures in surgery schedules
5. Understand the importance of medical terminology for service quality in the Operating Room

INTRODUCTION

Sterile Processing (SP) technicians require knowledge of medical terms to help them succeed on the job. Medical terminology is the language of medical professionals that allows healthcare workers to communicate more effectively. This special terminology is used to describe parts of the body, diseases, instruments and surgical procedures.

IMPORTANCE OF MEDICAL TERMINOLOGY

The Healthcare Profession

The Association of periOperative Registered Nurses (AORN) specifically states that "skilled and competent allied health care providers and support personnel are valued members of the perioperative care team, contributing to safe patient care and positive patient outcomes." As such, SP technicians must have a grasp of the medical terminology used by healthcare customers and fellow SP professionals. The American National Standards Institute (ANSI) and the Association for the Advancement of Medical Instrumentation (AAMI), in ANSI/AAMI ST79: 2017 (with 2020 amendments) *Comprehensive guide to sterilization and sterility assurance in health care facilities,* specifically states that SP technicians must be "knowledgeable and competent" to adequately perform their vital tasks. The Joint Commission (TJC) states that in order to maintain a reliable system for medical device processing, institutions must place an emphasis upon the "orientation, training and competency of health care workers" who are responsible for this task. Understanding medical terminology is part of the training and competency that SP technicians should possess.

Understanding the Operating Room

SP technicians must provide Operating Room (OR) personnel with the instruments and supplies needed for surgical procedures. As these needs are conveyed, SP technicians must also understand the terminology/language spoken to them in order to provide quality customer service and contribute to positive patient outcomes.

For example, if the OR calls for instrumentation needed for an emergency pericardial window, a knowledgeable SP technician will know that this is a cardiac (heart) procedure that involves cutting into the pericardium (a membranous sac that surrounds the heart) in order to drain fluid from the pericardial space into the pleural (chest) cavity. Also, if the OR calls for a case cart for a **STAT** repair of an abdominal aortic aneurysm (AAA), this request will be responded to immediately because the SP technician will understand that the patient is at risk of losing their life.

STAT Abbreviation for the Latin term *statim*, meaning immediately or at once.

Providing Quality Service to the Patient

It is through knowing and understanding medical terminology that SP technicians are able to understand what is being asked of them. This knowledge of medical terminology enables the SP technician to react appropriately when the OR or other medical staff makes a request; however, the opposite is also true. If the OR makes a request that is not understood, the productivity of the OR may be compromised. This interruption of the perioperative process can compromise the quality of service rendered to the patient and may cause a delay in treatment.

ANATOMY OF A MEDICAL TERM

SP technicians frequently encounter specialized medical terms in their daily work activities and each of those terms contains key elements to help staff better understand the word's origin and meaning. As technicians learn the meanings of these names, they will have a greater understanding of what their work entails.

Word Elements

The majority of medical terms are of either Greek or Latin origin. The word "pericardium," for example, is composed of two Greek **word elements**: peri (meaning "around") and kardia (meaning "heart"). The term refers to the membranous sac that surrounds the heart as well as the roots of the great vessels of the heart. The term "rigor mortis" is composed of two Latin word elements: rigor (stiffness) and mortis (meaning "of death"); the term refers to the stiffening of the body that occurs after death. Many terms combine both Greek and Latin word elements to form a single medical term. For example, the term "claustrophobia" (meaning fear of enclosed spaces) joins the Latin word element "claustrum" (enclosed space) to a Greek word element "phobia" (fear).

At first, medical terminology may seem daunting and overwhelming; however, after a working knowledge of these word elements is gained, it becomes easier to analyze and use the words effectively.

Medical terminology changes with the dynamics of evolving technology in healthcare. New terms, abbreviations and words are constantly being created to meet the needs of this new technology. Through word association and memorization of basic medical terms and word elements, SP technicians can establish a solid foundation upon which to build an extensive vocabulary. A SP technician's vocabulary must be in a constant state of growth, evolution and development.

Specialty Items

Medical terminology can seem difficult, if not impossible, to learn. Here are a few hints to make studying easier and more effective:

1. Become comfortable with the word elements before breaking down terms. Understanding the word elements helps students understand the more complex medical terms.
2. Write down the terms.
3. Record the words and then play them back.
4. Create flashcards and practice with classmates, colleagues, friends or family.

Prefixes, Roots and Suffixes

The anatomy of a medical word consists of three word elements:

- **Root word element** tells the primary meaning of a medical term, which can then be modified by either a prefix, suffix or both. Many roots signify a procedure, disease or body part. For example, the term "cardiology," the medical term for "heart," features the root "cardio" conjunction with the suffix "ology" referring to the study of the heart. The term "endocarditis" also features the root "cardio" but in this example, the root is modified by a prefix "endo" (meaning "within") as well as a suffix "itis" (meaning "inflammation"). When the entire word is analyzed, the word means "inflammation of the inner portion of the heart." The term "cardiothoracic" features two roots: "cardio" (meaning "heart") and "thoracic" (meaning "chest"); a cardiothoracic surgeon performs surgery on the heart, its major vessels and the lungs. The term "electrosurgery" also features a combination of two roots. While the root "electro" refers to the use of electrical current, the root "surgery" refers to the act of performing surgery and the use of electrical current to cut and cauterize during surgery.

- **Prefix word element** comes before the root. When added to a root (at the beginning of a word), the prefix can alter or modify its meaning. For example, the medical term for the prefix "around" is "peri"; the term "pericardial" means "around the heart." The term "perioperative" refers to the entire process surrounding a surgical procedure: before (preoperative), during (intraoperative) and after (postoperative). The prefix "peri" is also found in the surgical instrument "periosteal elevator," an instrument used to remove tissue from around a bone (the periosteum). Here, the prefix "peri" (around) is attached to the root "osteo" (bone). Even the term "abnormal" functions in this way. The "ab" functions as a prefix to negate the meaning of the root "normal." The prefix "ab" means "away from" meaning the word is away from "normal" or "not normal."

- **Suffix word element** comes after the root. When added to the root (at the end of a word), the suffix can also alter or modify its meaning. For example, the medical term for the suffix that means inflammation is "itis"; the term "pericarditis" refers to inflammation (itis) around (peri) the heart (cardio). The term "tonsillitis" refers to inflammation of the tonsils. Bronchitis refers to inflammation of the bronchi, which are the tubes extending from the trachea into both sides of the lungs. When the suffix "itis" is found at the end of a medical term (modifying a root word preceding it), it means inflammation is present.

Of special note: A **combining vowel** (typically an "o") is either added to a root or removed from it to ease the pronunciation of the word.

An easy way to remember the difference between prefix (which comes before the root) and suffix (which comes after the root) is to put the words in alphabetical order: prefix, root and suffix. This tells you that prefix is the first word element and suffix is the last word element. (See **Figure 2.1**)

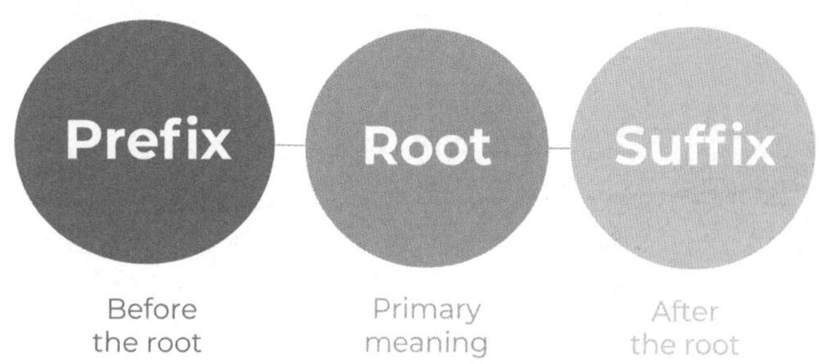

Figure 2.1

Note: Not all medical terms consist of all three word elements. A medical term may be formed by a root alone, combining two roots, a root and suffix, or a prefix and root. Some medical terms can even be formed by combining three roots.

Word elements Parts of a word.

Root word element Tells the primary meaning of a word; also called "base word element."

Prefix word element The word element that comes before the root word element.

Suffix word element The word element that comes after the root word element.

Combining vowel A letter (typically an "o") that is sometimes used to ease the pronunciation of a medical word.

The best way to learn the meaning of a medical term is to analyze and understand its components so that the word can be taken apart. Begin with the suffix (if present) since it most often gives a clue and meaning about the root and how it is being used. Then consider the root and prefix (if present). In other words, consider the overall relationship between each word element in the term. Medical terms can be a lot like building blocks; if one can figure out how they fit together, one can determine what they mean. (See **Figure 2.2**)

When analyzing medical terms, several suffixes meaning "pertaining to" may be encountered. **Figure 2.3** provides a list of these suffixes, examples of common words, and the meaning of those words.

Prefix	Root	Suffix	Word
hemi- half	arthro joint	-plasty surgical restoration	hemiarthroplasty surgical restoration of half of a joint, the femoral portion of the hip joint, and the proximal femur; a form of hip replacement surgery
hemi- half	gastro stomach	-ectomy surgical removal	hemigastrectomy removal of half of the stomach
hemi- half	colo colon	-ectomy surgical removal	hemicolectomy removal of half of the large intestine
para- beside, near	thyroid thyroid	-ectomy surgical removal	parathyroidectomy surgical removal of parathyroid glands
septo- dividing wall	rhino nose	-plasty surgical restoration	septorhinoplasty surgical restoration of the nose
chole- bile	cyst fluid-filled sac	-ectomy surgical removal	cholecystectomy surgical removal of the gallbladder
electro- electrical activity	cardio heart	-gram written record of	electrocardiogram written record of the electrical activity of the heart
electro- electrical activity	encephalo brain	-gram written record of	electroencephalogram (EEG) the tracing of brain wave activity

Figure 2.2 Combined word elements

Suffix	Example	Meaning
-ac	cardi-ac	pertaining to the heart
-al	derm-al	pertaining to the skin
-ic	hem-ic	pertaining to blood
-eal	esophag-eal	pertaining to the esophagus
-ary	pulmon-ary	pertaining to the lungs
-ous	cancer-ous	pertaining to cancer

Figure 2.3 Suffixes that mean "pertaining to"

Making medical terms conform to the basic rules of spelling and pronunciation may result in letters in the word element being changed, dropped or added. **Figure 2.4** shows some examples.

When analyzing a medical term, it is sometimes best to start with the suffix. In this way, one can readily identify if the word relates to a surgical procedure, a medical condition or a portion of the human anatomy. **Figure 2.5** lists some common suffixes.

Root	Suffix	Word	Letters Changed
procto rectum	-itis inflammation	proctitis	"o" is dropped
broncho bronchus	-itis inflammation	bronchitis	"o" is dropped
endo within	- oscopy visual examination	endoscopy	"o" is dropped
arterio artery	-ectomy removal	endarterectomy	"o" and "y" are dropped
fascia fibrous membrane	- otomy cutting into an organ	fasciotomy	"a" is dropped
chir hand	-plasty surgical repair	chiroplasty	"o" is added
herni rupture	-rrhaphy to suture	herniorrhaphy	"o" is added
hyster uterus	-pexy fixation	hysteropexy	"o" is added

Figure 2.4 Letters in word elements may be dropped or added.

Suffix	Meaning	Example	Combined Meaning
-algia	pain	neuralgia	nerve pain
-cide	kill	bactericide	substance that kills bacteria
		virucide	substance that kills viruses
		fungicide	substance that kills fungi
-cise	cut	excise	to cut out
		incise	to cut into
-ectomy	surgical removal	cystectomy	removal of a cyst
		tonsillectomy	removal of the tonsils
		pneumonectomy	removal of a lung
		laminectomy	removal of a portion of a lamina (part of the vertebrae in the spine)
		hysterectomy	removal of the uterus
		appendectomy	removal of the appendix
		thrombectomy	removal of a blood clot
		orchiectomy	removal of a testicle
		nephrectomy	removal of a kidney
		vitrectomy	removal of some or all of the vitreous humor from the eye

Suffix	Meaning	Example	Combined Meaning
		hemorrhoidectomy	removal of swollen or inflamed vascular structures in the anal canal
		bunionectomy	removal of a misaligned bone in the big toe
		discectomy	removal of a herniated disc in the spine
		microdiscectomy	minimally invasive removal of a herniated disc in the spine
		thyroidectomy	removal of the thyroid gland
-emia	blood	hyperglycemia	high blood sugar
		hypoglycemia	low blood sugar
-genic	origin	osteogenic	originating in the bones
		iatrogenic	adverse effect or complication originating from a physician
-gram	record/image of	mammogram	radiographic image of the breast for early detection of breast cancer
		cholangiogram	radiographic image of the bile ducts using contrast medium to check for a blockage (frequently done during a cholecystectomy)
		arthrogram	radiographic image of a joint after injection of a contrast medium
		angiogram	radiographic image of the inside (lumens) of blood vessels and organs of the body using a contrast agent
-itis	inflammation	tonsillitis	inflammation of the tonsils
		hepatitis	inflammation of the liver
		arthritis	inflammation of a joint
		bronchitis	inflammation of the bronchi
		meningitis	inflammation of the meninges (the membranous layer surrounding the brain and spinal cord)
-megaly	large or enlargement	cardiomegaly	enlargement of the heart
-necrosis	death of tissue	arterionecrosis	tissue death of an artery
-ology	study of	bacteriology	study of bacteria
		oncology	study of cancer
		neurology	study of the nervous system
		cardiology	study of the heart
		nephrology	study of the kidney
-oma	tumor	carcinoma	malignant (cancerous) tumor
		myoma	tumor consisting of muscular tissue

Suffix	Meaning	Example	Combined Meaning
		meningioma	tumor of the meninges (the membranous layer surrounding the brain and spinal cord)
		fibroadenoma	breast lump composed of fibrous and glandular tissue
		papilloma	benign tumor that grows on the skin or mucous membrane; can be caused by a virus
-oscopy	visual examination	laparoscopy	visual examination of organs in the abdomen
		arthroscopy	visual examination of a joint
		cystoscopy	visual examination of the bladder
		bronchoscopy	visual examination of the bronchi
		colonoscopy	visual examination of the large intestine
		thoracoscopy	visual examination of the thoracic cavity
		fluoroscopy	an imaging technique that provides live images of a surgical site during surgery
-ostomy	creation of an opening	colostomy	creation of an opening to the colon
		tracheostomy	creation of an opening to the trachea
		urostomy	creation of an opening for the urinary system
		nephrostomy	creation of an opening to the kidney
		ventriculostomy	creation of an opening within a cerebral ventricle for drainage
		ileostomy	creation of an opening to the ileum
-otomy	incision into	craniotomy	incision into the skull
		thoracotomy	incision into the plural space of the chest
		arthrotomy	incision into a joint
		osteotomy	incision into a bone
		faciotomy	incision into fibrous membrane (fascia)
		urethrotomy	incision into the urethra
		fistulotomy	incision into a fistula
		sternotomy	incision into/splitting of the sternum (breastbone)

Suffix	Meaning	Example	Combined Meaning
-pathy	disease	encephalopathy	disorder or disease of the brain
		cardiomyopathy	disorder or disease of the heart
-pexy	surgical fixation	orchiopexy	surgical fixation of an undescended testicle to the correct location
		hysteropexy	surgical fixation of the uterus
-plasty	surgical restoration	rhinoplasty	surgical repair of the nose
		arthroplasty	surgical repair of a joint
		cranioplasty	surgical repair of the skull
		tympanoplasty	surgical repair of the eardrum
		urethroplasty	surgical repair of the urethra
		kyphoplasty	surgical repair of a fractured vertebra
-rrhage	flow	hemorrhage	uncontrolled flow of blood
-rrhaphy	to suture	myorrhaphy	to suture a muscle wound
		herniorrhaphy	to suture a hernia
-tome	a cutting instrument	dermatome	instrument used for cutting skin
		osteotome	instrument used for cutting bone

Figure 2.5 Common suffixes

As can be seen by the brief listing of suffixes in **Figure 2.5**, medical terms can be complex and mean entirely different things, depending on how they are composed.

Figure 2.6 lists common roots found in medical terminology. Roots are base word elements that refer to the main body of a medical word.

Root	Meaning	Example	Combined Meaning
adeno	gland	adenoma	glandular tumor
aero	air	aerobic	requiring oxygen for growth
		anaerobic	not requiring oxygen for growth
arthro	joint	arthritis	inflammation of a joint
		arthroscopy	visual examination of a joint
		arthrocentesis	joint puncture for the aspiration of synovial fluid
		arthrodesis	surgical fusion of a joint
broncho	bronchus	bronchoscope	endoscope used to visualize the bronchi
cardio	heart	endocarditis	inflammation of the inner layer (endocardium) of the heart
		cardiomyopathy	heart muscle disease
		cardiopulmonary resuscitation (CPR)	emergency efforts to revive a person in cardiac arrest by means of chest compressions and rescue breaths
		myocardium	cardiac/heart muscle

Root	Meaning	Example	Combined Meaning
cerebro	brain	cerebrospinal	referring to the brain and spinal cord
chole	bile	cholecyst	referring to the gallbladder
chondro/io	cartilage	chondroma	cartilaginous tumor
colo	colon	colectomy	removal of part of the large intestine
costo	rib	intercosto	between the ribs
cranio	skull	craniotomy	surgical opening into the skull
cysto	bladder	cyst	a fluid-filled sac
cyto	cell	erythrocyte	red blood cell
derma	skin	dermopathy	skin disease
gastro	stomach	gastrointestinal	pertaining to the stomach and intestines
gyne	woman	gynecology	study of diseases affecting women
hema or hemat	blood	hemophilia	inability of the blood to clot
		hemostat	instrument used to control bleeding
		hematoma	collection of blood in tissue
		hemodialysis	filtration of the blood mechanically; occurring outside the body
hepat	liver	hepatitis	inflammation of the liver
herni	rupture	herniorrhaphy	surgical repair of a rupture
hyster	uterus	hysteropexy	abdominal fixation of the uterus
		hysteroscopy	visual examination of the uterus
leuko	white	leukocyte	white blood cell
		leukemia	form of cancer of the blood or bone marrow involving abnormal white blood cells
lipo	fat	liposuction	aspiration of fat cells
litho	stone	lithotripsy	crushing of a stone
mast	breast	mastectomy	surgical removal of a breast
nephros	kidney	nephritis	inflammation of the nephrons in the kidneys
		nephrosis	degenerative disease of the kidneys
oopher	ovary	oophorectomy	surgical removal of an ovary
osteo	bone	osteosynthesis	surgical reduction and fixation of a bone fracture
rhino	nose	rhinoplasty	surgical repair of the nose
stoma	opening	anastomosis	connection or reconnection of two separate tubular structures; for example, blood vessels or portions of intestines
thrombus	blood clot	thrombosis	formation of a blood clot inside a blood vessel obstructing the flow of blood (DVT= deep vein thrombosis)
tracheo	trachea	tracheostomy	creation of new opening to trachea

Figure 2.6 Common roots

Figure 2.7 lists common prefixes used in medical terminology. Prefixes are word elements that are placed before the root to alter or modify its meaning.

Prefix	Meaning	Example	Combined Meaning
a, an-	without	asepsis	without infection; sterile
		anesthesia	without sensation (local or general)
		atraumatic	not inflicting wound or injury
		analgesia	without pain
		atrophy	reduction in size of a body part (wasting away) due to poor circulation, poor nutrition or a disease process
ad-	toward (in the direction of)	addiction	toward dependence on a drug
ante-	before	antepartum	before the onset of labor
anti-	against	antiseptic	preventing sepsis (infection)
bi-	two/both sides	bilateral total hip reconstruction (THR)	two (both) total hip reconstructions
		bilateral myringotomy with tubes	incision into (both) eardrums (tympanic membrane) in order to place drainage tubes
		bilateral salpingo-oophorectomy	surgical removal of both fallopian tubes and ovaries
		bilateral strabismus repair	surgery performed on the extraocular muscles to correct eye misalignment
dis-	apart, away	hip dislocation	displacement of femur from pelvic joint
		disinfectant	chemical used to kill microorganisms
dys-	painful	dysentery	painful inflammation of the intestine
endo-	within	endotracheal	within the trachea
		endoscope	instrument used to visualize a joint or organ in the body
		endoscopy	visualization within and possible treatment of, a part of the body using an endoscope and endoscopic instrumentation
extra-	outside	extracorporal	outside of the body
hemi-	half	hemigastrectomy	surgical removal of half of the stomach
		hemiarthroplasty	form of hip replacement surgery
		hemicolectomy	removal of half of the large intestine
hyper-	above, excessive	hyperacidity	excessive acid in the stomach
		hypertensive	high blood pressure
		hypertrophy	excessive growth/size of a part of the body due to cellular enlargement
hypo-	below, deficient	hypoglycemia	low sugar content in the blood
		hypotensive	low blood pressure
inter-	between	intercellular	between or among cells
		interstitial	an empty space
		interdepartmental	between departments
		intercostal	between the ribs
intra-	within, inside	intravenous	in or into a vein
		intramuscular	located in or injected into a muscle

Prefix	Meaning	Example	Combined Meaning
		intraabdominal	within the abdomen
		intraoperative	during surgery
		intraarticular	within a joint
		intraocular	within the eye
		intracranial	within the skull
neo-	new	neonatal	newborn
para-	beside, near	parathyroidectomy	surgical removal of parathyroid glands
		paratracheal	beside the trachea
per-	through	percutaneous	through the skin
peri-	around, about	periosteal elevator	instrument used to remove tissue around the bone (the periosteum)
		perioperative	all aspects of the surgical process (before, during and after)
		pericardium	the serous (fluid-emitting) membrane that stretches around the heart and lines the mediastinum
		peritoneum	the serous (fluid-emitting) membrane that stretches around the abdominal cavity and is its lining
post-	after	postpartum	after delivery of a baby
		postoperative	after surgery
pre-	before	preoperative	before surgery
sub-	under, beneath	subcutaneous	beneath the skin
		subclavian	located under the clavicle
		subdural	located under the dura mater (the outermost membrane surrounding the brain)
supra-	above	suprapubic	above the pubis
		supracondylar fracture	fracture of the distal humerus above the elbow joint
trans-	across, through	transanal	through the anus
		transoral	through the mouth
		transesophageal	through the esophagus
		transurethral	through the urethra

Figure 2.7 Common prefixes

Understanding Usage

Learning medical terminology can be an almost endless process. As new surgical procedures are created, new medical terminology will also be created to refer to these procedures. SP technicians must understand the language spoken to them by the OR and medical staff to provide them with the goods and services needed for their procedures. Language frequently used by the OR utilizes abbreviations or acronyms to refer to various types of surgeries. **Figure 2.8** contains a list of some surgical procedure abbreviations or acronyms.

Abbreviation	Surgical Procedure	Meaning
AAA	Repair of an abdominal aortic aneurysm	Surgical repair of a weakening/ballooning area of the abdominal portion of the aorta
ACF	Anterior cervical fusion	Surgical fusion of vertebrae in the cervical spine; approached from the side of the patient's body
ACL	Anterior cruciate ligament	Reconstruction or repairing of the anterior cruciate ligament. In an ACL reconstruction, a graft is used to replace the ligament. In an ACL repair, the torn ligament is put back together.
AKA	Above the knee amputation	Surgical removal of the leg above the knee.
ALIF	Anterior lumbar interbody fusion	Spinal surgery in which bone grafts/implants are used to fuse vertebrae in the lumbar spine; approached from the front of the patient's body
AV Graft	Arteriovenous graft	Surgical connection made between an artery and a vein to allow hemodialysis access.
BKA	Below the knee amputation	Surgical removal of the leg below the knee
BMT	Bilateral myringotomy with tubes	Incision into both sides of the eardrum for drainage via tube placement
BSO	Bilateral salpingo-oopherectomy	Surgical removal of both fallopian tubes and ovaries
CABG	Coronary artery bypass graft	Creation of a new blood supply to an area of the heart with a clogged/ blocked artery using the patient's own blood vessel to function as the graft
CR	Closed reduction	Treatment of a fractured bone without a surgical incision
D&C	Dilation and curettage	Dilation of the uterine cervix and scraping of the inner lining
EGD	Esophagogastroduodenoscopy	Endoscopic procedure that visualizes the upper portion of the gastrointestinal tract up to the duodenum
ESS	Endoscopic sinus surgery	Use of endoscopic instrumentation to operate on the nose
EUA	Exam under anesthesia	The use of anesthesia to conduct a surgical examination of a sensitive part of the body
I&D	Incision and drainage	Incision into and drainage of pus/fluid from an abscess, boil, wound or infected area of the body
ICD	Implantable cardioverter defibrillator	Insertion/implantation of a battery-powered device that can deliver a jolt of electricity to treat cardiac arrhythmia
IMN	Intramedullary nail	Insertion/implantation of a nail or rod into the medullary cavity of a long bone, such as the femur or tibia.
IOL	Intraocular lens	Insertion/implantation of a lens within the eye to treat cataracts
IORT	Intraoperative radiation therapy	Use of therapeutic levels of radiation to treat exposed cancer tumors during surgery; frequently done during breast surgery
LAVH	Laparoscopic-assisted vaginal hysterectomy	A visualization and treatment of pelvic organs, followed by removal of the uterus through the vagina
L&B	Laryngoscopy and bronchoscopy	A visual examination of the larynx and the bronchi
LP	Lumbar puncture	A collection of cerebrospinal fluid (CSF) for diagnostic or therapeutic purposes, commonly referred to as a spinal tap
MIDCAB	Minimally invasive direct coronary artery bypass	Use of a small incision in the ribs (mini thoracotomy) to access the heart to bypass diseased coronary arteries

Abbreviation	Surgical Procedure	Meaning
MIS	Minimally invasive surgery	A type of surgery that uses endoscopic techniques and instrumentation to reduce trauma to the body during surgery
ORIF	Open reduction internal fixation	Treatment of a fractured bone with an incision and the use of plates and screws or pins to hold the fragments together
PAL	Power-assisted liposuction	Suction of fat cells by means of a motorized hand piece and cannula
PCI	Percutaneous coronary intervention	A procedure to open narrowed coronary arteries.
PDA	Patent ductus arteriosus	Repair of a congenital heart disorder in a neonate (newborn)
PEG	Percutaneous endoscopic gastrostomy	Insertion of a feeding tube (PEG tube) into the stomach through the abdominal wall
PICC	Peripherally inserted central catheter	Intravenous catheter inserted in a vein for long-term IV access
PLIF	Posterior lumbar interbody fusion	Spinal surgery in which bone grafts/implants are used to fuse vertebrae in the lumbar spine; approached from the back of the patient's body
STSG	Split thickness skin graft	Surgical removal of healthy epidermis and portions of dermis (skin) that is used as a skin graft elsewhere on the body.
TAH	Total abdominal hysterectomy	Surgical removal of the uterus through an incision in the abdomen
TEE	Transesophageal echocardiogram	Ultrasound image of the heart by using a probe/transducer inserted into the esophagus
THA	Total hip arthroplasty	Hip joint reconstruction by removing the bone and placing an implant in the hip socket, as well as the femoral head (the proximal femur), resulting in a completely rebuilt joint.
TKA	Total knee arthroplasty	Knee joint reconstruction by placing implants, resulting in a completely rebuilt joint
TURP	Transurethral resection of the prostate	Surgical removal of part of the prostate gland by inserting instruments across the urethra to reach the prostate internally
VATS	Video assisted thoracoscopic surgery	Use of endoscopic instruments to access the chest cavity, lungs or thorax
VP Shunt	Ventriculoperitoneal shunt	Surgical placement of a drain (shunt) to transfer excess cerebrospinal fluid (CSF) from the brain (ventricle) to the abdominal lining (peritoneum)
Wound VAC	Wound vacuum-assisted closure	A treatment that applies gentle suction to a wound to help it heal.
XLIF	Extreme lateral interbody fusion	Spinal fusion surgery approaching from the side of the patient using special instrumentation to reduce trauma on the patient's body

Figure 2.8 Abbreviations/acronyms for surgical procedures

Room	Start Time	Patient ID	Procedure	Comments
1	7:00	Abc123	Cystoscopy with left retrogrades, left stent insertion	C-arm
	TF	Xyz578	Transurethral resection of the prostate	
2	7:00	Nop482	Septoplasty, possible endoscopic sinus surgery	
	TF	Cde223	Tonsillectomy	
3	7:00	Bnm445	TAH with BSO	
	TF	Rty468	D&C	
4	7:00	Vbg368	TKA right – revision	Loaned instrumentation
	TF	Klm562	ORIF – left ankle	
	TF	Jkl628	CR, possible pinning right thumb	Possible ORIF
* TF means To Follow				

Figure 2.9 Sample surgery schedule

ANATOMY OF A SURGICAL PROCEDURE

Once SP technicians understand medical terminology with its numerous prefixes, roots and suffixes, they will be able to better understand the surgical procedures referred to in surgery schedules and the instruments and supplies that will be requested. Challenges arise when the OR is supplied with incorrect instrumentation and supplies for a surgical procedure. When the OR receives a case cart for a scheduled procedure with the incorrect instrumentation and supplies, the surgical team's attention is diverted away from the patient and to getting the correct items into the room.

PROCEDURE APPROACH AND PURPOSE

When reading surgery schedules and interacting with OR staff, SP technicians need to understand how procedure approach and purpose are identified. When a surgical procedure is referred to in a surgery schedule, the suffix attached to the primary medical term will indicate the purpose of the procedure. For example, "oscopy" will refer to visual examination of and possible treatment, "otomy" will refer to an incision into, "ectomy" will refer to removal of, and "plasty" will refer to repair/reconstruction of.

Another key element in how a procedure can be understood relates to the approach the surgeon will use when performing the surgery. The approach or method typically comes at the beginning of the surgical procedure term. The following are some examples:

- Laparoscopic cholecystectomy will remove the patient's gallbladder using laparoscopic instrumentation and techniques.
- Robotic-assisted prostatectomy will remove the patient's prostate by using robotic instrumentation and techniques.
- Bilateral myringotomy will make incisions for drainage into the patient's tympanic membrane (eardrum) on both sides.
- Anterior cervical fusion will fuse some of the patient's cervical vertebrae, approaching from the front of the patient's body.
- Posterior lumbar interbody fusion will fuse some of the patient's lumbar vertebrae, approaching from the back of the patient.
- Vaginal hysterectomy will remove the patient's uterus via the vaginal canal.
- Total abdominal hysterectomy will remove the uterus through an open incision in the abdomen.

Sterile Processing Technicians and the Surgery Schedule

SP technicians may be responsible for reading the OR surgery schedule to print pick lists, obtain the needed instrumentation and find/obtain instrumentation that is already in use in another surgical procedure. Surgery schedules are prioritized according to patient needs. **Figure 2.9** provides a basic example of a surgery schedule and terminology an SP technician might encounter.

CONCLUSION

Knowledge of medical terminology is essential for ensuring that SP technicians have a clear understanding of what the OR and other healthcare customers require for their procedures. Prefixes, roots and suffixes are vital tools that will allow SP technicians to communicate more proficiently.

RESOURCES

Association for the Advancement of Medical Instrumentation. ANSI/AAMI ST79:2017 & 2020 Amendments A1, A2, A3, A4 (Consolidated Text) *Comprehensive guide to steam sterilization and sterility assurance in health care facilities.*

The Joint Commission. *Hospital Accreditation Standards, IC-10.* 2022.

Centers for Disease Control and Prevention. *Guideline for Disinfection and Sterilization in Healthcare Facilities.* 2008.

Leiken JB, Lipsky MS, eds. *American Medical Association Complete Medical Encyclopedia.* Random House. 2003.

STERILE PROCESSING TERMS

STAT

Word elements

Root word element

Prefix word element

Suffix word element

Combining vowel

Chapter 3

Anatomy for Sterile Processing Technicians

Learning Objectives

As a result of successfully completing this chapter, the reader will be able to:

1. Review the structure, function, activities and roles of cells, tissues and organs in the body
2. Identify and describe the structure and roles of each major body system and identify common surgical procedures that involve each system
3. Explain how knowledge of anatomy can help with surgical instrument identification

INTRODUCTION

Many surgical interventions have been developed to treat the human body and enable it to heal. Sterile Processing (SP) technicians play an important role in the surgical support process by providing the instruments and supplies needed to perform specific surgeries. As members of the surgical team, developing a basic understanding of the human body can aid in communication with the Operating Room (OR) and can help facilitate requests.

The study of the human body requires an understanding of **anatomy** and **physiology**.

Anatomy The study of the structure and relationship between body parts.

Physiology The study of the functions of body parts and the body as a whole.

ANATOMICAL POSITION

Anatomical positioning is a system created to describe different body part positions and locations. It allows healthcare professionals to universally communicate those specific areas of the body to other professionals. Understanding anatomical positioning, terms and planes can help SP technicians gain a better appreciation for where, how and which instrumentation will be used for different surgical procedures. For example, in a total hip replacement procedure, different instrumentation is used for an anterior approach versus a posterior approach. **Figure 3.1** illustrates anatomical position, and **Figure 3.2** explains the meaning of common anatomical terms.

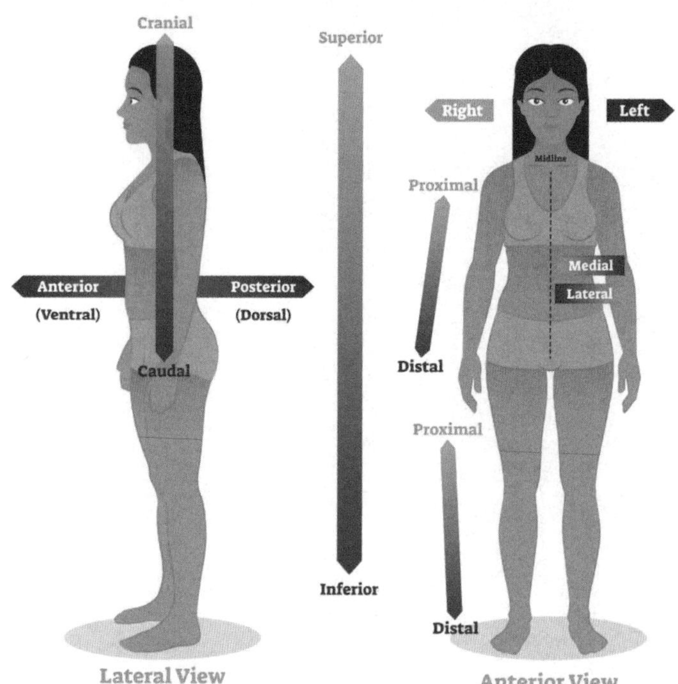

Figure 3.1 Anatomical position

Anatomical Planes

The use of anatomical planes is another method for describing portions of the body or the location of structures as they relate to other structures in the body. (See **Figure 3.3**)

Anatomical Term	Meaning	Example
Anatomical left	Refers to a structure on the patient's left side	Left tympanoplasty procedure
Anatomical right	Refers to a structure on the patient's right side	Right total knee procedure
Anterior	Toward the front or belly surface; ventral	The kneecap is on the anterior potion of the leg
Posterior	Toward the back; dorsal	Shoulder blades are located posteriorly
Midline	The imaginary line that divides the body into left and right halves	The spine is located in the midline of the body
Medial	Nearer the midline of the body	The sternum is medial to the shoulder
Lateral	Farther from the midline; toward the side	Ears are lateral to the nose
Distal	Farther from the origin of a structure or from a given reference point	The ankle is distal to the hip
Proximal	Nearer to the point of origin or to a reference point	Fingers are proximal to the wrist
Superior	Above; in a higher position; cranial	Eyebrows are superior to the eyes
Inferior	Below or lower	The mouth is inferior to the nose

Figure 3.2 Anatomical terms

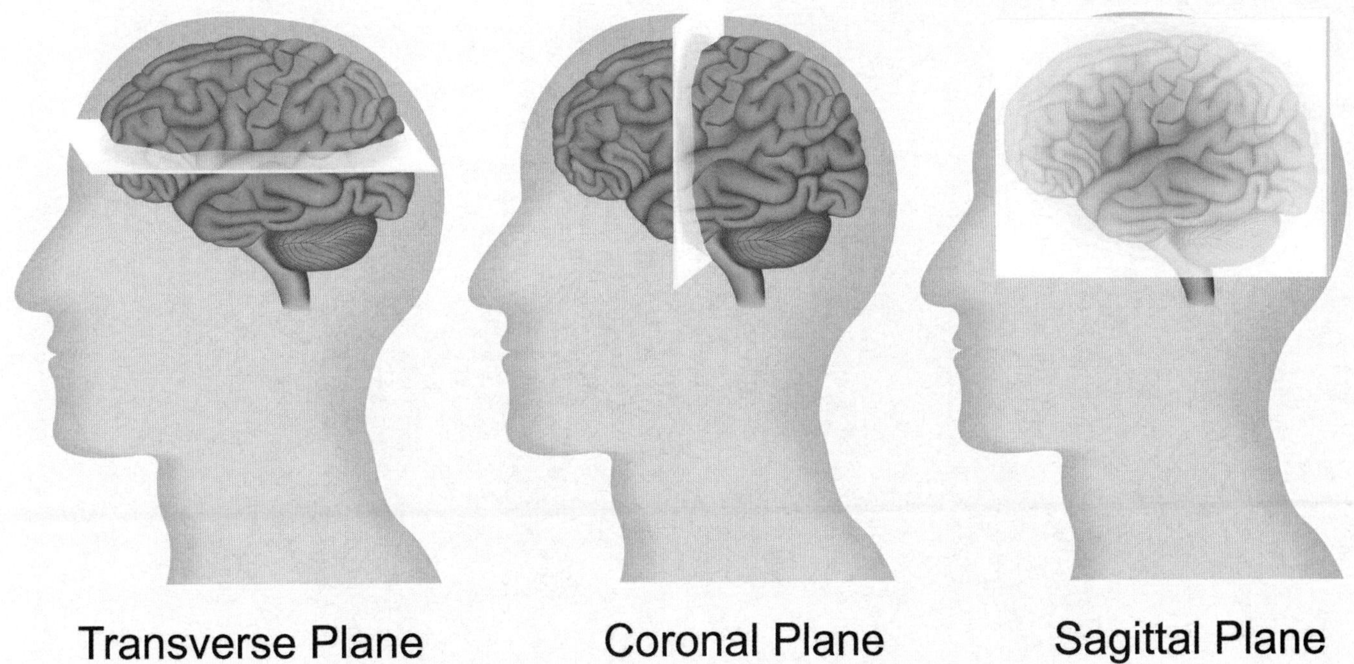

Figure 3.3 Anatomical planes

The following are three commonly used anatomical planes:

- Transverse plane – Passes through the body, organ or structure, dividing into upper (superior) and lower (inferior) sections.
- Coronal plane – Passes through the body, organ or structure, dividing into front (anterior) and back (posterior) sections.
- Sagittal plane – Passes through the body, organ or structure, dividing into left and right halves.

CELLS, TISSUES AND ORGANS

Cells

Here are some facts about **cells**:

- They are the basic living unit of life. The human body is comprised of more than 100 trillion cells.
- They vary in size, shape and function, depending upon their location in the body.
- They are so small that they can only be seen with a microscope.
- Within each cell are still smaller structures called organelles, microscopic organs that perform specific functions.
- Functions of the cell include respiration, nutrition, energy production, waste elimination, and reproduction.
- Living cells only come from other living cells.

Regardless of their size and shape, each human cell consists of three main parts: cell membrane, cytoplasm and nucleus.

- The **cell membrane** is porous and flexible and surrounds the cell to keep it separated from the outside environment. The cell membrane surrounds the cytoplasm and allows and controls the passage of materials in and out of the cell. Examples include the absorption of oxygen and food and the elimination of waste products produced by the cell. (See **Figure 3.4**)
- The **cytoplasm** is a clear, jelly-like substance that surrounds the nucleus and contains the cell fluid and organelles.
- The **nucleus** is surrounded and protected by the cytoplasm. This oval structure serves as the brain center of the cell to direct and control all activities, including duplication into two new cells.

Cell The basic unit of life; the smallest structural unit of living organisms capable of performing all basic functions of life.

Cell membrane The outer covering of a cell that regulates what enters and leaves it.

Cytoplasm The clear, jelly-like substance of a cell between the cell membrane and nucleus.

Nucleus The functional center of a cell that governs activity and heredity.

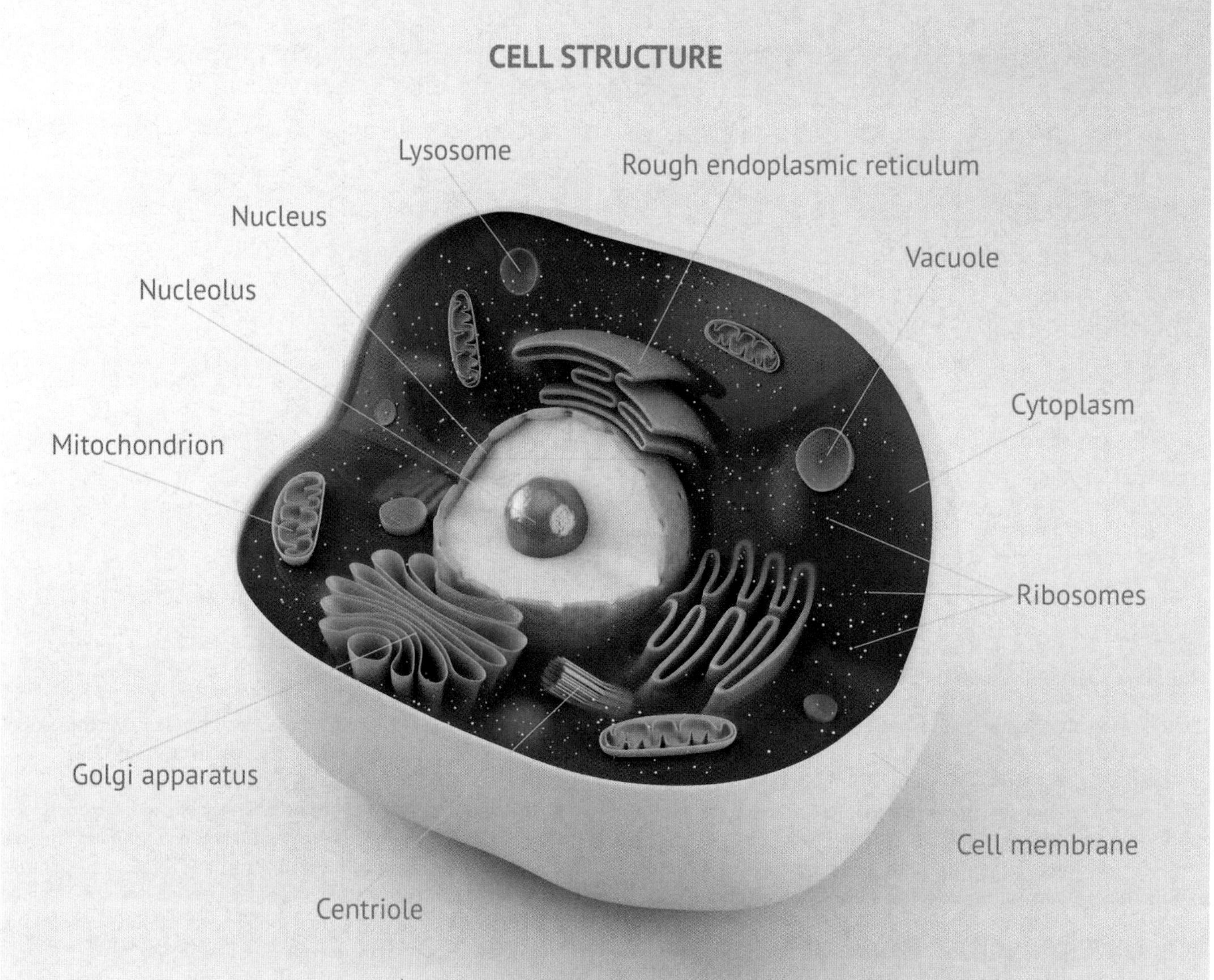

Figure 3.4

Tissue

Tissue forms when two or more cells that are similar in structure and function join together. The four primary tissues of the human body are:

- Epithelial tissue – Covers the body's external surface (skin) and the linings of body cavities (the mouth, ears, nose and throat).

- Connective tissue – Provides support, stores energy, and connects other tissues and parts. Examples of connective tissue include bone, fat, blood and cartilage. Bones provide protection, support and shape to the body as well as storage for calcium. Fat keeps the body warm, cushions organs and stores nutrients. Blood transports food and oxygen to all body parts and removes waste products. Cartilage provides framework and support to the human body.

- Muscular tissue – Shortens as it contracts. When attached to bone, these contractions make body movement possible. Muscle tissue also lines the inner walls of organs that contract to help food pass through the digestive system. As cardiac muscles contract, blood is pumped throughout the body.

- Nervous tissue – Located throughout the body. When stimulated, nervous tissue carries messages back and forth between the brain and every part of the body.

Organs

Organs are formed when two or more different types of tissues are grouped together to perform a specific function. Examples of organs include:

- Brain – The organ in the central nervous system that is the primary receiver, organizer and distributor of information in the body.

- Heart – Pumps blood throughout the body.
- Stomach – Part of the digestive system that helps digest food by mixing it with digestive juices and converting it into a liquid.
- Skin – The largest organ; serves as the body's outer covering.

Tissue A group of similar cells that perform a specialized function.

Organ A part of the body containing two or more tissues that function together for a specific purpose.

BODY SYSTEMS

A **body system** is a group of organs that work together to carry out a particular activity. While each body system provides a specific bodily function, none are independent of one another. Except for the reproductive system, each body system and its organs work together to help the body function as a total organism and maintain life. The remainder of this chapter will provide details about the body's major systems and common procedures performed to treat issues that can occur in those systems.

Skeletal System

Without the skeletal system (see **Figure 3.5**), the body would be an immovable mass. Approximately 206 bones comprise the body's skeletal system. They are arranged in an orderly manner and are fastened together by tough connective tissue known as **tendons** and **ligaments**. The five main functions of the skeletal system are to:

- Give the body shape and support
- Allow movement
- Protect vital organs
- Produce blood cells
- Store calcium

Most bones are made from **cartilage**, but through a process known as **ossification**, cartilage is sometimes replaced by bone. Cartilage is a flexible connective tissue that provides framework to the body. Its purposes include:

- Supporting body structures such as the ears and nose
- Connecting the ribs to the sternum
- Serving as a cushion between bones to prevent them from rubbing together at junctures and **joints**

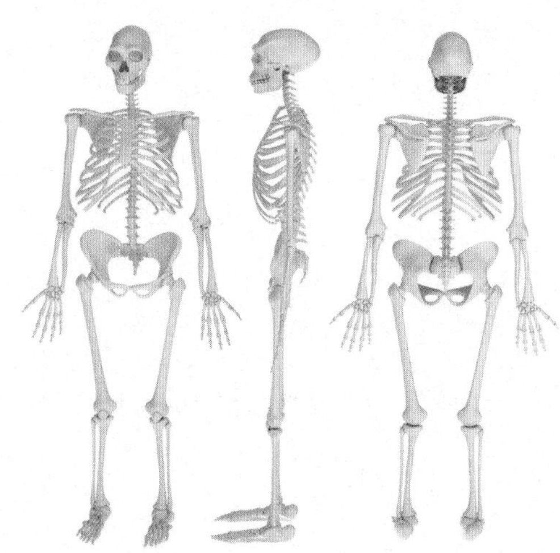

Figure 3.5

There are several types of joints:

- Gliding joints – Allow the head to lower as the vertebrae (bones in the spinal column) of the neck slide over one another.
- Ball and socket joints – Allow movements like swinging one's arm in a circle. Ball and socket joints consist of a bone with a rounded head that fits into a rounded cup of another bone (hips and shoulders).
- Pivot joints – Allow a turning motion such as the palm of the hand rotating from up to down.
- Hinge joints – Allow backward and forward bending motions like a door hinge (knees, knuckles and elbows).

A joint is a place where two bones meet. Some are immovable such as those found in the skull; others, such as the knee and elbow joints, are movable and allow the bones that they connect to move. **Figure 3.6** shows the location of some joints in the body.

Body system A group of organs that work together to carry out a specific activity.

Tendon A cord of fibrous tissue that attaches a muscle to a bone.

Ligament A band of connective tissue that connects a bone to another bone.

Cartilage A type of flexible connective tissue.

Ossification The process by which cartilage is replaced by bone.

Joint A place where two bones meet.

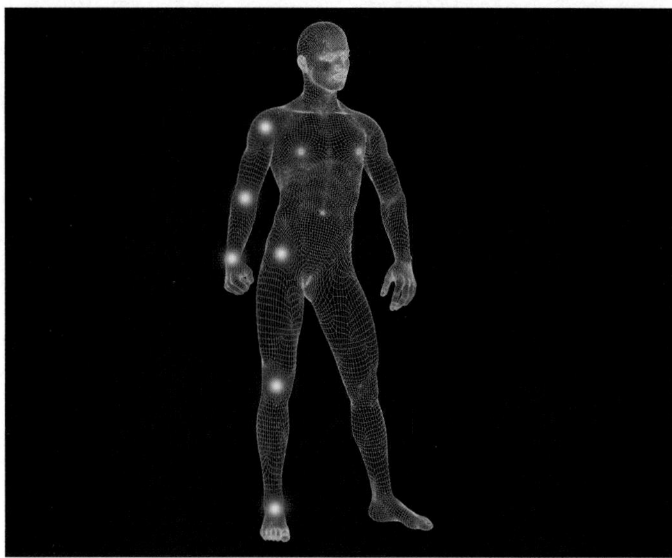

Figure 3.6

The overall covering or lining of a joint is called a synovial membrane. It secretes a fluid, called synovial fluid, to lubricate joint surfaces. (See **Figures 3.7** and **3.8**)

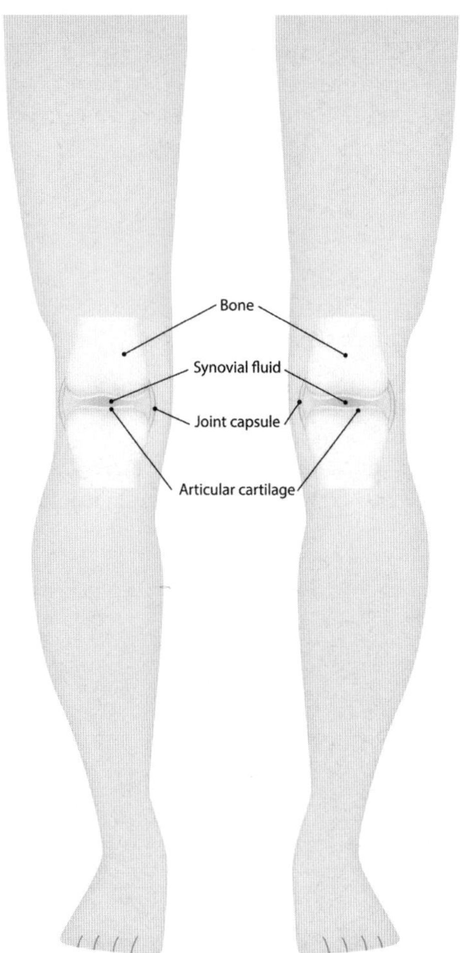

Figure 3.7

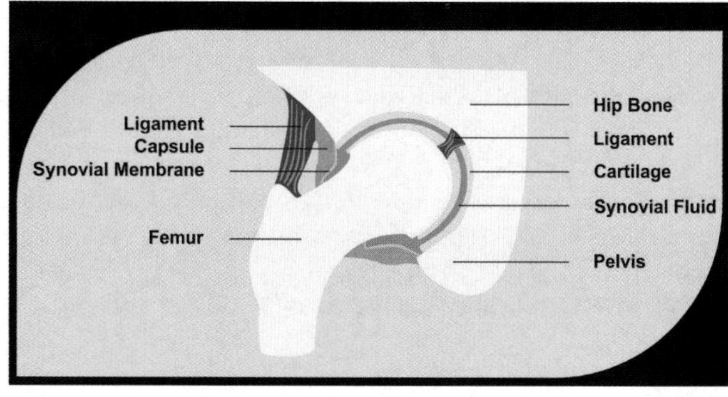

Figure 3.8 Hip joint

Bones are comprised of living tissue and their strength and hardness come from chemical substances called minerals. Bone consists of two principal materials:

- A hard outer material called cortical bone that is dense and strong and consists of calcium and phosphorous. This hard outer surface is surrounded by the periosteum, a tough membrane that contains bone-forming cells and blood vessels.

- The inner section, called spongy or cancellous bone, is porous.

Bones are filled with a material called marrow. A pipeline of blood vessels and nerves runs through the middle of thick bones. (See **Figure 3.9**)

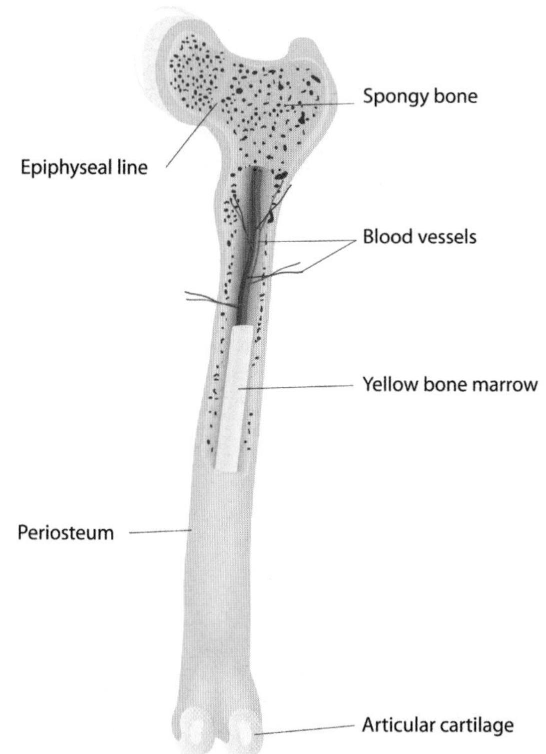

Figure 3.9

Examples of surgical procedures involving the skeletal system include:

- Craniotomy – Making an opening into the skull bone to access the brain.
- Anterior cervical fusion – Removal of disc tissue pressing on a nerve in the neck area by inserting a piece of bone between the vertebrae and fusing this area with plates and screws.
- Posterior lumbar interbody fusion (PLIF) – Removing disc tissue pressing on the lower spine area by inserting a piece of bone between the vertebrae and fusing this area with plates and screws.
- Open reduction internal fixation (ORIF) – Making an incision in the skin, realigning a fractured bone, and inserting screws and plates to ensure the bone ends do not move, so healing can be promoted. (See **Figure 3.10**)

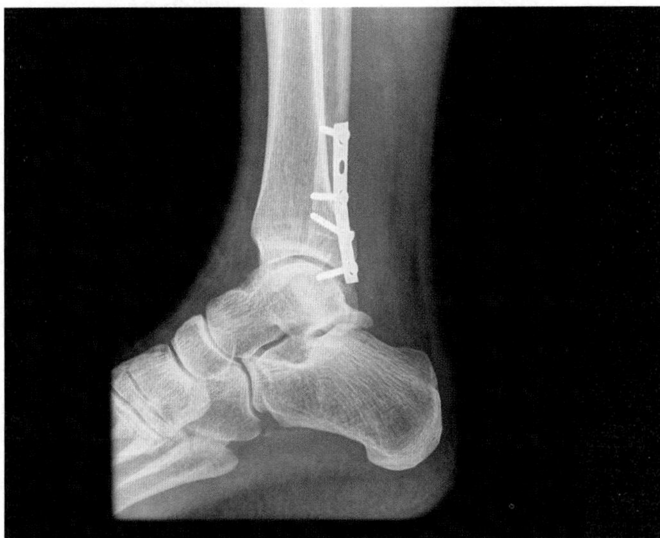

Figure 3.10

- Total knee arthroplasty (TKA) – Removing the bone at the distal (farthest) end of the femur and the bone at the proximal (nearest) end of the tibia and replacing them with implants. (See **Figure 3.11**)

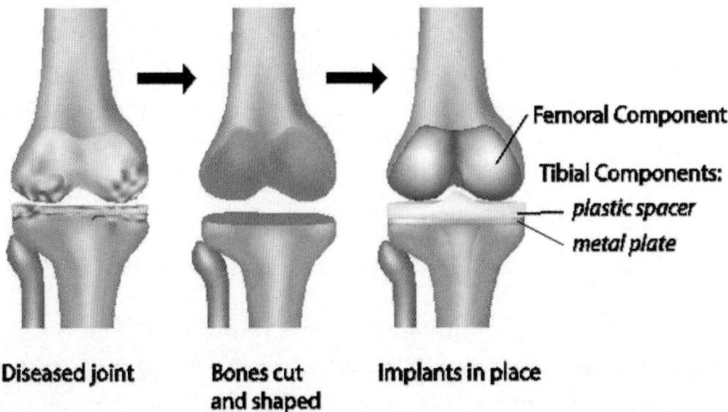

Figure 3.11

- Total hip arthroplasty (THA) – Removing the head of the femur and the socket where it fits in the hip bone and replacing these structures with metal, ceramic and plastic components. (See **Figure 3.12**)

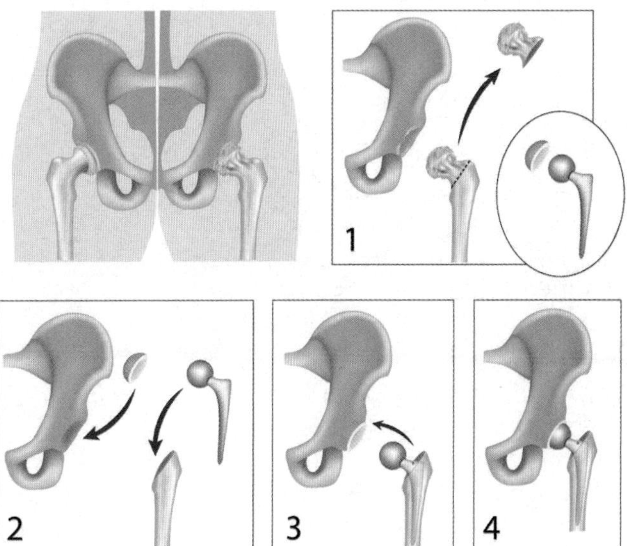

Figure 3.12

- External fixation – Treating fractures with extensive tissue damage with either an optimal frame (placing pins with connected tubes to create a frame) or modular external fixator (rod-to-rod construction) to hold the bones together. (See **Figure 3.13**)

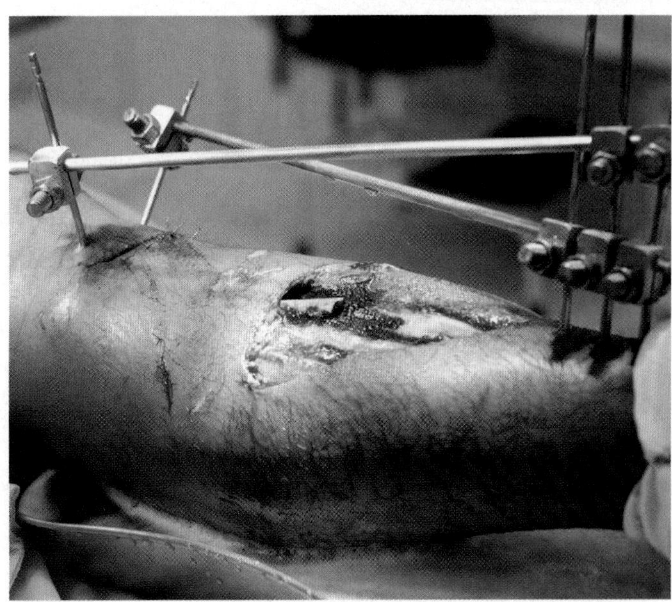

Figure 3.13

- Hip pinning – Stabilizing broken hip bones with surgical screws, nails, rods or plates. Also known as internal fixation of the hip. (See **Figure 3.14**)

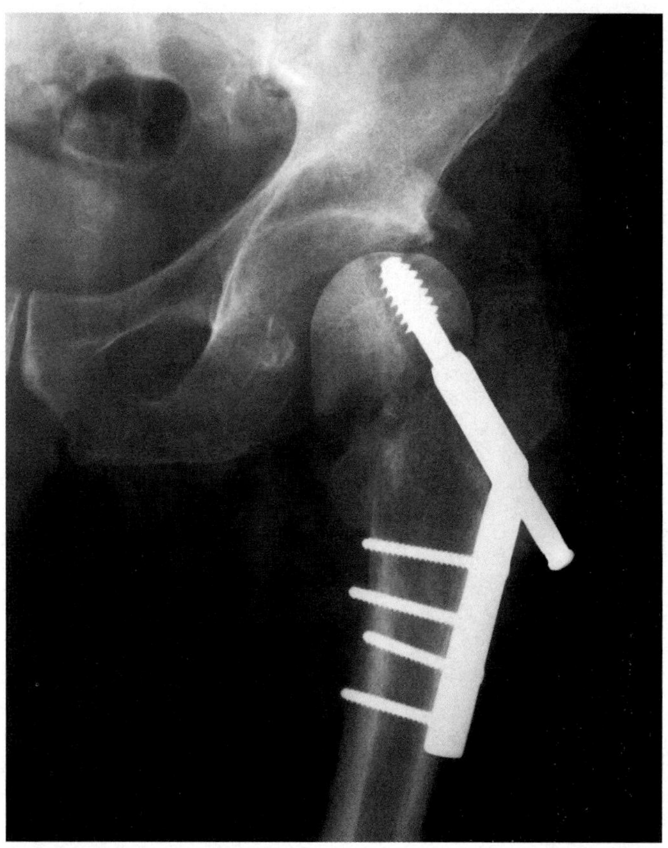

Figure 3.14

- Trigger finger release – Making a small incision in the palm, then cutting the tendon sheath tunnel to widen it and allow the tendon to slide through it more easily.

- Tibial osteotomy – A procedure to realign the knee by wedging open the upper shin bone (tibia) to reconfigure the knee joint. The weight-bearing part of the knee is shifted from degenerative or worn tissue onto healthier tissue.

Muscular System

The muscular system works with the skeletal system to enable movement of the body or materials through the body. (See **Figure 3.15**) Even as one sleeps, many of the more than 600 muscles in the body, including 400 that are skeletal, are actively at work. For example:

- Heart muscles contract to pump blood throughout the body.

- Chest muscles contract to move air in and out of the lungs.

- Muscles in the digestive tract move food and fluid through the body.

- Muscles throughout the body contract to produce heat and maintain the body's core temperature.

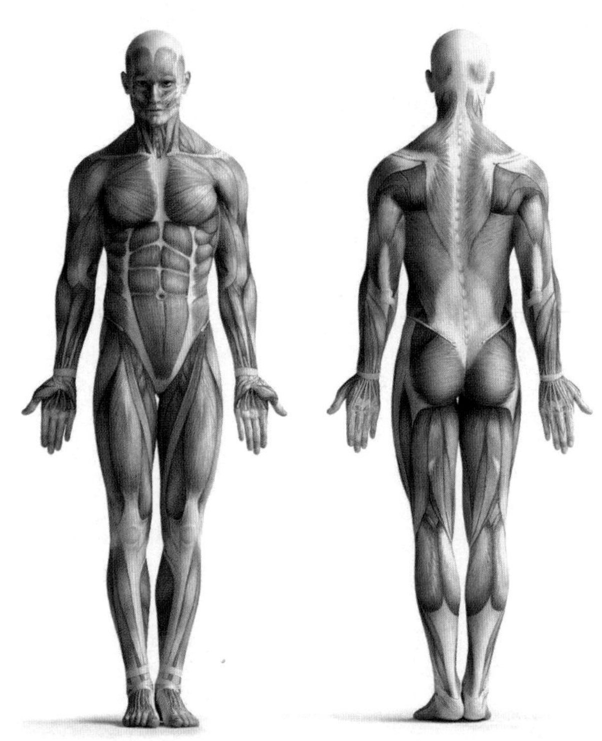

Figure 3.15

Muscles are comprised of long, thin cells or fibers that run parallel to one another and they are bundled together by connective tissue, called **fascia**. Muscle fibers have the ability to contract (shorten), and this contraction causes body movements.

Fascia Band or sheet of fibrous connective tissue.

There are three types of muscle tissue: skeletal, smooth and cardiac. (See **Figure 3.16**)

- Skeletal muscles – Attached to bones by tendons. As skeletal muscles contract, the arms, legs, head or other body parts to which they are attached move. Skeletal muscles are consciously controlled; they move only when we want them to move.

- Smooth muscles – Organized into thin, flat sheets of tissue. Smooth muscles are called involuntary or visceral muscles because they contract and function without conscious control. They control breathing and the movement of food and fluid in the digestive system, movement of blood throughout the circulatory system, and movement of urine through the urinary system.

- Cardiac muscle – Similar to woven mesh fibers that branch out through the heart to give it more strength to pump blood. These involuntary, durable muscle fibers contract and make the heart beat. In a healthy heart, these fibers typically do not tire.

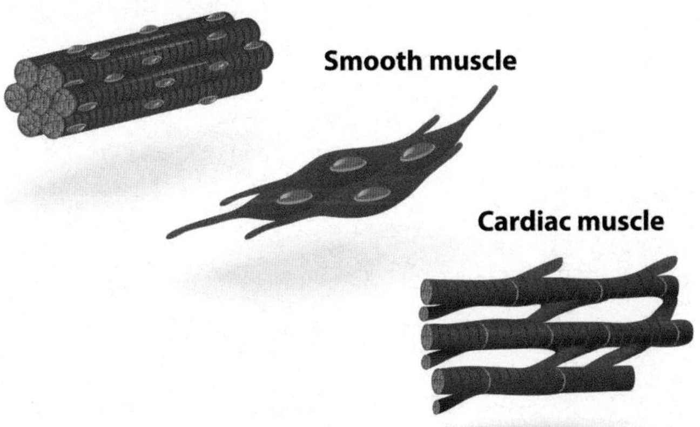

Figure 3.16

To function properly, these muscle fibers require energy (derived from consumed food) and oxygen (derived from the environment when we breathe). Their functions include movement and support, the maintenance of posture and body position, and the production of body heat.

Examples of surgical procedures involving the muscular system include:

- Fasciotomy – Making an incision into the fibrous membrane covering a muscle, usually to relieve pressure from an injured or swollen muscle.
- Herniorrhaphy – Repairing a cavity wall or muscle layer that is allowing all or part of an organ to project through the opening.
- Rotator cuff repair – Repairing the muscles and ligaments of shoulder joints. Frequently used methods are the Bankart, Putti-Platt, and Bristow procedures. (See **Figure 3.17**)

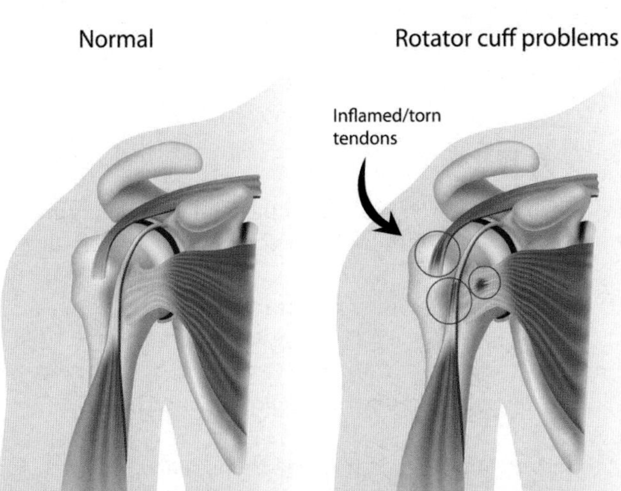

Figure 3.17

- Anterior cruciate ligament (ACL) repair – Rebuilding the ligament in the center of the knee with a new ligament from the patient's own body (or from a donor), usually by knee arthroscopy. In some cases, ACL repair is done by making an incision into the knee. (See **Figure 3.18**)

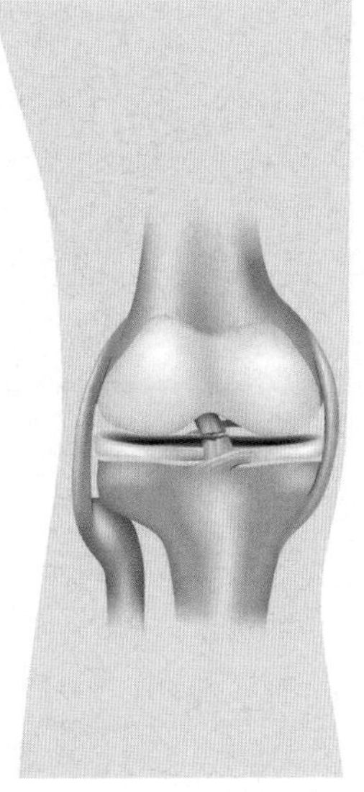
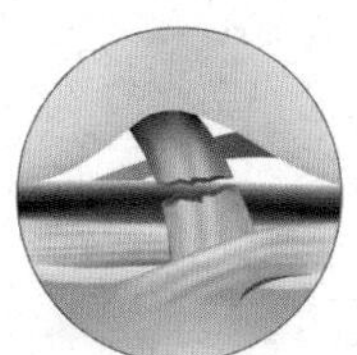

Figure 3.18

- Muscle biopsy – Removing a small sample of muscle tissue for testing in a laboratory.
- Tendon repair – Retrieves a torn tendon and reattaches it to soft tissue or bone with either a small incision or arthroscopic techniques.

Nervous System

The nervous system is a vast communication network. It coordinates and carries messages between all parts of the body and enables us to be aware of changes in the environment—and to react accordingly. A complex series of nervous tissues, somewhat like electrical wiring, runs from the brain and spinal cord throughout the entire body. (See **Figure 3.19**)

The nervous system controls all body functions and allows the body to respond to stimuli. Many reactions are automatic such as blinking when a foreign object approaches the eye. Nerve tissue carries electrical messages from the brain and spinal cord that signal muscles to contract. Other actions are more conscious and involve emotion, reason and memory. Like a computer, the brain stores information based on past experiences that can later be communicated to the body by the nervous system.

Anatomically, the nervous system is divided into two parts: the **central nervous system** (CNS) and the **peripheral nervous system** (PNS).

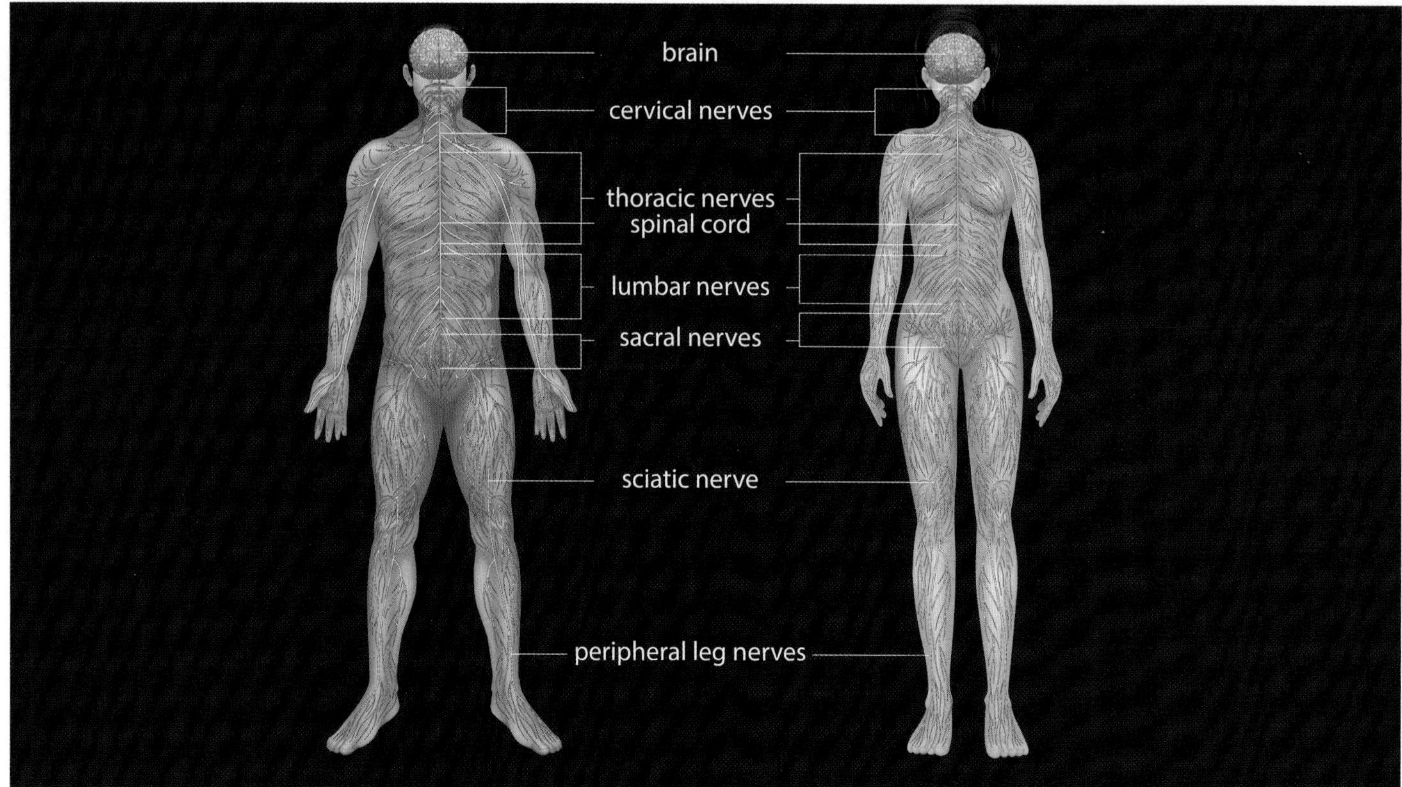

Figure 3.19 Human nervous system (male and female)

The CNS consists of the **brain** and spinal cord, which are covered by protective membranes called meninges. The CNS is the body's control center and storehouse for information about what is happening or has happened within or outside the body. The brain, a spongy and complex organ, is the main control unit of the CNS. It is comprised of more than 100 billion nerve cells. The brain is divided into three parts, each carrying out a specific function: **cerebrum**, **cerebellum** and **brain stem**. (See **Figure 3.20**)

Central nervous system (CNS) The part of the nervous system that includes the brain and spinal cord.

Peripheral nervous system (PNS) All nerve tissue outside the CNS.

Brain The main control unit of the CNS.

Cerebrum The largest part of the brain. It controls mental activities and movement.

Cerebellum The second largest part of the brain. It controls muscle coordination, body balance and posture.

Brain stem Controls many automatic body functions such as heartbeat and breathing.

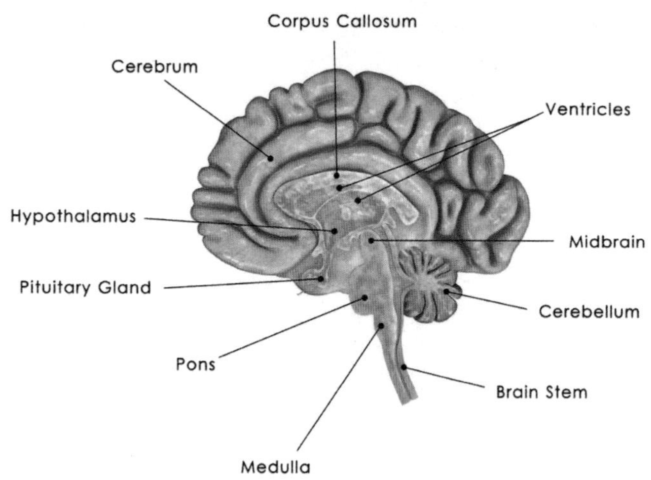

Figure 3.20

The cerebrum is the largest part of the human brain. It functions to:

- Manage the nerve impulses that allow us to think, speak and remember.
- Control most voluntary muscle contractions.
- Interpret information gathered by the senses.
- Influence the foundation of personality, emotions and attitudes.

The cerebrum is divided into two halves (hemispheres). Each half controls different mental activities and movement on the opposite side of the body. A series of nerve pathways run between each half to facilitate communication.

The cerebellum is located inferior (below) and posterior (behind) the cerebrum. It is the second largest part of the brain, and its role is to adjust the motor impulses that control muscular coordination, body balance and posture.

The brain stem is located at the base of the brain and is formed by bundles of nerves that extend from the cerebrum and cerebellum. The lowest part of the brain stem (the medulla oblongata) joins the brain to the spinal cord. It contains nerve centers that control many automatic body functions, including heartbeat and breathing.

The PNS involves the network of nerves and sense organs that branch out of the CNS and connect the CNS to other parts of the body. One part (the autonomic nervous system) controls all involuntary body processes, like heartbeat and **peristalsis**. Other nerves are under direct control of the conscious mind. When someone tells their hand to wave, for example, a message is sent from the brain, down the spinal cord, and through a peripheral nerve to the hand.

> **Peristalsis** The rippling motion of muscles in the digestive tract that mixes food with gastric juices to form a thin liquid.

Sense Organs

Sense organs (eyes, ears, nose, tongue and skin) are accessory structures of the nervous system that provide an impression of all that surrounds us. These organs house special sensory receptors that are message-carrying structures. Most sense organs respond to stimuli from outside the body, while others keep track of the body's internal environment. They respond to light, sound, taste, chemicals, heat and pressure.

Eyes

Eyes (See **Figure 3.21**) are the organs of vision. They produce images by focusing light rays that are interpreted by the brain. Eyes consist of three layers of tissue:

- Sclera – The white portion of the eye that serves as an outer coat to provide protection. At the center front of the sclera is a transparent protective shield called the cornea.
- Choroid – The middle layer of the eye that furnishes nourishment to the eye via blood vessels. The choroid layer includes the iris, a muscle that is the colored portion of the eye. A circular opening, called the pupil, is found at the center of the iris; it controls the amount of light entering the eye as it narrows or widens. Between the cornea and eye lens is the aqueous humor, a watery-like fluid that fills the anterior (front) compartment of the eye.
- Retina – The eye's third layer, located on the back surface of the eyeball. The eye lens focuses light onto the retina, which contains light-sensitive cells (receptors) that receive and transmit impressions to the brain through the optic nerve. The vitreous humor is a fluid-filled compartment of the eye that gives the eyeball its round shape.

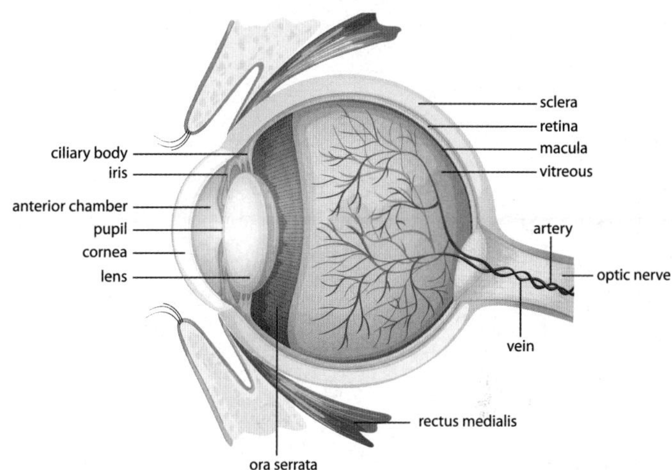

Figure 3.21 Anatomy of the human eye

Ears

Ears are the organs of hearing. They are comprised of three parts: the outer, middle and inner ear. (See **Figure 3.22**) Sound waves travel through the ear to the auditory nerve that transmits nerve impulses to the brain. The ear allows us to hear in the following ways:

- The outer ear serves as a funnel that gathers sound waves and passes them through the ear canal to the tympanic membrane (also known as the eardrum).

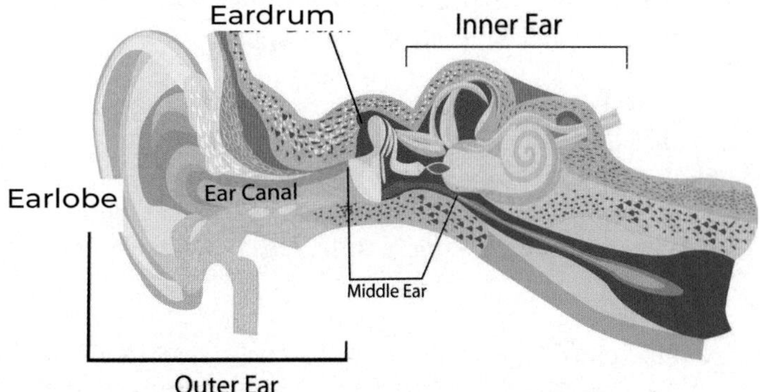

Figure 3.22 Anatomy of the human ear

- The eardrum consists of a tightly stretched membrane that separates the outer ear canal from the middle ear. Vibrations of the eardrum enter the middle ear, which contains three tiny bones: the malleus, incus and stapes.

- The sound vibrations are then passed through these bones into the fluid-filled inner ear. There, vibrations are channeled through the fluid into a spiral-shaped tube called the cochlea, which contains the receptors or nerve endings that transmit nerve impulses to the brain.

The inner ear also contains semi-circular canals consisting of three curved tubes filled with fluid. Body balance is regulated by this fluid as it shifts with body movement. As the fluid shifts, it presses against tiny hairs, stimulating nerve impulses that travel to the brain. The brain responds to these impulses by coordinating muscle movement.

Nose

The nose is the organ of smell and consists of many sensory receptors or cells. These receptors are located in the mucous membranes of the nasal cavity and are sensitive to chemicals carried through the air. The olfactory nerve endings extend to the receptors and are stimulated by different odors. Olfactory bulbs are the enlarged portion at the ends of the olfactory nerves.

Tongue

The tongue is the organ of taste and is covered with taste buds (sensory receptors). The sense of taste, like smell, is a chemical sense. Chemicals are carried by the saliva throughout the mouth. Taste buds located in different areas of the tongue can distinguish four kinds of taste: sweet, sour, bitter and salty. There are 80 different types of chemical odors, and the combination of taste and odors produces flavors.

Skin

The skin is the largest body organ and contains many nerve endings at and below its surface. Skin, therefore, acts as an important sensory organ. Touch receptors near the skin's surface allow us to distinguish textures and respond to heat and cold. Further below the skin's surface are receptors that respond to touch and pressure. The sense of pain stimulates nerves and sends messages of potential danger to the brain.

There are numerous surgical procedures involving the nervous system including:

- Craniotomy – Creating an opening in the skull to expose the brain to facilitate procedures, such as the removal of tumors and clots.

- Carpal tunnel repair – Removal of tissue or displaced bone in the wrist area to release pressure on the median nerve. (See **Figure 3.23**)

- Ulnar nerve transposition – Making an incision at the elbow area, allowing the ulnar nerve to be moved to an area that provides protection and comfort.

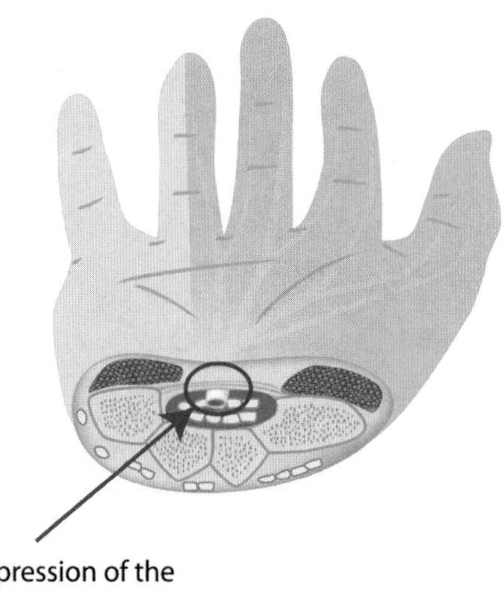

Figure 3.23 Carpal tunnel syndrome

- Cataract extraction with implant – Removing a clouded eye lens and replacing it with a clear, artificial lens. (See **Figure 3.24**)

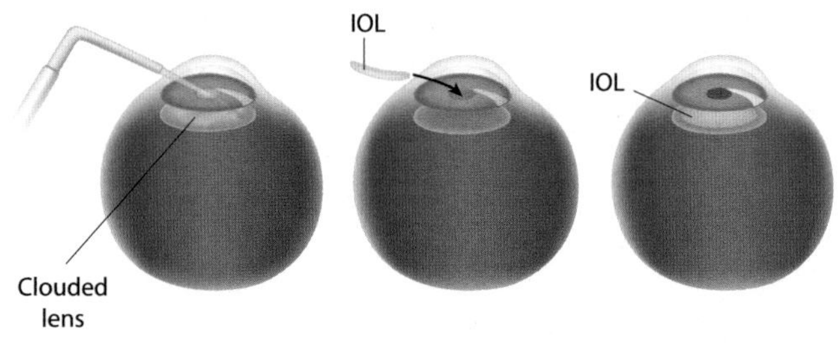

Figure 3.24 Cataract surgery

- Corneal transplant – Grafting corneal tissue from a donor eye to another to improve vision when the cornea is damaged or scarred.

- Bilateral myringotomy with tubes (BMT) – Making an incision into the tympanic membrane (eardrum) to permit fluid to drain. Small tubes are placed in the membrane to allow continuous drainage. The tubes fall out as the membrane heals.

- Stapedectomy – Removal of the stapes (an ear bone) when it has thickened and no longer transmits sound waves. It is replaced with an artificial implant to improve hearing.

- Tympanoplasty – Reconstructing the eardrum, so sound waves can be sent to the middle and inner ear.

- Split-thickness skin graft (STSG) – Cutting the skin (graft) from a donor site. The graft is then transplanted onto the surgical area.

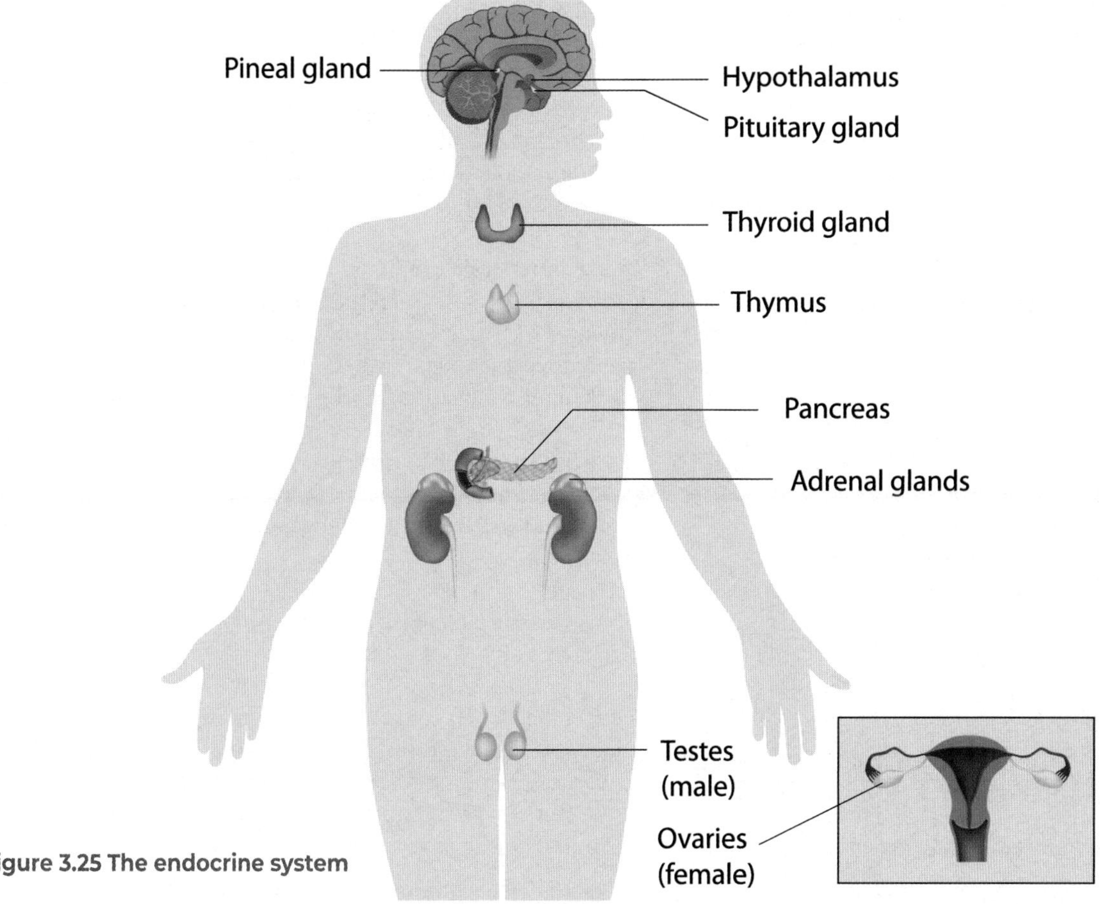

Figure 3.25 The endocrine system

Endocrine System

The endocrine system adapts to changes in the environment. During times of excitement, stress or when one feels threatened, how does the body react? Chances are muscles tense, the heartbeat quickens, and breathing rhythm changes. These rapid changes in bodily functions are set in motion by the **hormones** or secretions produced by the glands of the endocrine system. (See **Figure 3.25**) These glands and the substances they produce have a profound influence on bodily functions, such as **metabolism**, growth and personality.

Because hormones are distributed throughout the body, the endocrine glands that produce them are not necessarily next to the organs they control. Regardless of where hormones enter the bloodstream, they continue their journey through the circulatory system until they reach their targeted organ. Tissue cells and organs recognize and accept hormones made for them and reject others that are not.

The nervous system and endocrine system work together. When the brain interprets information as a threat, it rapidly sends nerve impulses that trigger certain endocrine glands to release their hormones into the bloodstream. In a fearful situation, the hormones cause heartbeat acceleration and prepare muscles for action. In this state, one is ready for fight or flight (to defend or run).

The major glands of the endocrine system include:

- Pituitary gland – A small, pea-shaped gland located at the base of the brain. It is considered the master gland because it helps control the activities of all other endocrine glands. Its secretions also stimulate skeletal and body growth, development of sex organs, regulation of blood pressure, the reproductive process, and muscle development.

- Thyroid gland – Located at the base of the neck, just below the larynx (voice box). Its hormones help regulate the rate of metabolism and maintain the body's levels of calcium and phosphorous.

- Parathyroid glands – Four pea-shaped glands located on (or sometimes in) the thyroid that control the blood's calcium level.

- Adrenal glands – During sudden stress, these glands, which are located on top of each kidney, release adrenaline that increases heart rate and physical strength. Adrenaline also enhances the ability to think and respond more quickly than usual in emergency situations.

- Pancreas – Located just below the stomach, this gland contains cells organized into groups, known as the islets of

Langerhans. Two primary hormones are produced by the pancreatic islets: **insulin**, which reduces the level of sugar in the bloodstream, and **glucagon,** which can increase the blood's sugar level.

- Ovaries – Female sex glands that produce two hormones: estrogen and progesterone. Estrogen is responsible for the development of female characteristics, and progesterone, together with estrogen, regulates the menstrual cycle.

- Testes – Male sex glands that produce the hormone testosterone that stimulates the development of masculine characteristics.

Hormones Chemical messengers that travel through the blood and act on target organs.

Metabolism The total chemical changes by which the nutritional and functional activities of an organism are maintained.

Insulin A hormone that reduces the level of sugar in the blood.

Glucagon A hormone that can increase the blood sugar level.

Examples of surgical procedures involving the endocrine system include:

- Thyroidectomy – Removal of all or part of the thyroid gland.

- Oophorectomy – Removal of an ovary.

- Orchiectomy – Removal of a testicle.

- Pituitary tumor resection – Removal of a tumor on the pituitary gland.

- Thyroid excision – Removal of nodules and/or goiters (enlargements) on the thyroid.

- Adrenalectomy – Removal of one or both (bilateral adrenalectomy) adrenal glands.

Reproductive System

Life begins as a single cell, formed when two other cells join in a process called fertilization. The male sex cell is produced by the male reproductive system and is called **sperm**. The female sex cell (egg) is called **ovum** (plural: ova) and is produced by the female reproductive system. Both sperm and ovum contain rod-shaped structures called **chromosomes** that are responsible for inherited characteristics passed on from parent to child. Each sex cell contains 23 chromosomes; therefore, a fertilized egg consists of 46 chromosomes, receiving 23 from the sperm and 23 from the ovum.

The male reproductive system consists of two **testes**. These oval-shaped glands are located in a skin-covered, pouch-like structure called the **scrotum**. Two tube structures are also in the scrotum. The **epididymis** is a tube that carries sperm cells from the testes to the **vas deferens** (a thick-walled tube structure approximately 18 inches long) where they mature. The vas deferens then carries sperm to a hollow chamber, called the **seminal vesicle**, located behind the bladder.

The seminal vesicle joins with the vas deferens to form the ejaculatory duct. The secretions of the seminal vesicle are called **semen**, which bathes and nourishes the sperm cells. In the **ejaculatory duct**, the semen-containing sperm enter the **urethra** which, upon ejaculation, transfers the sperm to the female's body.

The **prostate gland** is a partly glandular and partly muscular gland that surrounds the neck of the bladder. It secretes a fluid, which is part of the semen and stimulates sperm motility (movement).

The female reproductive system consists of the **vagina**, a muscular canal approximately 4½ inches long through which a baby passes during birth. It extends from an external opening to the **cervix** (neck of the uterus). The **uterus** is located between the rectum and urinary bladder and is a hollow, pear-shaped organ. It is lined with a fluffy vascular layer of tissue called **endometrium**. The fertilized ovum embeds itself into the endometrium, which sloughs off (separates) during menstruation if the ovum is not fertilized.

The **fallopian tubes** (oviducts) extend from two openings on each side of the anterior portion of the uterus. The distal (farthest) ends of the fallopian tubes are funnel-shaped, and finger-like projections, called **fimbriae**, extend from them. They are located near, but not attached to, the **ovaries**. The fimbriae draw the ovum into the fallopian tube where it travels to the uterus.

Examples of surgical procedures involving the reproductive system include:

- Orchiopexy – Relocating a non-descended testicle to the correct location in the scrotum.

- Transurethral resection of the prostate (TURP) – Removal of part of the prostate gland through the insertion of instruments across the urethra to reach the prostate internally.

- Radical prostatectomy – Removal of the prostate gland using an incision in the abdomen and the urinary bladder.

- Hysterectomy – Removal of the uterus.

- Bilateral salpingo-oophorectomy (BSO) – Removal of the fallopian tubes and ovaries.

Sperm Male sex cell.

Ovum Female sex cell (egg).

Chromosomes Rod-shaped structures responsible for inherited characteristics passed on from parent to child.

Testes Male reproductive gland that forms and secretes sperm and several fluid elements in semen.

Scrotum Sac in which testes are suspended.

Epididymis A tube that carries sperm cells from the testes to the vas deferens.

Vas deferens A duct that transfers sperm from the epididymis to the seminal vesicle.

Seminal vesicle A gland that produces semen.

Semen Mixture of sperm cells and secretions from several male reproductive glands.

Ejaculatory duct A duct formed by joining the seminal vesicle with the vas deferens, through which semen moves during ejaculation.

Urethra Tube that discharges urine.

Prostate gland Produces a fluid element in semen that stimulates the movement of sperm.

Vagina Muscular canal in a female that extends from an external opening to the neck of the uterus.

Cervix Lower end (neck) of the uterus.

Uterus Female organ within which the fetus develops during pregnancy.

Endometrium Lining of the uterus.

Fallopian tubes Slender tubes that convey the ova (eggs) from the ovaries to the uterus.

Fimbriae Finger-like projections extending from the fallopian tubes that draw ova (eggs) into the uterus.

Ovaries Female reproductive organs.

- Endometrial ablation – Scarring or removal of the inner lining of the uterus to treat abnormal bleeding.

- Dilation and curettage (D&C) – Widening of the cervix (opening of the uterus) to permit evacuation of the contents or scraping of the lining of the uterus.

- Ectopic pregnancy – Removal of a fertilized ovum growing in the fallopian tube to prevent complications, such as hemorrhage, shock and scarring of the fallopian tube.

- Pelviscopy – Visualization of the pelvic cavity (lower abdomen) using an endoscope for medical diagnosis or treatment of female reproductive organs.

- Tubal ligation – Cutting, burning, tying or applying a clip on the fallopian tubes to prevent future pregnancies. (See **Figure 3.26**)

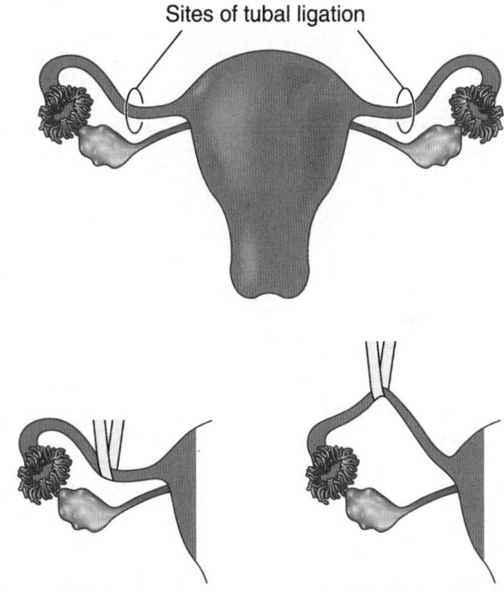

a) Fallopian tube is raised to create a loop

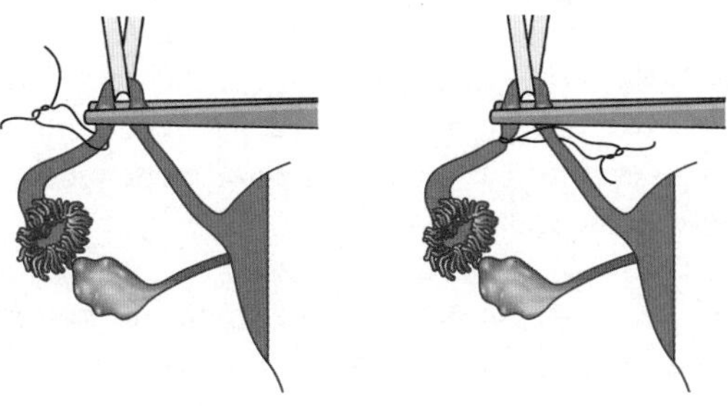

b) The loop is crushed with forceps, then ligated in a figure-of-eight

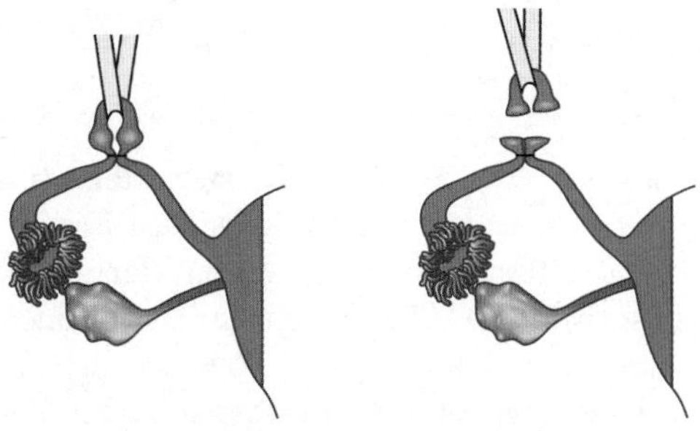

c) The loop is excised at the crushed zone

Figure 3.26

- Vasectomy – A surgical procedure for male sterilization and/ or birth control. (See **Figure 3.27**)

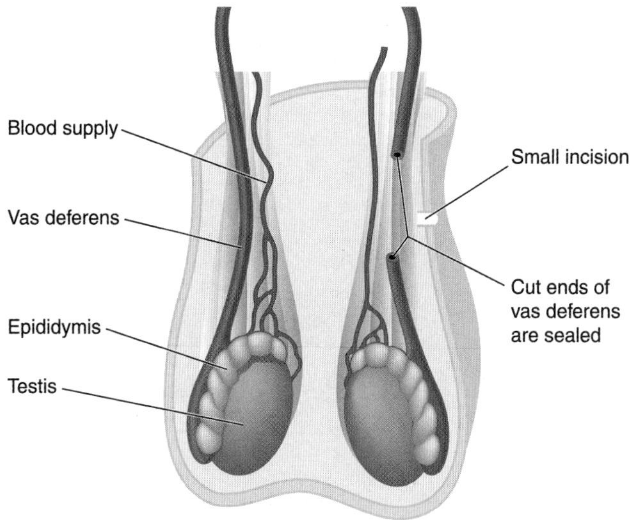

Figure 3.27

Urinary and Excretory Systems

The urinary system provides "pollution control" by eliminating bodily waste. This process takes place as blood is filtered by the urinary system. Urine is a water solution consisting of various waste substances that are products of metabolism. It obtains its color from excreted bile pigments and may be a shade of amber, pale yellow or clear. Depending on the amount of liquid intake or loss through perspiration, an average adult may excrete between 1000cc and 1800cc of urine during a 24-hour period. In males, the urinary and reproductive systems are closely related and comprise the genitourinary system. In females, however, the two systems are not interrelated.

Organs of the urinary system in both sexes (See **Figure 3.28**) include:

- **Kidneys** – Two bean-shaped organs that contain a vast network of vessels and tubules, called nephron, that act as a filter to remove excess water and waste from the blood to produce urine.

- **Ureters** – Two tube-like structures that extend from each kidney and connect to the urinary bladder. The peristaltic (automatic constriction and relaxation) action of the ureters moves urine from the kidneys to the urinary bladder.

- **Urinary bladder** – Serves as a reservoir for urine. It is a muscular, membranous sack located in the pelvis, just anterior (front) of the sigmoid colon and posterior to (behind) the pubis. The bladder is flexible, and its size depends on the amount of urine present (average capacity ranges from 300cc to 500cc in adults). As the amount of urine in the urinary bladder increases, it applies pressure on the bladder walls, sending an impulse to the CNS. As the bladder wall contracts, the sphincter muscle at the junction of the urethra relaxes and urine is released.

- Urethra – A membranous canal or tube that connects the urinary bladder to outside the body to eliminate urine. In males, the urethra is approximately 20cm long; it passes through the prostate gland and pelvic wall and extends through the **penis**. The female urethra is about 4cm long; it runs from the bladder through the sphincter muscle to the external meatus (opening) located at the anterior (front) of the vagina.

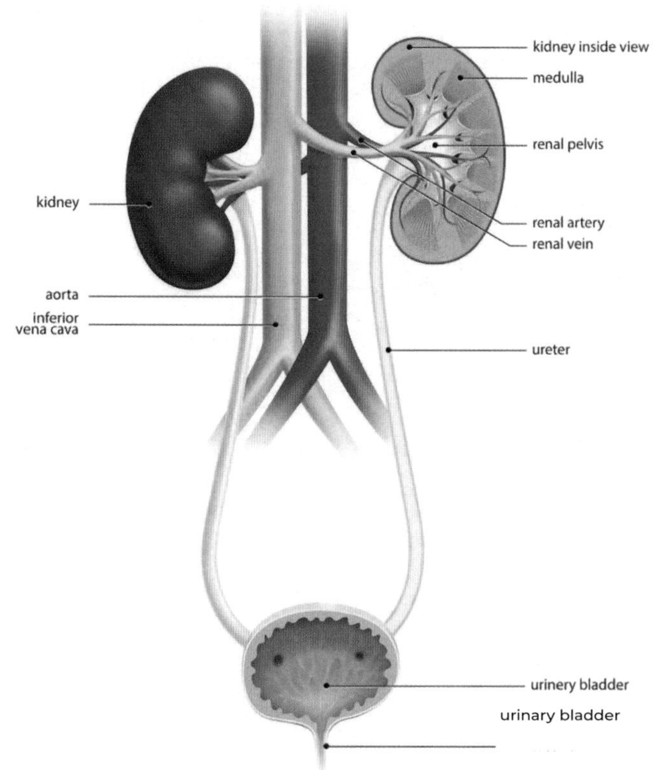

Figure 3.28

Kidneys Organs that remove excess water and waste substances from the blood in a process that yields urine.

Ureters Tube-like structures extending from the kidneys to the urinary bladder that move urine between these organs.

Urinary bladder The reservoir for urine.

Penis Male organ of urination and intercourse.

The excretory system removes toxic (poisonous) waste substances. The kidneys (urinary system) and lungs (respiratory system) also perform excretory functions, as do the **liver** and **skin**.

Liver An organ that filters the blood to remove amino acids and neutralize some harmful toxins.

Skin This organ contains sweat glands that, through the process of perspiration, produce and excrete sweat.

The liver is another filter for the blood. It removes amino acids and can neutralize some harmful toxins. It can also convert hemoglobin from worn-out blood cells into substances the body requires.

Skin contains sweat glands, oils, hair and nails. Sweat glands remove excess water, salt and other bodily wastes. These are located in the dermis (inner layer of skin) and consist of coiled tubes connected to pores in the skin's surface. The sweat glands, through the process of perspiration, produce and excrete sweat. Perspiration rids the body of waste and helps regulate the body's temperature by cooling its outside surface. The excretion of oil by the sebaceous glands keeps the skin soft and prevents hair from becoming too dry or brittle.

Examples of surgical procedures involving the urinary system include:

- Cystoscopy – Viewing the urinary bladder using an endoscope.
- Nephrectomy – Removal of the kidney.
- Lithotripsy (kidney stone shock wave treatment) – Serves to crush stones that form in the kidney and become stuck in a ureter. The procedure involves decreasing the size of the stones with a laser or shock waves or removing them using a long, flexible instrument called a stone basket. (See **Figure 3.29**)

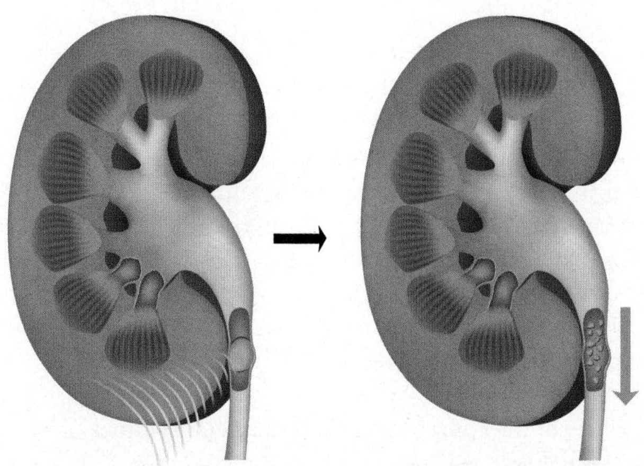

Figure 3.29 Kidney stone shock wave treatment

Respiratory System

The respiratory system (See **Figure 3.30**) supplies the body with oxygen and removes carbon dioxide.

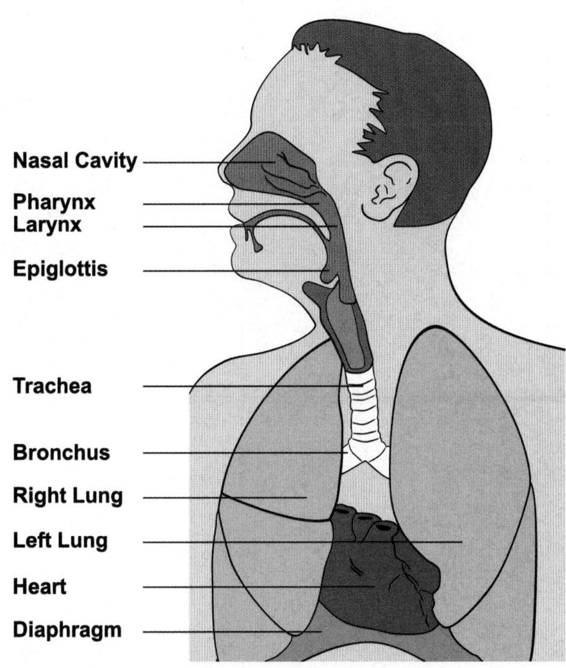

Figure 3.30 Respiratory system

This exchange of gases is accomplished automatically as one breathes in a two-step process: inspiration (inhaling air into the lungs) and expiration (exhaling air from the lungs). Air contains impurities, such as dirt, dust and microorganisms, and these are filtered out by the respiratory system.

The primary organs of the respiratory system are:

- **Nose** (nasal cavity) and **mouth** – During inspiration, air enters the nostrils (nasal openings) and mouth. Air in the nose is filtered, moistened and warmed.
- **Pharynx** – Air passes to the pharynx (throat), which is the crossroads of the nose, mouth, voice box and **esophagus**. Food continues down the esophagus, while air passes through the **larynx** (voice box) to the **trachea**.
- Trachea (windpipe) – The trachea divides into two tube-like structures, the right and left **bronchi**, that extend into the **lungs**.
- Lungs – Air continues through the bronchi to the bronchioles, a series of many smaller tubes extending from each bronchus (somewhat like branches of a tree). At the end of each bronchiole are small clusters of air sacs, called alveoli, that comprise the lungs' tissue. Alveoli and each alveolus are covered by a thin wall surrounded by a vast network of capillaries (tiny blood vessels). The blood then picks up oxygen from the inspired air and releases the waste gas, carbon dioxide, during expiration.

The right lung consists of three lobes. The left lung consists of two lobes to allow space for the heart.

The lungs are located in the thoracic cavity (chest), where they are covered by thin membranes, called pleura, and protected by the skeletal rib cage and sternum. The pleura secretes a lubricating fluid that permits smooth movement of the lungs during the respiratory cycle.

Nose Organ of smell; also filters the air we breathe.

Mouth Opening through which air, food and beverages enter the body; beginning of the alimentary canal.

Pharynx Throat.

Esophagus Connects the throat to the stomach.

Larynx Voice box.

Trachea Windpipe.

Bronchi The main passageway for air to travel from the trachea to the lungs.

Lungs Main organs of the respiratory system whose function is transporting oxygen into the blood and removing carbon dioxide from the blood.

- Diaphragm – A muscle located below the lungs. The diaphragm contracts and causes the chest cavity to expand to allow more space for air. During expiration, it relaxes and air is forced out of the lungs.

Examples of surgical procedures involving the respiratory system include:

- Thoracotomy – Making an opening into the thoracic cavity (chest) to give surgeons access to the lungs and heart.
- Thoracoscopy – Viewing the thoracic (chest) cavity with an endoscope for diagnosis or treatment.
- Pneumonectomy – Removal of a lung.
- Tracheotomy – Making an incision into the trachea. (See **Figure 3.31**)
- Lobectomy – Removal of a lobe of an organ, usually referring to the brain, lung or liver.
- Laryngectomy – Removal of the larynx (voice box).
- Bronchoscopy – Visualizing the bronchus with an endoscope.
- Septoplasty – Straightening or removing cartilage and/or bone in the nose when the nasal septum is deformed, injured or fractured.
- Endoscopic sinus surgery (ESS) – Removal of bone defects or inflamed tissue of the paranasal sinuses to allow the sinuses to drain.

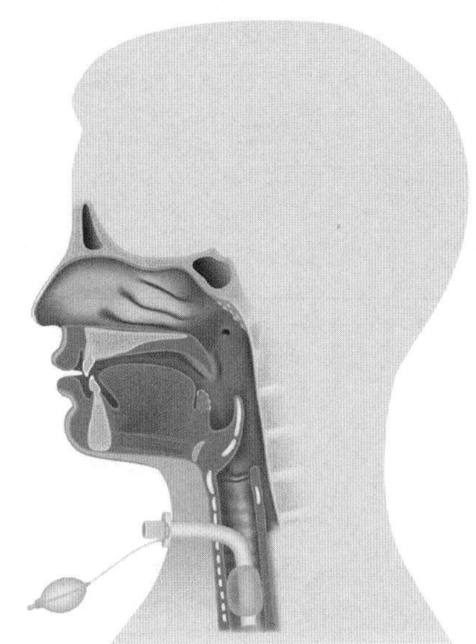

Figure 3.31 Tracheotomy

Digestive System

The human body, like any other complex piece of machinery, requires a source of energy or fuel to keep it functioning. The body gets its fuel from the chemicals (nutrients) in food.

The function of the digestive system (see **Figure 3.32**) is to convert food into energy for the body. The human body requires six basic categories of nutrients: proteins, carbohydrates, fats, water, minerals and vitamins. A well-balanced diet is important for keeping the body healthy and strong.

The process of digestion breaks food down mechanically and chemically so it can be absorbed by body cells or discharged as waste. The pathway that food takes through the digestive system is called the **alimentary canal** (digestive tract). The alimentary canal is approximately 30 feet long and consists of the mouth, esophagus, **stomach**, **small intestine**, **large intestine**, **rectum** and **anus**. The liver, gallbladder and pancreas are accessory organs of the digestive system. The salivary, gastric and intestinal glands are accessory structures to the digestive system that contribute to the process of digestion.

A review of the components of the alimentary canal allows us to study the digestive process:

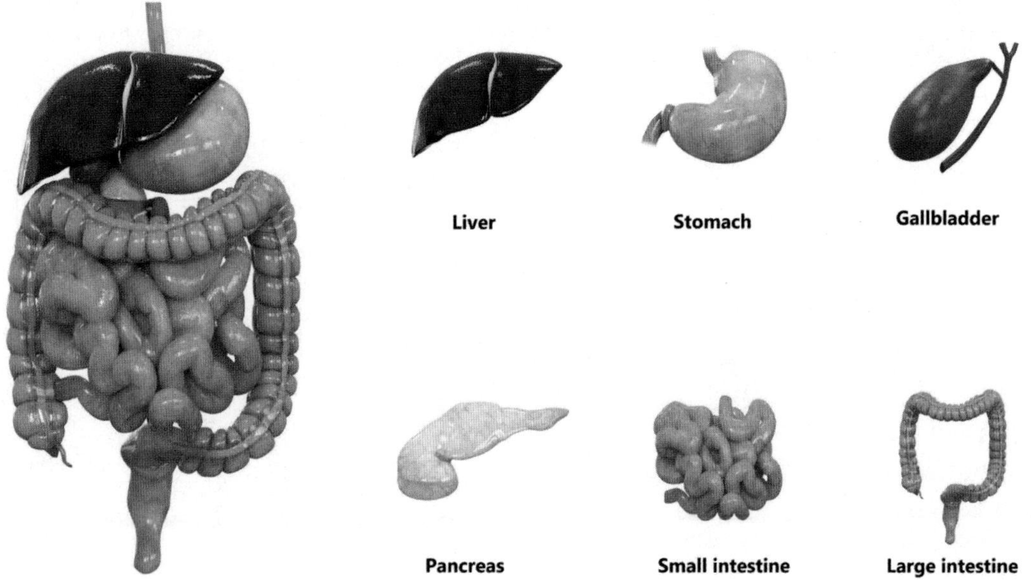

Figure 3.32 Human digestive system anatomy

- Mouth – The digestive process begins in the mouth. There, food is softened by saliva secreted by salivary glands located throughout the mouth. The teeth tear and grind the softened food into smaller particles that allow it to be easily swallowed. The food then passes through the esophagus.

- Esophagus – A somewhat flexible, muscular tube that produces peristaltic contractions, which move food into the stomach.

- Stomach – An elongated and muscular J-shaped pouch that serves as a reservoir for food as gastric gland secretions (mucin, hydrochloric acid and enzymes) convert the food into a semi-liquid material called chyme.

- Small intestine – From the stomach, the liquified food enters the small intestine (an organ approximately 20 to 23 feet long). This is where the greatest amount of digestion and absorption of nutrients into body cells occurs. The small intestine is divided into three portions: duodenum, jejunum and ileum. Bile (produced by the liver and stored in the gallbladder), along with pancreatic and intestinal juices, facilitates digestion in the small intestine.

- Large intestine (colon) – Material that is not absorbed by the small intestine enters the large intestine (colon), which is approximately five to six feet long. The first few inches of the large intestine are called the cecum, from which the appendix extends. The large intestine consists of six portions: ascending colon, transverse colon, descending colon, sigmoid colon, rectum and anus. Peristaltic action moves food through the large intestine where the absorption of water and electrolytes or salt occurs.

- Rectum and anus – The rectum is the last several inches of the large intestine where the remaining waste (feces) becomes dehydrated and is eliminated through the anus.

Alimentary canal The pathway that food takes through the digestive system; also called digestive tract.

Stomach A pouch that serves as a reservoir for food that has been consumed.

Small intestine The organ in the digestive system where the greatest amount of digestion and absorption of nutrients into the body cells occurs.

Large intestine (colon) The digestive organ that dehydrates digestive residues (feces).

Rectum The last several inches of the large intestine.

Anus The lower opening of the alimentary canal.

Examples of surgical procedures involving the digestive system include:

- Appendectomy – Removal of the appendix

- Parotidectomy – Removal of a salivary gland (parotid) because of tumor formation

- Gastrectomy – Removal of the stomach. Other procedures include removal of portions of the stomach (e.g., hemigastrectomy or gastric sleeve). (See **Figure 3.33**)

- Gastric bypass – Isolating a small portion of the stomach and suturing part of the small intestine to it to treat morbid obesity. Food intake is then limited to the small part of the stomach. (See **Figure 3.34**)

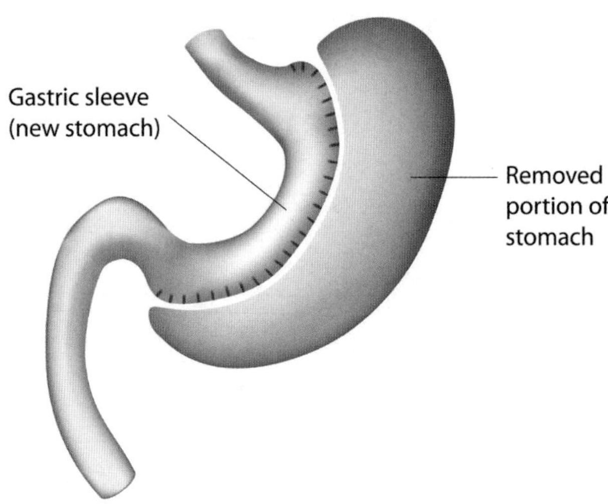

Figure 3.33 Vertical sleeve gastrectomy

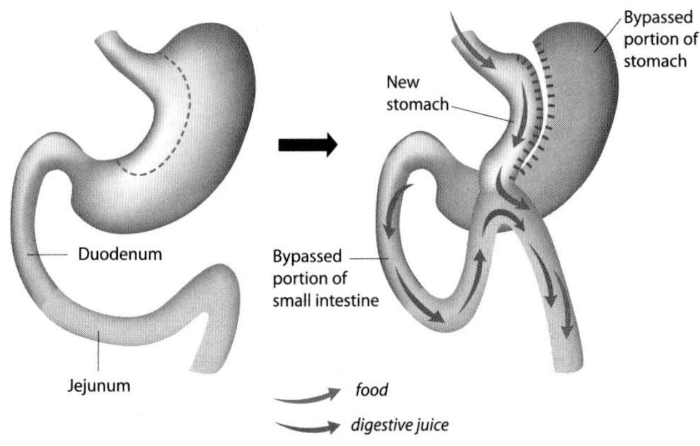

Figure 3.34 Mini-gastric bypass

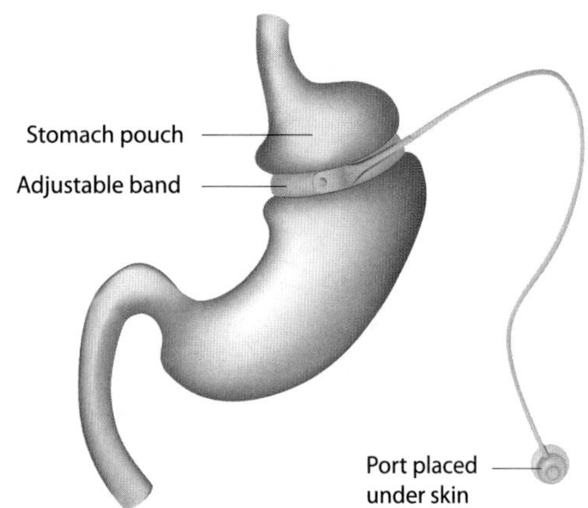

Figure 3.35 Adjustable gastric band (lap band)

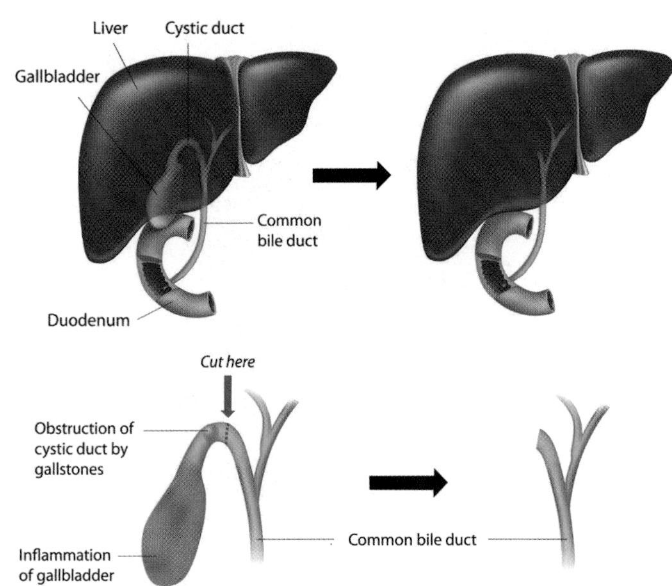

Figure 3.36 Cholecystectomy

- Gastric banding – An inflatable silicone device placed around the top portion of the stomach to treat obesity (see **Figure 3.35**)
- Cholecystectomy – Removal of the gallbladder with a surgical incision or by endoscopic surgery, called laparoscopic cholecystectomy (see **Figure 3.36**)
- Colectomy – Removal of all or part of the large intestine
- Laparoscopic cholecystectomy – Removal of the gallbladder with endoscopic instrumentation

Circulatory System

The circulatory system (see **Figure 3.37**) is the body's primary transportation network. It delivers nutrients and oxygen to body cells and carries away carbon dioxide and other harmful waste products. This is accomplished as blood is pumped through 60,000 miles of blood vessels in the body.

The lymphatic system (see **Figure 3.38**) is a subsidiary of the circulatory system and serves a vital role in the body's defense against disease. The lymphatic system consists of a series of tiny vessels located throughout the body that carry clear liquid fluid (lymph) that originates from blood plasma. Large numbers of lymph nodes (tissue masses containing special cells called lymphocytes) that filter bacteria and other harmful materials out of the lymph are located in the lymph and blood vessels. Lymph flows from the lymph vessels into two veins located in the neck region to return lost fluid back into the bloodstream.

Tonsils are one type of lymph node, and they are located on both sides of the base of the tongue in the throat. (See **Figure 3.39**)

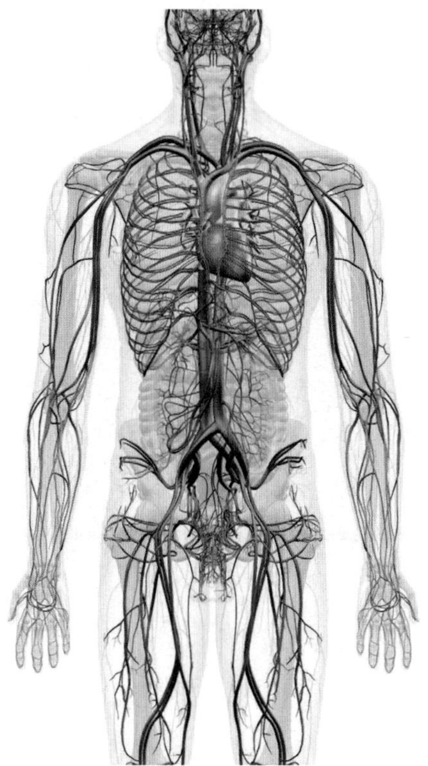

Figure 3.37 Circulatory system

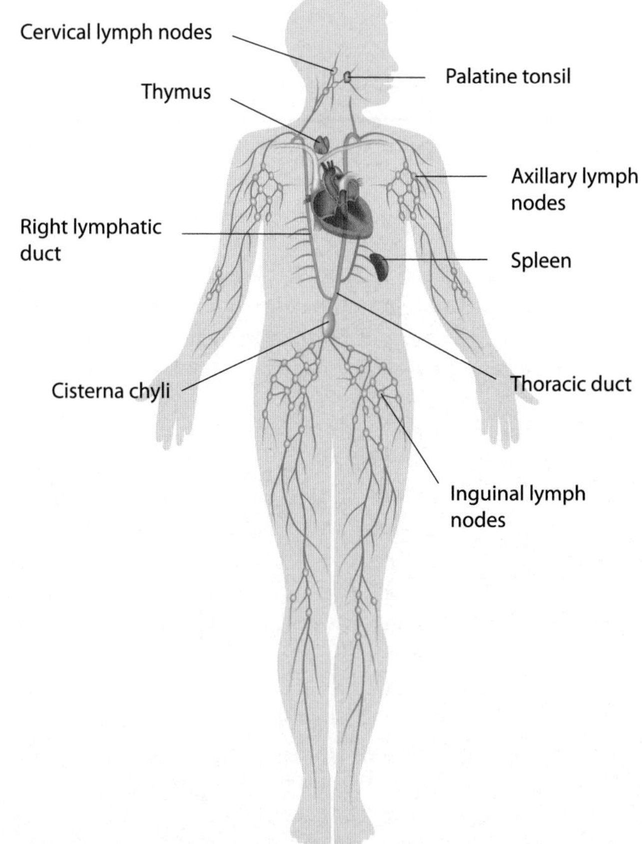

Figure 3.38 Lymphatic system

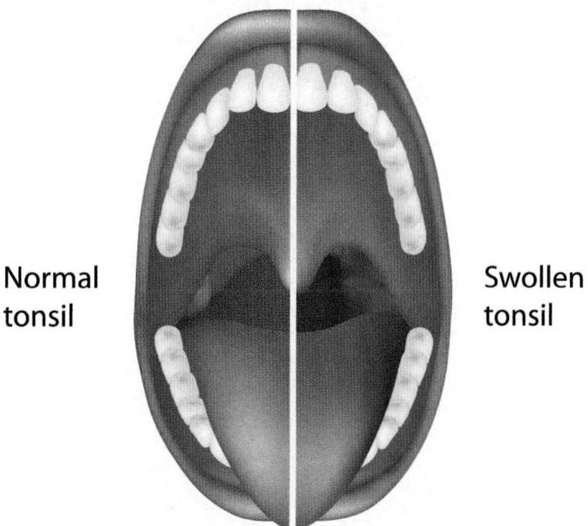

Figure 3.39 Tonsillitis

Sentinel lymph nodes are frequently identified during cancer surgery. The surgeon tries to find the first (sentinel) lymph node where the cancer cells have started to spread.

Blood is a type of connective tissue fluid that moves throughout the circulatory system and transports many important substances. The body contains an average of five to seven liters of blood. Blood is a mixture of plasma, red blood cells (erythrocytes), white blood cells (leukocytes) and platelets:

- **Plasma** – More than 55% of blood is made up of plasma, a yellowish liquid that is composed of water (92%) and proteins. Plasma serves as the vehicle of transportation for dissolved nutrients, enzymes, waste and other substances through the body.

- **Red blood cells** – These structures have thin centers that allow them to be pliable when moving through narrow capillaries. Red blood cells are rich in hemoglobin (an iron protein) that picks up oxygen in the lungs and transports it to all the body cells and then transports carbon dioxide back to the lungs. These cells are produced in the bone marrow and have a life span of approximately 120 days. Worn-out or damaged red blood cells are broken down in the liver and destroyed by the spleen.

- **White blood cells** – Some white blood cells are twice as large as red blood cells and their life span can range from hours to years. White blood cells are also produced by bone marrow and their purpose is to attack, destroy and digest disease-producing organisms that enter the body.

- **Platelets** – These tiny cell fragments detach from bone marrow and enter the bloodstream. They have no color or nucleus and last for a maximum of 10 days. Enzymes released by the platelets act on other blood components to create fibrin. This chemical weaves across cells in blood vessels and traps blood cells and plasma that will harden and clot.

Blood A type of connective tissue fluid that transports many substances throughout the circulatory system.

Plasma The largest component of the blood. Plasma transports nutrients throughout the body and helps remove waste from the body.

Red blood cells Blood cells that carry oxygen throughout the body.

White blood cells Blood cells that circulate in the blood and help defend the body against infection or foreign invaders.

Platelets Blood cell fragments whose function is to help the blood to clot.

Circulation in the body is a continuous process, traveling the same route throughout the body all the time. Blood moves from the **heart** to the lungs and then back to the heart where it is pumped to all the cells of the body through a system of vessels. Blood then returns back to the heart to be recirculated.

The vessels that carry blood away from the heart are called **arteries. Veins** are the vessels that carry blood back to the heart. **Capillaries** are the tiny vessels abundant throughout the body that serve as connections between veins and arteries.

The heart (see **Figure 3.40**) is a muscular organ, about the size of a fist, that pumps five liters of blood through the body every minute, while resting only between beats. Located in its upper right side is a "pacemaker" that signals the heart muscle to contract; this controls the heartbeat. Here's how the heart works:

- The heart consists of four hollow chambers, two on each side.
- A thick tissue wall, called the septum, separates the left and right sides of the heart.
- The upper chambers of the heart are called **atria,** and the lower chambers are called **ventricles**.
- Deoxygenated blood (blood that has had oxygen removed by the cells) returns to the heart and enters the right atrium.
- As the right atrium becomes full, a tissue flap (called a heart valve) opens. It allows blood to flow into the right ventricle.
- When the right ventricle is full, the valve closes to prevent backflow of blood.
- As the right ventricle contracts, blood is forced out of the heart through the pulmonary artery and into the lungs where it is oxygenated.

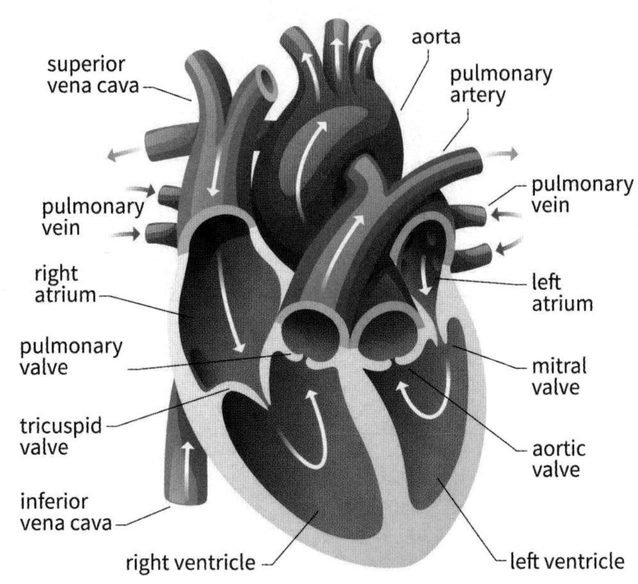

Figure 3.40

- The oxygenated blood leaves the lungs through the pulmonary veins and enters the left atrium.
- As the left atrium becomes full, the left atrium heart valve opens and the blood flows into the left ventricle. As the left ventricle becomes full, the left atrium valve closes, the left ventricle contracts, and oxygenated blood leaves the heart. As the heart contracts, blood is forced out of the left ventricle through the aortic valve into the **aorta**, the largest blood vessel in the body. The aorta is an artery that carries blood away from the heart and it branches out into a vast network of smaller arteries throughout the body. The left ventricle pumps blood throughout the entire body, working about six times as hard as the right ventricle, which only pumps blood a short distance.

Heart The muscular organ that pumps blood throughout the body.

Arteries Vessels that carry blood away from the heart.

Veins Vessels that carry blood back to the heart.

Capillaries Vessels that serve as connections between veins and arteries.

Atria The two upper chambers of the heart.

Ventricles The two lower chambers of the heart.

Aorta The largest blood vessel in the body.

Examples of surgical procedures involving the circulatory system include:

- Tonsillectomy – Removal of lymph tissue in the pharynx (throat)
- Adenoidectomy – Removal of tonsil tissue at the end of the soft palate (roof of the mouth)
- Arteriovenous (AV) fistula – Suturing the radial artery and cephalic vein together in the lower arm to allow the dilated (enlarged) vein to be used for large bore needle insertion for renal dialysis
- Aneurysm repair – abdominal aortic aneurysm (AAA) – Removing a weakened, balloon-like area in the aorta and replacing it with a synthetic product (see **Figure 3.41**)

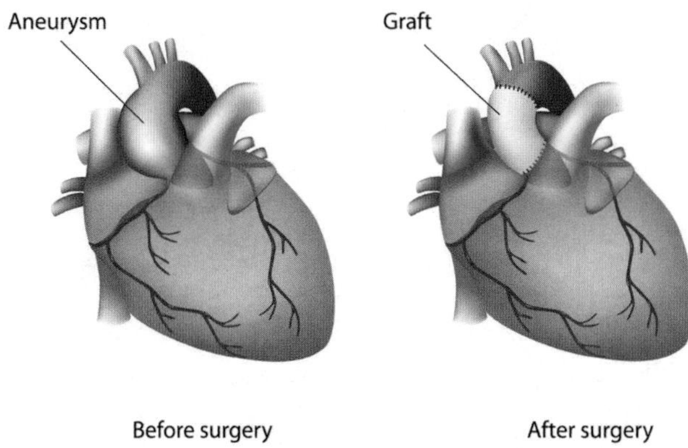

Figure 3.41 Ascending aortic aneurysm and surgical repair

- Pacemaker insertion – A small electrical medical device implanted in a patient to make the heart beat regularly (see **Figure 3.42**)

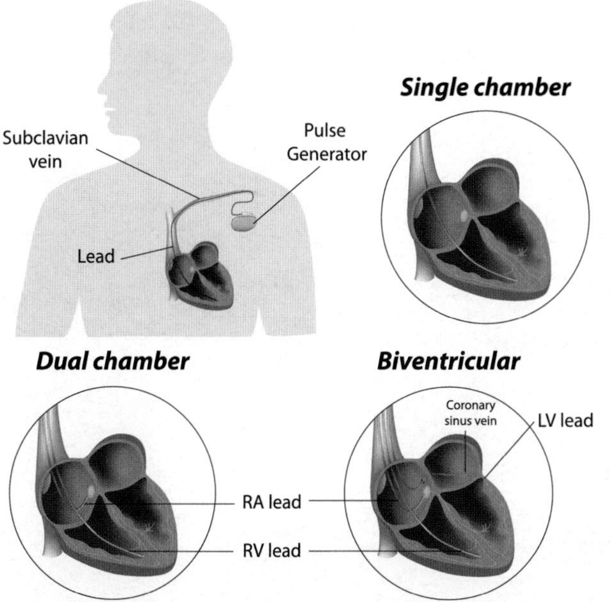

Figure 3.42

- Hemorrhoidectomy – Removal of swollen, inflamed veins from the anus
- Coronary artery bypass graft (CABG) – Removal of a vein, usually from a lower limb, to bypass the blocked section of the coronary arteries (see **Figure 3.43**)

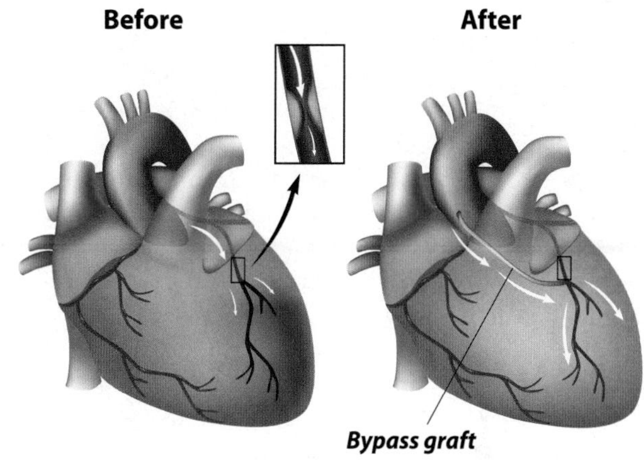

Figure 3.43 Coronary artery bypass surgery

- Carotid endarterectomy – A procedure to reduce the risk of stroke by removing plaque from the carotid artery that causes lack of brain oxygenation

ANATOMY AND INSTRUMENT NAMES

SP technicians who familiarize themselves with common aspects of human anatomy and physiology may find it easier to understand the need for specialized instruments to address a specific body system.

The names of many surgical instruments reflect the anatomical region for which they have been designed. For this reason, taking the time to learn how the body works will help SP technicians better understand the purpose of a particular instrument and help them remember its name.

Here are just a few examples of the hundreds of instruments that reflect the anatomical area from which their names are derived:

- Aortic compressor
- Vaginal speculum
- Adenotome
- Eyelid retractor
- Urethratome
- Bowel forceps

- Anal retractor
- Lacrimal duct probes
- Hip skid
- Uterine sounds
- Brain spatula

CONCLUSION

While SP technicians do not provide direct patient care, an understanding of basic anatomy and common surgical procedures can help improve communication with surgery and other procedural units and, therefore, improve patient outcomes. A basic understanding of anatomical terms can also increase instrument knowledge. Both enhancements make it easier to function in the role of surgical support.

The human body is incredibly sophisticated. With its many parts, networks and functions, it is amazing to wonder how these various systems must work together and how disease or injury can disrupt the body system symphony. By gaining a basic understanding of how the body works and the common surgical procedures that are performed to treat certain conditions, SP technicians can become more knowledgeable about the instruments and devices in their care and improve their ability to communicate with the surgical team.

RESOURCES

Brooks M. *Exploring Medical Language: A Student-Directed Approach. Fifth Edition.* Mosby Inc. 2002.

Davies J. *Essentials of Medical Terminology. Third Edition.* Delmar Publishers Inc. 2002.

Fremgen B. *Medical Terminology: An Anatomy and Physiology Systems Approach.* Prentice-Hall Inc. 1997.

Gylys B. *Medical Terminology Simplified: A Programmed Learning Approach by Body Systems.* F. A. Davis Company. 1995.

Gylys B. Wedding M. *Medical Terminology: A Systems Approach. Third Edition.* F. A. Davis Company. 1995.

Isler C. *The Patient's Guide to Medical Terminology. Third Edition.* Health Information Press. 1997.

Lillis C. *A Concise Introduction to Medical Terminology. Fourth Edition.* Appleton & Lange. 1997.

McCann Schilling J. *Medical Terminology Made Incredibly Easy.* Springhouse Corp. 2001.

STERILE PROCESSING TERMS

Anatomy

Physiology

Cell

Cell membrane

Cytoplasm

Nucleus

Tissue

Organ

Body system

Tendon

Ligament

Cartilage

Ossification

Joint

Fascia

Central nervous system (CNS)

Peripheral nervous system (PNS)

Brain

Cerebrum

Cerebellum

Brain stem

Peristalsis

Hormones

Metabolism

Insulin

Glucagon

Sperm

Ovum

Chromosomes

Testes

Scrotum

Epididymis

Vas deferens

Seminal vesicle

Semen

Ejaculatory duct

Urethra

Prostate gland

Vagina

Cervix

Uterus

Endometrium

Fallopian tubes

Fimbriae

Ovaries

Kidneys

Ureters

Urinary bladder

Penis

Liver

Skin

Nose

Mouth

Pharynx

Esophagus

Larynx

Trachea

Bronchi

Lungs

Alimentary canal (digestive tract)

Stomach

Small intestine

Large intestine (colon)

Rectum

Anus

Blood

Plasma

Red blood cells

White blood cells

Platelets

Heart

Arteries

Veins

Capillaries

Atria

Ventricles

Aorta

Chapter 4

Microbiology for Sterile Processing Technicians

Learning Objectives

As a result of successfully completing this chapter, the reader will be able to:

1. Define the term microbiology and explain why it is important for Sterile Processing technicians
2. Identify basic facts about microorganisms
3. Discuss methods to identify and classify microorganisms
4. Explain environmental conditions necessary for bacterial growth and survival
5. Provide basic information about non-bacterial organisms
6. Review basic procedures to control microorganisms

INTRODUCTION

Sterile Processing (SP) technicians are sometimes daunted by microbiology because much of its terminology is unfamiliar and deals with a world that cannot be seen without a microscope; however, microorganisms have a dramatic impact on the world. For example, everyone has become sick with infections like colds or the flu.

Some microscopic organisms can cause serious illness and even death. How can something so small have such massive power over the human body? Why can anyone, even the strongest and healthiest person, become infected by microorganisms? Why does the risk of infection increase in those whose immune systems or natural body defenses are compromised? This chapter will help answer these and related questions about how these unseen organisms affect everyone.

OVERVIEW OF MICROBIOLOGY

Most people have some understanding of **microbiology**. They know that it is not wise to eat food that falls on the floor, touch a sick person's soiled facial tissues or share eating utensils. They know they should wash their hands before eating and after using the restroom. They understand that taking these precautions helps to protect against germs. For the average person, this limited understanding of the world of microbes is typically enough; however, SP technicians must have a deeper understanding about microbiology for two reasons:

- They have the responsibility to protect patients from microorganisms in the healthcare environment.
- The nature of SP technicians' job duties may increase the risk of exposure to harmful microorganisms for themselves and their co-workers.

Microbiology The study of microorganisms. The scientific study of the nature, life and action of microorganisms.

Microorganisms are tiny organisms that can only be seen with a microscope. Examples of their small size can be seen in **Figures 4.1** and **4.2.**

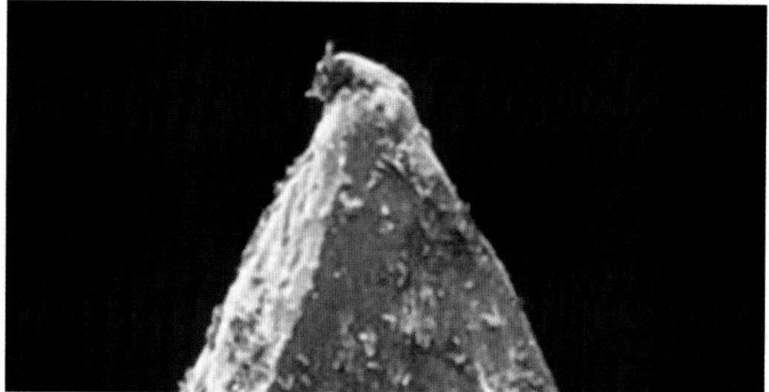

Figure 4.1 Contaminated needle under magnification

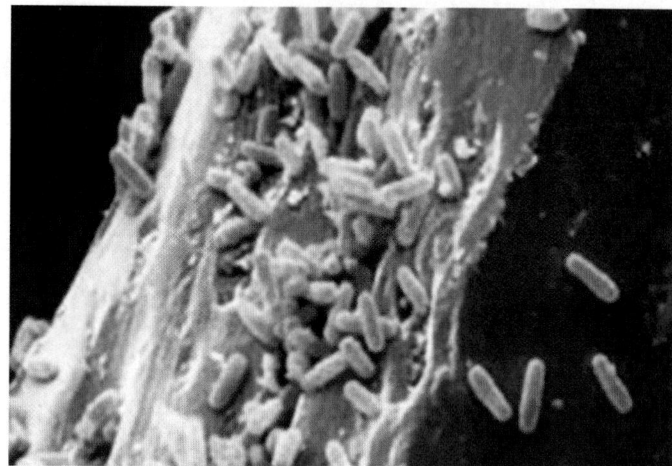

Figure 4.2 Magnified microorganisms as seen on a contaminated needle's surface

SP technicians should be able to recognize the conditions that favor the growth of microorganisms and recognize that even though microorganisms cannot be seen with the naked eye, they are present in the environment. (See **Figure 4.3**) The surgical instruments, equipment and utensils processed by SP personnel every day are **contaminated** with microorganisms that pose a threat to patients, SP technicians and other facility personnel.

Contamination The state of being soiled by contact with infectious organisms or other materials.

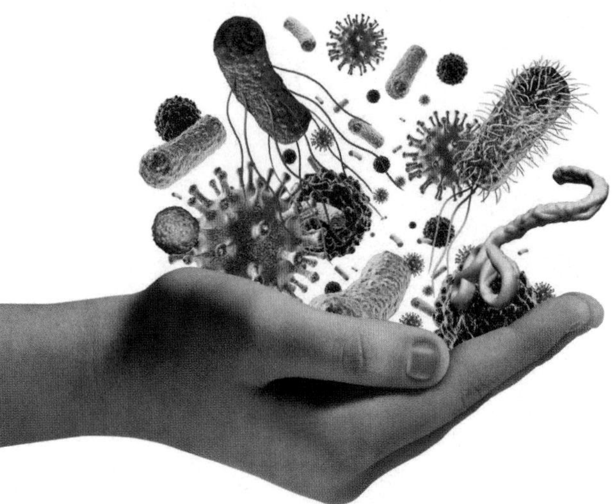

Figure 4.3

This chapter provides a broad overview of microbiology, including:

- Basic facts about microorganisms
- Beneficial versus dangerous microorganisms

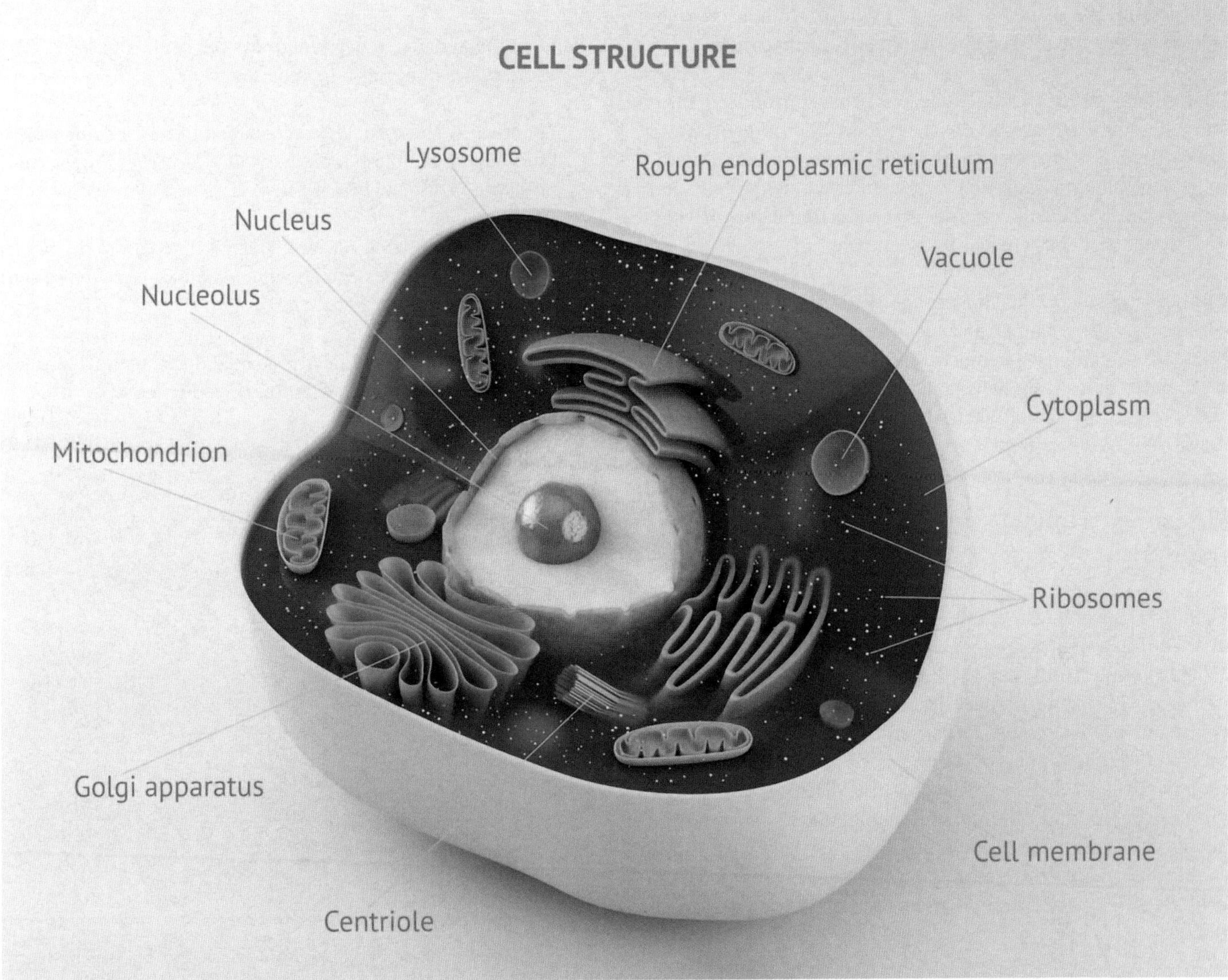

Figure 4.4 Components of a cell

- How microorganisms are identified and classified
- The conditions microorganisms need to grow and reproduce
- How microorganisms are transmitted
- How microorganisms can be controlled and eliminated

Basic Facts About Microorganisms

Cells are the basic units of all living organisms (plants, animals, protozoa and bacteria) and they are the smallest unit that can live, grow and reproduce. (See **Figure 4.4**) Cells differ in size and shape but they all have:

- A nucleus (the controlling unit of the cell)
- Cytoplasm (the material that fills the cell)
- Cell membrane (the outer membrane that allows some liquids and gases to seep in and out of the cell)

Bacterial cells differ from both plant and animal cells because they have no membrane to separate the nucleus from the cytoplasm. Plants and animals have a nuclear membrane surrounding many strands.

BENEFICIAL VERSUS DANGEROUS MICROORGANISMS

Many microorganisms, or microbes, are harmless. In fact, 95% of bacteria are beneficial and essential; they are everywhere in nature and necessary for the existence of humans, plants and animals. For example, microorganisms maintain the balance of chemical elements in the natural environment by breaking down dead matter and recycling carbon, nitrogen, sulfur and other elements. Microorganisms are also useful in sewage treatment to convert waste materials into soluble, odorless compounds for disposal.

Harmless microorganisms are also found on human skin and hair, in the intestinal tract, and in some bodily discharges.

Microorganisms can cause infections when introduced into a body site where they are not typically found. Microorganisms that can cause illness are called **pathogens**. Pathogens cause disease by producing powerful toxins that interfere with how body systems work. Their uncontrolled reproduction can overwhelm body systems or cause tissues to degenerate.

Pathogens are a specific concern for SP technicians, as disease-causing organisms can reside on instruments and devices used in patient care, leading to healthcare-associated infections (HAIs). It is estimated that each year 1.7 million patients acquire infections in the healthcare facility that have nothing to do with their initial illness, and 98,000 patients (one in 17) die due to these HAIs.

HOW MICROORGANISMS ARE IDENTIFIED AND CLASSIFIED

There is a prescribed method for naming microorganisms. The first word in a microorganism's name (always capitalized) is the genus, or tribe (family), of the microorganism; the second word is the specific name of the organism, also called the species. For example, *Pseudomonas aeruginosa*, can cause infections in the blood, lungs (pneumonia) or other parts of the body after surgery. *Escherichia coli* (*E. coli*) can cause diarrhea, urinary tract infections, respiratory illness, and pneumonia. Microorganisms, like all living things, are identified and classified according to certain characteristics. These organisms can be broken down into two categories: bacteria and non-bacteria.

Bacteria

Characteristics

Bacteria are incredibly small—so small, in fact, that a microscope that can magnify at least 900 times is necessary to view them. Bacteria are measured by **microns** and most bacteria are one to two microns in size.

The most common ways to identify and classify bacteria are by shape, color change and oxygen needs (**aerobic** or **anaerobic**).

Pathogen Capable of producing disease.

Micron 1/25,000 of an inch or 1/1,000 of a millimeter.

Aerobic Requiring the presence of air or free oxygen.

Anaerobic Bacteria that can live in the absence of atmospheric oxygen.

Shape

Shape of bacteria is determined by cell wall structure. The common shapes of bacteria include:

- Spherical – These bacteria are shaped like a circle or sphere (coccus). Examples include *Staphylococcus aureus* and *Streptococci*. (See **Figure 4.5**)
- Rod – These bacteria are shaped like rods or bricks (bacillus). Examples include *Pseudomonas aeruginosa* and *Enterobacteria*. (See **Figure 4.6**)
- Spiral – These bacteria are shaped like spirals (spirilla). *Helicobacter pylori* is an example. (See **Figure 4.7**)

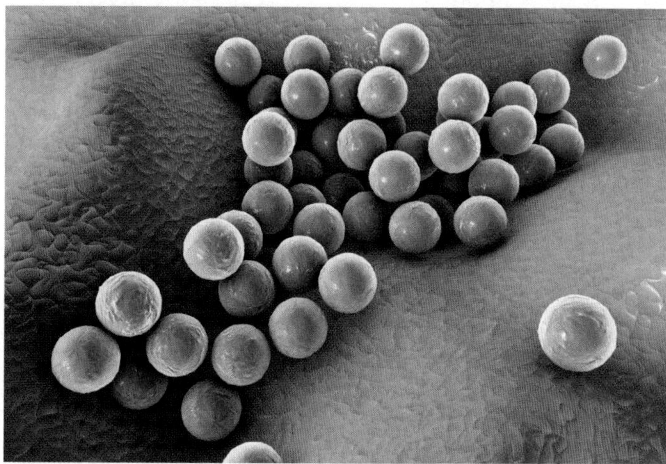

Figure 4.5

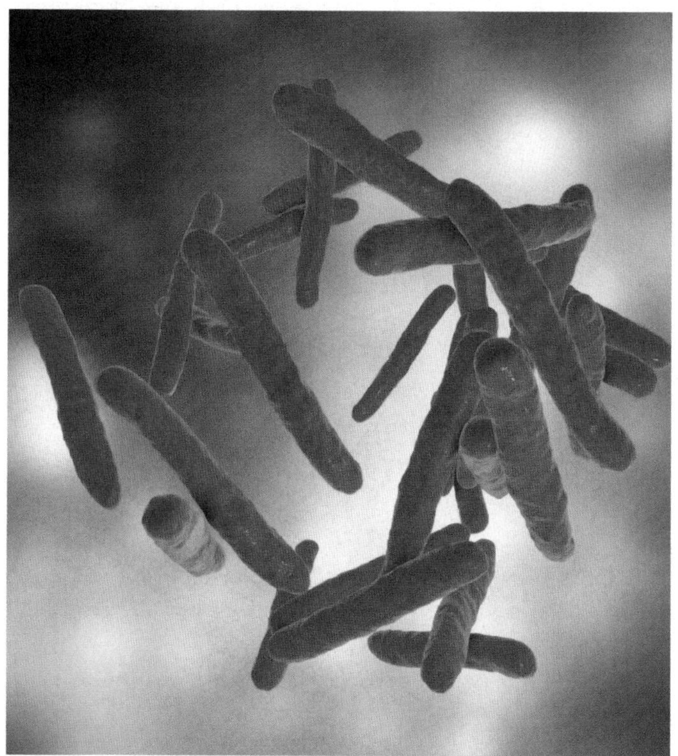

Figure 4.6

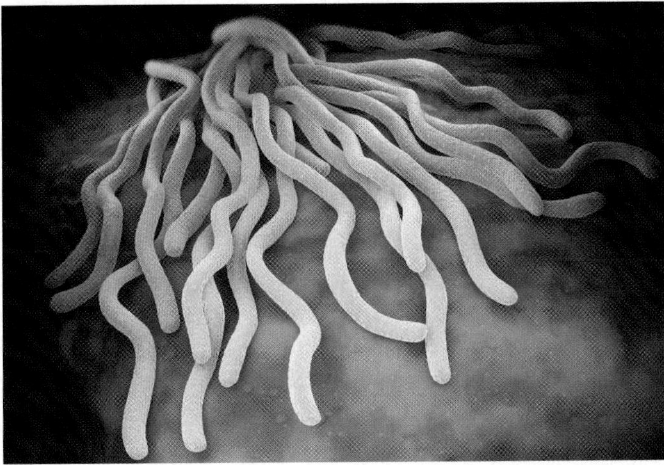

Figure 4.7

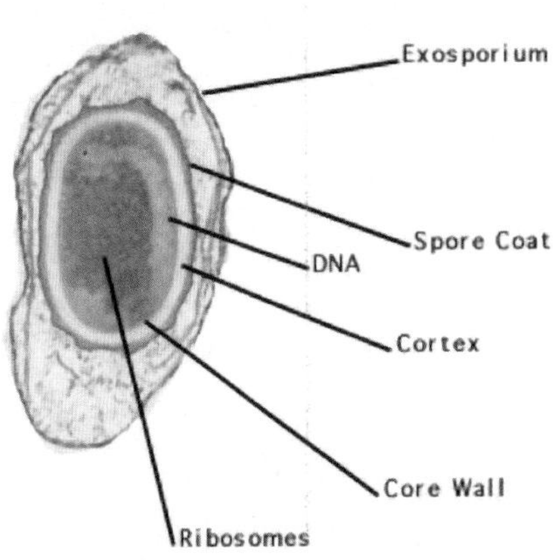

Figure 4.8 Bacterial spore diagram

Certain bacteria can change into a different form, called **endospores (spores)**, by developing a thick coat around the cell's nucleus when conditions required for growth are not adequate. These spores can become infectious and produce toxins once inside the body. For example, some spores (such as *Bacillus anthracis* that causes anthrax, and the *Clostridium* species that cause tetanus, botulism and severe diarrhea) are found in the soil, air and all over the body. (See **Figures 4.8** and **4.9**) Spores are highly resistant to disinfection and other conditions, such as heat, making them very difficult to kill.

Endospores (spores) Microorganisms capable of forming a thick wall around themselves, enabling them to survive in adverse conditions.

Color Change

Bacteria are typically clear and colorless organisms that cannot be seen unless they are dyed with a stain, allowing the shape of each individual organism to be viewed. There are two main types of staining processes used to identify the shapes and characteristics of bacteria.

Gram staining, a multi-step process using several stains and rinses, is used most frequently. The specimen is placed on a slide that is first stained purple with crystal violet; it is then stained with iodine, discolored using alcohol or acetone and, finally, stained with safranin.

***Clostridium difficile* spores**

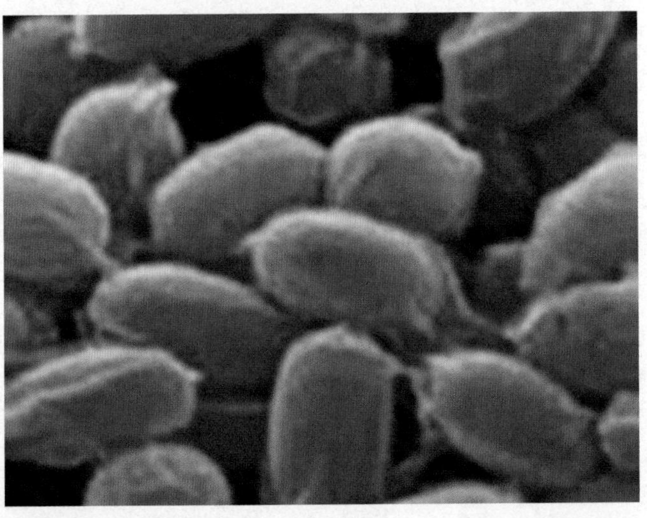

***Anthrax* spores**

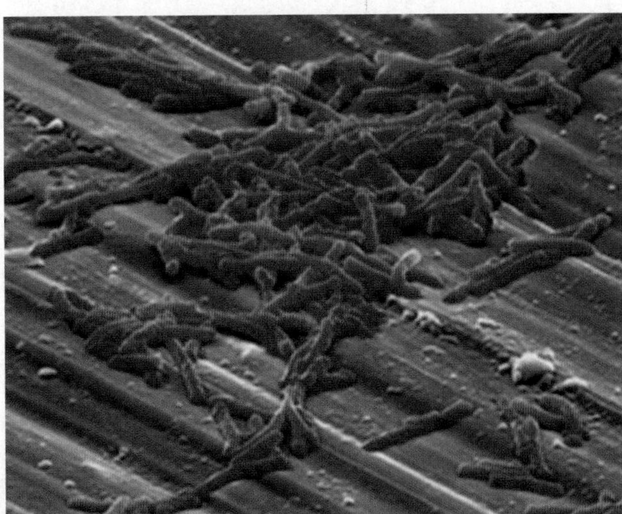

Figure 4.9 Examples of spores

Gram stain Differential stain used to classify bacteria as gram positive or gram negative, depending on whether they retain or lose the primary stain (crystal violet) when subjected to a decolorizing agent.

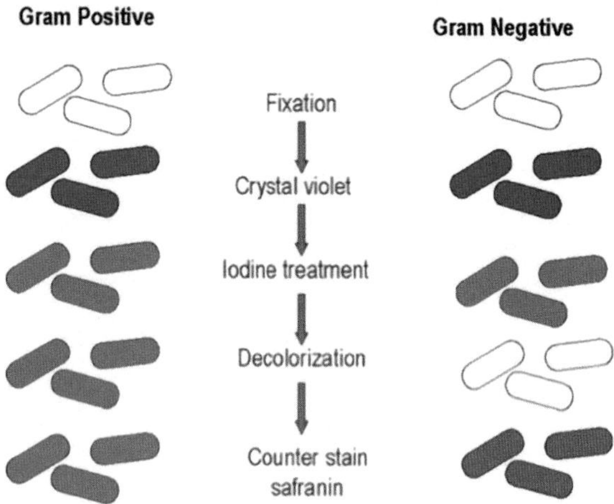

Figure 4.10 Gram stain

Gram-negative bacteria have an outer membrane that will not retain the purple stain after treatment with iodine; instead, they will stain pink. Gram-negative bacteria include *Pseudomonas aeruginosa* that cause urinary tract infections (UTIs), *E. coli* and *Salmonella* species that cause intestinal disease, and *Klebsiella* species that cause pneumonia. (See **Figure 4.11**)

Gram-positive bacteria have no outer membrane and will retain the purple stain, even if a decolorizer is used. Gram-positive bacteria include *Staphylococcus aureus,* which affect skin and mucous membranes, *Bacillus anthracis,* which causes anthrax, and *Clostridium difficile,* which causes diarrhea. (See **Figure 4.12**)

Figure 4.13 contains a list of common Gram-stain classifications.

Acid Fast (Ziehl-Neelsen Stain)

Some acid-fast bacilli are rod-shaped and very difficult to stain; however, once they are stained and heat or other agents are used, the bacteria will resist decolorization with a diluted acid-alcohol solution. (See **Figure 4.14**) This group includes mycobacteria, such as *M. tuberculosis,* which causes tuberculosis (TB), and *M. leprae,* which causes leprosy. (See **Figure 4.15**)

Escherichia coli (E. coli)

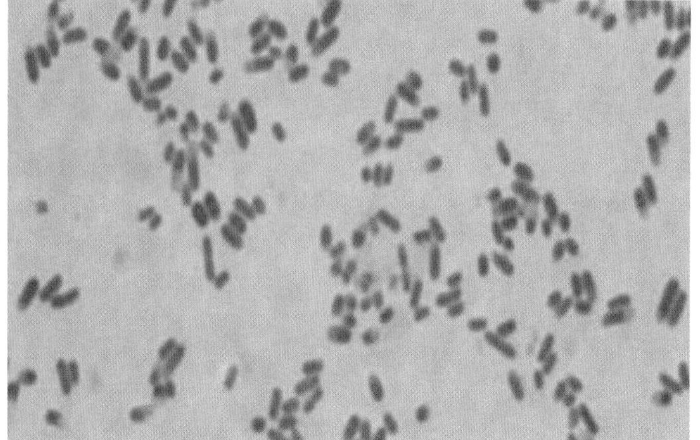

Pseudomonas

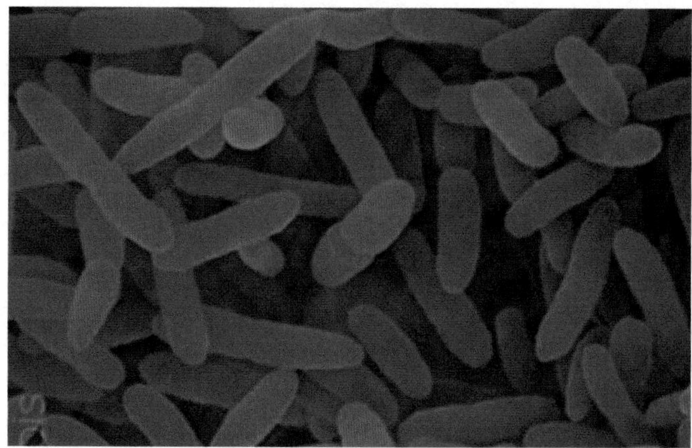

Figure 4.11 Gram-negative bacteria

Clostridium difficile

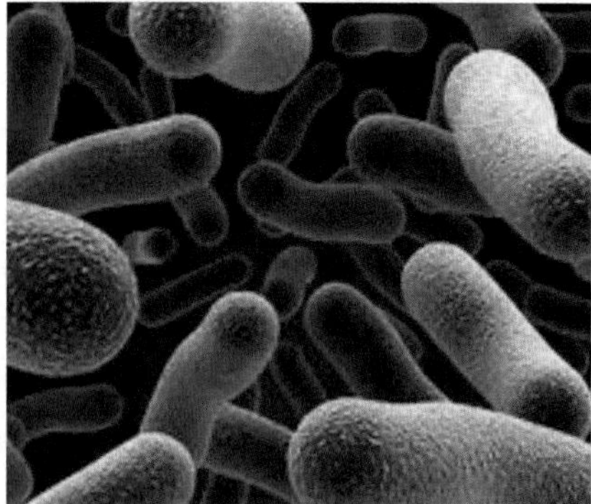

Bacillus anthracis

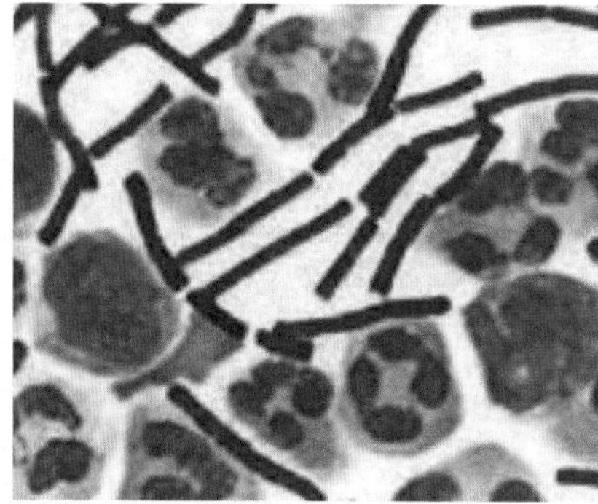

Staphylococcus aureus

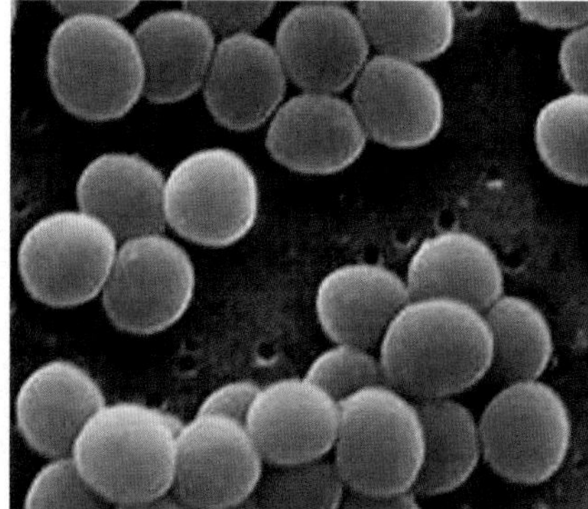

Figure 4.12 Gram-positive bacteria

Gram Stain Chart

Gram Stain Classification		
Bacteria	**Shape**	**Gram stain**
Staphylococcus	Cocci	Gram-positive
Streptococcus	Cocci	Gram-positive
Enterococcus	Cocci	Gram-positive
Mycobacterium tuberculosis	Bacillus	Gram-positive
Mycobacterium leprae	Bacillus	Gram-positive
Clostridium tetani	Bacillus	Gram-positive
Clostridium botulinum	Bacillus	Gram-positive
Clostridium perfringes	Bacillus	Gram-positive
Bacillus anthracis	Bacillus	Gram-positive
Geobacillus species	Bacillus	Gram-positive
Neisseria meningitis	Cocci	Gram-negative
Neisseria gonorrheae	Cocci	Gram-negative
Acinetobacter	Cocci	Gram-negative
Escherichia coli (E. coli)	Bacillus	Gram-negative
Proteus	Bacillus	Gram-negative
Klebsiella	Bacillus	Gram-negative
Pseudomonis	Bacillus	Gram-negative
Salmonella typhi	Bacillus	Gram-negative
Shigilla dysenteriae	Bacillus	Gram-negative

Figure 4.13

Ziehl-Neelsen Stain Process

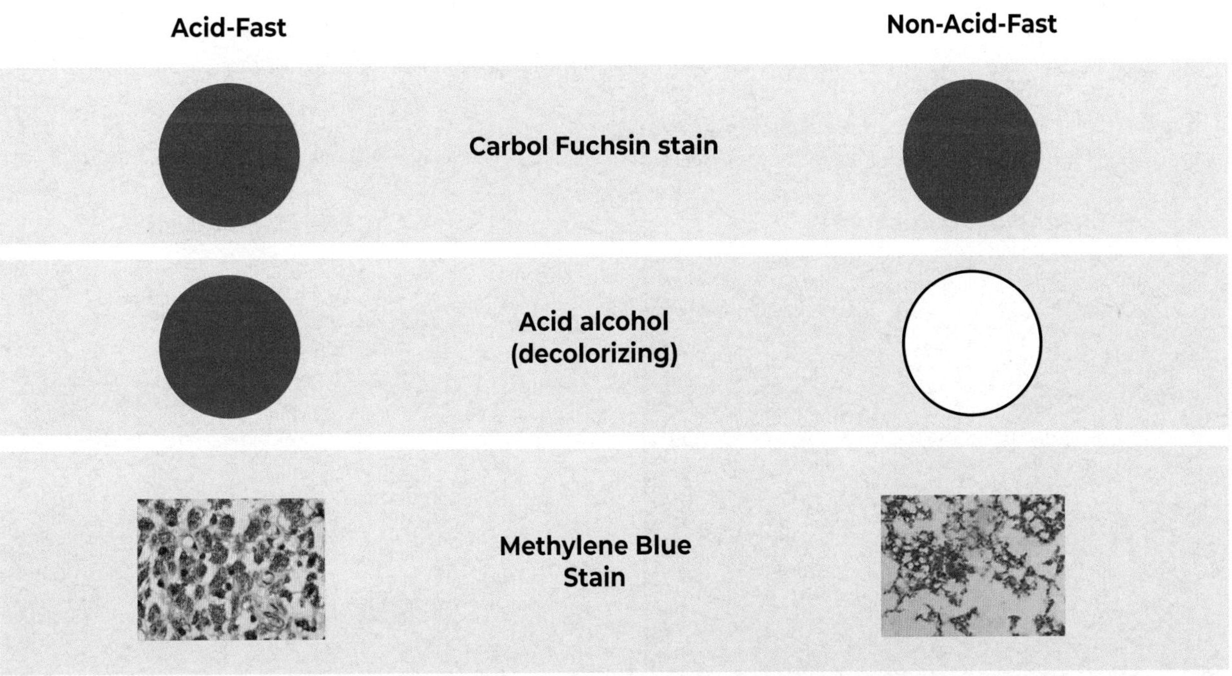

Figure 4.14

M. leprae

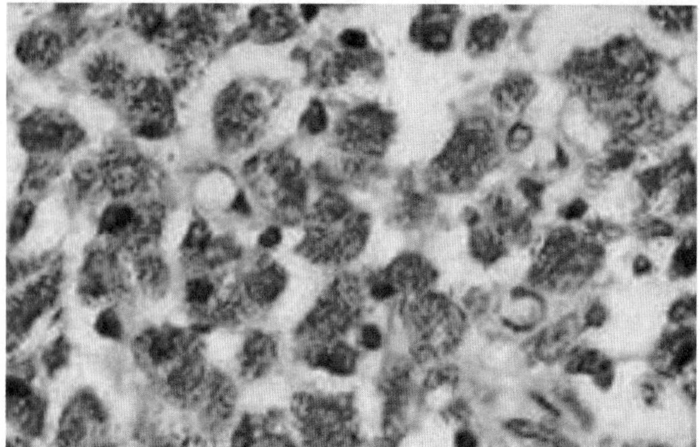

M. tuberculosis

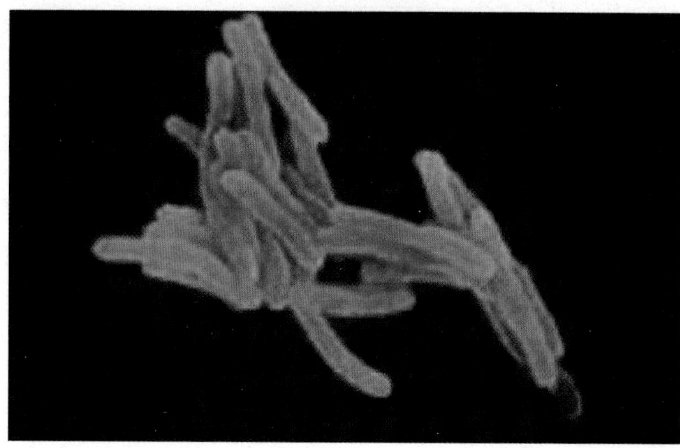

Figure 4.15 Acid-fast bacteria

Need for Oxygen

Bacteria can also be classified according to whether they need oxygen to grow. Aerobic bacteria require oxygen, just as humans do. They may grow in liquids, but the liquid must have oxygen dissolved in it because oxygen is needed for respiration and metabolism.

On the other hand, anaerobic bacteria, such as *C. tetani*, which causes tetanus, and *C. botulinum*, which causes botulism, must have oxygen eliminated from the environment in order to grow. (See **Figure 4.16**) When tetanus bacteria are introduced deeply into the flesh by a nail or similar object, and when the nail is removed, the tissue closes the wound, oxygen is removed from the environment, and the anaerobic bacteria can grow.

Conditions Microorganisms Need to Grow and Reproduce

Groups of microbes have specific requirements for growth and survival. This tends to limit where they may be found. Suitable environments for bacteria are as diverse as the bacteria themselves. For example, a microbe that lives and thrives in the soil may not grow well in the vital organs of humans. Suitable environments for bacteria can be broken down into nutritional needs, temperature, moisture/humidity, **pH** and light.

pH Measure of alkalinity or acidity on a scale of 0 to 14; pH of 7 is neutral (neither acid nor alkaline); pH below 7 is acid; pH above 7 is alkaline.

Pathogenic bacteria are most likely to thrive where their specific nutritional needs can be met. Some, like *Staphylococci*, can grow on and in many areas of the body, skin, blood and hair. Others, such as *Neisseria gonorrhoeae*, are more delicate and require a special environment, such as the mucous membranes of the reproductive system where they can live and invade deeper tissue.

Clostridium botulinum

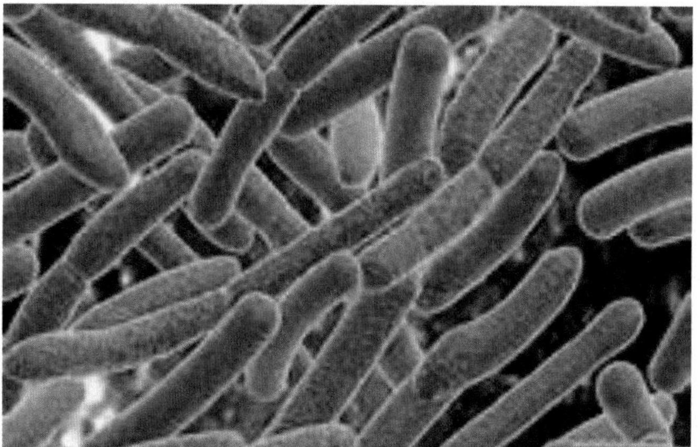

Clostridium tetani

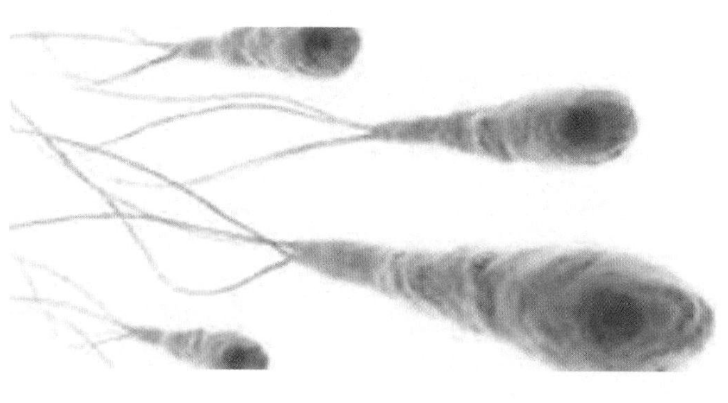

Figure 4.16 Anaerobic bacteria

Temperature requirements vary widely among bacteria as well. Some bacteria like cold temperatures (59°F to 68°F); some bacteria, like moderate temperatures, such as 68°F to 113°F; and others like warm temperatures of 122°F to 158°F. (See **Figure 4.17**)

Temperature Requirements for Bacteria	
Preferred Environment	**Optimal Temperature for Growth**
Cold Temperature	59° F to 68° F (15° C to 20° C)
Moderate Temperature	68° F to 113° F (20° C to 45° C)
Warm Temperature	122° F to 158° F (50° C to 70° C)
Bacteria pathogenic to humans prefer the moderate temperature (Mesophiles)	

Figure 4.17

Moisture and relative humidity play a major role in the growth and survival of microorganisms. Microorganisms that inhabit skin, bacteria that produce spores, and TB bacillus can survive for years in a dry state. Some other species cannot survive for more than a brief period when subjected to complete dryness.

Except for bacteria used in the fermentation process (such as beer), most species will not grow in an acidic pH of 4.4 or lower. Pathogenic microorganisms have an optimal pH range of 7 to 7.8, the same pH as blood.

Dark conditions are favorable to the growth of bacteria, while sunlight is lethal to many organisms in their actively growing or **vegetative stage**. When spores of gram-positive bacilli are in a resting stage, they are most resistant to sunlight. The most lethal light is ultraviolet light, which can be used, at the appropriate strength, to disinfect.

Vegetative stage State of active growth of microorganisms (as opposed to the resting or spore stages).

Bacteria are transmitted primarily by the droplet route, contaminated water or food, direct contact through wounds, airborne mode, and/or by disease-carrying animals.

How Bacteria Grow

Under optimal conditions, microorganisms reproduce every 20 minutes (approximately) in a process called **binary fission**.

Binary fission The typical method of bacterial reproduction in which a cell divides into two equal parts.

Multiple Drug-Resistant Organisms

In some cases, microorganisms adapt and change as a means of survival. For example, multiple drug-resistant organisms (MDROs) have become resistant to antibiotics used to treat bacterial infections. MDROs are increasingly found in hospitals, nursing homes and healthcare facilities of all sizes and are reducing the effectiveness of even the best antibiotics. Resistant pathogens can produce many types of infection in almost any body site.

- Methicillin-resistant *Staphylococcus aureus* (MRSA) lives on the skin and is known for causing severe infections. Staph infections are spread by direct contact with an infected individual or by touching contaminated surfaces. (See **Figure 4.18**)

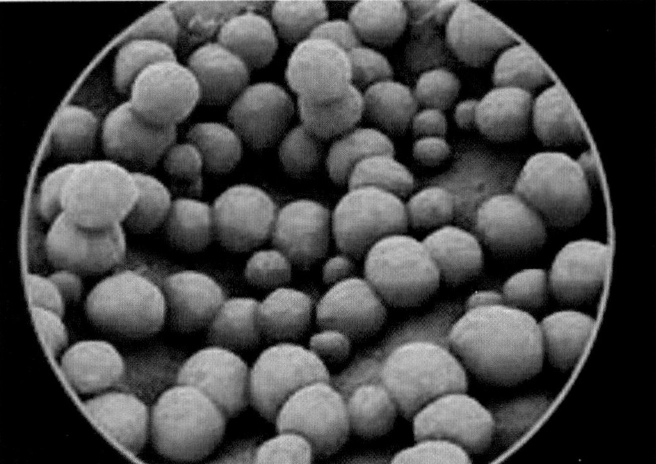

Figure 4.18 Methicillin-resistant *Staphylococcus aureus* (MRSA)

- Vancomycin-resistant *Enterococci* (VRE) lives in the bowels. This bacterium is transmitted when hands become contaminated from infected feces, urine or blood. It is also contracted by touching contaminated environmental surfaces. (See **Figure 4.19**)

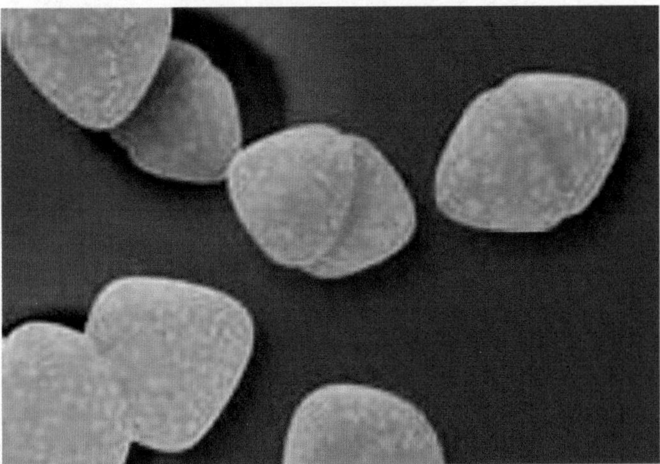

Figure 4.19 Vancomycin-resistant *Enterococci* (VRE)

- Vancomycin-resistant *Streptococcus pneumoniae* causes pneumonia in susceptible humans. Strep is transmitted through direct contact with infected droplets from coughing or sneezing or from contact with other infected fluids. (See **Figure 4.20**)

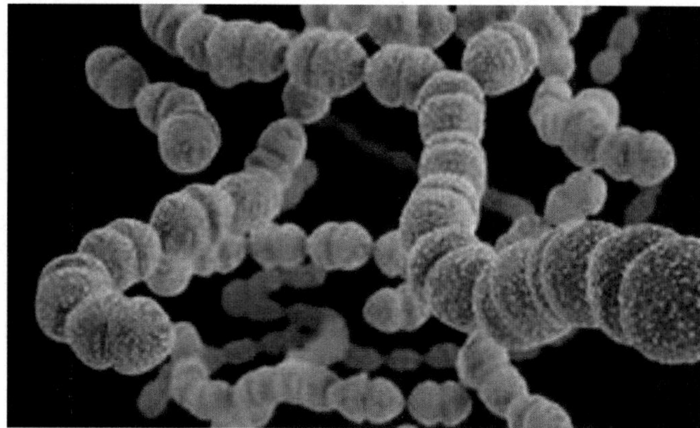

Figure 4.20 Vancomycin-resistant *Streptococcus pneumoniae*

- *Klebsiella* can be found on hands and in the intestinal tract. This bacterium causes pneumonia, nasal infections, urinary tract infections (UTI), wound, and bloodstream infections. *Klebsiella* is typically transferred through hand contact. (See **Figure 4.21**)

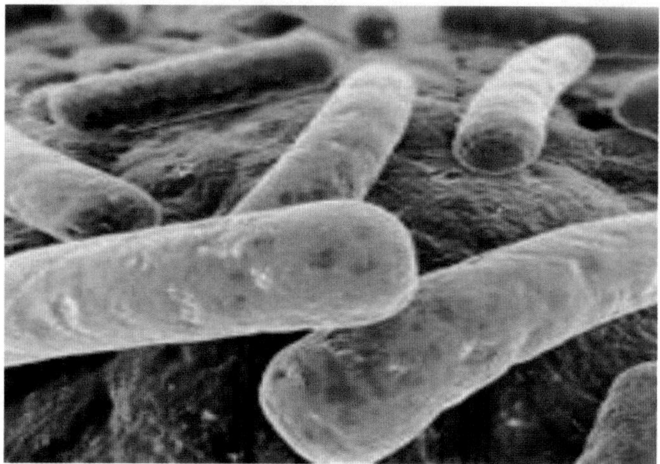

Figure 4.21 *Klebsiella*

- *Acinetobacter* is normally found in soil. This bacterium can cause various illnesses ranging from pneumonia to serious blood or wound infections, and the symptoms vary depending on the disease. *Acinetobacter* can be resistant to many of today's antibiotics. It is transmitted by person-to-person contact or by contact with contaminated surfaces. (See **Figure 4.22**)

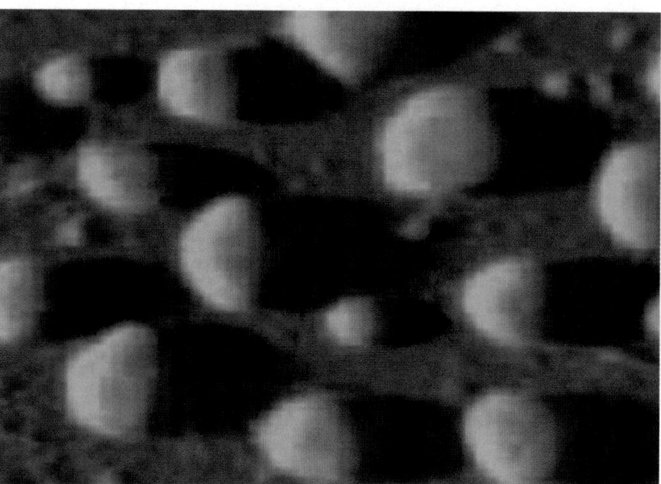

Figure 4.22 *Acinetobacter*

- *Pseudomonas aeruginosa* is frequently found in water and in soil. *Pseudomonas* infections include UTIs, respiratory system infections, dermatitis, soft tissue infections, bacteremia, bone and joint infections, gastrointestinal infections, and a variety of systemic infections. *Pseudomonas* is transmitted through hand-to-hand contact or contact with contaminated surfaces. (See **Figure 4.23**)

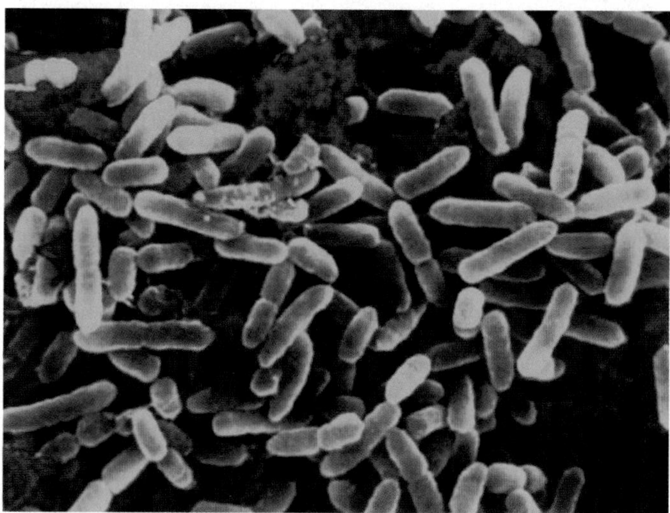

Figure 4.23 *Pseudomonas aeruginosa*

- Carbapenem-resistant *Enterobacteriaceae* (CRE) are a family of germs that are difficult to treat because they have high levels of antibiotic resistance. *Klebsiella* species and E. coli are examples of *Enterobacteriaceae*, a normal part of the human gut bacteria that can become carbapenem resistant. CRE infections have been associated with devices such as flexible endoscopes and ventilators. Some CRE infections are very difficult to treat and can contribute to death in up to 50% of patients who become infected.

Flu virus

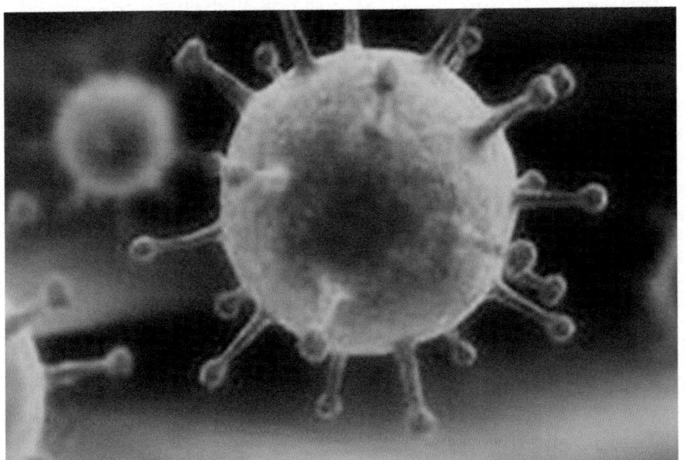

Chicken pox virus

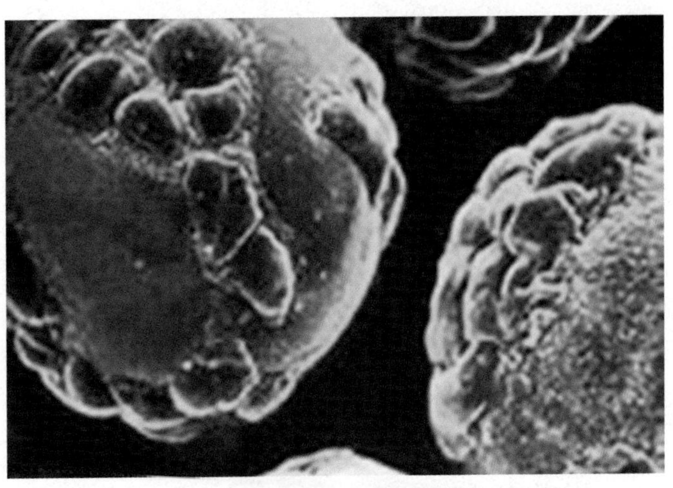

Figure 4.24 Viruses

Non-Bacterial Microorganisms

Viruses

Viruses are the smallest microorganisms and are about 1,000 times smaller than bacteria. A virus enters a living plant or animal cell and reproduces itself within the cell. It usually destroys the cell, then enters another cell to survive. The virus itself has no means of movement and depends on air, water, insects, humans or other animals to carry it from one host to another. (See **Figure 4.24**)

In the healthcare setting, several bloodborne viral pathogens are of significance: human immunodeficiency virus (HIV), hepatitis B virus (HBV) and the most prevalent chronic bloodborne infection today, hepatitis C virus (HCV). (See **Figures 4.25** and **4.26**)

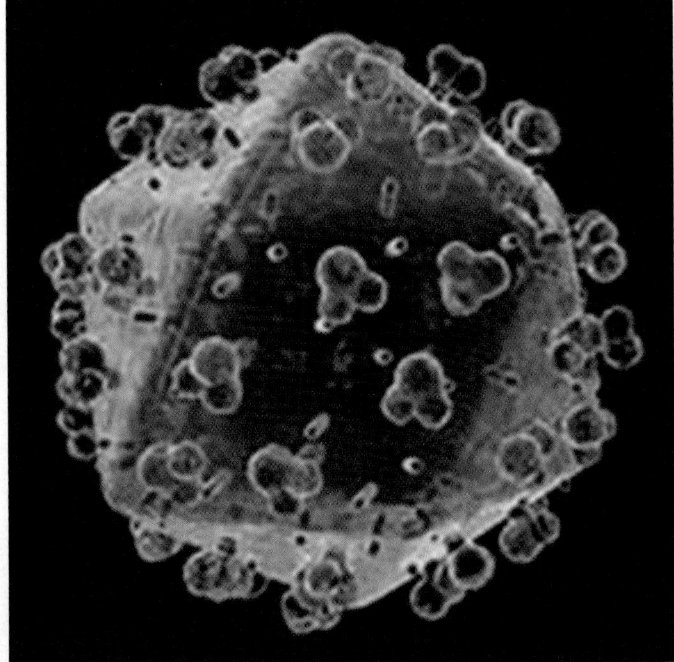

Figure 4.25 HIV

Hepatitis B virus

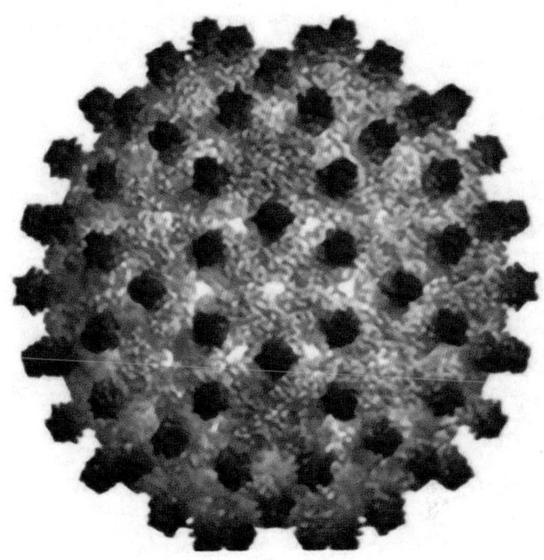

Hepatitis C virus

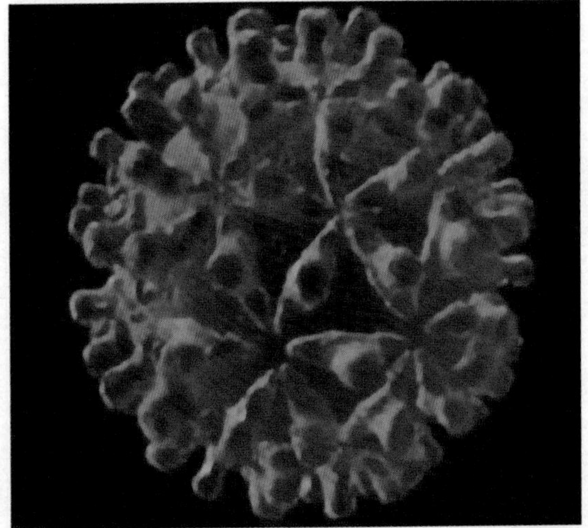

Figure 4.26 Hepatitis virus

Viruses are transmitted primarily by the airborne or droplet route and include chickenpox (varicella), shingles (zoster), measles (rubeola), influenza and the common cold.

Ebola virus (or Ebola hemorrhagic fever) is a viral disease caused by the filovirus species. This virus is contracted by contact with blood or body fluids of an infected animal or human. The incubation period ranges from two to 21 days after exposure. (See **Figure 4.27**)

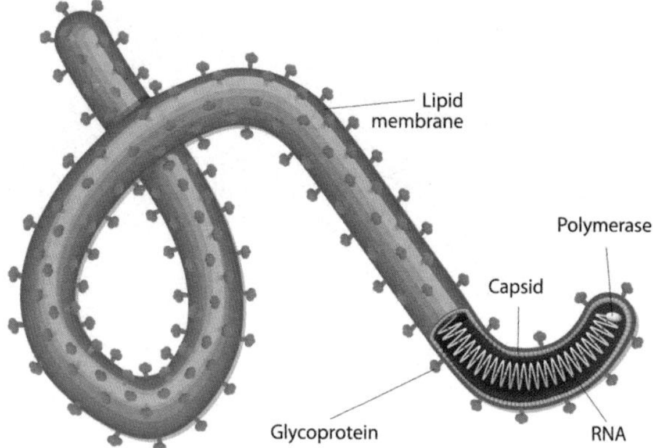

Figure 4.27 Ebola virion

Viruses transmitted by contaminated water or food include those that cause acute viral gastroenteritis such as rotavirus, Norovirus and noro-like virus. These often have symptoms similar to bacterial infections and spread through the four Fs: food, feces, fingers and flies. Another virus spread by food or water is hepatitis A; it is contracted by unwashed hands or eating raw or improperly cooked food.

Viruses that spread primarily by direct contact include cold sores (herpes labialis), genital herpes, genital warts, infectious mononucleosis, and rabies.

Viruses can also be transmitted through multiple routes [e.g., severe acute respiratory syndrome coronavirus 2 (SARS-CoV-2) more commonly known as COVID-19]. COVID-19 can be transmitted through direct contact, indirect contact, and airborne and droplet routes. (See **Figure 4.28**)

Like bacteria, some viruses can survive away from the host for many hours or days when in organic material such as scabs, blood and bodily waste. Some viruses, like the herpes simplex virus (HSV), can survive in a dry state for 1 ½ to four hours on toilet seats, up to 72 hours on cotton gauze, and 18 hours on plastic.

Standard cleaning protocols—with careful attention to cleaning processes—are usually sufficient to control these microorganisms.

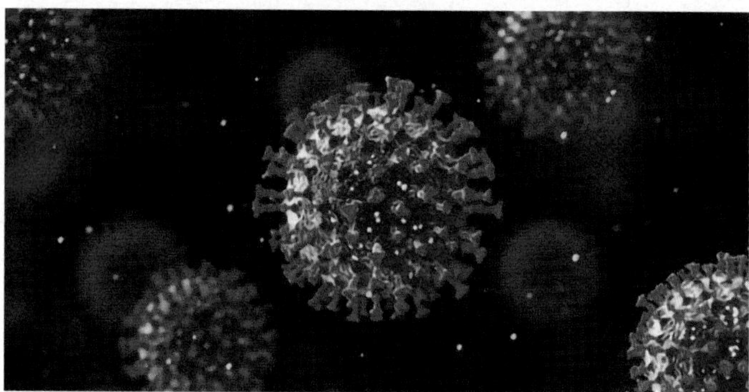

Figure 4.28

Protozoa

Protozoa are one-celled animal organisms that vary widely in size and shape and contain no cell walls.

Most protozoa live in moist habitats and are aerobic, but some species found in the human intestines are anaerobic. They are known for their ability to move independently, and some protozoa can form cysts and become pathogenic. Some protozoa may be spread by insects or direct contact.

The most frequently encountered pathogenic protozoa is *Entamoeba histolytica*. It is found in feces, intestinal ulcers and liver abscesses of infected people. *Cryptosporidium* is another protozoan that can cause diarrhea and abdominal pain. This organism can cause severe, life-threatening diarrhea in AIDS or cancer patients and organ transplant recipients. (See **Figure 4.29**)

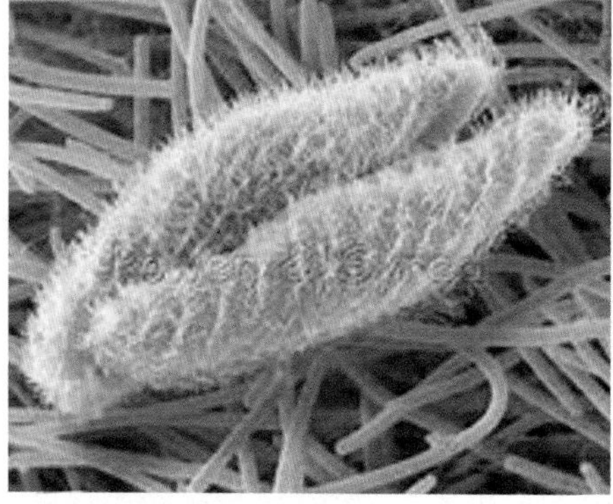
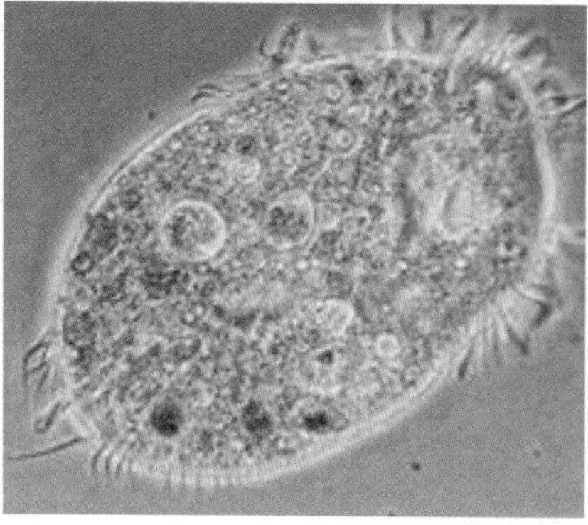
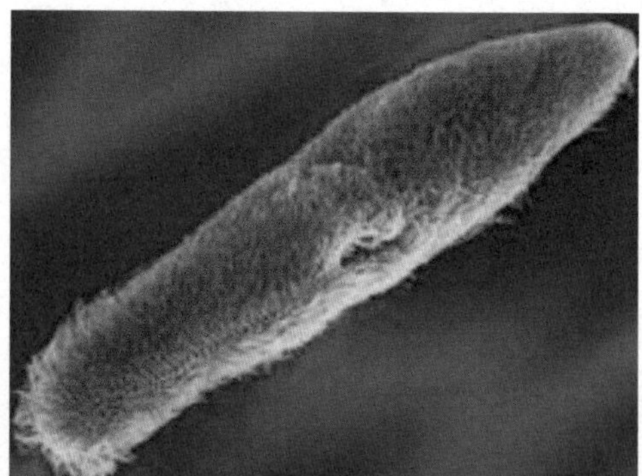

Figure 4.29 Protozoa

Penicillium

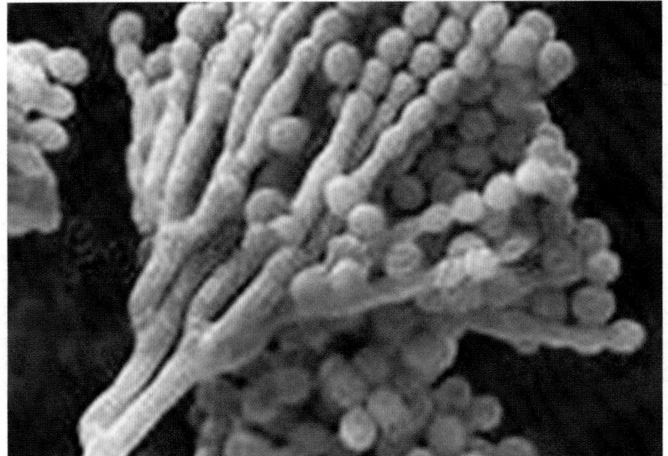

Candida

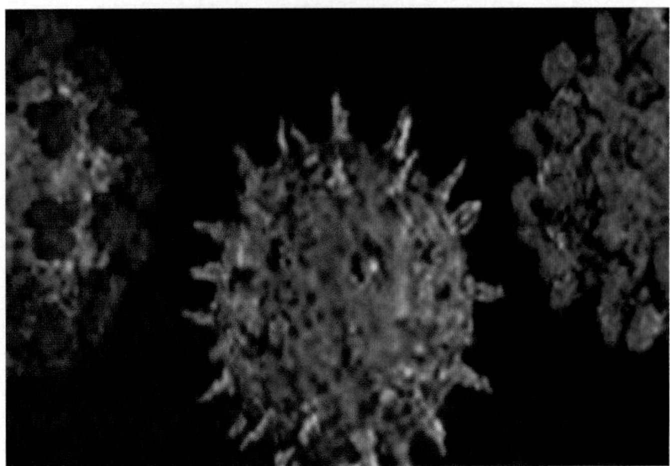

Figure 4.30 Fungi

Fungi

Fungi are a large group of plant-like organisms that include molds, mushrooms and yeasts. Fungi and bacteria are often found together in nature. While some fungi, such as yeast, occur as single cells that require a microscope to see, others, such as mushrooms, are quite large.

The vegetative structure of a fungus varies widely in size, shape and complexity. Fungi (except for yeasts) are identified and classified by their shape and distribution of their reproductive structures. Most fungi are aerobic.

Molds are composed of many-celled organisms that typically grow in compact masses of intertwining, branching and hair-like filaments.

Fungi have three major roles: to turn dead organic matter into usable substances through decay and mildew; to have a mutually symbiotic relationship with other organisms; and to be parasitic or pathogenic to plants or animals.

Fungi survive by feeding on living or dead organisms, and this process can be both beneficial and harmful. For instance, fermentation by fungi has been used for years to preserve food in places where refrigeration is unavailable. Fungi are necessary to produce bread, cheese, wine and beer, while other fungi, such as mushrooms, are used as food. Some fungi are used to produce pharmaceuticals, such as cortisone, the mold *Penicillium notatum* that produces penicillin, as well as the immunosuppressive agent cyclosporine. On the other hand, mold can produce toxins, spoil food and create illness. (See **Figure 4.30**)

Several fungus species can cause respiratory diseases in humans who acquire infections by inhaling spores from dust, bird droppings, soil and other sources.

Some fungi target the skin, hair, nails and mucosal surfaces and are called superficial fungi. Common examples are ringworm of the scalp, athlete's foot, and candida, such as thrush and vulvovaginitis.

Prions

Prions are abnormal, pathogenic agents that are transmissible and able to induce abnormal folding of specific normal cellular proteins. (See **Figure 4.31**) The abnormal folding of the prion proteins leads to brain damage and the characteristic signs and symptoms of prion disease.

> **Prion** An infectious protein particle that, unlike a virus, contains no nucleic acid, does not trigger an immune response, and is not destroyed by extreme heat or cold.

Creutzfeldt-Jakob Disease (CJD) is a specific type of prion disease. It is rare that SP technicians in the U.S. receive instrumentation exposed to CJD, but when they do, they must know and apply proper processing procedures.

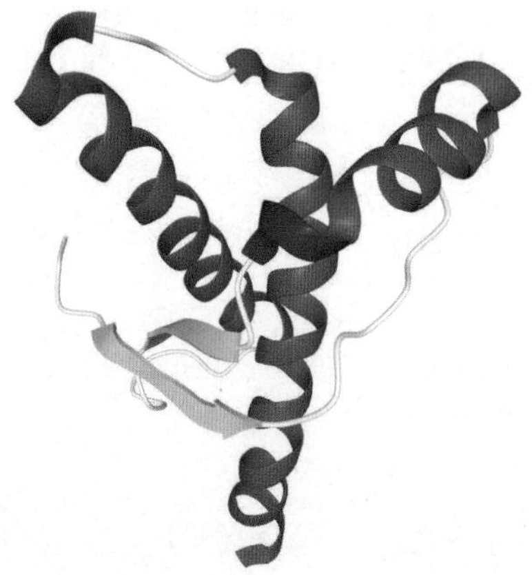

Figure 4.31

In infected patients, prions are most frequently found in the brain, dura mater (the tough membrane that encases the nerves of the spinal cord) and eyes. They are also detected less frequently in cerebrospinal fluid, the spleen, lymph nodes, kidney and liver. Seldomly, they are located in blood, urine, skin, muscle, bone, adrenal glands, heart, feces, peripheral nerves, nasal mucous, gingival, saliva, sputum, and tears. When a suspected CJD patient undergoes a procedure, all healthcare professionals involved with that patient must be notified prior to the procedure, and the facility's CJD policies and procedures must be followed.

Cleaning and sterilizing items contaminated with prions is a challenge because prions are difficult to remove or deactivate and standard cleaning/ sterilization procedures are ineffective against prions. Whenever a suspected CJD case is scheduled, the following should be performed:

Communication

- Inform the department's manager as soon as notification of a prion or potential prion procedure is received.

- Immediately contact Infection Prevention and Control to determine which cleaning and sterilization guidelines will be followed at the facility. Currently, recommended guidelines are published by the World Health Organization (WHO), the Centers for Disease Control and Prevention (CDC) and the Society for Healthcare Epidemiology of America (SHEA). Current guidelines are reviewed and updated as new knowledge regarding prions is gained.

Instrumentation

- Due to the difficulty in cleaning and sterilization, disposable instruments should be used whenever possible when managing patients with prion disease. All current guidelines suggest disposing of reusable instruments that have become contaminated with high-risk tissue (brain tissue, dura mater, spine and eye tissue). Reusable instruments will likely be damaged or completely destroyed during the stringent cleaning and sterilization protocols.

- Heat- and moisture-sensitive items should not be used because they would likely be destroyed during cleaning and sterilization.

Environmental surfaces

- Surfaces, such as countertops, that have become contaminated with prion material should be cleaned following the most current published protocols for CJD. Contaminated non-critical equipment should be cleaned following the most current published guidelines.

Note: Additional information about CJD can be found on the WHO and SHEA websites, in ANSI/AAMI ST79, Annex C, and from the CDC website (https:///www.cdc.gov/prions/cjd/infectioncontrol.html).

CONTROLLING AND ELIMINATING MICROORGANISMS

To prevent the spread of the microorganisms that can cause disease, healthcare settings must practice microbial control. The Infection Prevention and Control and Sterile Processing departments are vital to microbial control and patient safety. Every time an instrument or device enters a patient's body during an invasive or minimally invasive procedure, there is a risk of infection.

It is important to remember that microorganisms can pose a significant threat to humans. One can compare microorganisms to seeds and draw some comparisons. There are many varieties of seeds and each produces a different plant. Seeds must have the proper conditions to grow and continue living. Those in a paper envelope at the store will not germinate and grow (See **Figure 4.32**); however, when they are placed in the correct conditions with proper soil, water, fertilizer, warmth and sunlight they grow and develop. In the same manner, there are many varieties of microorganisms and each can produce a specific effect (an infection or disease) when they have the proper conditions for growth and reproduction.

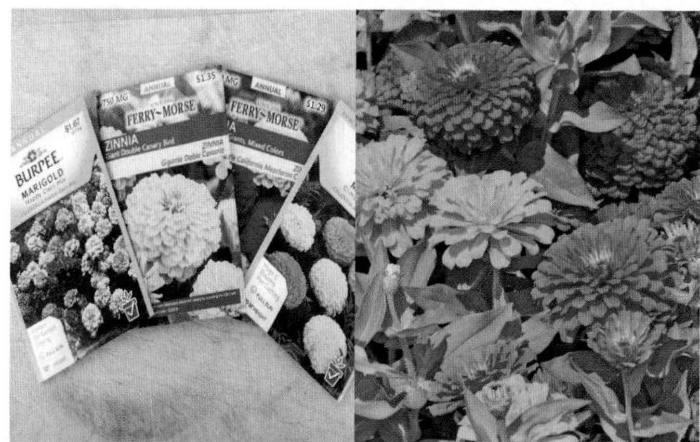

Figure 4.32 Like microorginisms, seeds need the proper conditions to grow.

Microbial control is a complicated endeavor. Just as microorganisms differ in their needs for growth and reproduction, they also die at different rates. The type of microbial control used against an organism varies according to the microbes' susceptibility. Some pathogens are more difficult to kill than others, and that is one reason why disinfection and sterilization processes are so complex. Microbial control can also depend on whether the goal is to kill a pathogen-causing infection through antibiotics, inactivate or kill microorganisms on the skin through antisepsis or—in the case of SP—kill pathogens on medical instruments or devices that will be used on patients. In addition to microbial susceptibility, the vast array of items that must be processed is another reason no single disinfection or sterilization process can kill all microorganisms.

SP technicians should be able to recognize the conditions that favor the growth of microorganisms and learn to "see" microorganisms in the workplace. For example, the decontamination workstation in the top image in **Figure 4.33** looks safe to the untrained eye; however, if microorganisms were as easy to see as plants, that same workstation might look like the photo on the bottom.

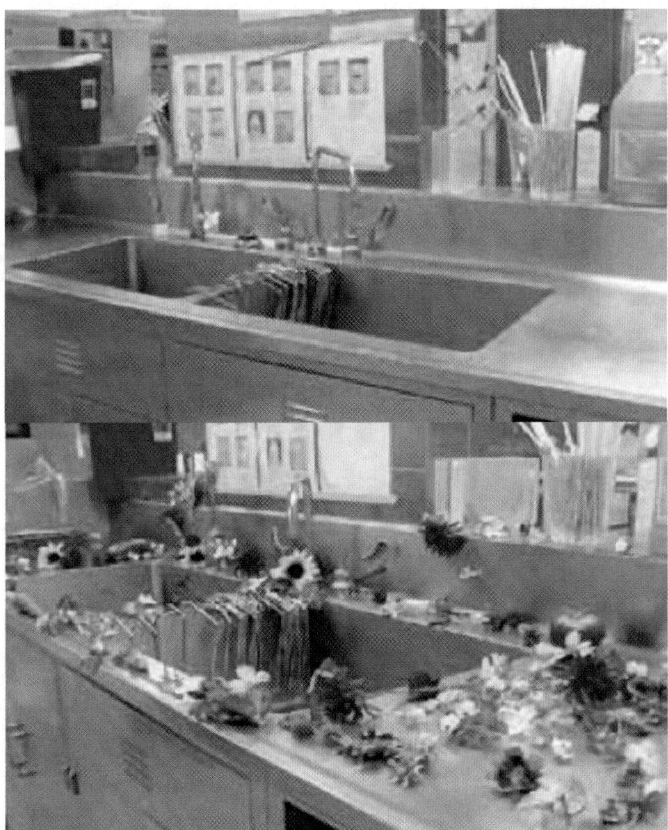

Figure 4.33 What if we could "see" what was growing on work surfaces?

CONCLUSION

Having a basic understanding of the principles of microbiology and learning about bacterial and non-bacterial organisms and how they can be transmitted helps SP technicians understand the important role they play in eradicating microorganisms and preventing infection.

RESOURCES

Needham C, Hoagland M, McPherson K, Dodson B. *Intimate Strangers: Unseen Life on Earth.* ASM Press. 2000.

Huys J. *Sterilization of Medical Supplies by Steam.* Vier-Turme GmbH Benedict Press. 2004.

Tierno P. *The Secret Life of Germs.* Pocket Books. 2003.

Centers for Disease Control and Prevention. *Guideline for Isolation Precautions: Preventing Transmission of Infectious Agents in Healthcare Settings.* 2007.

Alcamo E. *Cliffs Quick Review: Microbiology.* Hungry Minds Inc. 1996.

McCall D, Stock D, Achey P. *Introduction to Microbiology.* Blackwell Science Inc. 2001.

ANSI/AAMI ST79: 2017 & 2020 Amendments A1, A2,A3, A4 (Consolidated Text) *Comprehensive guide to steam sterilization and sterility assurance in health care facilities,* Annex C.

Chess B. *Foundations in Microbiology: Basic Principles, 9th Edition.* 2014.

Haque M, Sartelli M, McKimm J, Abu Bakar M. "Health care-associated infections – an overview." *Infect Drug Resist.* 2018;11:2321-2333 https://doi.org/10.2147/IDR.S177247

STERILE PROCESSING TERMS

Microbiology

Contamination

Pathogen

Micron

Aerobic

Anaerobic

Endospores (spores)

Gram stain

pH

Vegetative stage

Binary fission

Prion

Chapter 5

Infection Prevention

Learning Objectives

As a result of successfully completing this chapter, the reader will be able to:

1. Explain the role of Sterile Processing in the prevention of healthcare infections
2. Explain the principles, practice and importance of personal hygiene and attire, including personal protective equipment
3. Identify the hazards of bloodborne pathogens and how the Occupational Safety and Health Administration's requirements impact personal safety
4. Explain the rationale for the separation of clean and dirty and the environmental requirements for maintaining that separation
5. Discuss the chain of infection and the technician's role in breaking that chain

INTRODUCTION

The Sterile Processing (SP) technician plays a significant role in the prevention of **surgical site infections (SSIs)** and healthcare-associated infections (HAIs). When the importance of this role is understood, technicians recognize that their work practices can mean the difference between a patient's successful surgery or hospital stay and a negative outcome that could lead to infection or possibly death.

STERILE PROCESSING PROCESSES

Every step or process in the SP department (SPD) is carefully designed to prevent poor patient outcomes. Poor outcomes can be traced to many factors, including the condition of instruments, trays and other medical devices processed in the SPD.

SP technicians support infection prevention by:

- Cleaning contaminated medical devices to make them safe for handling and prepare them for a **biocidal** process
- Inspecting instruments to help ensure they are safe and functional
- Assembling and packaging instruments in a manner that facilitates the chosen sterilization method, and providing a barrier after sterilization
- Selecting and properly using the sterilization or high-level disinfection (HLD) method for each medical device
- Safely storing items until they are needed and delivering them using methods that protect the integrity of the sterile packages and items that have undergone disinfection
- Understanding how to apply infection prevention principles in sterile processing (e.g., preventing cross-contamination and recognizing hand hygiene moments)

> **Surgical site infection (SSI)** An infection that occurs after surgery in the part of the body where the surgery took place.
>
> **Biocidal** Process or ability to kill or control the growth of living organisms.
>
> **Chain of infection** The six-step process of an infection spreading from one host to the next.

While those tasks may appear easy, there are several steps to each process. Each requires attention to detail, understanding of specific protocols and process parameters, an understanding of each medical device's manufacturer's Instructions for use (IFU) and dedication to processing each item exactly as stated. Every medical device not processed according to the manufacturer's IFU has the potential to cause infection in both the patient and healthcare worker.

Cause for Concern

In 2015, the Centers for Disease Control and Prevention (CDC) reported that approximately one of every 31 hospitalized patients, or 687,000, contracted an HAI. Of those approximate 687,000, about 72,000 patients died as a result of their hospitalizations. Many of these infections may have been preventable. An SSI is an infection that occurs after surgery in the part of the body where the surgery took place.

The CDC reports that approximately 310 million major surgeries are performed around the world each year, with 40 to 50 million of those procedures performed in the U.S. Each involves the use of medical devices or instruments that have contact with a patient's sterile tissues or mucous membranes. Infection is a major risk in all of these procedures. Additionally, a growing number of microorganisms are becoming resistant to antibiotics or are naturally difficult to control. Many of these microorganisms may be easily transferred to other surfaces and people. Controlling these microorganisms and preventing their transmission is the number one responsibility of SP professionals.

From 2014 to the present, endoscope reprocessing has garnered significant media attention because improper processing of endoscopes has led to infection and, in some cases, death.

A January 2014 article published in *The Seattle Times* noted that more than 100 patients who had undergone colonoscopies at a Washington hospital between 2011 and 2013 were advised to be tested for HIV and hepatitis B and C after the hospital discovered equipment used in the procedures had not been properly cleaned.

In 2015, the *Los Angeles Times* reported that two endoscopy patients died and five more were infected by the *Carbapenem-resistant Enterobacteriaceae* (CRE) superbug after being exposed to contaminated endoscopes; 179 more patients who underwent procedures between October 3, 2014, and January 2015 were also advised to be tested.

In May 2016, nine newly reported cases involving the endoscopic retrograde cholangiopancreatography (ERCP) endoscope, more commonly known as the duodenoscope, were linked to nine patient infections, resulting in three deaths at a hospital in Colorado.

These incidents led to research into endoscope reprocessing.

Infection prevention principles and practices are based on knowledge of the nature and characteristics of disease-producing microorganisms; this includes an understanding about how they are transmitted in the healthcare environment and their place in the **chain of infection**. The way an item is used also plays a significant role in how it is processed. The more SP technicians know about microorganisms, the better equipped they are to prevent the spread of these organisms. **Figure 5.1** identifies the top HAI-causing pathogens, as identified by the CDC.

CDC Top HAI Causing Pathogens	
Acinetobacter	*Burkholderia cepacia*
Clostridium difficile	*Clostridium sordellii*
Enterobacteriaceae (Carbapenem-resistance)	Hepatitis
Human immunodeficiency virus (HIV)	Influenza
Methicillin-resistant *Staphylococcus aureus*	*Klebsiella*
Norovirus	*Mycobacterium abscessus*
Staphylococcus aureus	*Pseudomonas aeruginosa*
Vancomycin-intermediate *Staphylococcus aureus*	Tuberculosis (TB)
Vancomycin-resistant Enterococci (VRE)	Vancomycin-resistant *Staphlococcus aureus*

Figure 5.1 *Source: Centers for Disease Control and Prevention*

Protection from Pathogens

In the early 1970s, the CDC established the first practical recommendations for the isolation technique. The new recommendations categorized infections and communicable diseases based upon the likely mode of transmission. To protect healthcare staff and patients from infectious diseases, standard precautions were adopted; the basis of this is to treat all human blood, bodily fluids and other potentially infectious materials as infectious.

Standard precautions drive the infection prevention and control procedures that SP technicians must use because they are exposed to contaminated instrumentation and equipment. Failure to wear the appropriate personal protective equipment (PPE) increases the individual's risk of acquiring an infection.

The primary purpose of the SPD is to stop the spread of disease-producing microorganisms to patients from instruments and other medical devices. SP technicians must ensure that items used in patient care, including instruments, utensils, supplies and equipment, are made safe by either cleaning, disinfection or sterilization. This chapter addresses how SP technicians control the spread of microorganisms and prevent infection. Understanding **asepsis** in healthcare is an important piece of the basic knowledge required to work in the SPD.

PRINCIPLES OF ASEPSIS

Asepsis can be defined as the absence of microorganisms that cause disease. **Aseptic technique** includes any activity or procedure that prevents infection or breaks the chain of infection.

There are two types of aseptic technique:

- **Medical asepsis** (clean technique) – Procedures performed to reduce the number of microorganisms in order to minimize their spread. Examples include handwashing and equipment decontamination.
- **Surgical asepsis** (sterile technique) – Procedures to eliminate the presence of all microorganisms and/or introduction of microorganisms to an area [e.g., proper processing, storage and techniques performed in the Operating Room (OR) prevent contamination of sterile instruments and supplies].

Asepsis The absence of microorganisms that cause disease.

Aseptic technique Any activity or procedure that prevents infection or breaks the chain of infection.

Asepsis (medical) Clean technique; procedures performed to reduce the number of microorganisms and minimize their spread.

Asepsis (surgical) Surgical technique; procedures performed to eliminate the presence of all microorganisms and/or prevent the introduction of microorganisms to an area.

There are five basic principles of asepsis:

- Principle one: Know what is dirty. Items that have been used for patient care are considered contaminated. An item is either contaminated or not contaminated. For the SP technician, the terms "dirty" and "contaminated" mean the same thing. Microbial contamination cannot be seen with the naked eye; however, it can be present, even when it is not seen. Examples of contaminated items include opened surgical instrument trays, IV pumps, and suction machines that have been sitting in a patient room.
- Principle two: Know what is clean. Cleanliness is the basis of aseptic technique. Mechanical cleaning removes soil and most microorganisms. Any item that has been properly cleaned via manual or mechanical means is considered clean. If that item has been cleaned with a detergent disinfectant or a thermal decontamination process, it is considered clean and decontaminated. The physical task of washing/cleaning removes soil and most microorganisms.

- Principle three: Know what is sterile. Sterility is defined as the absence of all microbes. Sterility is impossible to see with the naked eye; one cannot look at a specific item and determine its sterility.

- Principle four: Keep dirty, clean and sterile areas separate. There must be separation between the three areas to allow a margin of safety. Clean or decontaminated items must not come in contact with dirty items. If they do, they must again be considered dirty. If sterile items come in contact with non-sterile items, they must also be considered non-sterile.

- Principle five: Remedy contamination immediately. When dirty, clean and sterile areas or items have not been separated, the situation must be corrected immediately. One who observes a procedure has as much responsibility for maintaining proper aseptic technique as the person who performs the procedure. There are times when only an SP technician will know or suspect that something may be contaminated. Even though processing the item may result in more work, this must be done to protect the patient.

A careless attitude may lead to an increased risk of infection, so SP technicians must always be aware of their actions. By adhering to the principles of asepsis, the risk of infection will be reduced for patients and the facility's employees. The responsibility of SP technicians to provide safe items for use should never be underestimated or compromised.

SP technicians must assume several important responsibilities in their facility's infection prevention and control efforts. The SPD's infection prevention and control goals are to:

- Eliminate or destroy all potentially infectious contaminants present on reusable instruments and equipment.

- Safely distribute reusable and single-use items required for the delivery of patient care.

- Establish and enforce standards for decontamination, disinfection and sterilization in various healthcare settings.

The importance of these responsibilities is clear. The use of medical devices that have not been properly handled, disinfected or sterilized can cause infections in patients and staff. SP technicians are responsible for providing safe items that support good patient outcomes.

PERSONAL HYGIENE AND ATTIRE

Preventing the spread of microorganisms and maintaining appropriate environments for clean and sterile items requires good self-management skills. Hygiene and adherence to dress code protocols are critical components of infection prevention in the SPD.

Personal Hygiene

Hand hygiene is a term that means either handwashing or using an approved antiseptic hand rub (such as an alcohol-based product). Hand hygiene is considered the single most important factor in reducing infections. Handwashing refers to the use of soap, water and friction to wash one's hands. (See **Figure 5.2**)

> **Hand hygiene** The act of washing one's hands with soap and water or using an alcohol-based hand rub.

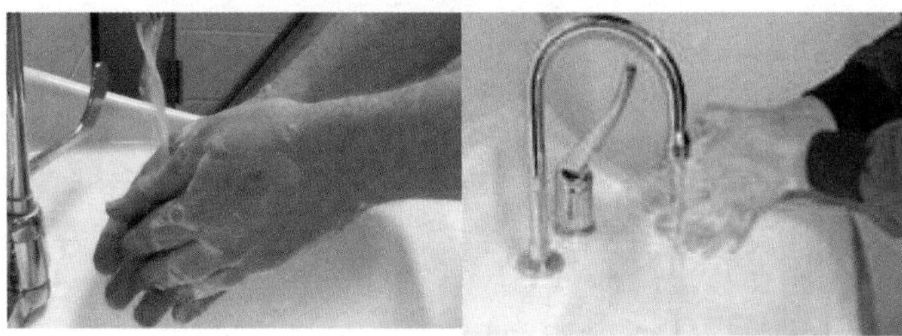

1. Remove all jewelry
2. Turn on faucet using a paper towel
3. Wet hands and apply soap
4. Work soap into a lather and scrub hands for at least 20 seconds*
5. Keep hands at a lower angle than elbows to prevent dirty water from running back onto arms
6. Interlace fingers to clean between them
7. Rinse hands thoroughly
8. Dry hands with clean disposable towels
9. Turn off the faucet using a clean disposable towel

Figure 5.2 *Source: Centers for Disease Control and Prevention*

SPDs should be equipped with handwashing sinks conveniently located for easy access. SP technicians should wash their hands only in dedicated handwashing sinks (not in sinks used for decontamination purposes).

Because fingernails harbor microorganisms, they should be kept clean and not extend beyond the fingertips. Long nails increase the risk of tearing gloves. Fingernail polish should not be worn in the SPD because nail polish may chip and fall onto an instrument set. Artificial nails should not be worn in the SPD because they also harbor microorganisms and may detach and fall into a tray, unnoticed.

Infection prevention begins at home. Personal hygiene is important for the prevention of infections. Bathing and shampooing regularly, wearing clean clothing and practicing good hand hygiene prepares SP technicians to continue this practice in the healthcare facility.

Personnel with open or weeping wounds or excessive skin irritations should refrain from handling any patient care equipment until the condition is resolved or medically evaluated.

Hand Hygiene

Hand hygiene should be performed prior to starting work, upon entering or leaving the work areas, before and after eating, using the restroom or whenever hands become soiled or contaminated. Hand hygiene should also be done before handling instruments and medical devices for sterilization packaging, contaminants, oils, and soils can be transferred to instruments from the hands of personnel compromising the sterilization process. Infection Prevention and Control experts recommend that hands be washed immediately and thoroughly if they become soiled with blood, bodily fluids, secretions or excretions. After contact with contaminated items without visible soil or after gloves are removed, an alcohol-based hand rub should be used according to the manufacturer's recommendations. Approved non-oil-based hand lotions may be used after handwashing to keep the skin healthy and to minimize skin irritation and excessive drying.

Attire

Most of the SP area is considered semi-restricted, and SP technicians must wear clean scrub attire provided by and laundered through the healthcare facility. The Association of periOperative Registered Nurses (AORN) states, "Home laundering is not monitored for quality, consistency or safety. Home washing machines may not have the adjustable parameters or controls required to achieve the necessary thermal measures (water temperature); mechanical measures (agitation); or chemical measures (capacity for additives to neutralize the alkalinity of the water, soap or detergent) to reduce the microbial levels in soiled scrub attire." Healthcare facility laundering protects the employee and other staff members, patients, family members, and the public.

Attire should be clean and not worn outside the facility. Technicians should change out of their street clothing and shoes (those worn at home) and into scrubs and shoes kept at the facility. Usually, there will be a locker space for personal belongings. At the end of the workday, scrubs must be left behind in the facility's laundry, protecting employees from infecting anyone at home or in the community. Jewelry, including necklaces, watches and rings, should not be worn in the department because it can harbor microorganisms, and some jewelry items may accidentally fall into instrument sets.

Lanyards, if used, should be left at the facility and cleaned on a regular basis. Personal electronics, including phones, should be stored and kept out of SP areas. Personal devices can harbor microorganisms and should be cleaned regularly. Other personal items, such as fuzzy pens, stuffed animals, and artificial plants should be left at home. Backpacks and purses should also not be brought into the work area. These items are difficult to clean and, like cellular devices, harbor microorganisms.

Basic attire should be worn in every area of the SPD and by everyone working in or visiting the department (this includes anyone entering to clean or perform repairs). (See **Figure 5.3**)

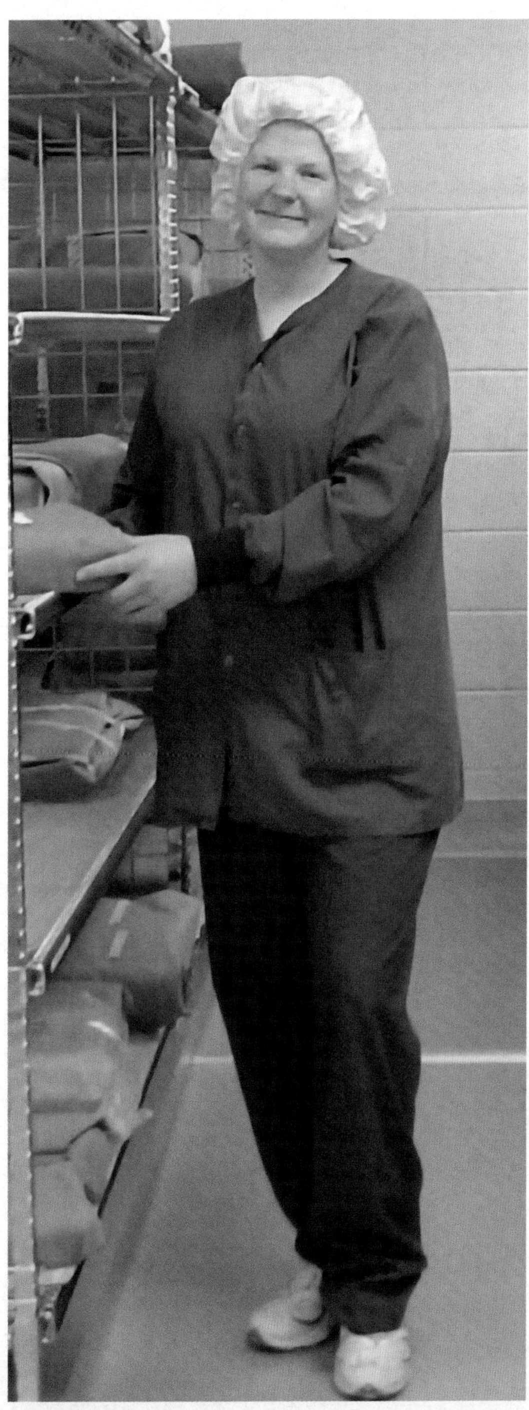

Figure 5.3

Scrub attire should always be donned (put on) just prior to starting work, and doffed (removed) before leaving work.

A disposable bouffant-type head covering should be worn in all areas of the department. Head covers should cover all head hair, except eyelashes and eyebrows. Reusable head covers, if allowed in the facility, should be covered with a bouffant cover to prevent contaminating the area with outside bacteria or with bacteria that may have multiplied on the caps due to improper cleaning. Skull-type caps are no longer suggested for use because they do not always fully cover head hair.

Beards and mustaches should be covered with an approved beard cover to prevent facial hair from shedding onto the items being processed.

Sturdy, closed-toe shoes with non-skid soles should be worn in the department. Shoes should be able to protect the feet from items that may inadvertently fall from work areas. It is good practice to have shoes dedicated to the area and not worn out of the facility.

A cover gown/lab coat may be used to protect the scrub attire when leaving the department for another area of the same facility (this depends on facility policy). Note: *Cover gown/lab coats are not meant to protect departmental attire while outside the building.*

- Scrub attire should be changed daily, anytime it becomes soiled, or as soon as it may have become contaminated. Scrub attire should at least consist of clean pants and a top. Some facilities provide long-sleeve jackets.

- T-shirts, if worn, should be completely covered by the scrub top. No part of the T-shirt should be visible outside the scrub attire.

- Some facilities allow outside visitors to wear disposable cover clothing, such as jumpsuits, instead of scrub attire. The disposable cover attire should also cover all outside clothing.

Decontamination attire: The decontamination area is a restricted area, and all individuals working in this area must comply with PPE/dress code requirements. This is required by the Occupational Safety and Health Administration (OSHA) and was established to help ensure workers are protected from potential pathogens. Decontamination PPE is required for anyone who enters the area, even if only for a very brief period.

Risk of exposure to pathogenic microorganisms can be reduced by diligently following dress codes in decontamination areas. For example, fluid-resistant gowns provide protection from splashes that may soak into and contaminate regular scrub attire. (See **Figure 5.4**)

All of the basic attire outlined previously, except the cover gown, should be worn in the decontamination area. Because of the nature of the work in the decontamination area (soiled and contaminated devices, water and chemicals) additional attire is required. **Figure 5.5** provides examples of PPE worn in the decontamination area. Decontamination PPE includes:

- Gloves approved for the decontamination area. To better protect the hands, these gloves are thicker than examination gloves. They also have longer cuffs (some are elbow length), so they can be placed over the gown cuff to keep fluids from flowing into the glove or up the gown sleeve.

- Fluid-resistant mask that fits around the ears or ties on the head to protect the nose and mouth.

- Level 3 fluid-resistant gown or jumpsuit to protect scrub clothes and skin. Fluid-resistant materials will keep fluids away from the skin, while standard fabrics will absorb fluids, allowing the skin beneath the fabric to become wet and contaminated.

- Goggles approved to protect the eyes.

Regular and Fluid-Resistant Fabric Comparison

Water on a regular fabric scrub top

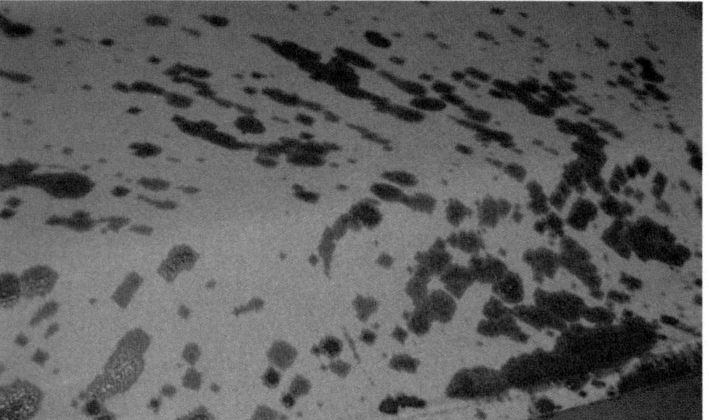

Water on a fluid-resistant gown

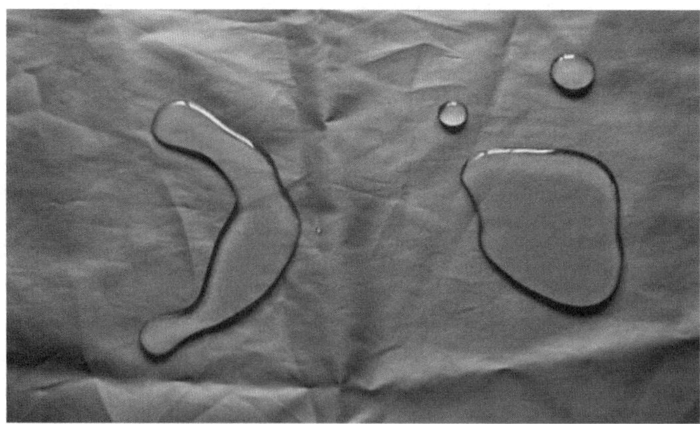

Figure 5.4

Examples of PPE Worn in the Decontamination Area

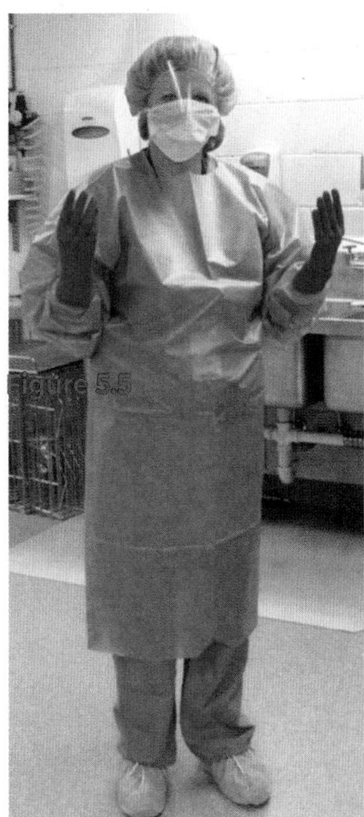
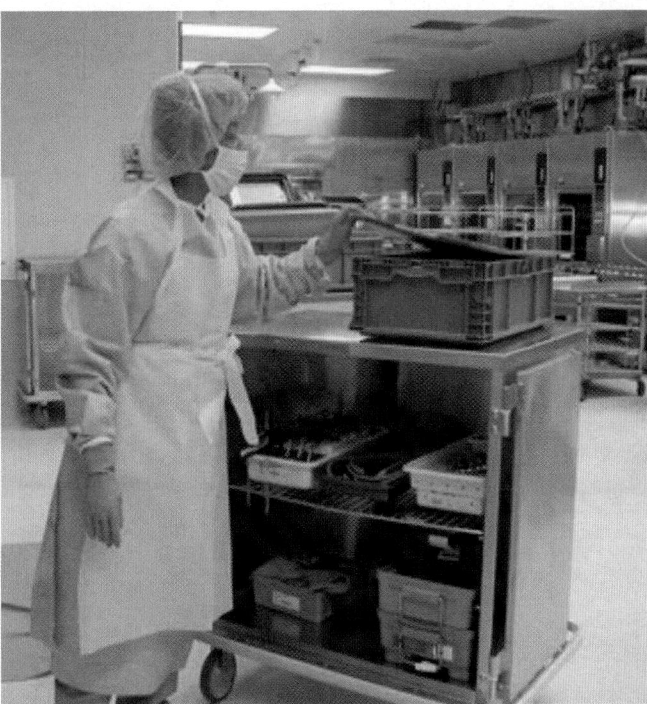
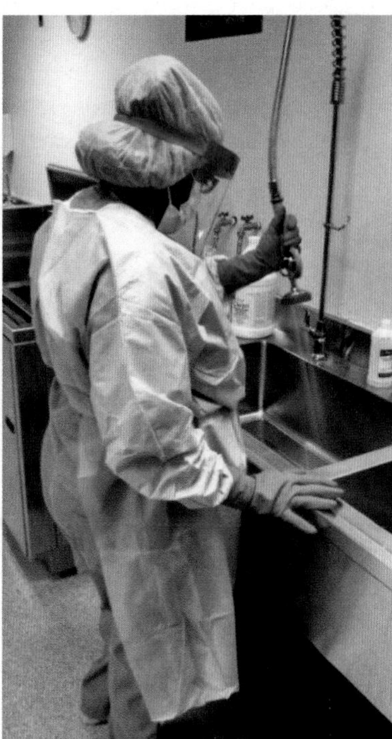

Figure 5.5

Type of PPE	Protects	Rationale
Level 3 fluid-resistant gown, apron, jumpsuit	Protect skin and scrubs	Provides a barrier against splash or spray
Fluid resistant mask	Protects mouth, nose, chin	Protects respiratory tract from airborne infectious aerosols
Goggles	Protects the eyes	Protects eyes from infectious aerosols
Face shield-full length and hoods	Protects eyes, nose, mouth, face and neck	Protects eye, nose, mouth, face and neck from sprays, splashes and infectious aerosols
Shoe covers	Protect shoes	Protects the shoes from spray
Gloves approved for the decontamination area	Protect hands	Protects hands from contaminated instruments

Figure 5.6 Types of PPE

How to Don (Put on) PPE		
*	Before beginning	Don surgical scrubs, a head cover and appropriate shoes and perform hand hygiene.
1.	Gown or jumpsuit	Don the fluid-resistant gown or jumpsuit. Tie, snap or zip completely
2.	Mask	Secure the earpieces around the ears or tie the strings on the head area. Fit the mask over the nose area, and ensure the nose and mouth areas are completely covered.
3.	Goggles or face shield	Don goggles or face shield and adjust to fit properly (goggles should wrap around the sides of the face).
4.	Shoe covers	Don shoe covers and ensure shoes are completely covered.
5.	Gloves	Don gloves and ensure gloves are over the gown cuff.

Figure 5.7

- Full face shields and hoods that protect the face, mouth, nose and other exposed areas such as the neck. *Note: Wearing a face shield does not replace the need to also wear a face mask.*

- Shoe covers to protect the shoes from contamination. Shoe covers should be worn even if the shoes are dedicated to department use only. Using boot-length covers (not required) will help protect the leg area as well.

Figure 5.6 provides a recap of basic PPE requirements and the reason each component is important. There is a proper way to don and doff PPE, and **Figures 5.7** and **5.8** give the proper sequence for both.

CDC recommendations for doffing (removing) PPE
1. Remove shoe covers
2. Remove gown and gloves (removed in combinations)
3. Remove goggles or face shield
4. Remove mask
5. Remove head cover
6. Wash hands

Figure 5.8 *Source: Centers for Disease Control and Prevention*

When wearing PPE, SP technicians should use safe work practices to protect themselves and limit the spread of contamination by:

- Keeping hands away from the face

- Changing gloves when torn or heavily contaminated

- Consistently performing hand hygiene before and after wearing PPE

MANAGING THE ENVIRONMENT TO PREVENT THE SPREAD OF BACTERIA

The first step in maintaining environmental integrity is to control the traffic that enters and passes through the SPD. As previously addressed, most areas of the SPD are considered semi-restricted and the dress codes apply to all who enter. Departmental dress standards for visitors (e.g., sales representatives, maintenance personnel and clinical engineering staff) vary between facilities. In some facilities, they must change into surgical scrubs; in others, coveralls or jumpsuits (worn over street clothes) are required. SP technicians must protect the integrity of the environment by enforcing traffic control guidelines. This may sometimes mean educating visitors about dress code and traffic control protocols.

Dress code requirements may change as SP technicians move from one area to another. For example, surgical scrubs and hair coverings may be appropriate for the clean assembly area whereas OSHA-required PPE is necessary for the decontamination area. (See **Figure 5.9**) Dress codes are an important part of traffic control; therefore, SP technicians must understand which attire is appropriate in different areas. *Note: If in an unfamiliar area and unsure of the attire requirements, ask before entering.*

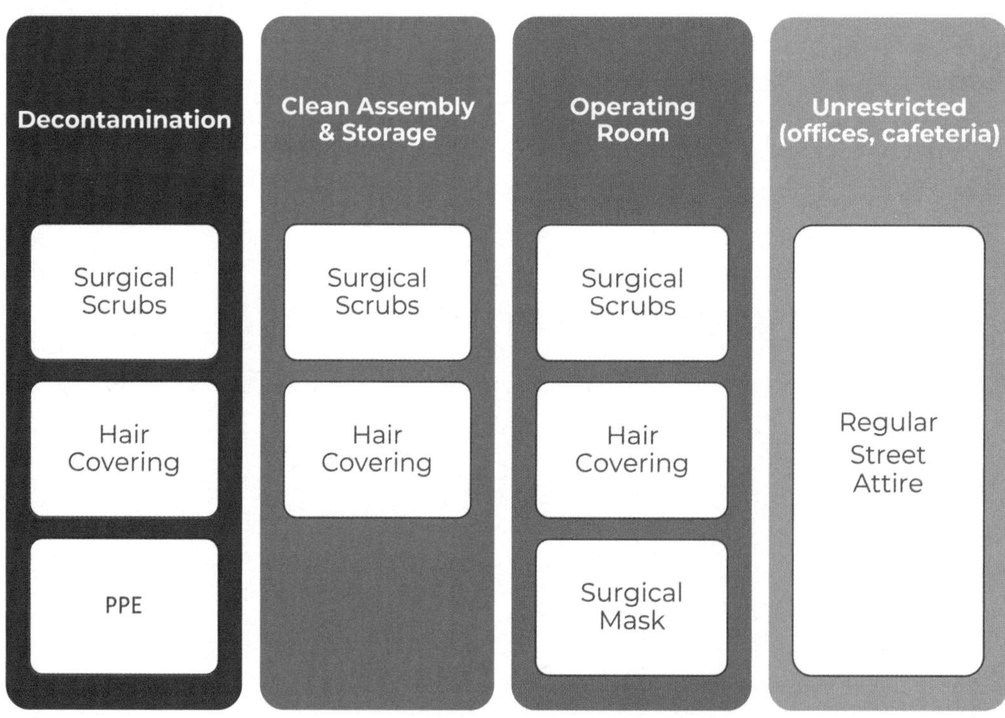

Figure 5.9

Examples of SP traffic control signs

ATTENTION:
Entering
Semi-Restricted
Surgical Area.
Surgical Scrubs, Hair
Covering REQUIRED.
NO Food or Beverage
Beyond This Point.

L716
DECONTAMINATION
ROOM
P.P.E. REQUIRED IN
DECONTAMINATION
ROOM

Airlock
to
Decontam
BIOHAZARD

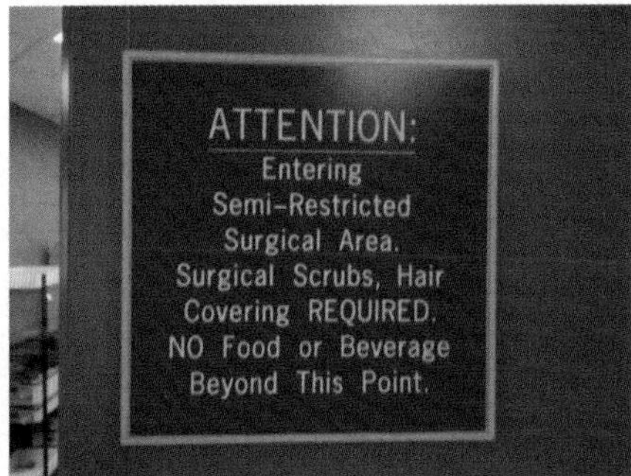

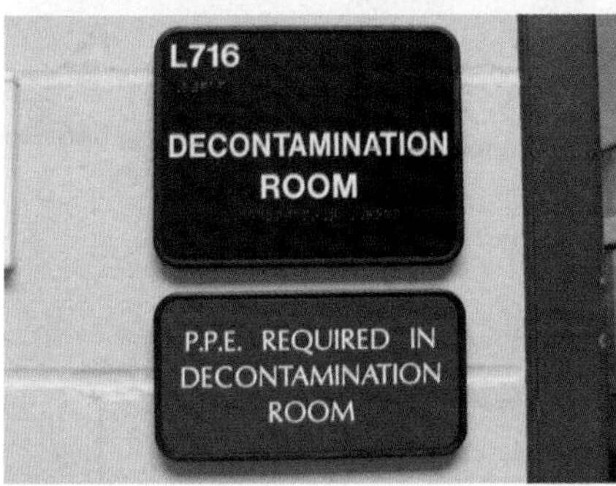

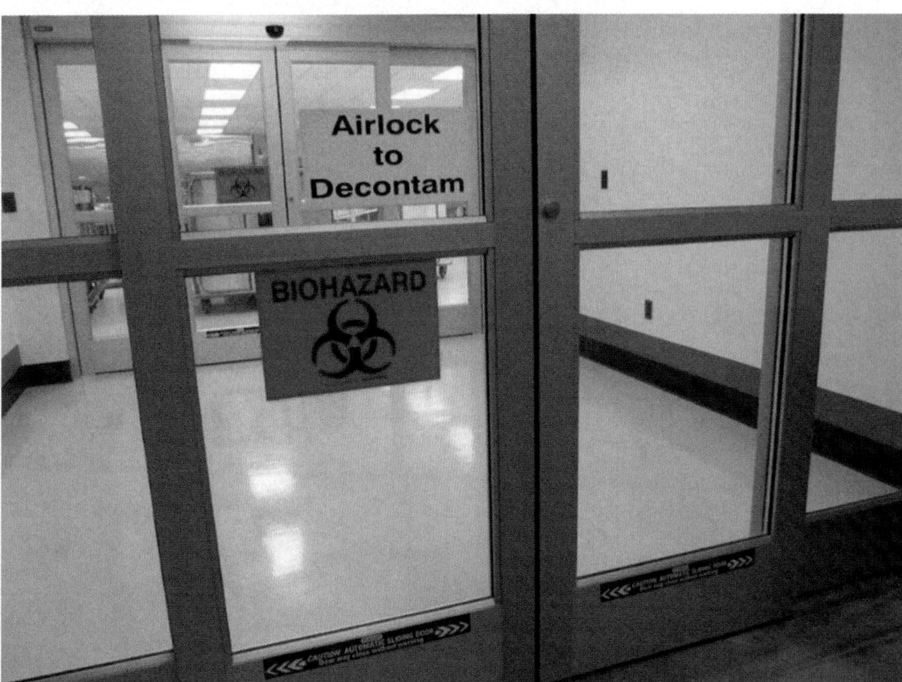

Figure 5.10 Common SP traffic control signs

Areas that SP technicians routinely travel through may have three separate traffic control/dress code requirements:

- Restricted – Areas where sterile surgical procedures are performed and the decontamination area of the SPD. Surgical scrub attire, hair coverings and masks are required in restricted areas. Those working within the sterile field (including surgeons, surgical technologists and nurses) are also required to wear a sterile surgical gown and gloves. *Note: Semi-restricted areas in the OR, such as access corridors to surgical suites, must follow restricted dress code.*

- Semi-restricted – These areas include peripheral support areas to the OR, SP clean assembly and sterile storage areas. Surgical scrub attire and hair coverings are required in these areas.

- Unrestricted – These areas include normal traffic areas such as hospital corridors, most offices, locker rooms and general public areas (e.g., cafeteria and waiting rooms). Street clothes may be worn in unrestricted areas.

SPDs use signage to assist in traffic control. All restricted and semi-restricted areas also have signage that informs people entering the area about the need for specific dress codes. (See **Figure 5.10**)

OSHA'S BLOODBORNE PATHOGENS STANDARD

OSHA is the primary federal agency charged with the enforcement of occupational safety and health legislation. In response to concerns, OSHA published the Bloodborne Pathogens Standard (29 CFR 1910.1030) to recognize the potential for occupational exposure to bloodborne diseases (hepatitis B and C; HIV). It places the responsibility for providing a safe work environment on the employer.

The standard requires a written exposure control plan (ECP) that summarizes the employer's program for the protection of workers from occupational exposure to bloodborne diseases. This plan includes:

- Implementation of various methods of exposure control, including following Standard Precautions (previously known as Universal Precautions) such as the proper use of PPE; the use of engineering controls to physically remove hazards; and the development of work practice controls.

- Policies and procedures to prevent occupational exposure and transmission of bloodborne pathogens.

- Housekeeping: Provision of a clean and sanitary working environment, including regularly scheduled cleaning using hospital germicides (disinfectants) approved by the U.S. Environmental Protection Agency (EPA).

- Hepatitis B vaccination

- Recordkeeping: Proof of training upon initial hire and annually thereafter. If significant changes are made to the ECP, additional training is required to address the changes. Medical records regarding any exposure must be maintained.

- The use of fluorescent orange or orange-red biohazard labels to identify contaminated items. (See **Figures 5.11** and **5.12**)

- Disposal of all sharp items in rigid, puncture-proof containers that are covered and properly labeled or color-coded. (See **Figure 5.13**)

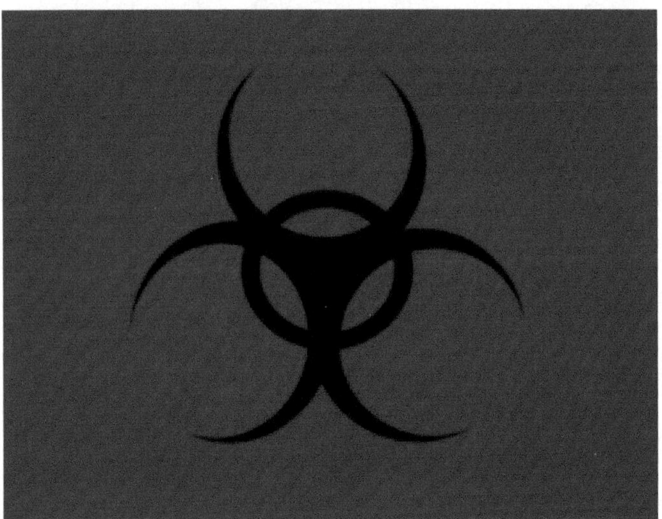

Figure 5.11

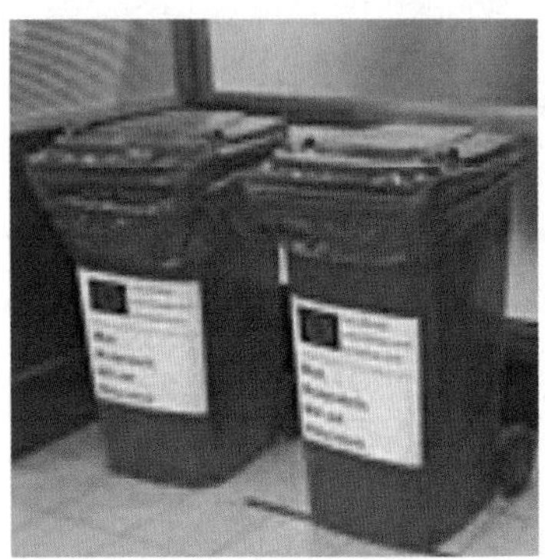
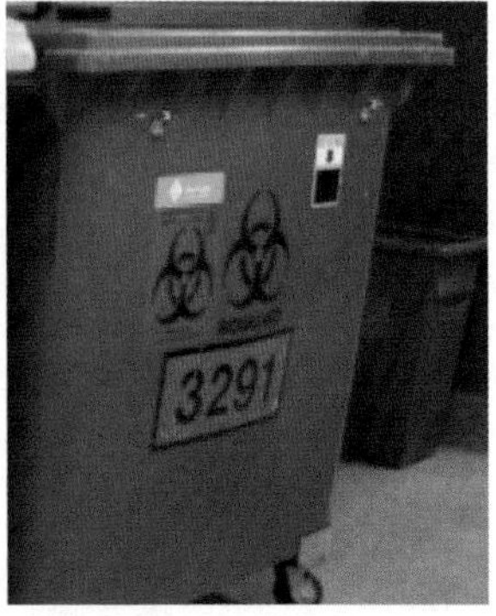

Figure 5.12 Biohazard waste containers

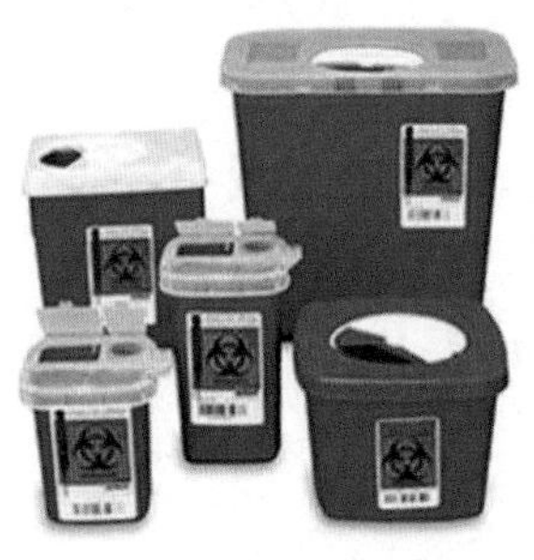
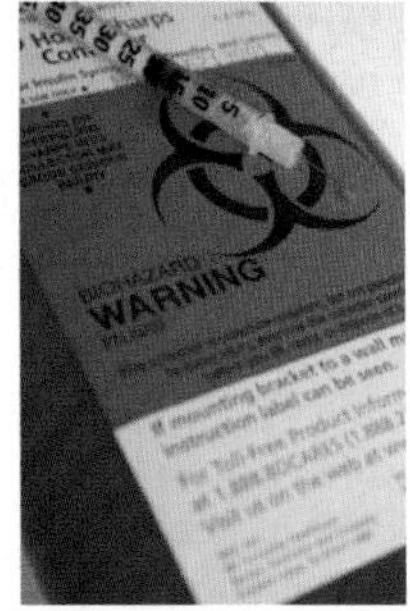

Figure 5.13 Biohazard sharps container

- Transport of reusable sharps in enclosed carts or hard-sided containers to prevent injury. (See **Figure 5.14**)

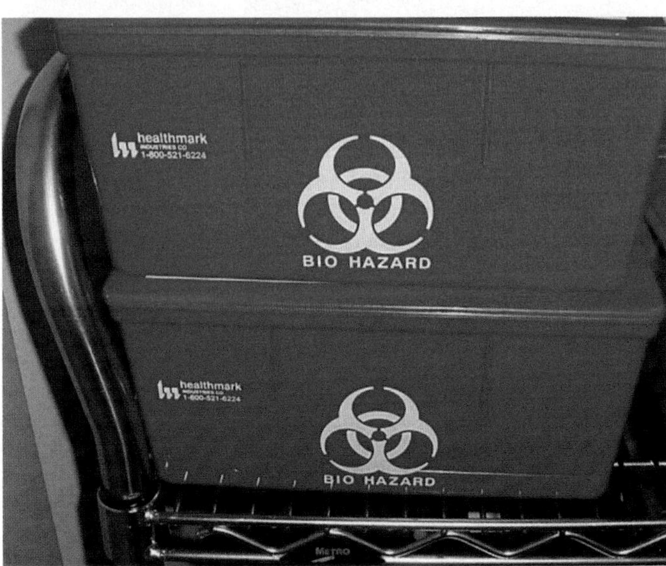

Figure 5.14 Biohazard transport bins

ENVIRONMENTAL CONCERNS IN STERILE PROCESSING AREAS

In addition to specific guidelines for dress codes and standard precautions, there are environmental tools designed to help SP technicians promote infection prevention. Some tools are evident; others, while not as evident, still play an important role in maintaining an environment that is safe for patients and employees.

Physical Design

An SPD's physical design should incorporate a clear separation of clean and dirty, and workflow patterns should be designed that create a one-way flow of goods from dirty to clean.

In addition to walls separating the decontamination area from the rest of the department, the area should be designed to reduce the likelihood that airborne bacteria can be transmitted from the decontamination area to the clean area. This is accomplished with use of positive and negative air pressure. The decontamination area has negative (lower) air pressure. This means that when a door or window is opened between the separate work areas, air flows from the clean (positive pressure) area to the dirty (negative pressure) area. This minimizes the risk of airborne bacteria in the decontamination area being carried to the clean area. **Figure 5.15** illustrates the airflow created using positive and negative air pressure. To maintain the balance necessary for air pressure systems to function correctly, windows and doors between the decontamination and clean areas must remain closed when not in use.

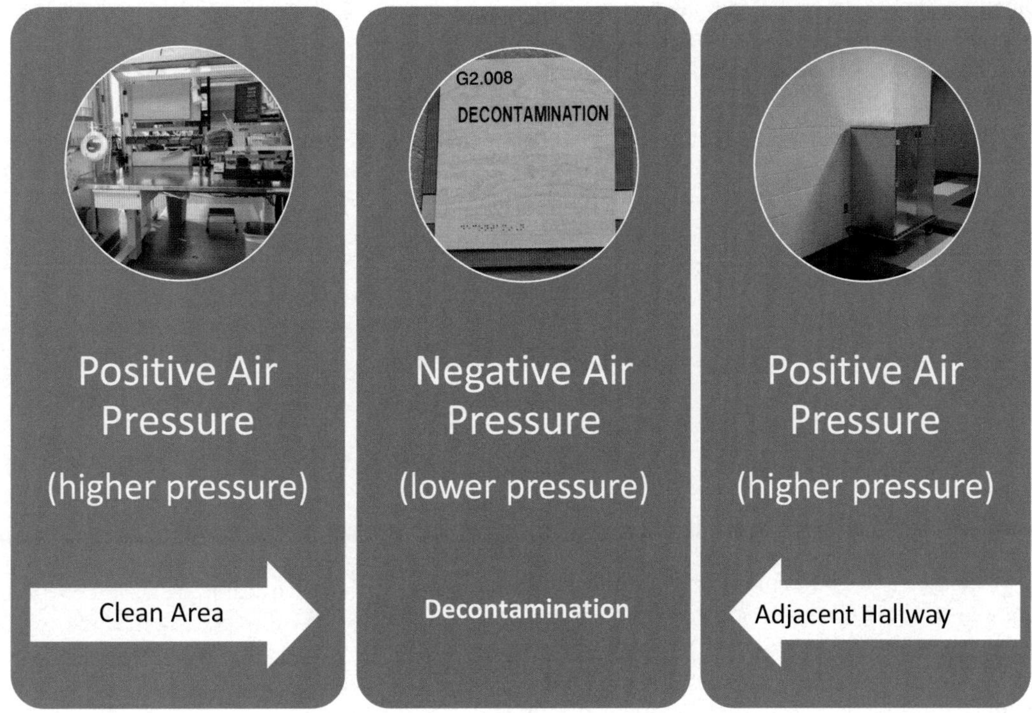

Figure 5.15 The use of air pressure to control airborne bacteria

In addition to the air pressure requirements, SP areas must meet specific temperature, humidity and air exchange requirements. These vary by work area, and SP technicians must be familiar with the requirements for each specific area and ensure that policies designed to manage airflow, temperature and humidity are followed at all times. SP temperature and humidity are controlled by the facility heating, ventilation and air conditioning (HVAC) system. The parameters for SP areas can be established by identifying which version of ANSI/ASHREA/ASHE 170 will be used based on when the HVAC system was initially installed or last upgraded.

Note: Some facilities may choose to use 20% for the lower humidity level. SPDs should check with their supply and equipment manufacturers to ensure that the lower humidity is acceptable for items stored in the area.

In many departments, SP technicians may be responsible for collecting data, such as temperatures and humidity and recording that data, as part of their department's formal documentation system.

Use of freestanding fans should not be permitted in any SP work area. Fans create highly turbulent air flow, which recirculates dust and microorganisms from the floor and work surfaces and interferes with airflow.

Work Area Cleanliness

The cleaner the work area, the more likely that the products prepared in SP areas will be safe for use in a sterile environment. Dust and lint particles do not only carry bacteria. In some cases, lint remaining in a sterile set may enter the patient's body during surgery and cause infection. SP technicians must minimize the amount of contaminants, such as dust, lint and bacteria, in all work areas.

Bacteria can be transmitted by contact with contaminated items. Inanimate objects that can transmit bacteria are called **fomites**. Common fomites that become contaminated in SP areas include door handles, computer pads, keyboards, telephones, work surfaces, and other items routinely handled by multiple people. SP technicians should know that by routinely cleaning these items and their general work areas (workstations), they can control the unwanted spread of bacteria within their workplace.

Fomite An inanimate object that can transmit bacteria.

Food and beverages should not be allowed in SP work areas. This standard is well understood for decontamination areas; however, this rule is also necessary in clean areas of the department for the following reasons:

- Beverages should not be allowed because they may spill and contaminate sterile items, or they may spill onto items that need to be sterilized and impact sterilization outcomes. Spilling may also contaminate items being assembled for sterilization or damage count sheets, reference books and other items on the workstation.

- Food should not be allowed because it may also contaminate items. SP technicians should not eat in their work areas because their hands may become soiled and they could transmit bacteria. Snack foods can leave an oily residue on hands that can adhere to instruments being packaged for sterilization. This oil may impede the contact of the sterilant with the entire surface of the instrument. Food and beverages also attract insects and other pests, and may increase the chance of such creatures invading the work area.

OSHA regulations prohibit the consumption of food and drink in areas in which work involving exposure or potential exposure to blood or potentially infectious material exist or where the potential of contaminated work surfaces exists as it does in SP areas.

Environmental cleaning (housekeeping), often referred to as Environmental Services (EVS), is a vital component in the SPD's overall infection prevention and control process. Procedures used in SP cleaning should be the same as those used in the OR and delivery rooms. Environmental cleaning should be based on an assessment of risk in each SP area. A team consisting of EVS and SP personnel should define the type of cleaning requirements for each area, including the surfaces to be cleaned (with responsibility assigned), and discuss the cleaning and disinfectant chemicals to be used and the frequency of cleaning. EVS and SP staff should follow these specific cleaning guidelines:

- Floors should be cleaned (wet mopped) at least daily. Floors should never be swept or dust mopped because dust will rise and fall on items, such as instruments, in the area. When sterile packages are opened, the dust that has accumulated on them may fall onto the package contents.

- The decontamination area should have separate and dedicated cleaning equipment such as mops and buckets. Items used to clean the decontamination area should not be used elsewhere.

- Horizontal work surfaces, such as counters and worktables, should be cleaned at least daily and, preferably, every shift.

- Light fixtures or their covers and air vents should be cleaned at least every six months or as necessary. This function is usually performed by another department such as EVS or Facilities Maintenance.

- Other surfaces (including walls, cabinets and racks) should be cleaned on a regularly scheduled basis.

- Trash should be emptied as needed and at least daily when areas are in use.

Although many SP housekeeping functions are performed by EVS personnel, routine cleaning of sterile storage cabinets, carts and racks is usually the responsibility of SP technicians who have been trained to properly handle sterile items and who know specific product names and locations.

A cleaning schedule and checklist should be established for each area, and cleaning verification tools should be utilized as part of an audit system to measure the adequacy of cleaning performed.

Other Environmental Cleaning Requirements

Fixtures and furnishings in the SPD must be constructed of materials that can be cleaned; such cleaning should be performed on a regularly scheduled basis.

The area designated for sterile storage may consist of either open (rack) or closed (cabinet) storage units. The decision about the type of storage used is based on the types of items to be stored and the amount of traffic in the area. For example, closed cabinets may be used in high-traffic areas, and open shelving (racks) may be used in more controlled, low-traffic areas. Open-rack systems should have a solid bottom, so items stored on the lower shelves are protected from contamination during housekeeping tasks.

Technicians in the SPD work with items at all stages of the decontamination, sterilization, storage and distribution processes, so they must understand the basic infection control principles. To ensure the workflow is maintained and items are handled properly at each stage in the processing cycle, technicians must understand and practice the principles of asepsis.

An Important Concern

Some microorganisms are becoming resistant to antibiotics or are naturally very difficult to control. Many of these resistant microorganisms can be transferred easily to other surfaces and people. Controlling these microorganisms and preventing their transmission is the number one responsibility of the SPD.

Understanding the way microorganisms can be transmitted is the key to helping stop cross-contamination.

ELEMENTS OF TRANSMISSION AND THE CHAIN OF INFECTION

Infection transmission is a complicated process that involves many factors for a pathogenic microorganism to result in disease or illness. According to the CDC's *Guideline for Isolation Precautions: Preventing Transmission of Infectious Agents in Healthcare Settings, 2007*, the transmission of infectious agents in a healthcare setting requires six elements: a **causative agent**, **reservoir**, **portal of exit**, **mode of transmission**, **portal of entry**, and **susceptible host**. This infectious disease process is better known as the chain of infection. (See **Figure 5.16**)

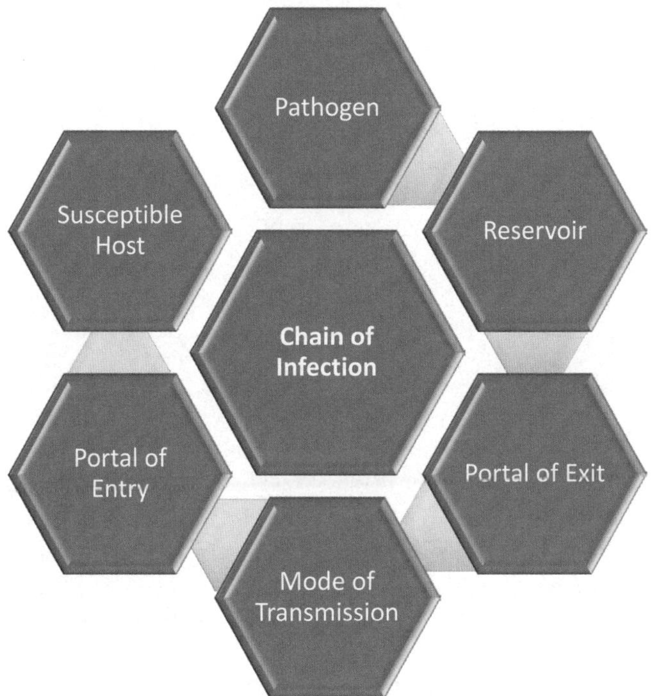

Figure 5.16

CHAIN OF INFECTION ELEMENTS

Causative agent Microorganism (pathogen) that causes an infectious disease.

Reservoir Place where an infectious agent (microorganism) can survive.

Portal of exit Path by which an infectious agent leaves the reservoir.

Mode of transmission Method of transfer of an infectious agent from the reservoir to a susceptible host.

Portal of entry The path used by an infectious agent to enter a susceptible host.

Susceptible host Person or animal that lacks the ability to resist an infection by an infectious agent.

Causative Agent

The first link is the causative agent (the pathogenic microorganism): bacteria, virus, fungi, protozoa or prion. The characteristics that make the organism capable of causing disease include:

- Invasiveness – An organism's ability to invade the host and cause damage
- Pathogenicity – An organism's ability to gain entry into the host and cause disease
- Virulence – Degree of pathogenicity
- Infectious dose – Quantity of organisms required to cause disease
- Viability – Organism's ability to survive outside the host
- Antimicrobial resistance - Ability to develop resistance to antimicrobial agents

The only way to interrupt the transmission of a causative agent is to eliminate it. This can be done by promptly initiating the appropriate processes, such as using aseptic technique to avoid cross-contamination, physically removing the contaminated substances through cleaning, and using effective disinfection and sterilization processes.

Reservoir/Source

The second link in the chain of infection is the reservoir or source of the agent, a place in which an infectious agent can survive. In the healthcare setting, the most common reservoirs are human sources such as patients, healthcare personnel, family and visitors; however, inanimate objects, including environmental surfaces, surgical instruments and devices, have also been implicated, as have contaminated food, water, or intravenous fluids.

Those with active infections but without obvious symptoms, and those who are **carriers**, represent the greatest risk to other patients and healthcare workers because the presence of disease-producing organisms may go undetected.

Carrier A person who is infected with an infectious disease but displays no symptoms. Although unaffected by the disease themselves, carriers can transmit the disease to others.

Good personal hygiene and health habits, the use of appropriate housekeeping measures, and proper cleaning and sterilization of hospital equipment can eliminate reservoirs.

Portal of Exit

The third link is the portal of exit or the path by which an infectious agent leaves the reservoir. Portals of exit associated with humans and animal reservoirs include:

- Respiratory tract (coughing and sneezing)
- Genitourinary tract (urine, vaginal secretions, or semen)
- Gastrointestinal tract (vomit or stool)

- Skin/mucous membrane (mucous or wound drainage)
- Blood (blood transfusions or contact with blood)
- Transplacental (through the placenta from mother to baby)

Common ways SP technicians can block the portal of exit include covering the nose and mouth when sneezing/coughing, disposing facial tissues immediately after use, performing proper hand hygiene, disposing of trash, and effectively using PPE.

Mode of Transmission

The fourth link is the mode of transmission or how a pathogenic organism is spread. This can vary by the type of organism and its route of transmission.

Direct contact occurs when microorganisms are transferred directly from one infected person to another via blood or other blood-containing bodily fluids. Indirect contact occurs through a contaminated object or person such as through inadequately cleaned or sterilized instruments, the hands of healthcare personnel, or contaminated PPE. Some infections transmitted by contact include herpes simplex virus (HSV), *Staphylococcus aureus*, respiratory syncytial virus and *Clostridium difficile*.

Droplet transmission occurs when an infected person coughs, sneezes or talks during procedures such as endotracheal intubation or suctioning. Infectious droplets can travel short distances to the susceptible person's mucous membranes of the eyes, nose and mouth. Some of the diseases spread in this manner include influenza virus, COVID-19, group A Streptococcus, adenovirus, and some types of meningitis.

Airborne transmission occurs when very small droplet particles are dispersed in the air over long distances by air currents and are then inhaled by susceptible individuals. Infectious agents transmitted by this route include Mycobacterium tuberculosis (TB), spores of Aspergillus spp, and varicella-zoster virus (chickenpox).

Common vehicle transmission occurs when infectious agents are present in a vehicle, such as food (salmonella), blood (HIV) or water (pseudomonas).

Vector-borne transmission rarely occurs in U.S. hospitals. Agents can be carried on insects (e.g., on the feet or wings of flies) or by the bites of insect or arthropods (mosquitoes, ticks and fleas).

Pathogenic transmission can be interrupted through proper hand hygiene, cleaning, decontamination, disinfection and sterilization, standard and isolation precautions as well as proper food handling, proper water treatment and maintenance of HVAC systems.

Portal of Entry

The fifth link in the chain of infection is the portal of entry or the path used by an infectious agent to enter a susceptible host.

Patients are particularly vulnerable to transmission in areas where the usual defense mechanisms are bypassed. Portals of entry associated with a human host include:

- Respiratory tract
- Genitourinary tract
- Gastrointestinal tract
- Skin/mucous membranes
- Transplacental
- **Parenteral**

> **Parenteral** Something that is put inside the body but not by swallowing (e.g., an injection administered into the muscle).

Safe protocols include maintaining clean or sterile techniques during patient care procedures. Proper hand hygiene can alter access of an infectious agent to a susceptible host. Other practices involve using only properly disinfected/sterilized equipment for invasive procedures and safe handling and disposal of sharps.

Susceptible Host

Most of the factors that influence whether a person acquires an infection are related to the sixth and final link: whether the individual is a susceptible host and lacks the ability to resist infection. Some who are exposed to an infectious agent will become severely ill and die, while others never develop symptoms at all. Some may progress from **colonization** to symptomatic disease shortly after exposure to the pathogen, while others will become temporarily or chronically colonized and never have symptoms.

> **Colonization** A process that occurs when microorganisms live on or in a host organism, but do not invade tissues or cause damage.

Whether or not an individual becomes susceptible to a microorganism can be influenced by various factors:

- Age (very young or very old)
- Disease history/underlying disease, such as cancer, diabetes and heart disease

- Medications and treatments that can compromise the immune system, including chemotherapy, radiation and steroid.
- Trauma (the injury itself and the treatment of the injury can increase the risk of infection)

Some measures to boost the ability to fight disease include treating the primary disease (e.g., keeping blood sugar under control in diabetics), administering vaccines (such as pneumonia and influenza) and recognizing that patients are at high risk for infection.

From an SP perspective, there are many opportunities to interrupt the chain of infection and play an active and important role in preventing and controlling infectious diseases. **Figure 5.17** provides an example of how the chain of infection can be impacted by the SPD.

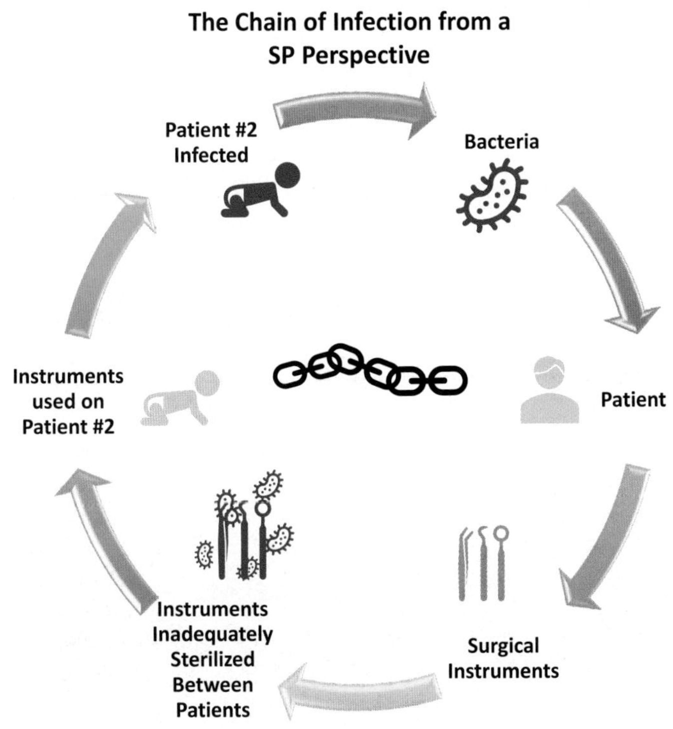

Figure 5.17

CONCLUSION

SP technicians face the ongoing challenge of ensuring that the instruments and equipment they process are safe for patient use. Advances in technology and the emergence of new microbiological challenges have increased the difficulty in meeting this challenge. Every SP technician must appreciate the importance of infection control and prevention and thoroughly understand their role in the process.

RESOURCES

Centers for Disease Control and Prevention. www.cdc.gov/nchs/fastats/insurg.htm.

Centers for Disease Control and Prevention. http://www.cdc.gov/HAI/organisms/organisms.html.

Dobson G. P. (2020). Trauma of major surgery: A global problem that is not going away. *International journal of surgery (London, England)*, *81*, 47–54. https://doi.org/10.1016/j.ijsu.2020.07.017

Association of periOperative Registered Nurses. *AORN Perioperative Standards and Recommended Practices 2022, Recommended Practice: Surgical Attire.*

Association of periOperative Registered Nurses. *AORN Guideline for Perioperative Practice. Guideline: Sterilization Packaging Systems.* 2022.

ANSI/AAMI ST79:2017 & 2020 Amendments A1, A2, A3, A4 *Comprehensive guide to steam sterilization and sterility assurance in health care facilities.*

Occupational Safety & Health Administration. *Bloodborne Pathogens (29 CFR 1910.1030).*

Terhune C. "Hospitals Grapple with Safety of Scopes after UCLA Outbreak." *Los Angeles Times.* Feb. 20, 2015.

Bartley N. "Children's Patients May Be at Risk of Infection after Colonoscopies." *The Seattle Times.* Jan. 22, 2014.

Leary, K. (2016, May 10). "Scope used in Colorado hospitals linked to infections." *Nine News.* https://www.9news.com/article/news/health/scope-used-in-colorado-hospitals-linked-to-infections/73-184766960

Ofstead C, et al. "New Research Suggests Medical Instrument Processing Personnel May Be Exposed to Tissue, Blood and Patient Fluid Despite the Use of Personal Protective Equipment." *AJIC.* Arlington, Va. Dec. 2, 2021.

ANSI/AAMI PB70:2012 *Liquid barrier performance and classification of protective apparel and drapes intended for use in health care facilities,* Section 4.2.3.6.

STERILE PROCESSING TERMS

Surgical site infection (SSI)

Biocidal

Chain of infection

Asepsis

Aseptic technique

Asepsis (medical)

Asepsis (surgical)

Hand hygiene

Fomite

Causative agent

Reservoir

Portal of exit

Mode of transmission

Portal of entry

Susceptible host

Carrier

Parenteral

Colonization

Chapter 6

Regulations and Standards

Learning Objectives

As a result of successfully completing this chapter, the reader will be able to:

1. Explain the difference between regulations and standards
2. Provide basic information about government and regulatory agencies
3. Explain the roles and responsibilities of the regulatory agencies that impact how the Sterile Processing department functions
4. Discuss how organizations and associations that develop regulations and standards affect Sterile Processing

INTRODUCTION

Regulations and **standards** impact every healthcare professional, including those working in the Sterile Processing department (SPD). These regulations and standards establish minimum levels of quality and safety. When regulations and standards are not followed, the results can vary from legal consequences to poor patient outcomes. This chapter will explain regulatory requirements that must be followed, as well as guidelines that are recommended.

> **Regulation** Rules issued by administrative agencies that have the force of law.
>
> **Standard** A uniform method of defining basic parameters for processes, products, services and measurements.

Industry, nonprofit organizations, trade associations and others develop standards. Generally, standards are not law; however, they may be incorporated into law by governmental bodies.

SP technicians are affected by regulations and standards. SP technicians must be familiar with applicable regulations and standards for the following reasons:

- Regulations must be followed and failure to comply with them may result in legal consequences to the healthcare facility.
- Regulations and standards may include workplace safety issues, which may help protect SP technicians from exposure to infectious agents and toxic substances.
- Regulations and standards may include disinfection and sterilization practices.
- With careful compliance with regulations and standards, patient safety is at its highest level of quality of care.

Regulations and standards are issued by federal, state and local governing agencies. Standards are also issued by professional organizations and provide significant assistance to healthcare personnel because they are developed according to **best practice**.

> **Best practice** A method or technique that has consistently shown results superior to those achieved by other means.

REGULATORY AGENCIES

U.S. Food and Drug Administration

The U.S. Food and Drug Administration (FDA) is responsible for ensuring that medical devices are safe and effective for patient care.

The FDA regulates the manufacture of all medical devices. It also regulates sterilants, high-level disinfectants, packaging materials, sterilizers, and quality monitors such as biological indicators (BIs).

Medical Device Classification

The level of regulation placed on any device depends upon how the FDA classifies that device:

- Class I devices – Low-risk devices, such as most handheld surgical instruments, hospital beds and ultrasonic cleaners. These items are subject to "general controls," which include registration and device listing, medical device reporting, and quality system regulation and labeling.
- Class II devices – Devices considered to pose potential risks great enough to warrant a higher level of regulation. Class II devices include most types of sterilization equipment, BIs and chemical indicators (CIs). Class II devices are usually subjected to performance standards, postmarket surveillance studies and specific guidelines or special labeling.
- Class III devices – The most stringently regulated devices, including heart valves, pacemakers and other life-sustaining devices. Manufacturers of new Class III devices must obtain a **premarket approval (PMA)** from the FDA to demonstrate product safety and efficacy.

> **Premarket approval (PMA)** The FDA process of scientific and regulatory review to evaluate the safety and effectiveness of Class III medical devices.

Premarket and Postmarket Requirements

FDA regulations help ensure medical devices are safe for patients and healthcare workers, including SP technicians; the agency requires the manufacturer to provide instructions for use (IFU) with the product. The IFU should contain detailed instructions on how to properly process and use the product. This includes disassembly, cleaning, assembly, disinfection and sterilization instructions. (See **Figure 6.1**)

Medical Device Reporting Requirements

Medical device reporting regulations require user facilities (i.e., hospitals, ambulatory surgical facilities, nursing homes and outpatient treatment facilities) to report suspected medical device-related deaths to the FDA and device manufacturers within 10 days of the event. User facilities must report medical device-related **serious injuries** only to the manufacturer within 10 days of the event. If the manufacturer is unknown, the injury should be reported to the FDA.

Manufacturer's Instructions for Use

Hard Copy

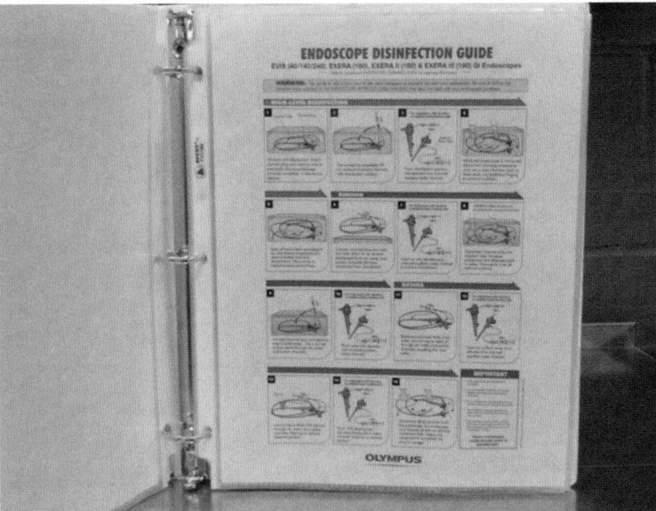

Online Access

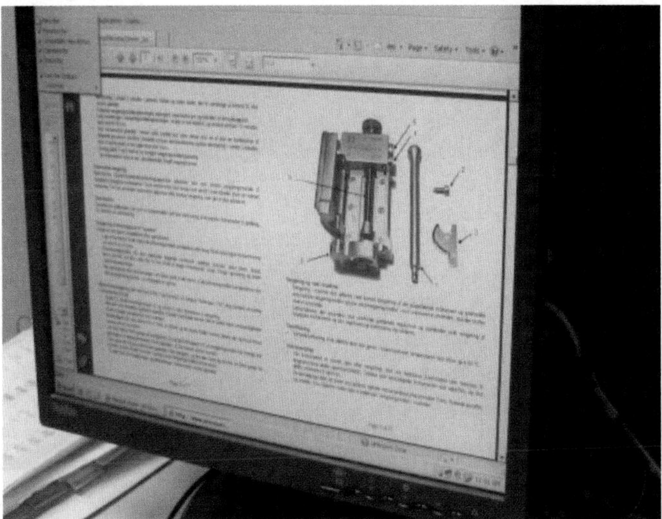

Figure 6.1 IFU

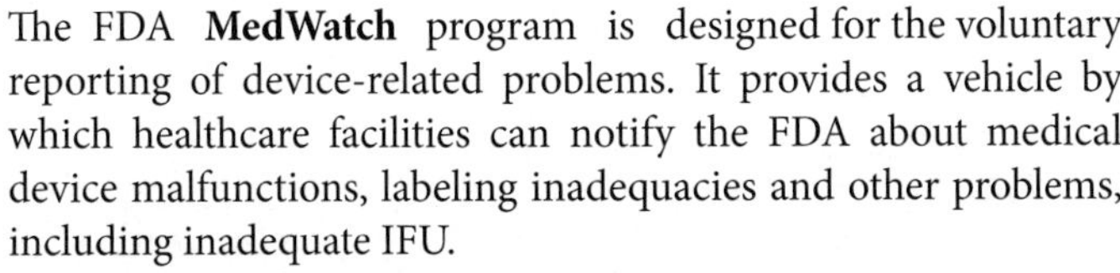

The FDA **MedWatch** program is designed for the voluntary reporting of device-related problems. It provides a vehicle by which healthcare facilities can notify the FDA about medical device malfunctions, labeling inadequacies and other problems, including inadequate IFU.

Serious injury An injury or illness that is life-threatening, resulting in permanent impairment of a bodily function or permanent damage to a body structure, or necessitates medical or surgical intervention to preclude permanent impairment of a body structure.

MedWatch The U.S. Food and Drug Administration's safety information and adverse event reporting system that serves healthcare professionals and the public by reporting serious problems suspected to be associated with the drugs and medical devices they prescribe, dispense or use.

In recent years, the FDA has used both voluntary and mandatory reporting programs to collect information about specific potential problems. Forms to report either voluntary or mandatory device issues may be obtained from the FDA website at www.fda.gov/safety/medwatch.

Medical Device Recalls

A recall is an action taken to address a problem with a medical device. This action can be initiated when a device is defective and/or poses a health risk. Recalls can be instituted voluntarily by the manufacturer, distributor or other interested party, or they can be mandated by the FDA. A recall does not always mean the affected product can no longer be used. Instead, it could mean that the product must be checked or repaired. For example, if an implant, such as a pacemaker, is recalled, it may not have to be removed from the patient; however, the risks of the removal decision should be discussed with the patient. The FDA monitors all mandated recalls to ensure the actions taken by the manufacturer are adequate to protect the public.

There are three categories of FDA recalls:

- Class I: High Risk – Means there is a reasonable chance the product will cause serious health problems or death. The manufacturer must notify customers and direct them to notify the product recipients. The notification must include the name of the device being recalled, the lot or serial numbers, the reason for the recall, and instructions to correct, avoid or minimize the problem. The manufacturer must also issue a press release to notify the public. In addition, the FDA may issue its own press release or public health notice. The FDA posts applicable information on its medical device recalls website at www.fda.gov/safety/recalls.

- Class II: Less Serious Risk – Means there is a possibility that the product will cause a temporary or medically reversible adverse health problem, or there is a remote chance that the device will cause serious health problems. The manufacturer must notify customers and sometimes ask them to inform the product's recipients. Generally, neither the FDA nor the manufacturer issues a press release.

- Class III: Low Risk – Means the use of a product is not likely to cause adverse health consequences. The manufacturer must notify customers, and neither the FDA nor the manufacturer will issue a press release.

Note: Be careful not to confuse FDA medical device classes with the FDA recall classes. FDA recall Class I is the most stringent recall whereas the medical device Class I is the least stringent category.

FDA Labeling Document

The FDA has expressed concern about the potential for the transmission of infectious diseases caused by improperly reprocessed medical devices. The FDA released a document, "Labeling Reusable Medical Devices for Reprocessing in Healthcare Facilities," which requires manufacturers to comply with certain criteria—mostly involving reprocessing instructions—when they submit medical device applications to the FDA for evaluation. The FDA holds both the manufacturer and user responsible for safe and effective reprocessing of medical devices. This is because reprocessing requires the manufacturer to provide IFU that the healthcare facility must follow.

The manufacturer is responsible for:

- Supporting the claim of reuse with adequate labeling and complete reprocessing instructions.
- The validation and documentation of tests, which show that the instructions are adequate and can be reasonably executed by users.

Users are responsible for confirming they have the facilities and equipment to execute the instructions and ensuring the instructions are followed.

FDA Enforcement Requirements for Healthcare Facilities Reprocessing Single-Use Devices

The FDA requires anyone who processes single-use devices (SUDs) to obtain and comply with FDA 510(k) directives to reprocess SUDs.

To obtain approval, the facility must prove it can properly clean and sterilize the product to the original manufacturer's standards each time the product is reprocessed. The facility must also show it is able to test the product to prove the standards have been met in all reprocessing areas, including decontamination, disinfection and sterilization. For more information, visit www.fda.gov.

Emergency Use Authorization

Emergency Use Authorization (EUA) allows the FDA to help strengthen the nation's public health protections against chemical and biological threats, including infectious diseases, and other threats, by facilitating the availability and use of medical countermeasures (MCMs) needed during public health emergencies.

During the COVID-19 pandemic, EUA was implemented to decontaminate some SUDs, like N95 face masks, because they were a critical item used to prevent the spread of COVID-19 and were in short supply.

The EUA is only authorized during a designated time period. Once the FDA has deemed that the emergency or shortage has ended, the EUA is removed. In the earlier example of decontaminating single-use N95 face masks, once the single-use N95 face mask shortage was resolved, the FDA revoked the face mask EUA, meaning healthcare facilities could no longer decontaminate them.

For more information about the FDA, visit www.fda.gov.

Centers for Disease Control and Prevention

The Centers for Disease Control and Prevention (CDC) is a federal agency that works to promote health and quality of life by preventing and controlling disease, injury and disability and by responding to health emergencies.

CDC personnel developed the first practical recommendations for isolation techniques and guidelines for infection control. Although CDC guidelines are not considered regulatory, other agencies rely heavily on them and review healthcare facilities for compliance. Many CDC guidelines are incorporated into the national standards.

In 2008, the CDC released its document *Guideline for Disinfection and Sterilization in Healthcare Facilities*. This document is widely used by other agencies and healthcare facilities, including SPDs.

For more information about the CDC, visit www.cdc.gov.

U.S. Department of Transportation

The U.S. Department of Transportation (DOT) is a federal government agency dedicated to ensuring a fast, safe and efficient transportation system. Laws relating to healthcare include those concerning the transportation of minimally processed instrumentation for repair or reprocessing and the transportation of hazardous and radioactive wastes. The DOT inspects and cites organizations for statute violations.

When soiled instrumentation is transported between healthcare and repair facilities, DOT regulations for labeling and packaging must be followed. These requirements include proper biohazard labeling and containment. SPDs should contact their state's DOT for specific requirements.

Note: State or local regulations may be more restrictive than federal regulations. In all cases, regulations with the most stringent provisions apply.

For more information about the DOT, visit www.transportation.gov.

U.S. Environmental Protection Agency

The U.S Environmental Protection Agency (EPA) is the regulatory agency responsible for minimizing greenhouse gases and toxic emissions, regulating the reuse of solid wastes, controlling indoor air pollution, and developing and enforcing chemical regulations.

Every disinfectant and sanitizer manufacturer must obtain an EPA registration number for every covered product. The manufacturer must submit data relating to labeling claims, efficacy and safety. If the data is approved and accepted, a registration number is issued. All EPA-approved products must contain the following label information:

- Product ingredients
- Directions for use
- Product precautions and warnings
- Directions for storage and disposal
- EPA registration number
- Expiration date (if applicable)

SP technicians must always read and consistently follow the information provided on all chemical labels.

The EPA regulates emission standards for ethylene oxide (EO) sterilization. Several states have developed standards for the allowable amount of EO a facility may emit into the atmosphere. To date, there are no national emission standards for EO sterilization within the healthcare industry.

Since the EPA regulates disinfectants, all disinfectants used in the SPD and other instrument reprocessing areas must be EPA-approved.

For more information about the EPA, visit www.epa.gov.

Occupational Safety and Health Administration

The Occupational Safety and Health Administration's (OSHA) primary role and responsibility is to protect workers from occupationally caused illnesses and injuries. Many of OSHA's regulations and standards are represented in laws passed by U.S. Congress. SP technicians should be aware of OSHA regulations pertaining to their work areas.

The Occupational Exposure to Bloodborne Pathogens Standard

This comprehensive OSHA guideline outlines employee safety in all areas of the facility as they relate to potential exposure from bloodborne pathogens. *Note: Non-compliance with this standard, such as not following the guidelines for transportation of contaminated instruments or not complying with the personal protective equipment (PPE) requirements, carries heavy fines.*

General Duty Clause of the Occupational Safety and Health Act

This act requires that each employer provide each employee with a place of employment that is free from recognized hazards that are causing or are likely to cause death or serious physical harm to employees.

OSHA may intervene in a matter of worker protection, even if there is no specific regulation that covers the situation. OSHA personnel conduct announced and unannounced facility inspections. The need for inspections is based on complaints through OSHA's Whistleblower Protection Program, the rate of workplace accidents, high-hazard targets, referrals, and follow-ups from previous visits. Some OSHA penalties are as follows:

- An employer who "willfully or repeatedly violates the requirements of section five of this Act" or rules promulgated under section six of this Act may be assessed a penalty "of not more than $70,000 for each violation, but not less than $5,000 for each willful violation."
- An employer who received a citation for a serious violation under section five of this Act or rules promulgated under section five shall be assessed a "penalty up to $7,000 for each such violation."
- An employer who received a citation for violating section five or six and is not one of "a serious nature" may be assessed a penalty up to $7,000 for each violation.

A repeat violation refers to a violation of any standard, regulation or rule where, upon reinspection, a substantially similar violation is found. Failure to abate refers to the failure to correct a prior violation, which may result in high financial penalties.

OSHA representatives may enter a facility for a specific reason; however, once inside the facility, they have the right and obligation to investigate any violation they may find in any department. Recent penalties and citations may be viewed by accessing the OSHA website and listing search criteria, such as zip code, facility size or citation type.

For more information about OSHA, visit www.osha.gov.

Centers for Medicare and Medicaid Services

The Centers for Medicare and Medicaid Services (CMS) is responsible for the operation of **Medicare**, **Medicaid** and the State Children's Health Insurance Program. CMS is also one of the agencies that administers the standards of the **Health Insurance Portability and Accountability Act (HIPAA).** HIPAA is the act that established national standards to protect patients' medical records and other personal health information. Violating HIPAA rules may result in loss of employment and associated fines to the healthcare facility.

Medicare A federal medical insurance program that primarily serves those older than 65 years (regardless of income), people under 65 with certain disabilities, and people of all ages with end-stage renal disease.

Medicaid A federal and state assistance program that pays covered medical expenses for low-income individuals. It is run by state and local governments within federal guidelines.

Health Insurance Portability and Accountability Act (HIPAA) The HIPAA Privacy Rule provides federal protections for individually identifiable health information held by covered entities and their business associates and gives patients an array of rights with respect to that information.

CMS is important to SP technicians because the agency performs both announced and unannounced surveys of hospitals, long-term care facilities, ambulatory surgery centers, and laboratories. Failure to follow CMS standards may result in the loss of all federal funding to a facility, including Medicare and Medicaid payments.

In 2008, CMS stopped reimbursing hospitals for patients that acquired any of the specific infections or events while in the hospital. These infections or events may include:

- Foreign object retained after surgery
- Surgical site infection

Non-payment for the amount of time the patient is in the hospital due to a healthcare-associated infection (HAI) means fewer operating funds for the facility.

For more information about CMS, visit www.cms.gov.

State Regulatory Agencies

State agencies may also be involved in the regulation of healthcare facilities and the SPDs within them.

- Department of Health Services (DHS) – Many states look to their DHS to establish local health safety standards that may mirror federal standards or be more stringent. A few states include DHS surveyors in the survey process. DHS surveys are often random and unannounced.

- DOT – Several states have their own regulations for transporting healthcare wastes from the facility to landfills or other final disposal sites.

- EPA – Some states have EPA offices that regulate biohazardous waste and drain discharge. This is important to SP technicians because the EPA offices monitor chemicals poured into the main sewer lines, and there may be regulations against pouring blood and disinfectants into drains in SP decontamination areas.

- OSHA – Approximately 25 states and two territories have state OSHA offices. These offices typically follow the same penalty criteria as those at the federal level.

Standards and regulations of state agencies may be more restrictive than, but cannot be less restrictive than, those of their federal counterparts. SP technicians must be aware of and consistently comply with state and other localized standards and regulations.

PROFESSIONAL ASSOCIATIONS

Professional associations may develop and promote voluntary standards that provide a foundation for processes and practices performed in SP. Some surveying agencies incorporate these standards into their survey requirements.

Association for the Advancement of Medical Instrumentation

The Association for the Advancement of Medical Instrumentation (AAMI) is a nonprofit voluntary consensus organization whose membership is comprised of healthcare technology professionals. AAMI committees and workgroups research and develop new **standards** and **technical information reports (TIRs).**

Standards (AAMI) Voluntary guidelines representing a consensus of AAMI members that are intended for use by healthcare facilities and manufacturers to help ensure that medical instrumentation is safe for patient use.

Technical Information Reports (TIRs) Reports developed by experts in the field that contain valuable information needed by the healthcare industry.

AAMI publishes many standards and TIRs, many of which address functions that affect the SPD, including cleaning, sterilization, packaging, and equipment testing.

ANSI/AAMI ST79:2017 with 2020 Amendments *Comprehensive guide to steam sterilization and sterility assurance in health care facilities* is one of the most widely used documents in SP. Although the title states the document is related to steam sterilization, many sections address processes that affect all types of sterilization, such as cleaning, packaging, indicators, product verification, education, and departmental workflow and design. This document became more important to SPDs when surveyors began referencing ST79 during facility surveys. The document is periodically reviewed, so it is important that the facility has and references the most current version.

Although AAMI is a voluntary organization, AAMI standards are considered a key resource for healthcare guidelines, as many of their documents have been approved by the American National Standards Institute (ANSI). Noncompliance with these standards is cited by regulatory and voluntary organizations that inspect healthcare facilities. SP technicians should be familiar with current AAMI standards that address processing and sterilization practices.

Examples of AAMI Standards and TIRs That Affect Sterile Processing

ANSI/AAMI ST58 *Chemical sterilization and high-level disinfection in health care facilities*

ANSI/AAMI ST79 *Comprehensive guide to steam sterilization and sterility assurance in health care facilities*

AAMI ST90 *Processing of health care products—Quality management systems for processing*

ANSI/AAMI ST91 *Flexible and semi-rigid endoscope processing in health care facilities*

AAMI TIR34 *Water for the reprocessing of medical devices*

AAMI TIR63 *Management of loaned critical and semi-critical medical devices that require sterilization or high-level disinfection*

AAMI TIR67 *Promoting safe practices pertaining to the use of sterilant and disinfectant chemicals in health care facilities*

AAMI TIR68 *Low and Intermediate Level Disinfection in Healthcare Settings for Medical Devices and Patient Care Equipment and Sterile Processing Environmental Surfaces*

For more information about AAMI, visit www.aami.org.

American National Standards Institute

ANSI's primary mission is to "enhance the global competitiveness of U.S. business and American quality of life by promoting and facilitating voluntary consensus standards.

For more information about ANSI, visit www.ansi.org.

Association of periOperative Registered Nurses

The Association of periOperative Registered Nurses (AORN) is a professional organization consisting of perioperative nurses and others who are dedicated to providing optimal care to the surgical patient. AORN's committees are comprised of AORN members and allied association members who develop nationally recognized guidelines. AORN's *Guidelines for Perioperative Practice* currently have several sections devoted to topics directly affecting the SPD, including cleaning, disinfection, packaging, endoscope processing, and sterilization. AORN is not a regulatory agency; however, regulatory officials look for compliance with AORN guidelines, and surveying agencies also refer to them when reviewing SP areas. Therefore, SP technicians should be aware of AORN recommended practices and guidelines.

Pertinent AORN Guidelines

Manual Chemical High-Level Disinfection

Processing Flexible Endoscopes

Care and Cleaning of Surgical Instruments

Sterilization Packaging Systems

Sterilization

Surgical Attire

Environmental Cleaning

For more information about AORN, visit www.aorn.org.

Association for Professionals in Infection Control and Epidemiology

The Association for Professionals in Infection Control and Epidemiology (APIC) is a voluntary organization whose members work to prevent HAIs. APIC members work in conjunction with other agencies, such as the CDC, to adopt standards for infection and disease prevention. SP technicians may interact with their facility's infection preventionist when they conduct departmental surveys to ensure compliance with standards, practices and guidelines. Infection preventionists may also be in the SPD to collect data relating not only to HAIs, but also employee health issues, or to provide inservice education. The Joint Commission (TJC), for example, holds the Infection Prevention and Control department, in conjunction with SP management, responsible for cleaning and sterilization outcomes within the SPD.

For more information about APIC, visit www.apic.org.

International Organization for Standardization

The International Organization for Standardization (ISO, commonly referred to as the International Standards Organization) is a non-governmental, international organization that brings together experts to develop voluntary, consensus-based standards. International standards give state-of-the-art specifications for products, services and good practice, helping to make the industry more efficient.

For more information about ISO, visit www.iso.org.

Accreditation Organizations

Healthcare facilities undergo accreditation surveys to demonstrate the level of quality in that facility. Accreditation demonstrates that the healthcare facility follows the current healthcare regulations and standards. Insurance companies and other third parties take that into account when determining whether to reimburse healthcare insurance claims because accreditation may be a condition of reimbursement.

Accreditation is in the best interest of any healthcare facility. Some of the accrediting agencies that perform on-site surveys include: The American Association for Accreditation of Ambulatory Surgery Facilities (AAAASF), which focuses on the quality of healthcare in outpatient facilities; the Accreditation Association for Ambulatory Health Care (AAAHC), an American organization that accredits its ambulatory healthcare facilities; the TJC, which develops standards and surveys healthcare facilities; the Accreditation Commission for Health Care (ACHC), whose surveyors use an educational approach to help facilities enhance the quality of services provided and improve operational efficiencies; and DNV GL Healthcare, which is part of Det Norske Veritas, a global independent foundation dedicated to safeguarding life, property and the environment. DNV accredits acute care and critical access hospitals and also provides Comprehensive as well as Primary Stroke Center certification.

The Joint Commission

TJC is a private, independent, nonprofit organization that develops standards for healthcare facilities. TJC personnel evaluate healthcare organizations and programs in the U.S. by conducting on-site surveys at least every three years. TJC teams arrive unannounced at a facility and spend two to five days studying virtually every aspect of care within the facility. TJC-accredited healthcare facilities are recognized as those that are dedicated to quality practices. TJC standards are voluntary but nonetheless carry significant weight. Failure to comply with these standards as evaluated through the TJC survey process may result in loss of accreditation by federal and state governments. This, in turn, may result in the forfeiture of millions of dollars in Medicare and Medicaid program payments.

For more information about TJC, visit www.jointcommission.org.

National Fire Protection Association

The National Fire Protection Association (NFPA) is an international organization that works to reduce the burden of fire and other hazards around the world. NFPA develops codes and standards that influence building safety. NFPA is important to SP technicians because of the fire safety standards used for the buildings in which they work. NFPA standards address the fire burden of all disposable packaged items.

For more information about NFPA, visit www.nfpa.org.

United States Pharmacopoeia–National Formulary

The United States Pharmacopoeia-National Formulary (USP-NF) creates and revises standards for the purity of medicines, drug substances and dietary supplements. The USP is important to SP technicians who work with purified water or sterilizing water for irrigation.

For more information about USP-NF, visit www.usp.org/uspnf.

World Health Organization

The World Health Organization (WHO) is an agency that works to further international cooperation in improving health conditions. Its major task is to combat disease, especially key infectious diseases, and to promote the general health of people worldwide.

For more information about WHO, visit www.who.org.

Society of Gastroenterology Nurses and Associates

The Society of Gastroenterology Nurses and Associates (SGNA) is a nonprofit organization dedicated to the safe and effective practice of gastroenterology and endoscopy nursing. SGNA collects information and establishes standards and guidelines related to the processing of flexible endoscopes.

For more information about SGNA, visit www.sgna.org.

American Society of Heating, Refrigerating and Air-Conditioning Engineers

The American Society of Heating, Refrigerating and Air-Conditioning Engineers (ASHRAE) is responsible for ANSI/ ASHREA/ASHE Standard 170, Ventilation of Health Care Facilities. This standard identifies the operating parameters for healthcare heating, ventilation and air conditioning (HVAC) systems.

For more information about ASHRAE, visit www.ashrae.org.

Standards in Other Countries

Other countries have their own standard organizations for healthcare medical device processing. For example, the Canadian Standards Association (CSA) is a nonprofit organization that develops standards for industry, government and healthcare for all Canadian provinces. Standards in other countries may not be the same as those in the U.S.

CONCLUSION

Standards and regulations are designed to keep both patients and employees safe. SP technicians should become familiar with the agencies and organizations that develop the requirements that impact their jobs and they should strive to keep abreast of changes as they happen, while ensuring all SP technicians have ready access to the most current versions. Doing so will help create an environment of safety and competency.

RESOURCES

U.S. Food and Drug Administration. *Code of Federal Regulations, Title 21, Part 813 — Medical Device Reporting, Subparts A, B, C.* U.S. Government Printing Office. 2000.

U.S. Environmental Protection Agency (EPA). *Clarification of HIV (AIDS Virus) Labeling Policy for Antimicrobial Pesticide Products.* Federal Register 54, No. 26:6288-6290.

EPA. *National Emission Standards for Hazardous Air Pollutants for Source Categories,* Code of Federal Regulations, Title 40, Part 63, Subpart 0 (Updated 1996).

Centers for Disease Control and Prevention. *Guidelines for Disinfecting and Sterilizing in Healthcare Facilities.* Guidelines for Handwashing and Hospital Environmental Control. 2008.

Occupational Safety and Health Administration (OSHA). *Occupational Exposure to Formaldehyde.* Federal Register 52, No. 233:46168- 46312. Code of Federal Regulations, Title 29, Part 1910. 1987.

OSHA. *Occupational Exposure to Ethylene Oxide.* Federal Register 49, No. 122: 25734-25809. Code of Federal Regulations, Title 29, Part 1910.1047.1984.

OSHA. *Occupational Exposure to Ethylene Oxide.* Federal Register 53, No. 66: 53:11414-11438. Code of Federal Regulations, Title 29, Part 1910.1047. 1988.

OSHA. *Hazard Communication Standard.* Code of Federal Regulations, Title 29, Part 1910.1200.

OSHA. *Occupational Exposure to Bloodborne Pathogens: Final Rule.* Federal Register 56, No. 235: 56:64004. Code of Federal Regulations, Title 29, Part 1910.1030. 1991.

OSHA. *Occupational Exposure to Bloodborne Pathogens: Final Rule.* 29 CFR Part 1910.1030. 1992.

OSHA. *Occupational Exposure to Bloodborne Pathogens; Needlestick and Other Sharp Injuries: Final Rule.* Amended and effective April 18, 2001; and 29CFR 1910.1035 *Occupational Exposure to Tuberculosis, Proposed Rule.* October 17, 1997.

STERILE PROCESSING TERMS

Regulation

Standard

Best practice

Premarket approval

Serious injury

MedWatch

Medicare

Medicaid

Health Insurance Portability and Accountability Act (HIPAA)

Standards (AAMI)

Technical information report (TIR)

Chapter 7

Decontamination: Point-of-Use Treatment and Transport

Learning Objectives

As a result of successfully completing this chapter, the reader will be able to:

1. Understand the importance of soiled item treatment and transport
2. Identify the sources of contaminated items
3. Explain the importance of point-of-use treatment
4. Review basic procedures to transport soiled items from user areas to the Sterile Processing decontamination area
5. Discuss safety guidelines for transporting soiled items to the Sterile Processing decontamination area
6. Identify basic sources for education and training information applicable to the transport of contaminated items

INTRODUCTION

Reusable instruments and other medical devices processed in the Sterile Processing department (SPD) are transported to patient care and treatment areas where they are used in a wide variety of procedures and applications. After use, they must be transported back to the decontamination area to be processed for reuse. Sometimes, the transport distance is only a few feet, but other items may need to be transported a great distance between facilities. Whether the distance is only a few feet between the user department and the SPD or a long distance between facilities, consistent handling of soiled instruments is a must. This chapter reviews recommended protocols and requirements for these transportation activities.

IMPORTANCE OF POINT-OF-USE TREATMENT AND TRANSPORT

Sterile Processing (SP) should be aware of the goals of point-of-use treatment and transport. These include:

- Removal of **gross soil** – Gross soil left on instruments not only makes them more difficult to clean but can damage instrumentation. (See **Figure 7.1**)
- Prevention of damage – Soiled items must be treated in a manner that will prevent damage during transport to the decontamination area of the SPD.
- Prevention of cross-contamination – Soiled items must be safely transported from point-of-use to the decontamination area without cross-contaminating the environment between those areas.
- Timeliness – The prompt return of soiled or contaminated items to the SPD is essential for cleaning and processing.
- Keeping others safe – Soiled items must be contained and labeled to help ensure that all individuals who may come in contact with contaminated items remain safe during the transportation process.

> **Gross soil** Tissue, body fat, blood and other body substances.

SOURCES OF CONTAMINATED ITEMS

Reusable medical devices, such as instruments and equipment, are used in numerous locations throughout the healthcare facility. The Surgery department generates a high volume of contaminated items, but other ancillary areas such as Labor & Delivery, the Emergency Department, Endoscopy, Cardiac Care Services and other procedure-based areas also generate contaminated items. Although ancillary users of instrumentation may not generate the same volume as surgical departments, it is extremely important that users of reusable instrumentation receive focused education and training prior to instrument pretreatment and transport activities.

In many facilities, the SP decontamination area is located close to the Operating Room (OR). That is the logistical location because surgery is the source of most soiled items transported to the SPD. Enclosed carts filled with contaminated instruments, equipment and utensils can be easily, quickly and safely transported to the decontamination area through a connecting hallway. If the SPD is located on another level of the facility, items can be transported between floors using a dedicated elevator or dumbwaiter system used exclusively to transport contaminated items. In some healthcare systems, the SPD is centralized to one facility, requiring the contaminated instrumentation to be transported by vehicles. (**Figure 7.2** provides an example

Examples of Gross Soil

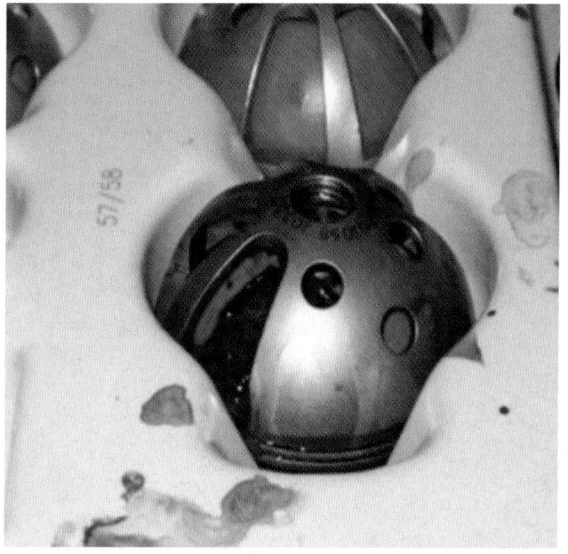

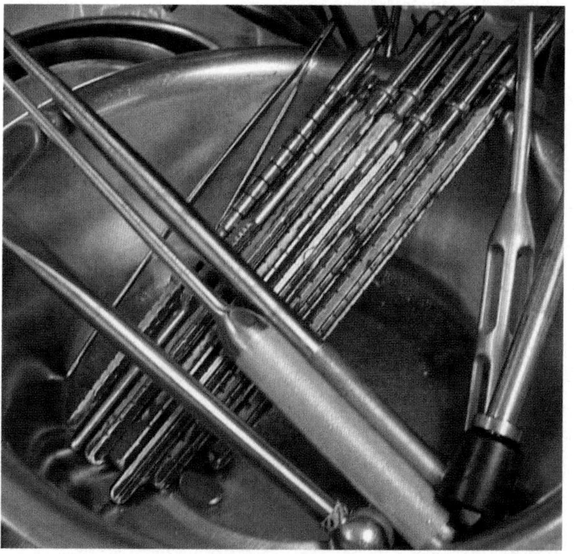

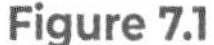
Figure 7.1

of a dedicated elevator used to transport contaminated items.) When using dedicated elevators or dumbwaiters to transport contaminated items, facilities should establish routine cleaning schedules and procedures.

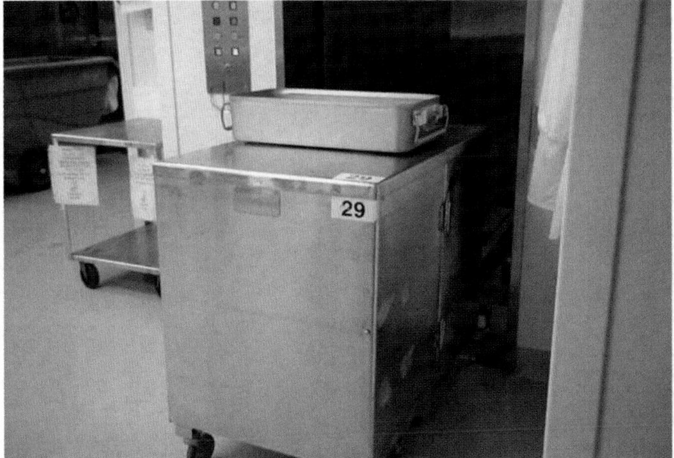

Figure 7.2 Dedicated soiled elevator

Contaminated items may be returned to the SP decontamination area during scheduled soiled pick-up rounds or upon request from a user department. Sometimes, soiled items may be delivered to the decontamination area by employees of the user department. For example, surgical staff return case carts to the decontamination area after surgical procedures. Generally, however, contaminated items are placed in a designated holding area to be picked up by SP technicians at designated times.

Holding Items Until Return to Sterile Processing

All departments that use and store reusable items for later transport to the Sterile Processing department need a designated holding area for contaminated items until they can be retrieved. These areas should be clearly designated with **biohazard signage** (see **Figure 7.3**) and should not be accessible to visitors or other unauthorized personnel. The contaminated holding area should have contaminated trash, linen receptacles, sharps container, a dedicated handwashing sink, and personal protective equipment (PPE) available.

Biohazard signage Notices posted in easily seen locations that alert people in the area about the presence of harmful bacteria, viruses or other dangerous biohazardous agents or organisms.

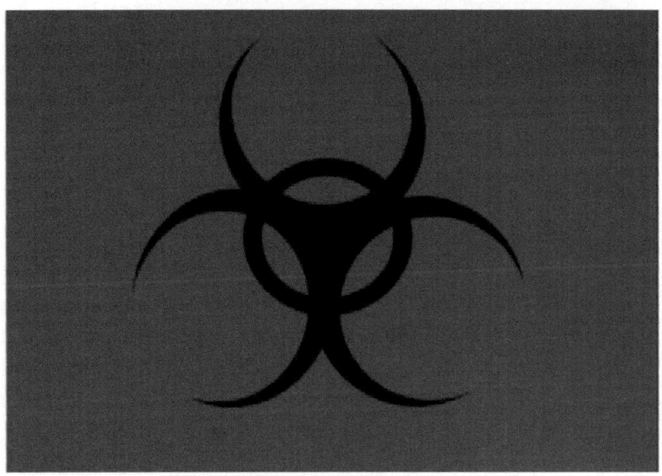

Figure 7.3 Biohazard signage

POINT-OF-USE TREATMENT

Instrument decontamination begins at the point of use. When the procedure is complete, instruments should be prepared in a manner that will help to ensure that they can be transported safely to the SP decontamination area for complete cleaning. SP professionals must enlist the help of user departments to ensure that instruments and equipment are correctly prepared for the decontamination process immediately after use. Some facilities have SP technicians assigned to the OR to assist with instrument setup and breakdown, so it is important to know proper point-of-use instrument handling.

Reasons for Point-of-Use Treatment

There are several important reasons that the point-of-use treatment process should begin in the user department (at the point of use):

- Point-of-use treatment helps prolong instrument life. Common substances to which instruments are exposed during procedures, such as blood and saline, can break down devices' protective finish and accelerate decomposition.
- Dry soil and debris, especially in instruments with lumens and hard-to-reach crevices, are much more difficult to remove than moist soil and debris.
- Soil and excess moisture promote the formation of biofilm colonies. **Biofilm** is highly resistant to cleaning and disinfecting chemicals, so removing the causes of biofilm is essential.

Biofilm A collection of microorganisms that attach to surfaces and each other and form a colony. The colony produces a protective gel that is very difficult to penetrate with detergents and disinfectants.

- When soil dries, instruments require more aggressive cleaning methods, and instruments with dried soil also take longer to clean.

The proper care and handling of instruments and equipment is the responsibility of everyone who comes in contact with them, and that begins with personnel at the point of use.

Personnel responsible for handling instruments at the point of use must keep in mind that those instruments are precision devices that can have a negative impact on patient care if not managed properly. Instruments should be handled with care throughout the procedure and be prepared properly for transport according to facility policy. **Figure 7.4** provides an example of an instrument setup in an OR.

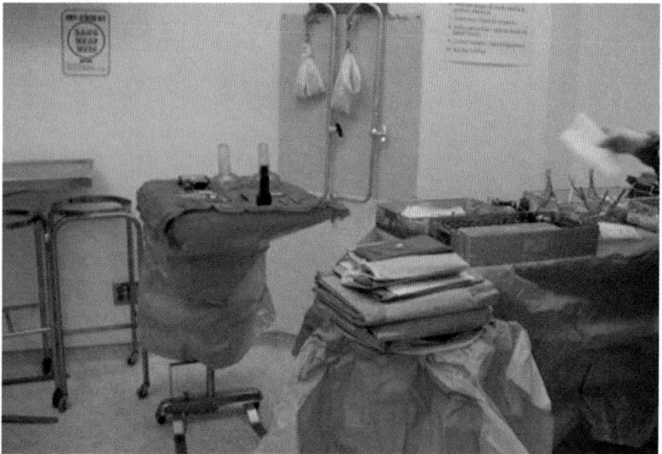

Figure 7.4

Point-of-Use Treatment Guidelines

Point-of-use treatment does not replace the cleaning process; instead, its purpose is to begin the cleaning process through precleaning and preparation activities. The following guidelines should be followed when users prepare items for transport to the SP decontamination area:

- All individuals performing point-of-use treatment should receive education, training and have competencies completed for the task being performed.

- Remove gross soil from instruments. Wear appropriate PPE while preparing instruments for transport.

- Follow the manufacturer's instructions for point-of-use treatment, which can include pre-cleaning and preparation activities.

- Separate reusable **sharps** from other instruments. Place instruments with sharp points or edges, such as cutting edges and skin hooks, in a separate container to reduce the risk of injuries from sharps.

> **Sharps** Cutting instruments, including knives, scalpels, blades, needles, and scissors of all types. Other examples include chisels and osteotomes, some curettes, dissectors and elevators, ronguers and cutting forceps, punches, saws and trocars.

- Protect delicate instruments from damage during transport by segregating them into different containers or placing them on top of heavier instruments.

- Separate reusable linen. Reusable linen should be removed and placed into an appropriate bag or container. Users should take extra caution to ensure that small instruments are not mistakenly included with the linen.

- Remove disposable components, such as blades, disposable tubing and canisters. Sharp items should be placed in a hard-sided container labeled biohazard. Separating disposable from reusable components reduces the amount of contaminated items that must be transported, and it also reduces the risk of injury from sharps such as knife blades and needles. When separating disposable items, watch closely to ensure that reusable items are not removed and discarded with disposable components. (e.g., metal drape clamps are sometimes left attached to disposable drapes).

- Open hinged instruments, disassemble multi-part instruments, and place instruments in the appropriate instrument tray in an orderly manner. Opening and disassembling instrumentation allows pre-treatment solutions to reach all areas of the instrument. Place heavy instruments on the bottom of the tray, with lighter instruments on top. Handle cords, endoscopes and cameras with care. Do not place any items on top of them. The SPD should be notified if some instruments are not being returned with the set for any reason. **Figure 7.5** provides an example of instruments that have not been properly prepared for transport.

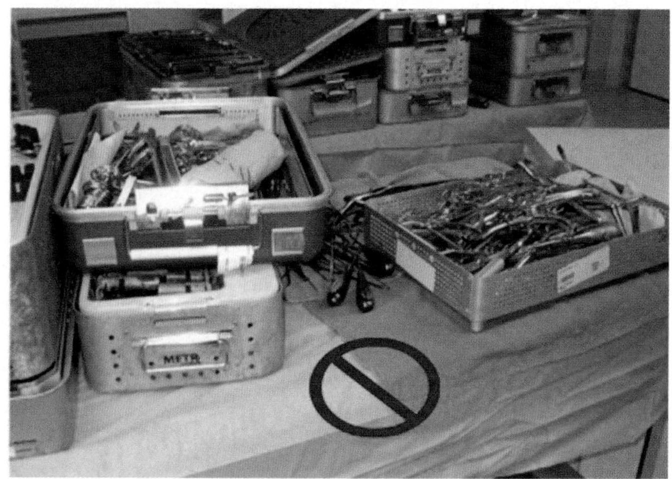

Figure 7.5

- Keep items together. Instrument sets or multi-part items should be kept together for their transport to the SP decontamination area. If items are separated or left behind, reassembly will be delayed. Failure to keep items together also increases the risk that components will be misplaced or lost. Keep instruments moist to prevent soil from drying on their surface. (See **Figure 7.6**) This can be accomplished by using commercial foams, gels or spray products, or placing a water-moistened towel over them. *Note: If instruments are placed in a soak basin or solution, they should not be exposed to the solution for an extended period of time because this may damage the instruments' surface. Review manufacturers' instructions for use (IFU) for recommended soaking times. The soak solution must be discarded before transport to reduce the risk of spills. Care should be taken not to contaminate the outside of the tray or container.*

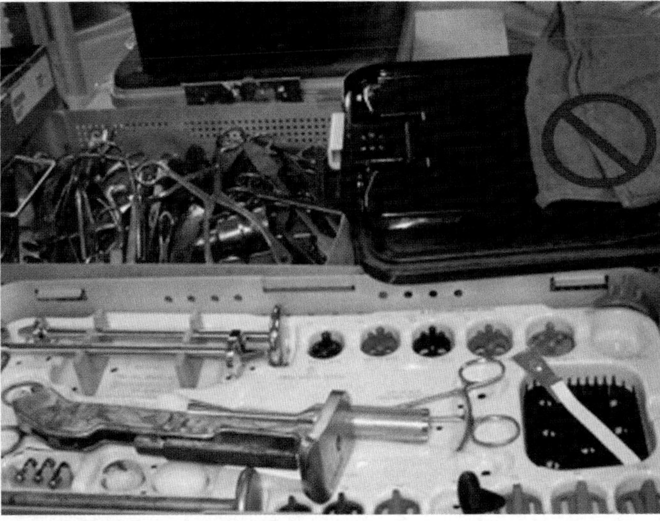

Figure 7.6 Dried blood on instruments makes them more difficult to clean.

> ### Working Smarter, Not Harder
>
> When there are big cases that require multiple instrument sets, keeping instruments together in the same set can be a challenge. Why is this important? Consider that in a busy decontamination department that processes 50 or 60 surgical procedures a day, there can be hundreds of trays processed. If instrumentation from one case is scattered between four different trays in the OR, it can be several hours before each tray is cleaned and makes its way to the assembly side of the SPD. On the assembly side, the time spent looking for and sorting out instrumentation can slow down productivity and be a frustrating process. Finding a process to keep instrumentation together prior to receipt in decontamination can help improve productivity and employee satisfaction.

- Empty fluids from containers. If a contaminated device has a reusable fluid container, bottle or receptacle, the fluid should be removed and disposed of according to the facility's protocols. Disposable fluid containers should also be handled according to required facility procedures.

- Third-party reprocessing items should be removed and properly contained or separated and sent to the SPD per facility protocols.

- If reusable instruments were used during a case with suspected or known Creutzfeldt-Jakob Disease (CJD), notify SP and Infection Prevention and Control. Follow hospital procedures for initial cleaning and containment for transport to the SP decontamination area.

- Notify the SPD about items needing repair. If instruments or equipment require repair, they should be identified or tagged, so they can be removed from service and sent for repair or refurbishing. (See **Figure 7.7**)

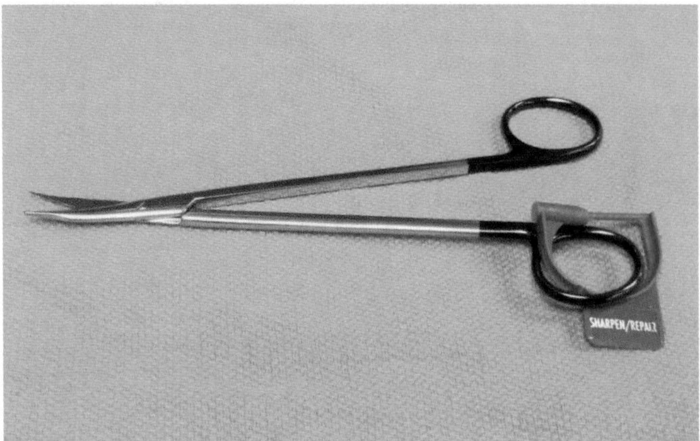

Figure 7.7 Tagged instrument

- Notify the SPD about items requiring **turnover/turnaround** for another case; do not automatically assume the department has this information.

> **Turnover/turnaround** Term used to describe instruments or equipment that must receive priority processing in order to be made available for another procedure.

SP professionals must work together with end users to ensure that point-of-use treatment is carried out according to manufacturers' IFU. In many cases, departments will need to develop joint procedures for the handling of used items to ensure that everyone involved understands their role in the process.

TRANSPORT OF SOILED ITEMS

Contaminated items should be contained before transport through the facility to minimize airborne or contact spread of microorganisms and reduce the risk of cross contamination and infection. The best way to transport soiled instruments is in enclosed carts. (See **Figure 7.8**) If an open transport cart is used, the cart must have a solid bottom shelf to prevent drips and spills, and the cart must be covered during transport. Smaller numbers of instruments from other departments can be transported in dedicated transport containers or in plastic bags that are clearly labeled biohazard. Large items, such as suction units and other types of patient care equipment, can be transported in special carts designed for soiled item transport. (See **Figure 7.9**)

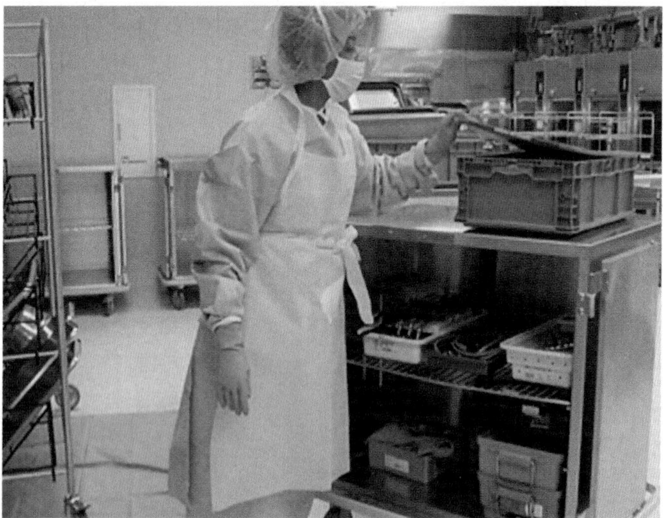

Figure 7.8

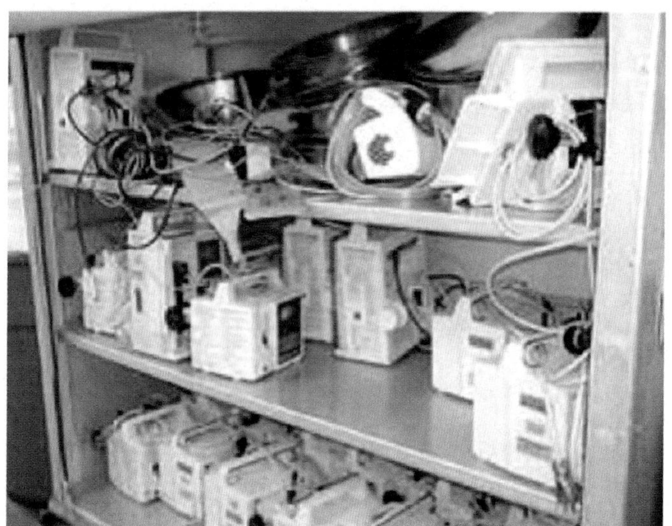

Figure 7.9 Large item transport cart

The goal of all soiled transport is to transfer the contaminated items to the SP decontamination area while minimizing the risk of cross-contamination. All transport devices must be free from external gross contamination, such as blood, before transport to reduce the risk of environmental contamination and personnel exposure. Contaminated items should be handled as little as possible to reduce the risk of exposure to employees and patients.

Place instrument sets securely in the cart. Sets should be placed so they do not slide or fall during transport. Metal trays and containers should not be placed on top of more fragile plastic trays and containers. (See **Figure 7.10**) Do not mix unopened sterile and soiled instruments in the same cart because this will contaminate sterile items.

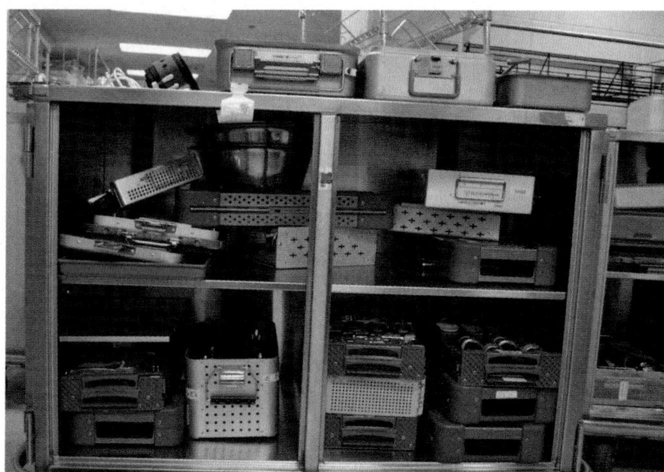

Figure 7.10 Incorrectly loaded case cart

Personnel transporting contaminated items should be educated, which includes training and competencies, and must consistently follow safe handling procedures. These include methods to safely load transport devices to avoid spillage and to ensure items are securely contained. (See **Figure 7.11**)

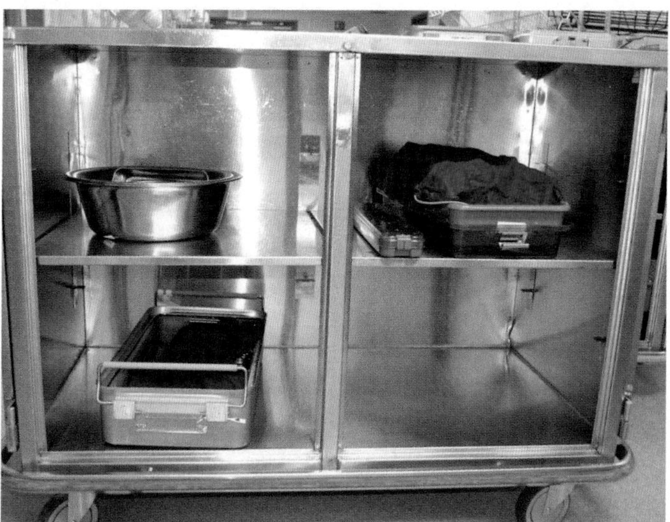

Figure 7.11 Cart correctly loaded for transport

When transporting instruments, contaminated items should remain physically separated from their clean and sterile counterparts. Containers and carts used for transporting contaminated items should not be used to transport and deliver clean items, unless they are thoroughly decontaminated between use. Surgical case carts used to transport soiled instruments from surgery to the decontamination area must be decontaminated before they can be used to transport sterile packages back to surgery.

Ideally, soiled devices will be transported to the SP decontamination area immediately after use. This reduces the opportunity for soil to dry on the instruments. The longer instruments remain unclean the greater the risk for biofilm formation. Returning instruments quickly allows the items to be returned to service in a timely manner.

Contaminated items from other departments are often placed in a holding area for pickup on a scheduled basis by SP technicians who then return them to the decontamination area for processing. These soiled pick-up rounds should be conducted as scheduled because failure to perform soiled item pickups can lead to equipment and instrument shortages. All healthcare facilities have limited numbers of instrument sets and patient care equipment. The instrument and equipment replenishment system relies on items moving through the system in a timely manner.

SAFETY GUIDELINES FOR SOILED ITEM TRANSPORT

All instruments, utensils and equipment used in patient care and treatment processes should be considered contaminated. SP technicians who transport contaminated items should wear appropriate PPE. After loading the cart, PPE should be removed, and hands should be washed.

Transporting equipment and carts through corridors can pose significant safety concerns. SP technicians must always maintain control of transport carts and should not move them at excessive speeds. Patients, visitors, healthcare providers and movable equipment share the same hallways as transport carts, and excessive speed or inattention could lead to accidents. SP technicians should maintain control of their carts and pay particular attention to hallway intersections and doors that may open into the path of the cart. Many facilities install safety mirrors at hallway junctions to help prevent accidents. (See **Figure 7.12**) Carts containing soiled items should never be left unattended.

In addition to maintaining safe control of their transport carts, SP technicians should always yield to patients and visitors in hallways and at elevators. In any healthcare facility, the routine transport of soiled items never takes precedence over the transport of patients.

Prior to transporting, SP technicians should be aware of ergonomic principals. Completing tasks that require lifting, bending, twisting, pushing and pulling incorrectly can cause injury. Applying ergonomic principles can help technicians avoid workplace injuries such as **musculoskeletal disorders** that cause back pain, tendonitis, carpal tunnel syndrome, and even bone fractures.

Musculoskeletal disorders Injuries or disorders of the muscles, nerves, tendons, joints, cartilage, and spinal discs.

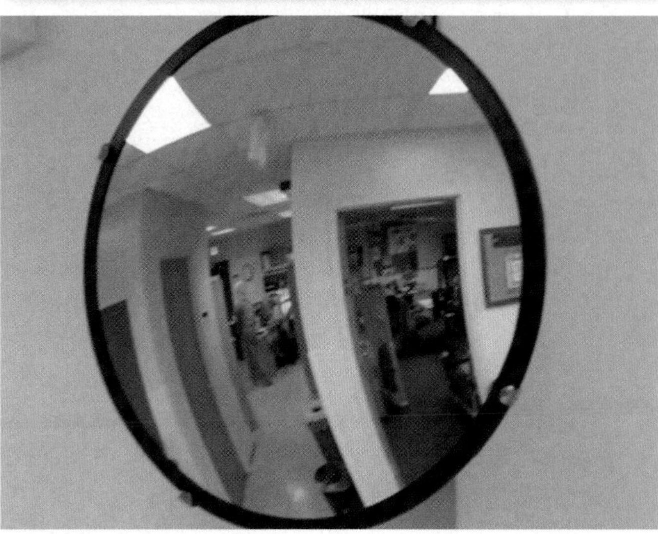

Figure 7.12 Safety mirror

OFF-SITE PROCESSING

Sometimes, contaminated items may need to be transported between buildings or to a central off-site processing center. When it is necessary to transport contaminated items using a truck or van, facility personnel must consult U.S. Department of Transportation (DOT) guidelines and follow applicable state and local requirements for the safe transport of biohazard materials.

When preparing items for off-site transport, care should be taken to protect the instruments from damage during transport. Instruments should be placed in their containers in a manner that will shield the instruments from movement that could lead to damage. Instrument trays should be placed securely in a transport cart, which can then be secured inside the transport vehicle to prevent accidental spills or contamination. Clear separation of clean and dirty should be established. Instruments should be transported as soon as possible after the procedure to reduce the risk of the soil drying, which makes instruments more difficult to clean. Policies and procedures should be defined to address the following:

- Route and road conditions – The quickest and safest route should be established.
- Temperature and humidity – Extreme temperatures and humidity can contaminate sterile supplies or degrade packaging.
- Separation of clean and dirty – Well-defined boundaries must be established to separate clean and dirty items to prevent cross-contamination.

- Establish cleaning procedures – Routine cleaning of the vehicle should be performed after transporting soiled items.
- Education, training and competencies – All individuals involved in transporting activities must be educated and have competencies kept on file.

EDUCATION AND TRAINING

When performed improperly, the transport of contaminated items can pose a threat to the safety of patients, visitors and employees. Carefully thought-out procedures must be developed to help ensure that all contaminated items are appropriately handled. The development of these procedures should be done with the input and support of the facility's Infection Prevention and Hazardous Materials committees.

Recommended practices for contaminated item transport are provided by the Association for the Advancement of Medical Instrumentation (AAMI). Procedures should also reflect Occupational Safety and Health Administration (OSHA) regulations. Additional information regarding soiled instrument treatment and transport can be obtained from the Association for periOperative Registered Nurses (AORN).

Anyone who may have contact with contaminated items must be educated about the dangers associated with biohazardous items. In addition to education and training for SP technicians, Environmental Services employees, courier and transport technicians and drivers should be included in education pertaining to transport and handling of contaminated items. This education should include proper handling of biohazardous items and the correct application and use of PPE.

CONCLUSION

Instrument point-of-use treatment and proper transport to the SPD requires interdepartmental teamwork. Good communication and training can help personnel in all departments protect their facility's instruments and better serve patients. By understanding and following the recommended guidelines for the point-of-use treatment and transport of contaminated items, SP technicians help protect patients, visitors and healthcare workers.

RESOURCES

ANSI/AAMI ST79:2017 & 2020 Amendments A1, A2, A3, A4 (Consolidated Text) *Comprehensive guide to steam sterilization and sterility assurance in health care facilities.*

Association of periOperative Registered Nurses. *Guidelines for PeriOperative Practice: Instrument Cleaning.* Guidelines for PeriOperative Practice. 2022.

Occupational Safety and Health Administration. *CFR 1910.1030. Bloodborne Pathogens Standard.*

Phillips N. *Berry & Kohn's Operating Room Technique, 11th Ed.* 2007.

Centers for Disease Control and Prevention. *Work-Related Musculoskeletal Disorders & Ergonomics.* 2020.

STERILE PROCESSING TERMS

Gross soil

Biohazard signage

Biofilm

Sharps

Turnover/turnaround

Musculoskeletal disorders

Chapter 8

Cleaning

Learning Objectives

As a result of successfully completing this chapter, the reader will be able to:

1. Define cleaning and identify challenges associated with cleaning medical devices
2. Discuss the purpose and set up of the decontamination area
3. Identify the importance of personal protective equipment and Standard Precautions
4. Explain the role of common cleaning tools
5. Discuss mechanical cleaning processes
6. Discuss the use of chemicals in the decontamination area
7. List steps in the cleaning process

INTRODUCTION

Cleaning is the cornerstone of instrument processing. Items that have not been cleaned properly cannot be sterilized or made safe for patient use. The cleaning processes performed in the Sterile Processing department (SPD) are very different than the cleaning processes carried out in other situations. When cleaning is performed outside the healthcare facility (for example, in home settings), the definition of clean can vary with the individual. When cleaning is performed in the healthcare facility, it must be performed consistently and to the highest level. Improper cleaning can cause infections and even death. This chapter will examine the cleaning process—from the tools required to perform cleaning to the basic steps necessary to carry out a successful process.

WHAT IS CLEAN?

Cleaning is defined as the removal of all visible and non-visible soil and other foreign material from medical devices being reprocessed. When faced with the complex configurations of today's medical devices, the cleaning process becomes quite challenging. Some soils are easy to see and remove; others are not. The goal of the cleaning process in the decontamination area is to remove all soils and residues, not just ones that are easy to see and remove.

Proper cleaning requires the correct tools and technique and attention to detail. A medical device may appear clean at first glance but may harbor soils that are not readily visible. The following photographs (**Figures 8.1** through **8.4**) provide some examples of the challenges associated with cleaning medical devices. **Figure 8.1** provides a look at the inside of a bulb syringe that was mistakenly assumed to have been cleaned. It is extremely difficult, if not impossible, to properly clean any area that cannot be seen. Lumens and other areas that do not provide good access for cleaning pose a significant challenge to Sterile Processing (SP) technicians. **Figure 8.2** provides a look inside an arthroscopic shaver using a borescope. The configuration of this instrument makes it difficult or even impossible to see all areas for cleaning. Borescopes should be used to view the internal surfaces of these types of instruments.

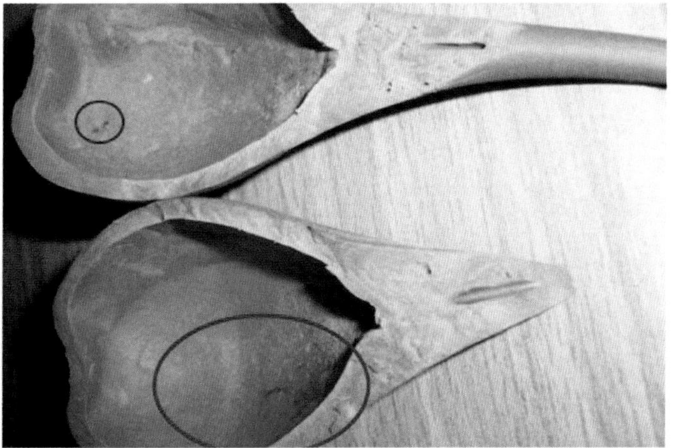

Figure 8.1 Soil inside a bulb syringe illustrates the difficulty of cleaning what cannot be seen.

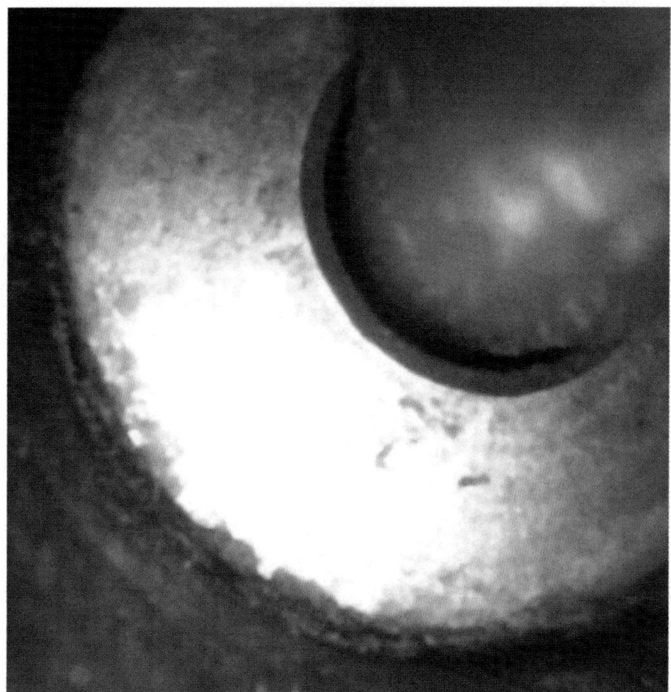

Figure 8.2 View of an improperly cleaned shaver using a borescope

Even when item surfaces are clearly visible, inadequate cleaning can occur. **Figure 8.3** provides a look at a common clamp that has undergone fluorescence-based protein detection testing to detect residual protein soil. Although the clamp appears visibly clean, several areas of concern are identified. The yellow and orange areas indicate residual soil. **Figure 8.4** provides a look at common biopsy forceps that have undergone fluorescence-based protein detection testing to identify residual protein soil.

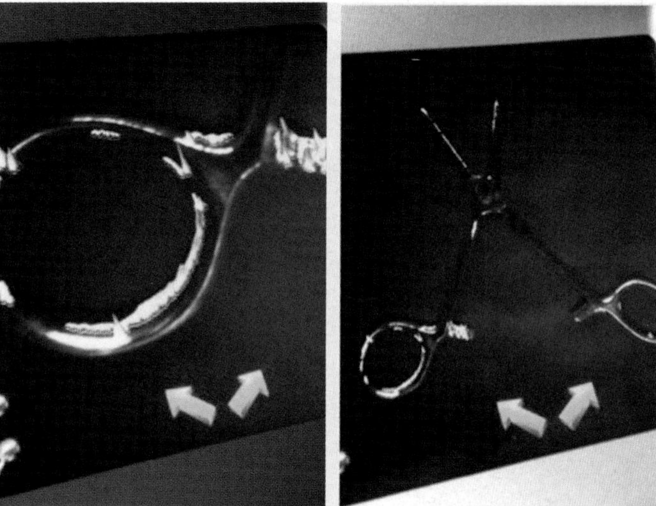

Figure 8.3 Residual protein soils detected by fluorescence-based protein detection testing

These examples illustrate that even simple instruments can pose a significant cleaning challenge. Every item that undergoes the decontamination process has the potential to harm a patient or present a danger to healthcare workers. That is why SP technicians assigned to the **decontamination area** must have the

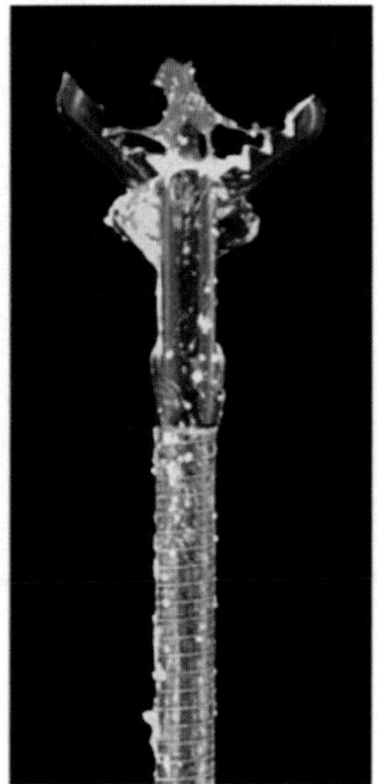

Biopsy forceps prior to reprocessing. Bioburden can clearly be seen in this laboratory photo.

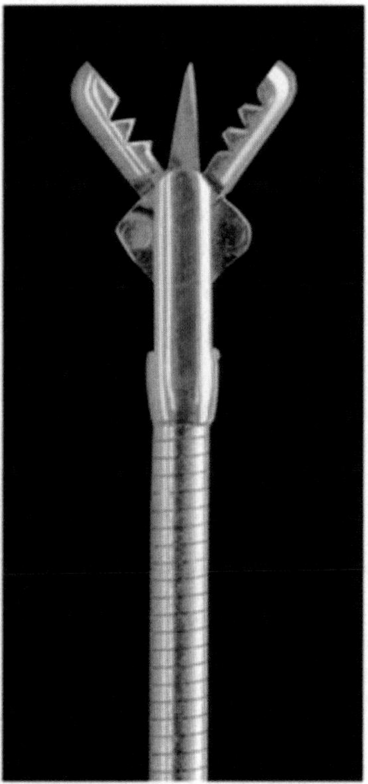

After reprocessing, this same instrument appears to be clean to the naked eye.

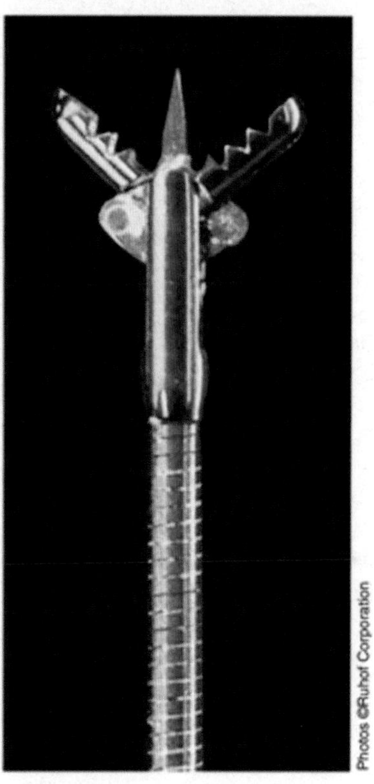

In some cases, residual bioburden remains after reprocessing, as seen in this laboratory photo.

Figure 8.4

proper cleaning tools, understand the correct cleaning technique for every item and always pay close attention to detail as they perform their duties.

Decontamination area The location within a healthcare facility designated for the collection, retention and cleaning of soiled and contaminated items.

INTRODUCTION TO THE DECONTAMINATION AREA

This section provides an overview of the decontamination area and the equipment and processes needed to accomplish thorough cleaning.

Design and Location of the Decontamination Area

The process of cleaning and decontamination begins long before even one soiled instrument arrives in the decontamination area. A great deal of planning and preparation goes into the design and set up of the work area and the acquisition of cleaning equipment, tools and supplies. SP technicians assigned to the decontamination area should be aware of the processes and safeguards used to facilitate the cleaning of soiled items, reduce the spread of microorganisms and ensure the safety of patients and employees.

Decontamination areas are unique because of their purpose and design. Soiled instruments should only be cleaned in a designated decontamination area. The decontamination area serves as a receiving area for soiled instruments and, in many cases, other medical devices and equipment from surgery and other areas of the healthcare facility. Several design-related factors must be considered as the decontamination area is planned. It is more cost effective to centralize the decontamination function to one area of the healthcare facility. If the decontamination area is not centralized, inconsistent practices and additional expenses will be incurred for duplicate equipment and space.

The location of the decontamination area should factor in the need to transport contaminated devices from the point of use. Proper transportation of contaminated devices is necessary to reduce the risk of cross-contamination and exposure to bloodborne pathogens. (See **Figure 8.5**) In many cases, the decontamination area is located near the Operating Room (OR) because most soiled instruments are generated there.

Enclosed carts

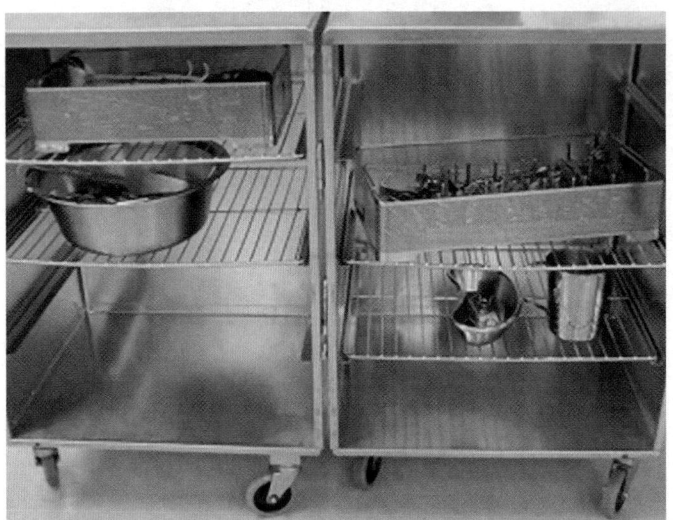

Covered bins

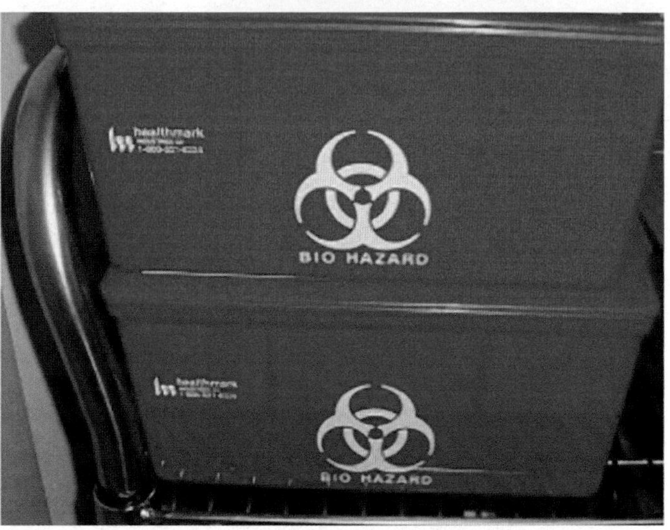

Figure 8.5 Examples of containment devices for soiled instruments

Decontamination Engineering Controls

Spills and splashes are a common occurrence in the decontamination area and create the need for frequent surface cleaning and disinfection. Specific engineering controls are designed to make the work area safe and efficient. Floors and walls in the decontamination area should be constructed with materials that can tolerate cleaning chemicals. Walls should not be constructed of particulate or fiber-shedding materials. Maintaining the decontamination environment is important to the cleaning process.

The healthcare organization monitors room temperature and **humidity** based on the version of ANSI/ASHRAE/ASHE 170 that was current at the time the heating, ventilation and air conditioning (HVAC) system was initially installed or last upgraded. The healthcare facility should have a process for monitoring HVAC performance parameters and a mechanism for identifying and resolving variances. The ventilation system should allow for no less than 10 air exchanges per hour, and the decontamination area should be under **negative pressure** in relation to other areas adjacent to the decontamination area. Negative air pressure inside the room is lower than the air pressure outside the room, causing the air to flow into the room with lower (negative) air pressure.

Lighting is essential to a safe work environment and is a key element in the cleaning process. Instrument cleaning requires attention to detail, and lighting must be adequate for technicians to perform inspections associated with the cleaning process. Detailed inspection of instrumentation may require a higher level of illumination than activities performed in other areas of the department. Lighting should be installed to avoid shadows and allow the maximum light over the inspection area.

Humidity Amount of water vapor in the atmosphere; expressed as a percentage of the total amount of vapor the atmosphere could hold without condensation.

Negative pressure Air pressure inside the room that is lower than the air pressure outside the room, causing the air to flow into the room with the lower (negative) air pressure.

An emergency eyewash/shower station (see **Figure 8.6**) should be accessible within 10 seconds or 30 meters of areas of potential chemical exposure. Eyewash stations cannot have their access blocked and cannot be placed in a decontamination sink.

Eyewash/shower stations should be activated weekly for a period long enough to verify they are performing to standards. This routine testing should be documented.

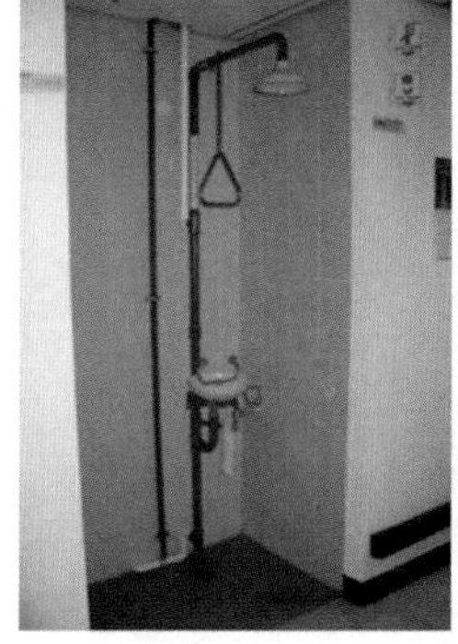

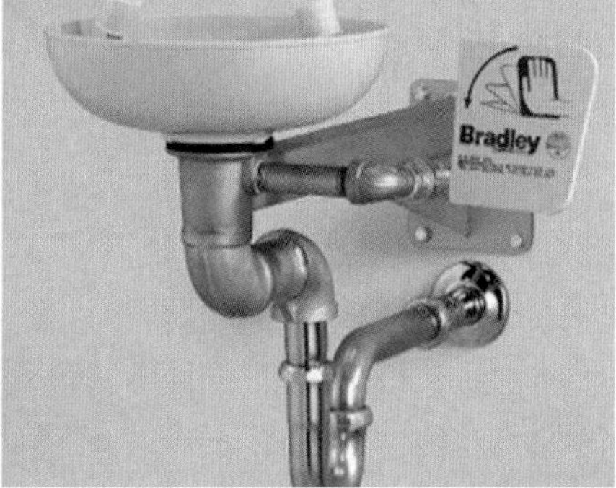

Figure 8.6

The decontamination area is the central point for handling contaminated devices, and a high microbial count will be

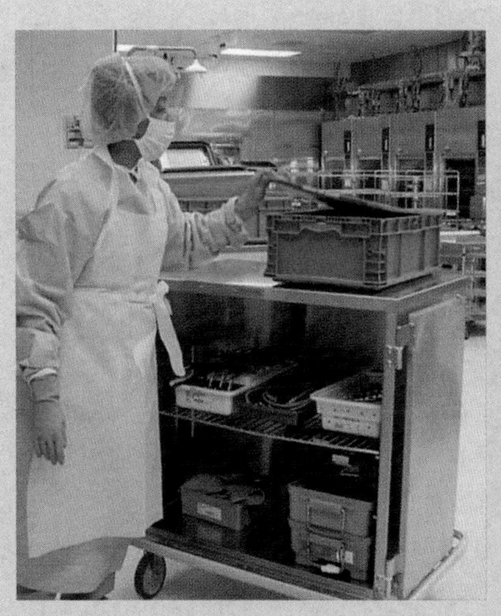

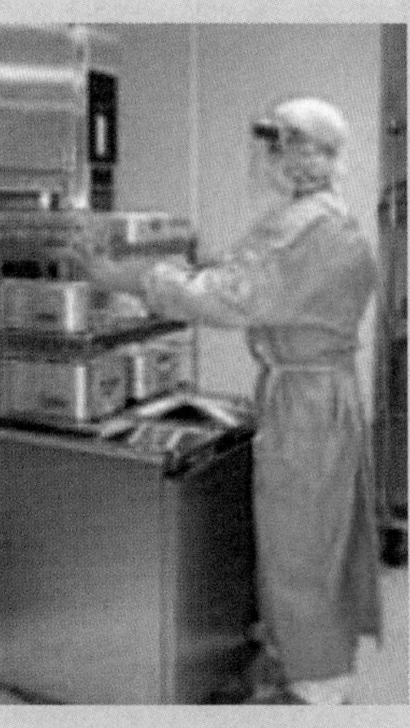

Personal protective equipment (PPE)

- Hair covering
- Eye protection, such as goggles or eyeglasses with solid side shields, or a chin-length face shield
- Fluid-resistant face mask
- A gown with reinforced cuffs and a front that acts as a barrier to fluids
- Strong general-purpose utility gloves that cover the cuffs of the reinforced gown and can resist cuts and tears
- Skid-resistant decontamination shoe covers
- Employer-provided cloth scrub attire that is changed at the end of each shift or when wet or soiled

Figure 8.7

present in the environment. The first line of defense for reducing contaminates is maintaining as clean a work area as possible. Special attention should be given to the cleaning procedures in the work area. For example:

- Horizontal work surfaces should be cleaned and disinfected at least at the beginning or end of each shift and as needed.
- Spills should be spot cleaned immediately.
- Floors should be cleaned and disinfected at least daily.
- All trash and soiled linens should be removed per facility policy.
- Sinks should be cleaned and disinfected per facility policy.
- **Biohazardous waste** should be removed per facility policy.
- Adequate storage for equipment used to clean the decontamination area should be available and tools, such as mops, used in this area should not be used in other areas of the department.

Biohazardous waste Waste containing infectious agents that present a risk or potential risk to human health.

Employee safety is always an important concern. Since SP technicians do not know the origin of the contamination, they must assume that every item received in the decontamination area can pose a potential risk. For these reasons, following personal protective equipment (PPE) requirements is essential. (See **Figure 8.7**)

The space for donning and doffing PPE should be in a designated area, preferably outside of the decontamination work area, adjacent to the decontamination room.

Handwashing and frequent use of appropriate hand germicidal agents are required. Whenever SP technicians remove PPE, they should properly wash their hands. A sink dedicated to hand hygiene should be provided within the decontamination area and it should be separated from sinks used to sort and prepare instruments for processing.

Before any new staff member is assigned to the decontamination area, they must receive a thorough and comprehensive orientation.

Effective, ongoing education and training is critical to the safe processing of medical devices. Following all safety protocol is the ongoing responsibility of both the employer and all SP technicians.

Traffic Control and Environmental Management

Technicians assigned to the decontamination area should be constantly vigilant of their surroundings. Traffic should be restricted to personnel working in the area, and access to the area should be controlled. (See **Figure 8.8**) Traffic control is imperative due to the potential for exposure to bloodborne pathogens and hazardous chemicals.

Work Area Setup

Preparation of the work area is an essential first step in promoting safety and efficiency in the decontamination area.

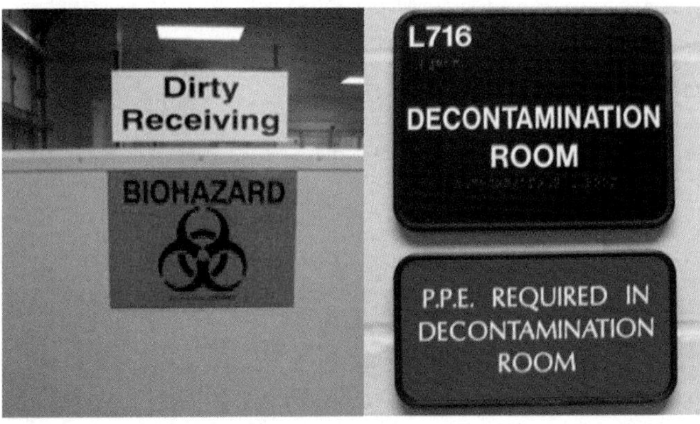

Figure 8.8 Decontamination areas must have restricted access.

Sinks

Ideally, each workstation will have three sink bays for washing, intermediate rinsing and final rinsing. If three bays are not available, the cleaning process must be modified. (See **Figure 8.9**) The workflow should always move from dirty to clean.

A three-sink arrangement used for manual cleaning should consist of:

- A wash sink with water and detergent or enzymatic solution. Fill water should have a temperature range of 80°F to 110°F (27°C to 44°C). Temperature monitors should be used to verify that the cleaning solution maintains the correct temperature. Water hardness, pH, temperature, and the type of soil present on instrumentation impact the effectiveness of enzyme cleaners and detergents. *Note: The detergent manufacturer's instructions for use (IFU) must always be followed.*

- All cleaning chemicals must be mixed per the manufacturer's instructions. Marking the sink to indicate gallon levels can help ensure that solutions are mixed to the proper dilution ratios. (See **Figure 8.10**) Cleaning solutions should be changed frequently for maximum cleaning.

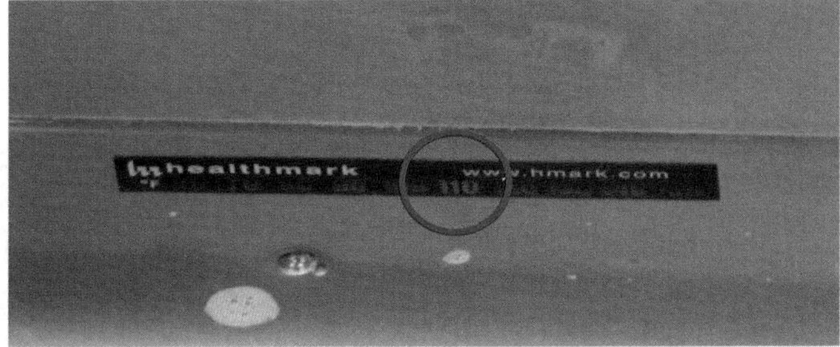

Figure 8.10

- A second sink (intermediate rinse) that contains **utility** or **critical** water. After cleaning, devices should be thoroughly rinsed to further assist in removing debris and detergent residue. This rinse water should be changed frequently, so the cleaning chemicals do not build up and reattach to the instruments being rinsed.

- A third sink (final rinse) that contains critical water. This helps prevent instrument spotting, rinse off cleaning chemical residues and prevent the redepositing of minerals and microbes.

Utility water Water as it comes from the tap that may need further treatment to achieve the required specifications. This water is mainly used for flushing, washing and rinsing.

Critical water Water that is extensively treated to ensure that microorganisms and organic and inorganic material are removed.

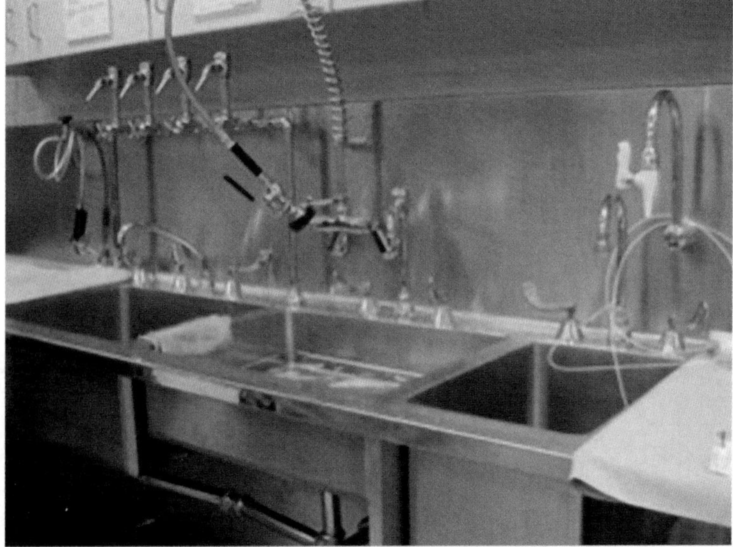

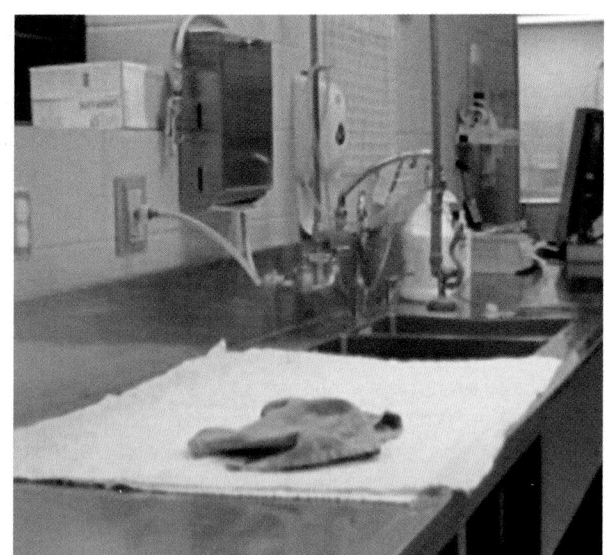

Figure 8.9 Examples of decontamination workstations

Effective cleaning of soiled devices is critical to decontamination. Cleaning and rinsing should result in decreased pathogens and no visible bioburden, which is essential to the effectiveness of disinfection and terminal sterilization.

Cleaning Tools

Water

Although water is frequently taken for granted and not often considered a tool, water quality makes a significant difference in instrument and equipment cleaning outcomes. Poor water quality can impact the performance of chemicals used for cleaning and disinfection and it can also affect the rinse phase by leaving deposits on items that have been cleaned.

There are many impurities in water, even in tap water treated at a municipal water treatment plant. Water from any source typically contains minerals, dissolved solids, particles, gases and organic and inorganic chemicals. Some water sources also contain bacteria, algae and parasites. These contaminants may impede the cleaning and **biocidal** processes and, in some cases, contaminants may shorten the life of instruments by harming their finish.

> **Biocide** A substance or microorganism that kills or controls the growth of living organisms.

Critical water is extensively treated, typically by a multi-step treatment process that may include a carbon bed, softening, and **reverse osmosis (RO)** and that process can be followed by either **deionization (DI)** or **distillation** to ensure that the microorganisms and inorganic and organic material are removed from the water. There are chemical performance qualification levels of water quality for medical device processing that should be monitored by the Facilities Engineering department.

> **Reverse osmosis (RO)** A water purification process by which impurities are removed from water using a semipermeable membrane.
>
> **Deionized (DI) water** Water that has had all ions removed through an ion exchange process.
>
> **Distilled water** Water that is heated to steam, then allowed to cool and condense.

Critical water should be used as a final rinse in any cleaning process to reduce or eliminate unwanted chemicals and pathogens. Water test sampling should be performed at each site where critical water is used as a final rinse.

Knowing the condition of the water used to process instruments allows facilities to make appropriate choices in the selection of cleaning and disinfection chemicals. Many chemicals used in the decontamination process require specific pH ranges. **Figure 8.11** provides a comparison of pH levels to common household items.

pH	
14	Liquid drain cleaner, Caustic soda
13	bleaches, oven cleaner
12	Soapy water
11	Household Ammonia (11.9)
10	Milk of magnesium (10.5)
9	Toothpaste (9.9)
8	Baking soda (8.4), Seawater, Eggs
7	"Pure" water (7)
6	Urine (6) Milk (6.6)
5	Acid rain (5.6) Black coffee (5)
4	Tomato juice (4.1)
3	Grapefruit & Orange juice, Soft drink
2	Lemon juice (2.3) Vinegar (2.9)
1	Hydrochloric acid secreted from the stomach lining (1)
0	Battery Acid

Figure 8.11 pH level comparison

Manual Cleaning Tools

Decontamination requires a combination of manual and mechanical cleaning processes; therefore, the area will have equipment for both types of cleaning. This section provides information about manual cleaning tools.

Brushes

Brushes are available in many diameters and lengths. Some must be rigid, and others must be flexible to properly clean the many different lumens, channels and crevices in instruments. (See **Figure 8.12**) Brushes used for cleaning usually have nylon bristles. Brushes are also available with sponge tips and other configurations.

Ideally, disposable brushes should be used. If reusable brushes are used, they should be decontaminated per the IFU to ensure they are not a source of contamination. Abrasive brushes should never be used because they can scratch the surface of the instrument and accelerate corrosion. Metal or wire brushes should only be used if indicated in the instrument's IFU.

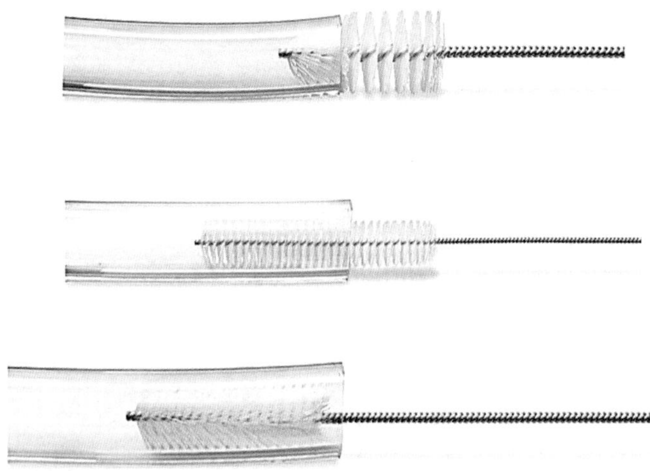

Figure 8.12 Brush size is important when cleaning lumens.

Correct brush size is also critical. In fact, it is essential that during the review of new instrumentation for purchase or evaluation, the IFU should be reviewed for the correct size and type of brush to use. Consider lumen cleaning, for example: if the brush is too large, it will not fit into the lumen. If the brush is too small, it will not have complete contact with the lumen walls and will not clean them thoroughly. The brush must also be long enough to pass through the lumen. (See **Figure 8.13**) Brushes that are worn should be discarded. (See **Figure 8.14**)

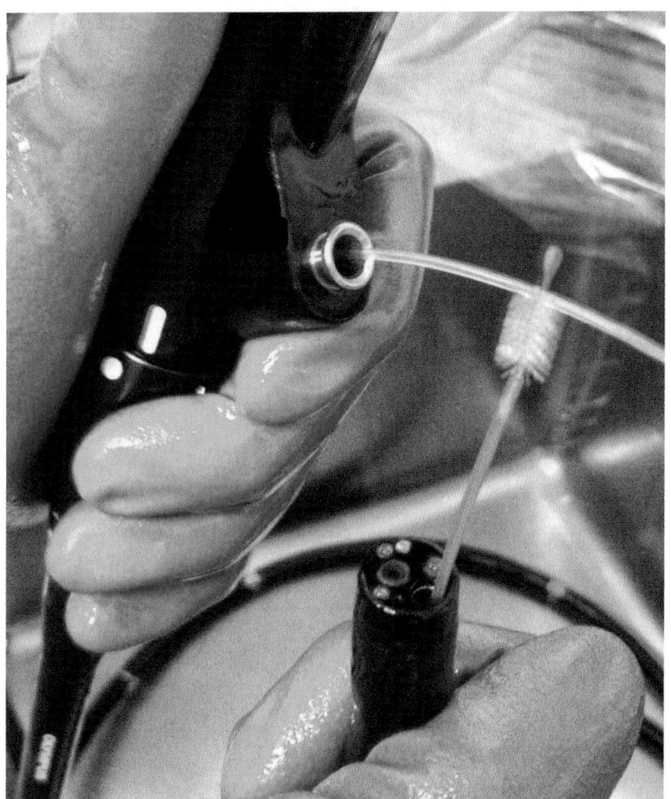

Figure 8.13 Correct brush length is critical.

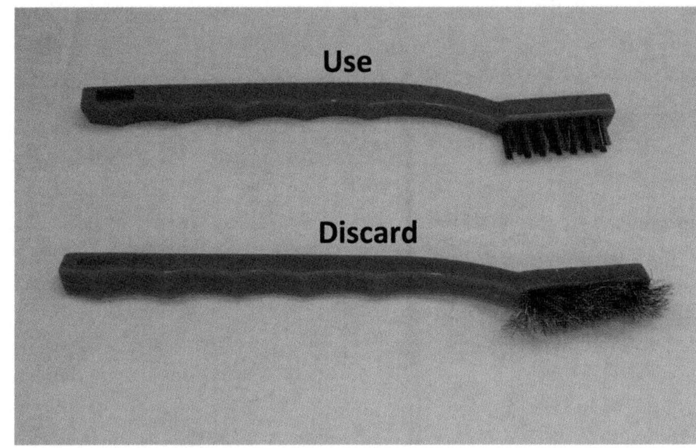

Figure 8.14 Discard brushes when worn.

Cleaning Cloths

Use of a non-linting cloth is recommended because it reduces the risk of lint fibers being left on instruments. Cloths should be changed regularly or when visibly soiled or stained.

Sponges

Sponges can be used to clean some medical devices. Some sponges are impregnated with detergents and should be used according to the manufacturer's IFU. The sponge's structure makes it virtually impossible to completely clean, so sponges must be discarded and replaced at least daily or after each use (according to the manufacturer's IFU). (See **Figure 8.15**)

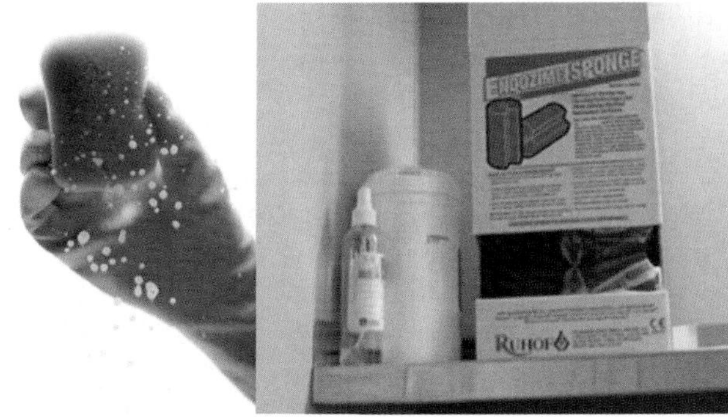

Figure 8.15 Sponges cannot be cleaned and should be replaced at least daily.

Water Irrigation and Instrument Air Devices

Water irrigation devices (see **Figure 8.16**) and instrument air devices should be checked to ensure they are in working order and have all of the necessary attachments. Adapter tips should be available to attach to different-sized lumened devices. The adapter tips should be cleaned and disinfected on a regular basis and when visibly soiled. Care should be used to direct air and water spray away from employees.

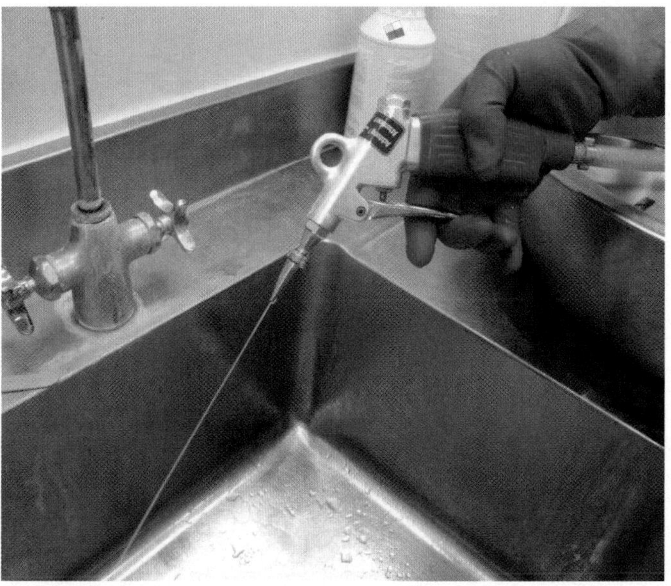

Figure 8.16

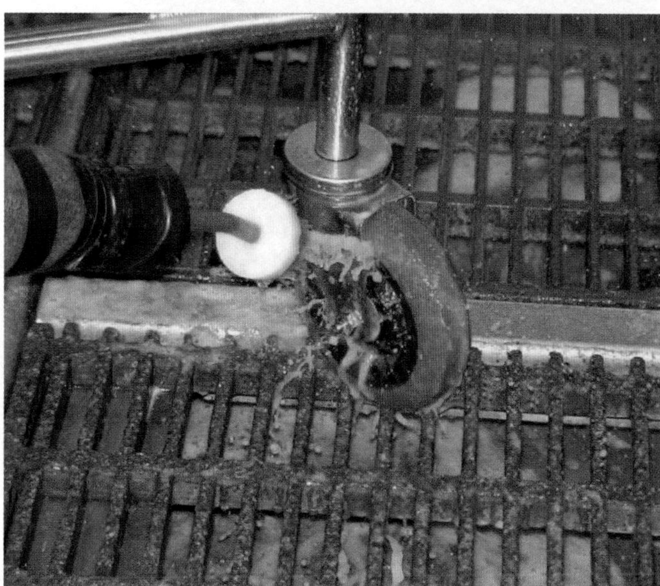

Figure 8.17

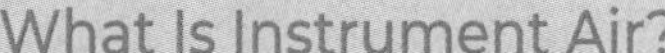

What Is Instrument Air?

Instrument air is compressed air that has had dust, dirt and other pollutants removed. In healthcare, instrument air is used to power some medical devices such as pneumatic drills and saws. Instrument air is also used to dry medical devices after cleaning and decontamination. To qualify as instrument air, air must be free of oil, water, hydrocarbons and other contaminates that could cause infection.

Automatic Dosing Units and Irrigators

Dosing units are used to deliver a specific and consistent amount of detergent to water to produce the cleaning solution. Dosing units deliver the precise dose of cleaning chemistries required for manual cleaning. Some types of dosing units also have irrigation capabilities to mechanically irrigate lumened devices. These units (and their tubing) should be cleaned and disinfected per the IFU. The unit should be routinely verified for correct dosing, and undergo calibration.

Floor Drains and Spray Nozzles

Many decontamination areas are equipped with a spray nozzle and floor drain/grate that provides drainage when manually cleaning bulkier items that do not fit into the cleaning sinks. The spray nozzle system is also used for cleaning the wheels of mobile equipment that cannot be sent through an automatic process. (See **Figure 8.17**)

Additional Tools

Specific instruments may require certain tools to perform cleaning and decontamination. For example, flexible endoscopes may require leak testing devices. Specific cleaning tools should be purchased at the same time as the instrument(s) and replaced as necessary. All SP technicians assigned to the decontamination area should be trained on the proper use of special cleaning tools.

MECHANICAL CLEANERS

Several mechanical options are available to assist with decontamination. Mechanical cleaning facilitates the decontamination process by removing soil and microorganisms using an automated cleaning process. When functioning correctly, these machines operate consistently and reduce time and labor. The cycles on mechanical cleaners should not be shortened as a cleaning failure can result. *Note: The use of mechanical cleaners does not completely replace the need for manual cleaning.*

Some units reduce microbial contamination through a multi-step approach using a combination of cleaning solutions, hot water, rinsing, lubrication and drying; others provide only a cleaning function. Mechanical devices commonly found in the decontamination area include ultrasonic cleaners, irrigating sonics, washer-disinfectors, cart washers, and pasteurizers. SP technicians should not use any type of mechanical equipment without receiving proper training and a competency review.

This section provides an overview of common equipment found in the decontamination area.

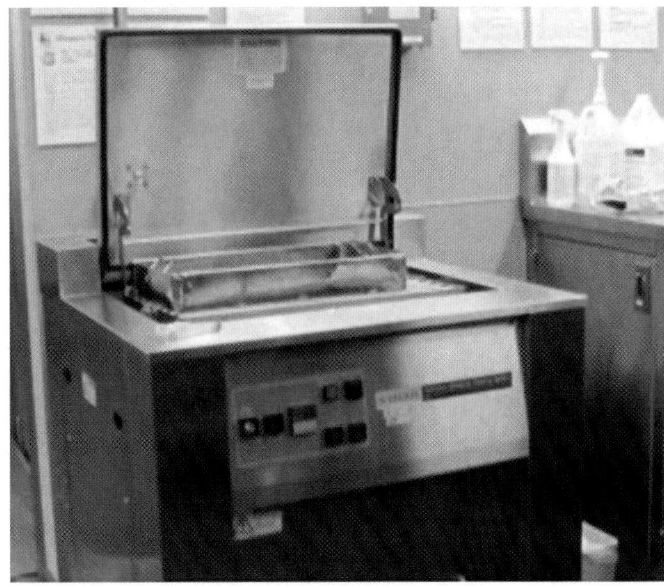

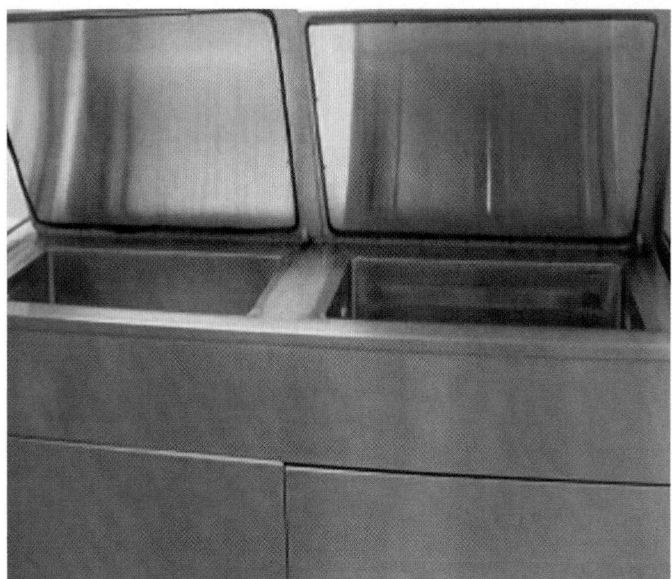

Figure 8.18 Examples of ultrasonic cleaners

Ultrasonic Cleaners

Most ultrasonic (sonic) cleaners are used for fine cleaning, not for disinfection or sterilization. They are used to remove soil from joints, crevices, lumens and other areas that are difficult to clean by other methods.

The term "ultrasonic" is an appropriate name for this type of mechanical cleaner. "Ultra" means beyond and "sonic" means sound. When an ultrasonic wave passes through a liquid, it makes the liquid vibrate. The vibrations are transmitted through the detergent bath and create **cavitation**. The molecules of the solution are set in rapid motion and small gas bubbles develop. As the bubbles grow larger, they become unstable until they collapse (implode). This implosion creates a vacuum in the solution that draws minute bits of foreign matter (including microorganisms) from cracks and crevices, such as hinges and serrations on instruments. This vacuum action results in cleaning of hard-to-reach areas.

> **Cavitation** The process used by an ultrasonic cleaner in which low-pressure bubbles collapse (implode) and dislodge soil from instruments.

After cavitation, rinsing is necessary to remove any residue, including detergents that remain on the instruments. It is important to routinely clean the tank according to the manufacturer's instructions.

An ultrasonic unit may have one, two or three chambers. When using a single-chamber unit, it is necessary to know whether the rinsing function is automatic. If the unit does not have a rinse cycle, it is important to manually rinse instruments after removing them from the sonic cleaner. Listed below are the different types of ultrasonic cleaners that may be in an SPD. (See **Figure 8.18**)

- Basic ultrasonic cleaners – The basic ultrasonic cleaner is the simplest design, consisting of one or more chambers. Some models have automated processes consisting of several phases: filling with water, adding a cleaning agent, degassing, rinsing and draining. Simpler models are completely manual, with the user performing all the functions of filling, rinsing and draining.

- Ultrasonic irrigators – This type of ultrasonic cleaner is designed to clean devices with lumens, flushing the inside of instruments as well as exterior surfaces. The cavitation process is used along with the addition of flushing and irrigation to remove bioburden from lumens, channels, box locks, and other crevices. These types of ultrasonic cleaners contain water ports with hoses and special adapters to connect to various devices such as laparoscopic, robotic and other instrumentation.

- Ultrasonic irrigator cleaner – Some ultrasonics have enhanced cleaning capabilities, allowing them to clean external surfaces and interior lumen channels using rapid-flow, high-pressure irrigation. This equipment provides programmable cleaning cycles.

- Ultrasonic irrigator cleaner disinfectors – Cleans internal lumens and channels through high-pressure irrigation and detergent solution washing and has an optional lubrication and thermal disinfection cycle.

Solution temperatures for cleaning instruments should be between 80°F and 109°F (27°C and 43°C), unless otherwise specified by the equipment or detergent manufacturer. Temperatures above 140°F (60°C) will coagulate protein, making it more difficult to remove. Water should be changed when it is visually soiled and at regularly scheduled intervals to prevent soiled particles from redepositing on instruments. The unit's tank should be cleaned, and the drain should be checked for debris per the IFU.

How to De-Gas an Ultrasonic Cleaner

Water must be degassed each time it is changed in the sonic cleaner. Excess bubbles in the water are formed during filling, and these gas bubbles reduce the energy released during implosion. To de-gas a unit, fill the sonic cleaner, close the lid and run it for five to 10 minutes. Degassing should only be done after the tank is filled (not while it is being filled) to avoid damaging the equipment. Some ultrasonic cleaners will automatically de-gas the solution when the chamber is filled. The lid of the sonic cleaner should be closed at all times when the unit is operating to prevent aerosols from being dispersed.

When using ultrasonic cleaners, there are some important factors to remember, including the following:

- Instruments must be precleaned prior to placing them in a sonic cleaner.
- When using ultrasonic cleaners, it is important to use the correct amount of low-foaming detergent.
- Instruments should be placed in trays designed for use in ultrasonic cleaners and for each specific model. Some ultrasonic models may require specific types of trays.
- All lumens must be completely filled with the cleaning solution, so the cavitation process can be effective inside the lumen.
- All instruments must be completely submerged in the solution, so they are exposed to the cavitation process.
- Hinged instruments placed in the sonic cleaner should be opened.
- Trays must not be overloaded. Check the ultrasonic IFU for load limitations.
- Lumened instruments should be connected to flushing ports by tubing and adapters.
- Heavy items should be placed on the bottom of the tray to prevent damage.

Ultrasonic energy can loosen the tiny screws of delicate instruments and degrade the sealants in other devices. Items that should not be placed in a sonic cleaner include:

- Chrome-plated and ebonized instruments and those made of plastic, cork, glass, wood, chrome and/or rubber
- Silicone mats
- Needles, unless approved for the process by the needle manufacturer's IFU
- Instruments that contain fiber optic components

Stainless steel instruments should not be mixed with aluminum, brass or copper instruments in a sonic cycle. Placing instruments made of dissimilar metals in the ultrasonic cleaner can cause the transfer of ions from one instrument to another (known as **electroplating**) and can result in etching and pitting of the instrument. Damage to the finish of the instrument can create surface imperfections that may harbor microorganisms and debris. Users should also be aware that some sonic detergents may change or dull the color of anodized aluminum.

As with all processing equipment, the sonic cleaning equipment manufacturer's operating and maintenance recommendations should always be carefully followed.

Electroplating A process that uses electrical current in a solution to produce a metallic coating.

Detergents for Ultrasonic Cleaners

Only detergents that have been specially formulated for ultrasonic cleaners should be used. Detergents must be low foaming to prevent interference with the cleaning process.

Washer-Disinfectors

Washer-disinfectors (washers) have been used for many years in SPDs and they are effective for cleaning instrumentation, instrument containers and utensils. Most are designed to perform multiple cleaning functions automatically. *Note: Automated mechanical washers are not appropriate for washing electrical, battery-powered or pneumatic devices unless otherwise stated in the device's IFU.*

Washers work on the principle of **impingement** and are an effective means for cleaning and disinfecting instruments because of their spray force.

Impingement The spray-force action of pressurized water against instruments being processed to physically remove bioburden.

In some ways, impingement washers work like a dishwasher; they rely on a combination of water temperature, special detergent and a spray-force action to remove soil from devices being processed. (See **Figure 8.19**) To clean effectively, items must be prepared properly and positioned in a manner that facilitates the mechanical cleaning process.

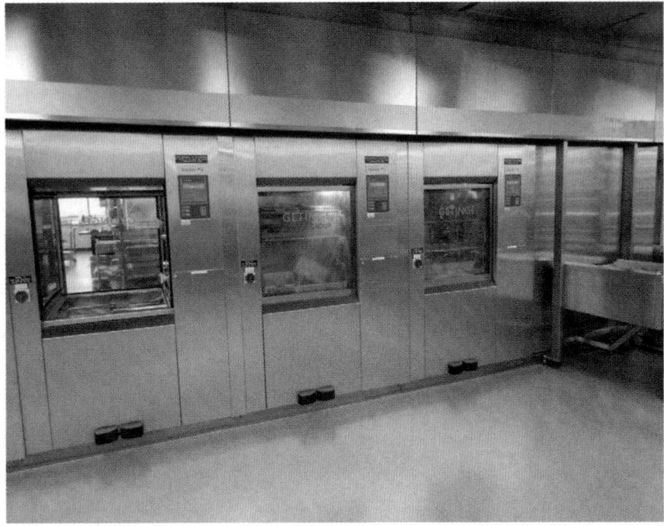

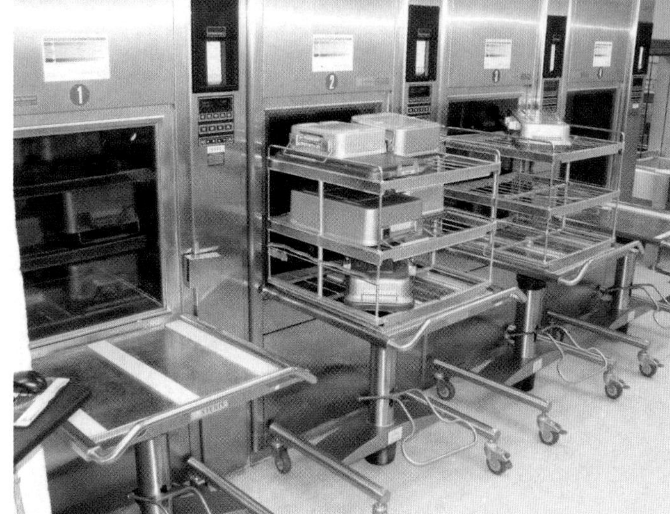

Figure 8.19 Examples of mechanical washer-disinfectors

Mechanical washer-disinfectors may be a single-chamber model or an indexed model. In single-chamber models, all cleaning functions are performed in one chamber, whereas the index model moves the instrument trays into separate chambers for each function. Many washer models have multiple types of cycles, including gentle, orthopedic instrument and glass, as well as the regular instrument cycle.

Washers are only effective when used and serviced according to the manufacturer's recommendations. Operator manuals and detailed instructions about the basic operation and loading of instrument racks should be provided, and SP technicians must understand and comply with these instructions. Cycles should never be shortened. Important factors to remember when using a washer-disinfector:

- All disposable items, such as chemical indicators and filters, must be removed because they can clog the washer, preventing full cleaning action.
- Silicone and rubber mats should be removed from sets to permit full impingement action.
- Washer racks should never be overloaded, and spray arms should move freely during operation. Instruments that are sticking up and/or out of their perforated baskets must be relocated away from the spray arms.
- Instruments should be disassembled, and their small parts should be placed inside an approved containment device for processing in the washer. (See **Figure 8.20**)
- Hinged instruments should be opened to permit direct contact with the water and detergent. (See **Figure 8.21**)

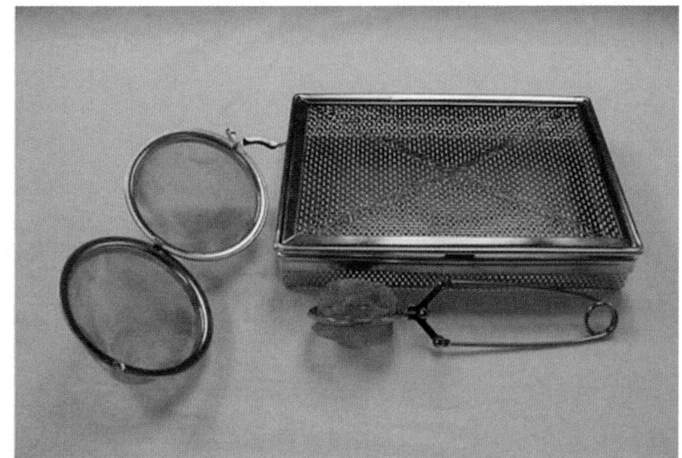

Figure 8.20 Examples of small part holders

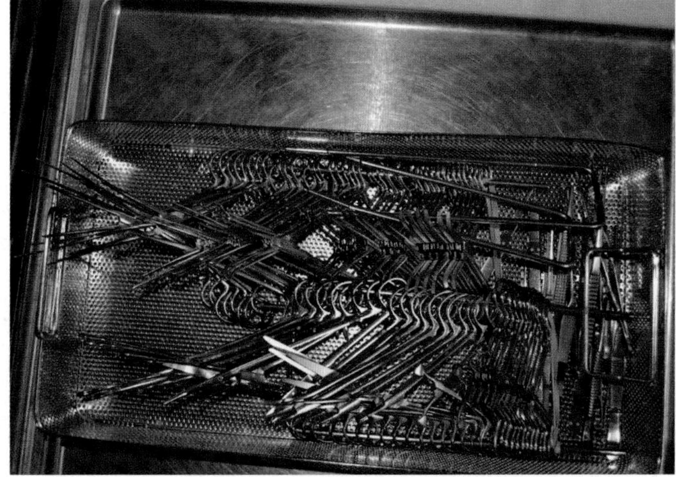

Figure 8.21

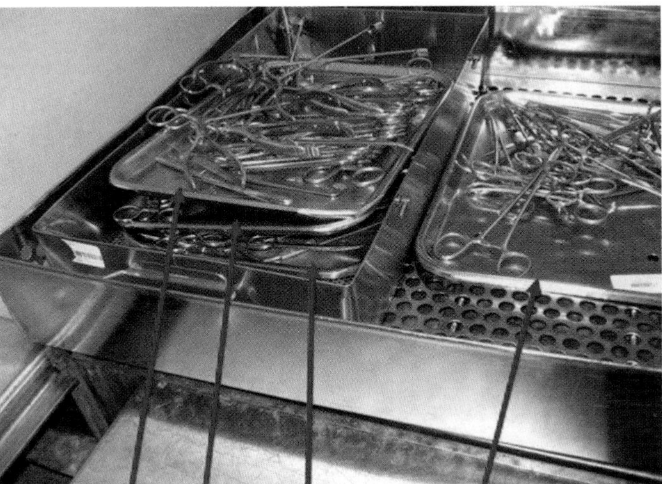

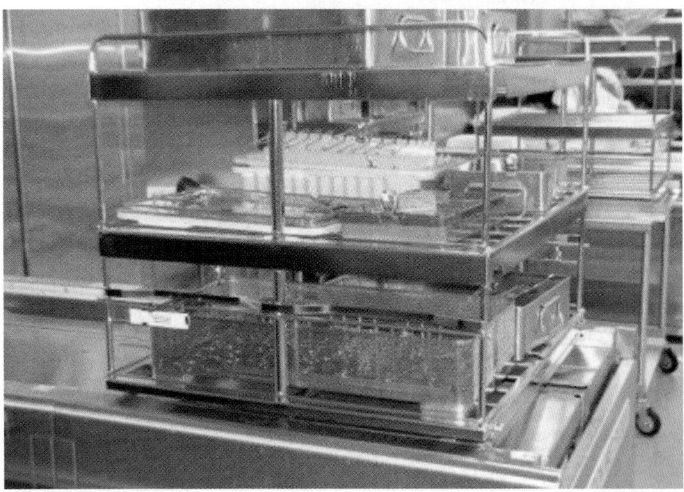

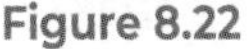

Figure 8.22

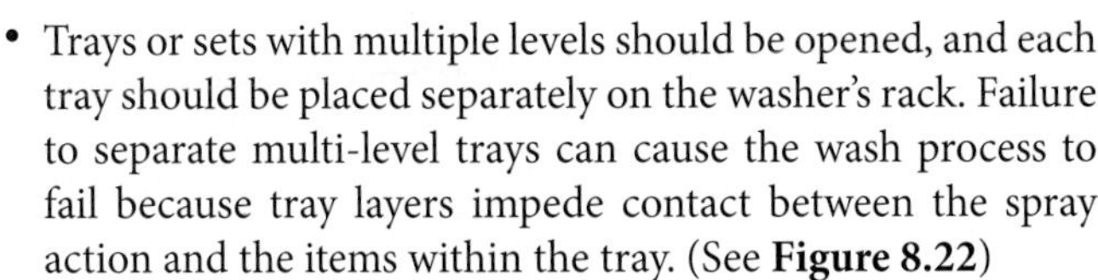

- Trays or sets with multiple levels should be opened, and each tray should be placed separately on the washer's rack. Failure to separate multi-level trays can cause the wash process to fail because tray layers impede contact between the spray action and the items within the tray. (See **Figure 8.22**)
- Trays with lids/covers should be opened, so contents may be exposed to the washer spray.
- Delicate instruments may be dislodged from the racks due to the blunt force of the spray action. These instruments should be confined in approved small, perforated baskets with approved lids.
- Use hold-down screens or other retaining systems to prevent instruments from shifting.
- Concave items, such as basins, should be placed so the spray can reach all surfaces and the water can easily drain.
- Connect lumens to lumen irrigator ports, if available.

Instrument washer racks and conveyor systems should be inspected daily. Routine cleaning of washers should include inspection and cleaning of spray arms and washer jets. (See **Figure 8.23**) Mineral buildup will hinder spray action and disrupt cleaning efficacy. Washer traps/screens need special attention and should be inspected for debris at least daily and cleared of any obstructions. Washer detergent levels should be monitored frequently. If detergent drums are allowed to run dry, a column of air may enter the detergent feed lines and affect the delivery of replacement detergent.

It is important to keep the chamber walls clean so the washer can perform at maximum efficiency. If white scale is seen in the chamber, it should be removed immediately with an approved descaler because scale can fall on instruments and clog pumps, motors and spray arms. (See **Figure 8.24**)

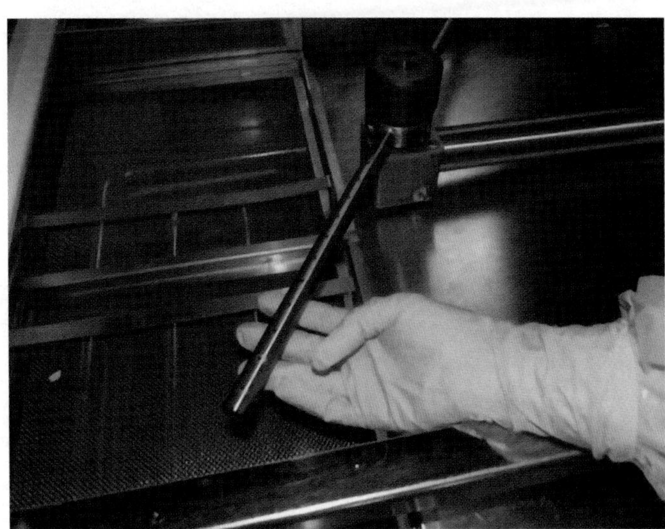

Figure 8.23

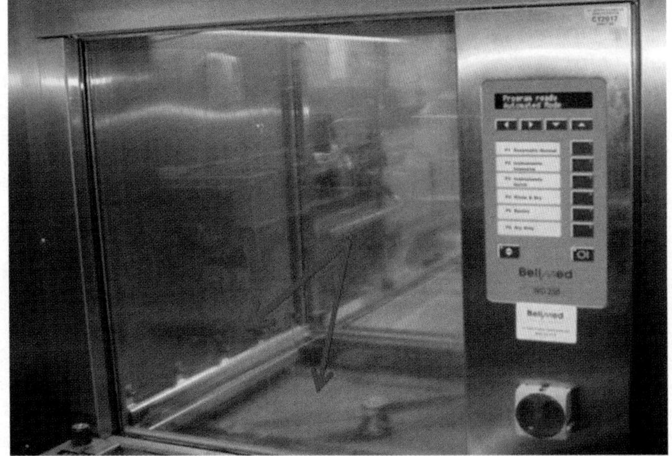

Figure 8.24 Example of a washer with white scale

Automated washers have preset, factory-installed cycles for use in different cleaning situations. Instrument cycles generally are the longest cycle because they have multiple rinse, wash, lubrication and drying times to meet the instruments' cleaning needs. Basins

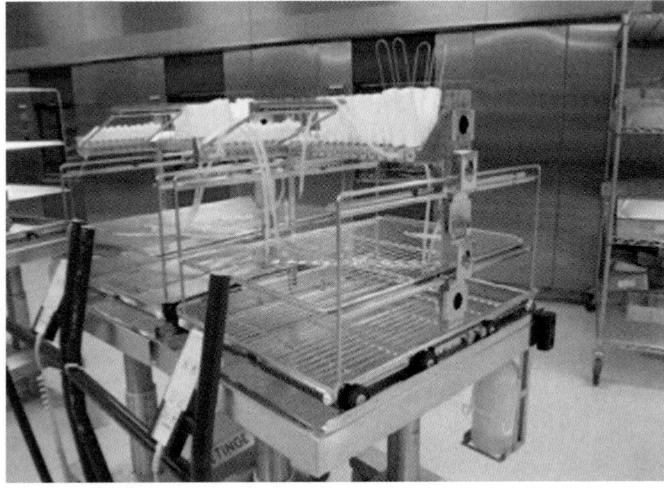

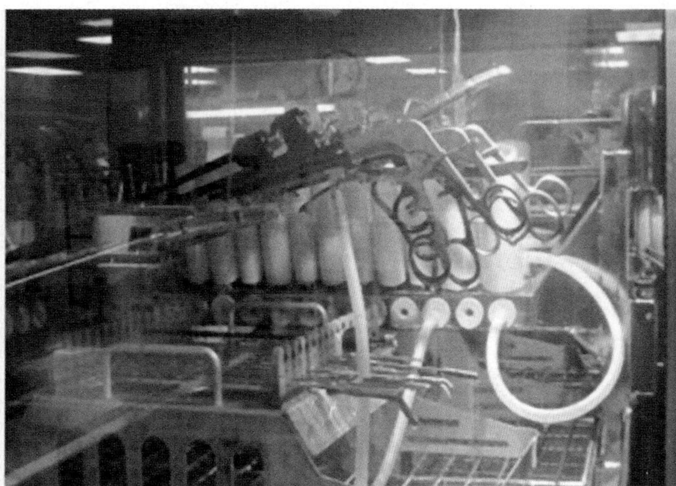

Figure 8.25 Examples of flushing mainifolds for mechanical washers

and containers are commonly run on a utensil cycle. Some washer manufacturers offer special cycles for delicate instruments. When running a mixed load of containers and instruments, the instrument cycle should be utilized for maximum cleaning. SP technicians should be familiar with different washer cycles and able to select the appropriate cleaning cycle for the items to be processed.

Some washer racks (manifolds) are equipped with irrigation lines that can be connected to certain complex instruments to add a channel flush to the mechanical cleaning process. (See **Figure 8.25**) Washer-disinfectors have a **thermal disinfection** cycle at the end of the cleaning /rinsing process.

> **Thermal disinfection** Use of heat to reduce the amount of microorganisms (excluding spores) on a medical device.

Automated Cart Washers

Cart washers were originally designed to clean carts used for transport of various supplies and instruments. (See **Figure 8.26**) Some cart washers are designed to process rigid containers and other miscellaneous items; other models have validated instrument cycles designed to clean instrumentation. Several manufacturers offer cart washers with design features and special washer racks to facilitate the processing of some durable medical equipment. (See **Figure 8.27**)

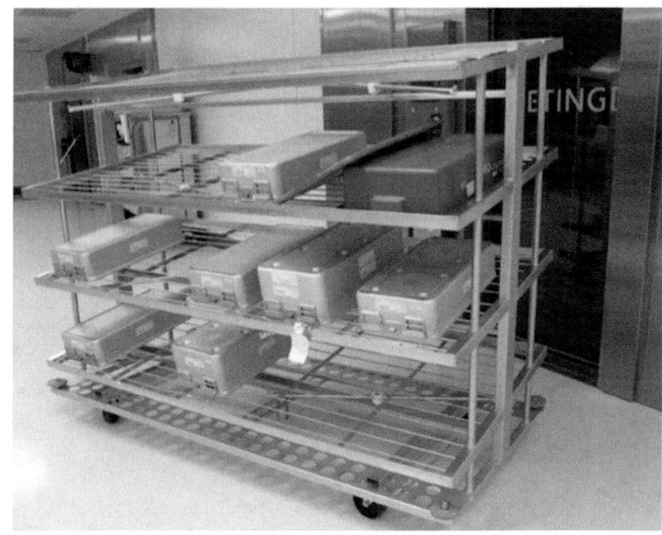

Figure 8.27 Example of a cart washer container rack

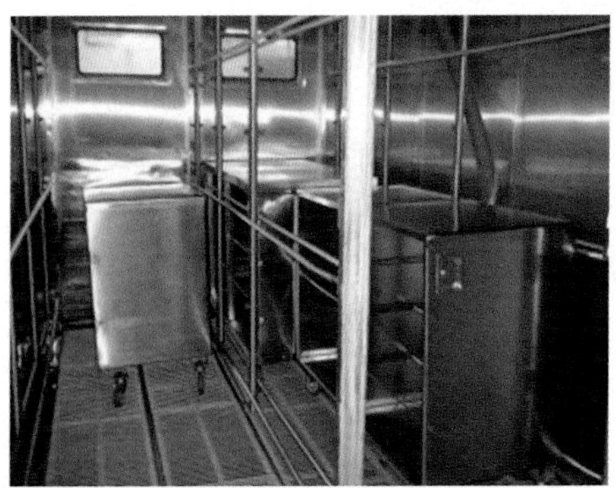

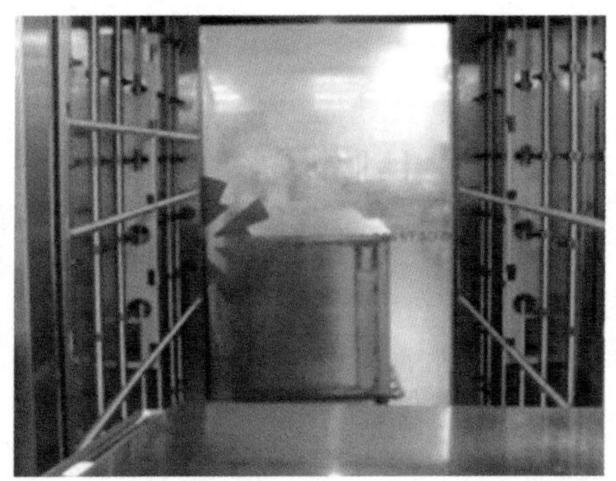

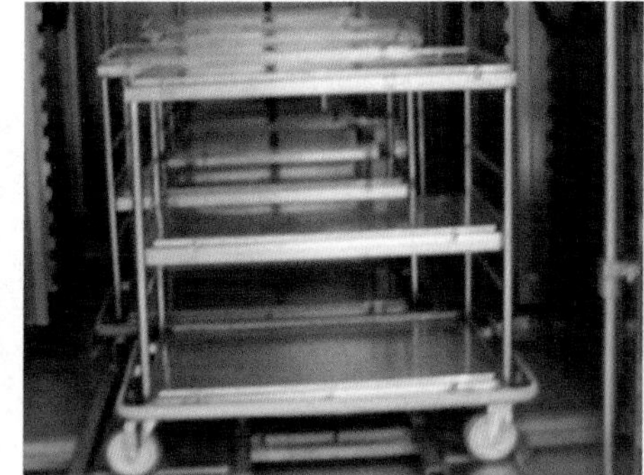

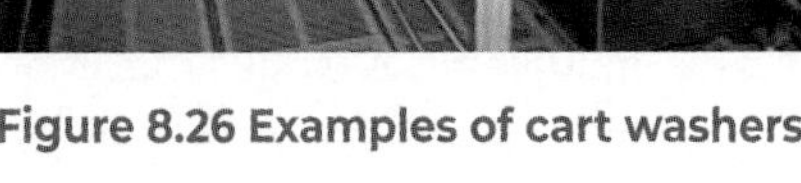

Figure 8.26 Examples of cart washers

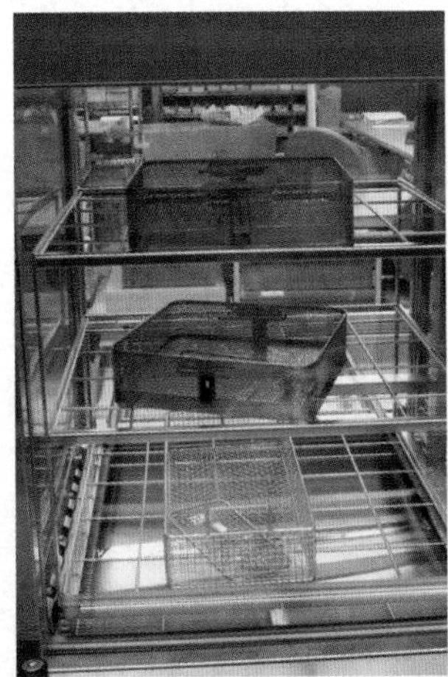

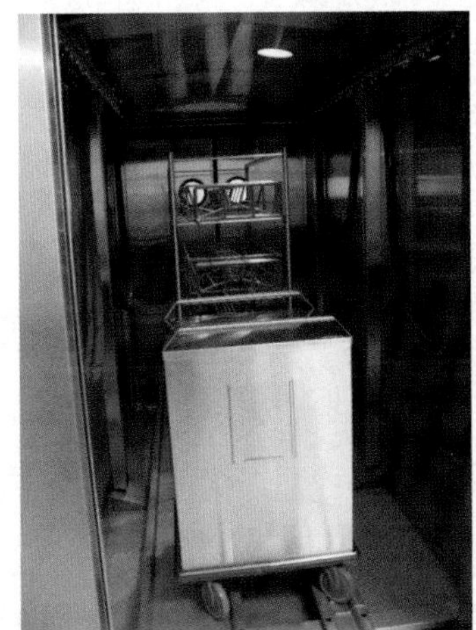

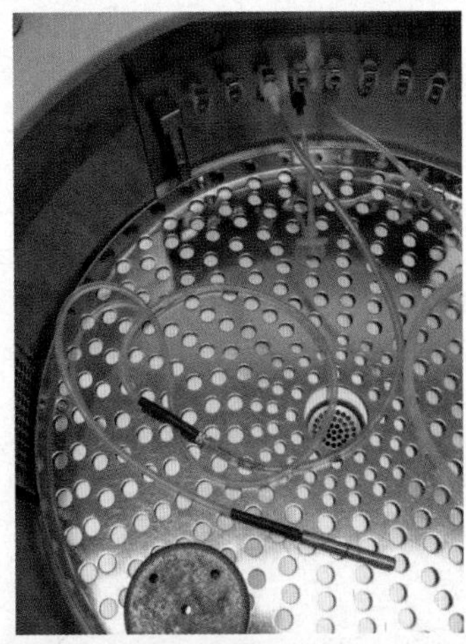

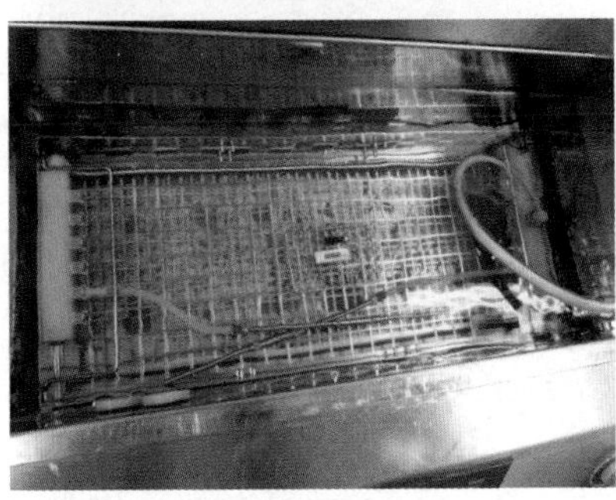

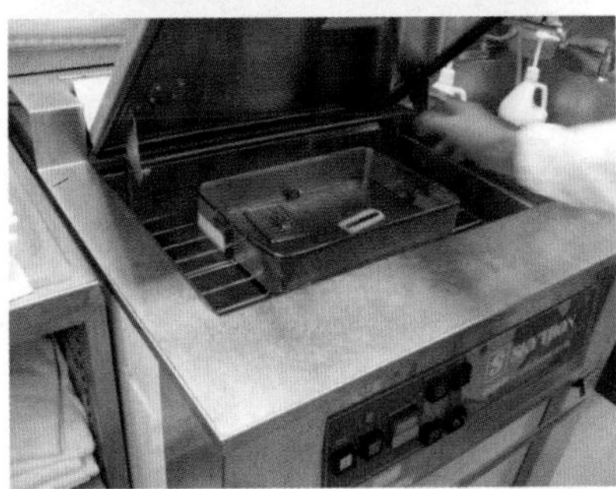

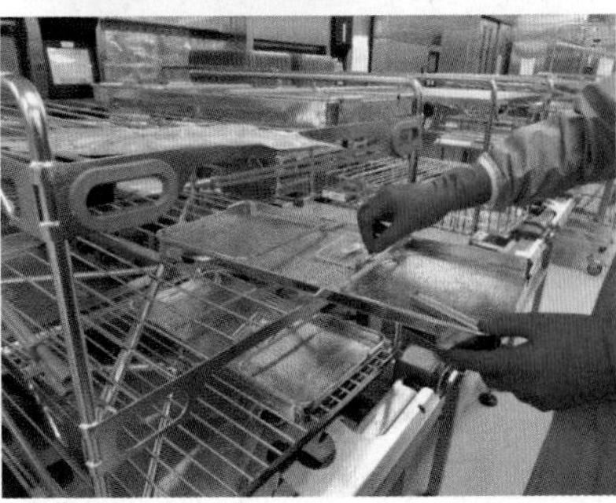

Figure 8.28 Mechanical cleaning equipment should be tested to ensure it is working properly.

Cart washers operate in a manner similar to automated instrument washers but on a larger scale. Spray arms deliver high-temperature water and detergent, and successive steps provide rinse water and hot air-drying cycles. Cart washers resemble automated car washes in their cleaning process. Most cart washers do not have multiple phase cycles like washer-disinfectors but include a high-temperature process to reduce bacteria and facilitate drying. Detergents selected for cart washing should be formulated for use in cart washers. Important factors to remember when using a cart washer:

- When cleaning enclosed carts, ensure they are approved to be cleaned by a cart washer.
- When opening cart doors, ensure they are secured in the open position.
- Do not process instruments in a cart washer that is not designed for that purpose.
- Do not process items inside carts. The walls of the cart will prevent cleaning solution and rinse water from reaching the items inside.
- Do not process items unless there are IFU.

EQUIPMENT TESTING

ANSI/AAMI ST79 *Comprehensive guide to steam sterilization and sterility assurance in health care facilities* recommends a quality assurance program to ensure that the mechanical equipment is working properly. Commercially prepared products can be obtained to verify the cleaning effectiveness of the equipment. (See **Figure 8.28**)

If the mechanical cleaner has a printout, the printout should be reviewed and initialed after each cycle to ensure the cycle reached the expected parameters.

Mechanical cleaners can save time and labor, while producing a consistent process; however, it is important that SP technicians remember that human factors play a significant role in mechanical cleaning. In other words, mechanical cleaners are only as good as their operators.

CLEANING CHEMICALS AND LUBRICANTS

Many types of soil can be present on reusable devices. When soil, especially blood, is allowed to dry prior to cleaning, it becomes difficult to remove. (See **Figure 8.29**) Blood flows into instrument joints, hinges, grooves and other difficult-to-clean areas; it then coagulates and dries to create a significant challenge to cleaning. Soil adheres to microscopic irregularities in the surface of instruments and must be manually and mechanically scrubbed away or chemically treated; otherwise, the formation of biofilm can result. Using proper chemicals in the correct concentrations rehydrates and loosens the soil and helps to properly clean the devices.

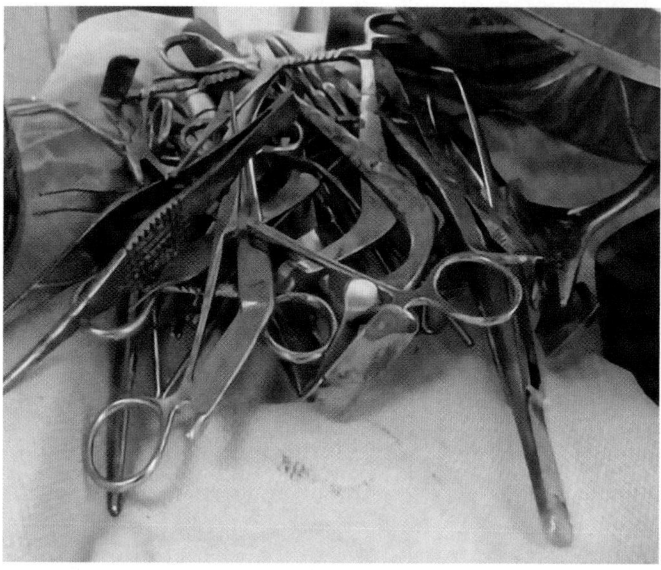

Figure 8.29 Dried soil is more difficult to clean.

Each chemical used should be compatible with both the medical device and the cleaning equipment. Different types of chemicals are used in the cleaning process, including enzymatic products, detergents and presoaks (precleaning agents). Each has a specific purpose in efficiently processing reusable items.

Enzymatic Products

Enzymatic cleaners are biodegradable, nontoxic cleaning agents used to break down soils, stains and other debris on heavily soiled instruments. They are very helpful for processing difficult-to-clean devices such as instruments with lumens. They are also used to keep instruments moist and begin breaking down the soil on instruments immediately after a procedure. Enzymes are very specific in their action (for example, a protein enzyme will not affect fat/lipase molecules) and there are different types of enzymatic products available. Some can be used at the point of use to moisten and loosen soil on instruments, and others are used in manual or automatic washing processes.

Popular enzymes used in SPDs include:

- Protease enzymes (protein) that break down blood, mucous, feces and albumin
- Lipase (fat) enzymes that break down fatty deposits, such as bone marrow
- Amylase enzymes that catalyze (change) starch into sugars

Elements in soil can gradually degrade enzymes during use and reduce their cleaning efficacy. Soil that has dried on a device must be rehydrated before enzymes that facilitate its removal can be effective. Point-of-use treatment (keeping the instruments free of gross soil) can reduce these problems. After precleaning, the instrument should remain moist to keep soil from drying, and hydration should be maintained to optimize the enzyme's efficacy.

Enzyme Effectiveness for Specific Soils	
Enzyme	**Effective against**
Protease	Proteins
Lipase	Fats
Amylase	Starches

Figure 8.30

Many enzymatic products used in the decontamination process are single enzyme products, so it is important to know the type of soil being cleaned. Multi-enzymatic products contain more than one type of enzyme. Detergents take longer to clean if they are not used in conjunction with enzymatic products.

Monitoring for proper temperature is critical when dealing with enzyme-based products. Temperatures should not exceed 140°F (60°C), unless otherwise stated by the enzyme manufacturer.

Detergents

Water is not an effective cleaning agent; therefore, detergents are used to enhance its cleaning ability. Detergents contain **emulsifiers, surfactants** and **chelating agents** to increase their cleaning efficacy. Chelating agents have an ionic charge that allows soils with the opposite charge to break away and attach to the chelating agent. An emulsifier surrounds these particles to prevent them from reattaching and they also help break bonds that oils can create to trap soil.

Emulsifier Any ingredient used to bind together substances that typically do not combine such as oil and water.

Surfactant A substance that lowers the surface tension of the water and increases the solubility of organic compounds.

Chelating agents Chemicals that hold hard water minerals in solution and prevent soap or detergent from reacting with the minerals.

When used properly, detergents penetrate and remove soil from instruments and keep soil in suspension so it does not reattach to the instrument. Remember that detergents do not kill microorganisms (unless they contain a biocide). Instead, they help to clean the instrument by removing bacteria-laden soil.

Detergents are designed to perform specific tasks. In the home setting, there are different detergents for washing dishes, doing laundry, and cleaning floors. In a similar manner, detergents for decontamination in the healthcare facility are formulated for different applications. Some detergents work in hard water, some are low-foaming varieties that do not hinder the operation of the mechanical cleaning equipment, and others are developed specifically for a certain type of equipment, like those formulated for ultrasonic cleaners.

Detergents also come in several forms. Liquid detergents can be purchased in small quantities for use at a sink or in large quantities for use in mechanical washers. (See **Figure 8.31**)

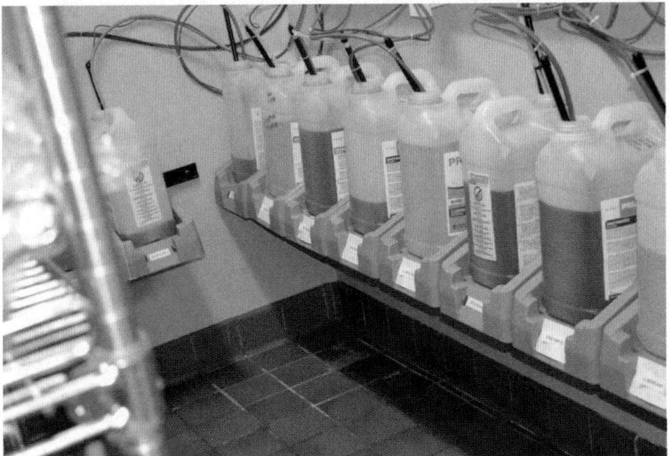

Figure 8.31

Detergents are selected at each facility, based on the items' and facility's specific cleaning needs, the quality of the water, and the types of soil present. Several types of detergents can be used for cleaning surgical instruments. Each has its advantages and disadvantages, so it is important to know how each type of detergent functions and how to properly use different detergents.

Neutral detergents are the most commonly used type in the U.S. Neutral detergents have a pH value of 6 to 8.

- Advantages – Neutral-pH detergents are effective on organic and inorganic soils and are safe to use on aluminum products.

- Disadvantages – Neutral-pH detergents are not very effective in hard water. They produce more foam and are more difficult to rinse than other types of detergents.

Alkaline detergents are highly effective at removing organic soils (blood, fat and oils). Alkaline detergents range in pH from 8 to more than 11. Prior to using an alkaline detergent, refer to the medical device and equipment manufacturer's IFU.

- Advantages – Alkaline detergents remove a wider range of soil than any other type of detergent.

- Disadvantages – Alkaline detergents require thorough rinsing because they can leave a powdery residue on the instrument's surface. Alkaline detergents cannot be used on devices made of bronze, copper or aluminum.

Acid detergents are primarily used to remove mineral deposits such as hard water, urine, minerals and scale. Acid detergents have a pH of 1.6 to 3.

- Advantages – Acid detergents are excellent for removing mineral deposits and urine. They work well on inorganic soils, neutralize alkaline residues and make stainless steel shine.

- Disadvantages – Acid detergents can damage the surfaces of stainless steel and aluminum, bronze and glass. Disposal into drains and sewer lines may be restricted in some states.

Review of Common Chemicals Used in the Decontamination Area

During the course of any shift, SP technicians must select and properly use several different chemicals. While initial selection of chemicals to be used in the department is done by managers, the technician must select the proper chemical for the job from the chemicals available in the decontamination area. *Note: Each chemical is different and cannot be substituted for another.* Technicians must read labels carefully and ask questions if any information is not understood. (See **Figure 8.32**)

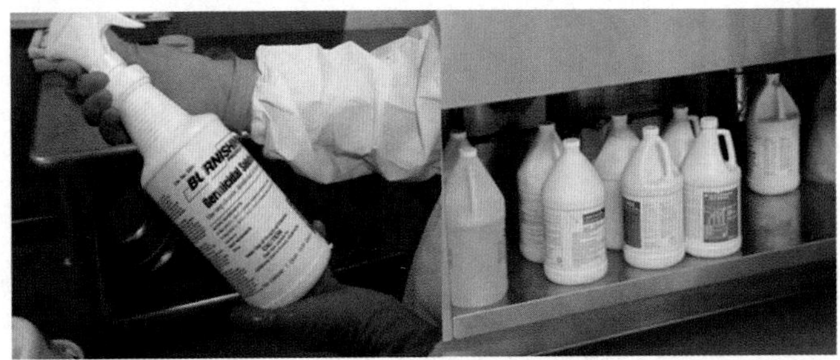

Figure 8.32 Chemicals are different; read labels carefully.

The following is a review of chemicals commonly found in the decontamination area:

- Precleaning chemicals are used in the first step in the decontamination process. Some commonly used precleaning agents include detergent solutions, enzymatic detergents and combination enzyme-germicide detergents.

- Precleaning should begin immediately after completion of any invasive procedure. Blood and other visible debris, if left on an instrument, serve as a reservoir for microbial growth and may damage an instrument's finish. If not removed, the corrosive agents in blood and body tissue can penetrate the protective outer layer of an instrument and cause rusting or pitting of the stainless steel. The manufacturer's instructions must be followed when using these precleaning products. Exceeding the time allowed for the instruments to be immersed in the solution can damage and corrode instruments and shortening the immersion time from what the instructions recommend can cause precleaning products to be ineffective.

- Precleaning chemicals are applied at the point of use but they may also be used in the decontamination area to keep soil moist and loosen dried soil. They must be removed prior to the cleaning process.

- Manual cleaning chemicals, when mixed properly, penetrate under the soil and break the bond that attaches the soil to the instruments. These cleaning products' main function is to remove soil, not kill microorganisms. Low-foaming and free-rinsing manual cleaners should be used. The manufacturer's IFU should be followed for proper dilution and to determine the proper water temperature for their use. Manual cleaners are usually neutral or alkaline products.

- Mechanical cleaning chemicals are specially designed for use in mechanical cleaning processes. They are low foaming and designed to work with the specific mechanical cleaning equipment (for example, an ultrasonic cleaner), so careful attention must be paid to the manufacturer's IFU.

- Descalers are not typically required if the water quality and detergent mixtures are correct and the equipment is operating properly. Still, problems can go unnoticed until a chalky, powdery, hard-to-remove substance appears in equipment and sinks. When this occurs, an acidic detergent or descaler is needed to remove the scale. It is important to use a descaling product when scale is detected in the cleaning equipment because scale can interfere with the equipment's cleaning ability.

- Lubricants (often called "instrument milk" because of their milky appearance) are an important part of the instrument maintenance program because they help maintain the integrity of instruments and keep them in good working order. Instruments require different types of lubricant depending on the design of the device or the sterilization method. Lubrication is performed after cleaning as one of the final steps in the mechanical wash process (or it can be applied manually in the clean assembly area using a spray bottle). In the past, instrument baths (pans filled with instrument lubricating solution) were commonly used. This process is now discouraged because of increased risk of contamination. SP technicians must always use lubrication according to the manufacturer's instructions to ensure proper contact time and dilution. It is also important to ensure the lubricant is designed for use with the instruments to be cleaned and compatible with the specific sterilization process that will follow.

- Stain and rust removers are used when the normal cleaning process does not remove stains on an instrument. Stains and rust typically result from improper care such as soaking the instruments in saline. Stain and rust remover can be used after instrument cleaning to restore the luster to stainless steel instruments. These chemicals remove hard water deposits, rust scale and discoloration from instrumentation and processing equipment. Most stain and rust removers are acid-based compounds (0 to 6.9 pH) that react with minerals and iron on the instruments. They remove mineral and detergent buildup, leaving the surfaces bright and shiny, and the instruments moving freely. Because these chemicals are acid-based, the IFU must be carefully followed to prevent instrument damage. After using a stain remover, the instruments should be recleaned.

When using any cleaning chemical, temperature is an important factor. Most cleaning chemicals deactivate if the temperature is higher than 180°F (82°C). Unless specified by the manufacturer, cleaning chemicals should never be combined with other chemicals.

To prevent instrument damage, the following chemicals should not be used to clean instruments (unless recommended by the device manufacturer):

- Abrasive cleaning compounds
- Saline
- Buffered iodine (such as povidone iodine)
- Hydrogen peroxide
- Bleach
- Any chemical not specifically recommended by the medical device manufacturer

INSTRUCTIONS FOR USE

Knowing and following the manufacturer's IFU are critical components of the decontamination process. Medical device IFU have undergone a scientific validation that provides the specific steps that must be taken to decontaminate each device. IFU are provided with every newly purchased item. The SPD should have a copy of all IFU, either as a paper or digital copy. SP technicians must understand how to follow each medical device's IFU and also clearly understand the IFU for any equipment and chemical they use. Failure to follow IFU can result in a failed decontamination process and damage to instruments and equipment.

STEPS IN THE DECONTAMINATION PROCESS

Point-of-Use Treatment

The process of decontamination begins with the end user, at the point of use. OR staff should take the time to ensure that the required point-of-use treatment process is performed. Following point-of-use treatment, the Association for the Advancement of Medical Instrumentation (AAMI) and the Association of periOperative Registered Nurses (AORN) recommend that instrument users take time to properly prepare instrumentation for transport to the decontamination area.

Soiled Receiving

If soiled items are hand-delivered to the decontamination area, the person delivering the items should place them on a cart or countertop designated for receipt of items into the decontamination area. (See **Figure 8.33**)

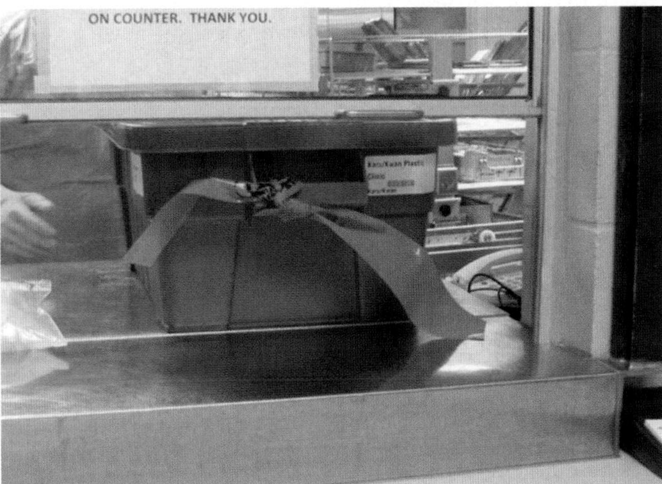

Figure 8.33 Soiled receiving for hand-delivered items

When carts loaded with soiled items are received, proper body mechanics must be used when handling the heavy carts. When loading and unloading carts from dumbwaiters or elevators, the weight of the cart should be checked. It is also critical to ensure that the wheels are aligned and that they will roll over door spaces or uneven edges. If the cart is too heavy to move easily, some items should be removed to lighten the load.

If items are in a closed cart or transport container, the lid or doors must be carefully opened because items may have shifted during transport. Items should be removed from the cart or container carefully and placed on a flat surface near a sink. The following guidelines should be followed during the unloading process:

- Fluids should be disposed of or contained at the point of use. If transported, fluids should be in a leak-proof container. Dispose of any fluids, per facility policy.
- If possible, disposable items and reusable textiles should be removed at the point of use. If this is not feasible, the items should be bagged and sent to the decontamination area. They should not be transported unless contained. (See **Figure 8.34**)
- Reusable sharps, including scissors and chisels, should be separated and safely contained at the point of use. (See **Figure 8.35**)
- Disposable sharps, such as scalpel blades and trocars, should be removed and discarded at the point of use. If disposable sharps are found in the transport device or in any tray, they should be removed and discarded in an approved sharps container. Misplaced sharps should be reported to the immediate supervisor per the hospital policy. *Note: Every sharps injury should be reported in accordance with facility policy and protocols.*

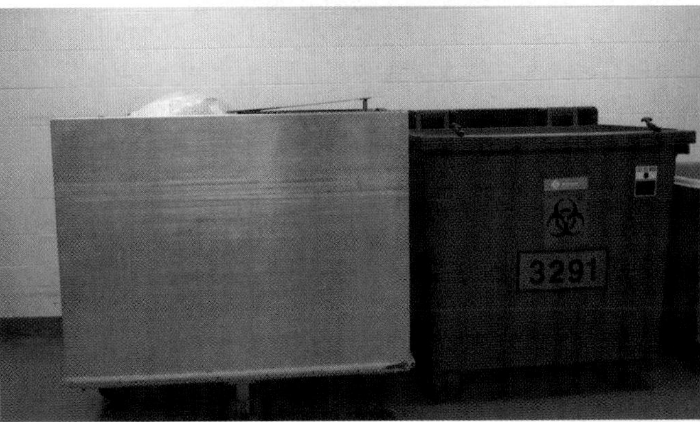

Figure 8.34

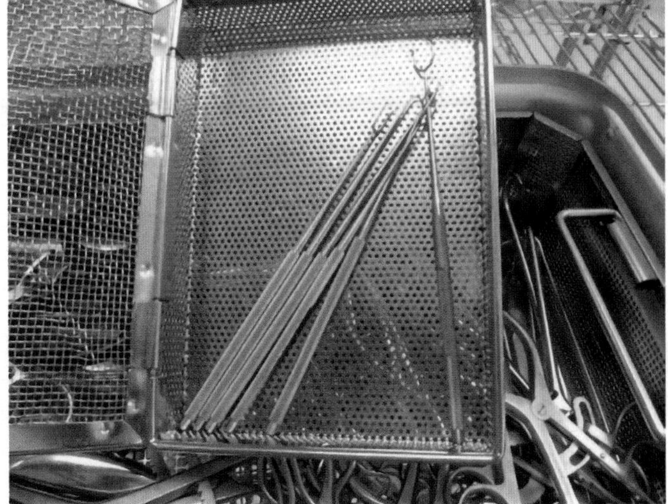

Figure 8.35

- Items for third-party reprocessors should be placed into their specific container. These disposable items will be sent out of the facility for reprocessing by a company that has been cleared by the U.S. Food and Drug Administration (FDA) for this type of reprocessing. Examples of these types of items include pulse oximeter sensors, deep vein thrombosis (DVT) sleeves, and laparoscopic instruments.
- Carefully remove all tray liners, indicators, filters, tip protectors and other disposable items left inside instrument trays.
- Remove the filter retention plates from rigid containers. Containers and lids should be cleaned without the retention plate or reusable filter in place. Discard disposable filters and clean reusable filters per the manufacturer's instructions.
- If the container system has valve-type closures, the valves should be inspected and cleaned following the manufacturer's instructions. Improper cleaning of container valves can

prevent the sterilant from reaching the instruments and may also lead to contamination of the instruments after sterilization.

- Interior baskets should be removed from inside the container. Instruments may be mechanically cleaned inside the interior tray after manual preparation.

- Ensure the transport container or the case cart is completely empty, then clean per the manufacturer's IFU.

Cleaning

Cleaning instruments and other medical devices is the primary function of the decontamination area. It is obvious that instruments should be cleaned after use; however, there are also other times when instruments should be cleaned. **Figure 8.36** lists some circumstances when instruments should be sent to the decontamination area for cleaning.

Clean Instruments:
After use
After they have been opened, placed on the sterile field, but have not been used
When new instruments are received at the facility
When used instruments return from repair or refurbishing
When instruments are pulled from back-up stock
When instruments are inadvertently contaminated
When loaned instruments are received

Figure 8.36

Thorough cleaning and adherence to IFU is important because cleaning process failures put patients and staff at risk. There are several types of cleaning methods:

- Precleaning (this process should occur at the point of use).

- Manual cleaning (also known as cleaning by hand).

- Mechanical cleaning (cleaning items using specialized cleaning equipment).

The method of cleaning selected should follow the device manufacturer's IFU.

Precleaning

Instruments must be precleaned to remove gross soil, such as blood and tissue debris, prior to mechanical cleaning. Gross debris must be removed from instruments undergoing mechanical cleaning; otherwise, it will circulate through the washer and be deposited onto the other instruments, which will block the cleaning action. For washing to be effective, all surfaces of the device should have contact with the cleaning solutions.

Precleaning solutions can interfere with the following cleaning steps, therefore all presoak chemicals must be completely removed before moving instruments to mechanical cleaning cycles. This can be accomplished either manually or mechanically.

Manual Cleaning

Manual cleaning is done to remove soil that was not removed or was only softened during the precleaning process; this is achieved by the use of friction and specialized cleaning chemicals.

Manual cleaning may be performed:

- Before the item is mechanically cleaned to ensure precleaning chemicals, blood, protein and other soil is removed

- When the decontamination area does not have a mechanical method of cleaning

- To clean items that cannot be immersed in water

- For instruments with lumens

- For delicate or complex medical devices such as microsurgical and robotic instruments

- For all items that require manual cleaning as part of their IFU

Manual Preparation and Cleaning Processes

The work area should be set up to accommodate the type of items to be cleaned. For example, for instruments that can be immersed, the sink should be filled with the appropriate cleaning solution. Each instrument set should be cleaned in a fresh cleaning solution. Place heavier instruments in the sink first, followed by lighter, more delicate items. Items should be placed gently into the sink. SP technicians should not "dump" them into the sink because instruments can damage easily.

Items should be placed in the sink in the following manner:

- Hinged instruments should be fully opened when placed in the sink.

- Multi-part instruments should be disassembled per manufacturer's instructions so all parts of the instrument can be exposed to the cleaning solution. (See **Figure 8.37**) Keep all parts near each other during the cleaning process.

- Lumen/cannulated items should be fully submerged, then flushed with fresh cleaning solution; this will force air bubbles

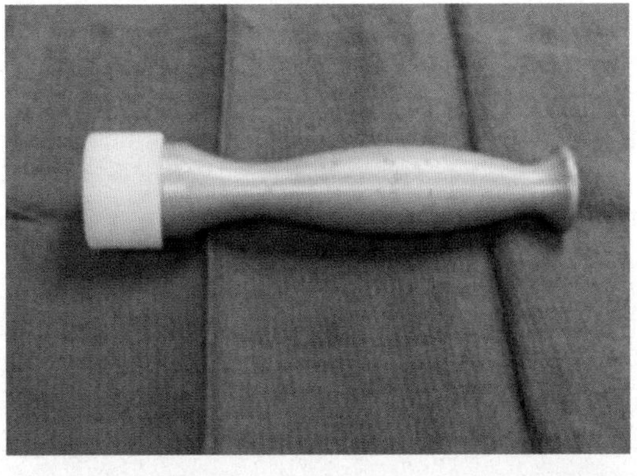

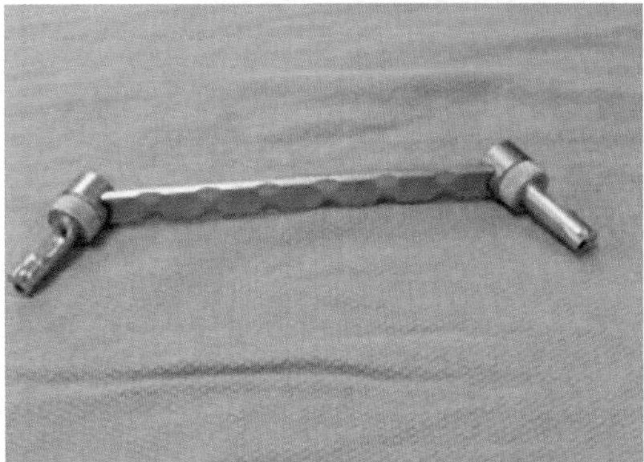

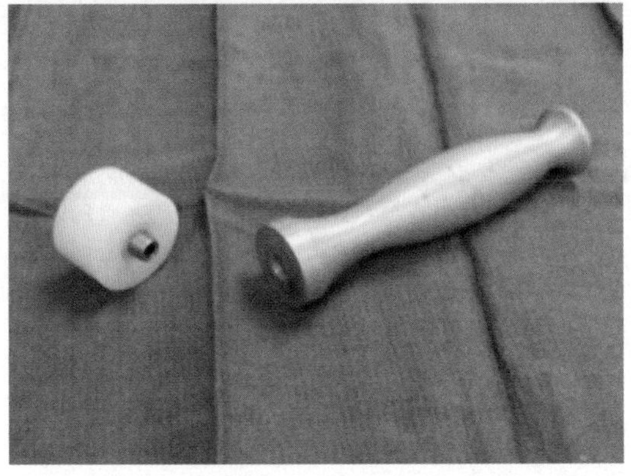

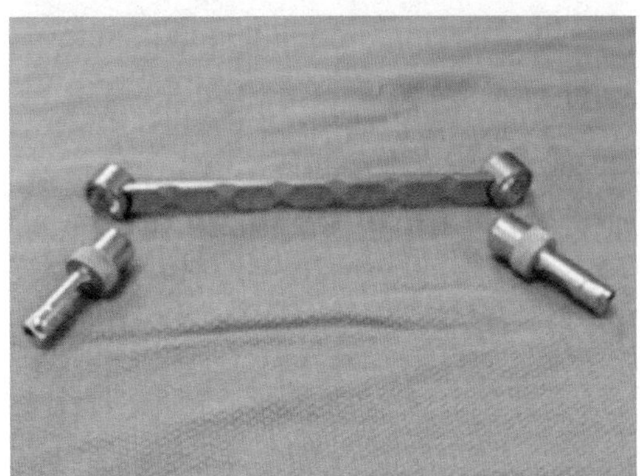

Figure 8.37 Disassemble multi-part instruments.

out of the lumen and ensure all the inner surfaces are in contact with the cleaning solution. If available, placing lumened items in a vertical soaking cylinder also helps ensure air bubbles are not inside the lumens. (See **Figure 8.38**)

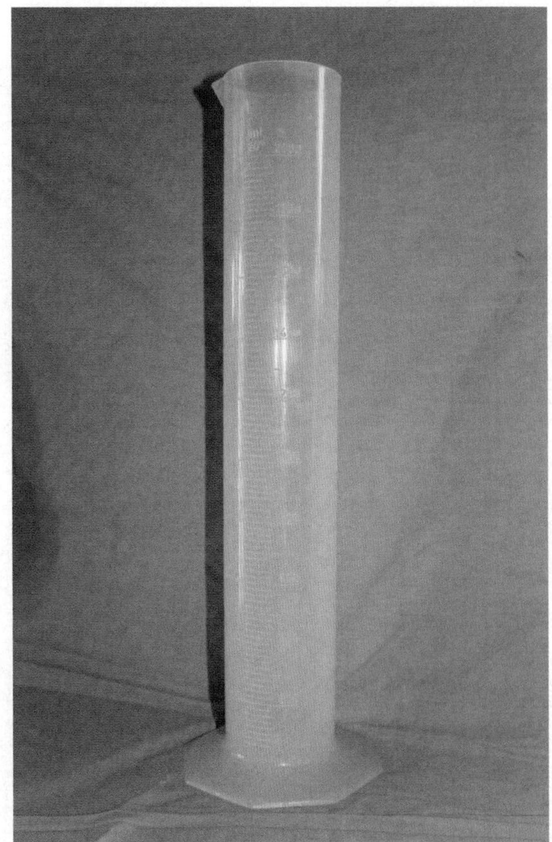

Figure 8.38

Ensure detergent can reach every part of the device being cleaned. If the detergent cannot reach every part of the instrument, the instrument cannot be thoroughly cleaned. Some IFU specify the amount of time an item must be soaked.

Items that cannot be immersed, like power equipment and many cables and cords, should be set aside and processed separately. Many SPDs have a sink area designated for cleaning these non-immersible items.

All instrument surfaces and cleaning efforts must be focused and performed consistently. Instruments should be brushed in a to-and-fro motion under the water's surface. Brushing under the water's surface prevents aerosolization. (See **Figure 8.39**) Aerosolization occurs when ultramicroscopic particles are released into the air. This is a concern because the cleaning solution contains contaminates from the instruments being cleaned. When cleaning, pay special attention to hinges and the tips of the instruments because these areas harbor the most soil. All serrated, toothed and creviced areas should be brushed to ensure the instrument is properly cleaned.

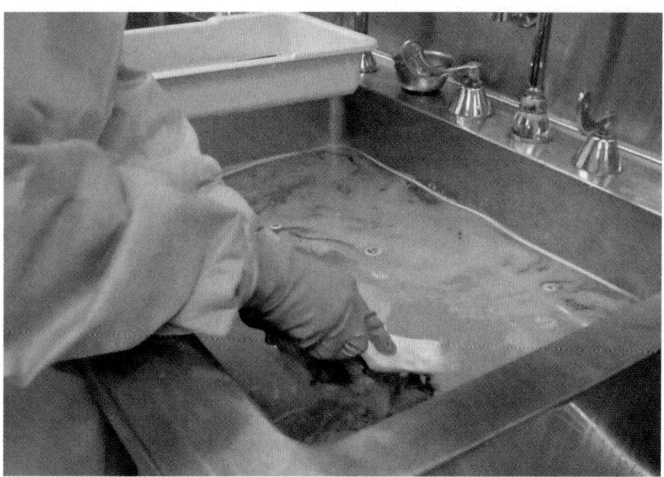

Figure 8.39

Lumened instruments should be cleaned carefully with a brush after soaking in the cleaning solution. Select a brush that fits into the lumen and touches all inner surfaces. With the lumened instrument under the surface of the water, gently push the brush through the lumen several times. As the brush comes out of the lumened device, it should be examined for debris and cleaned, and then pulled through the lumen to further clean the lumen. Brushing should continue until the debris is removed and no longer seen during examination. (See **Figure 8.40**) The lumen should be checked for cleanliness by using a clean brush or an approved, non-linting pipe-cleaner-type product or a borescope.

Because curettes, Kerrison and other rongeurs, and other orthopedic instruments can conceal bone and other bioburden, removing material with bristle brushes should be an initial step in the cleaning process. All crevices should be checked carefully because blood and bone may be in other areas of the instrument, not just the biting or cutting section. (See **Figure 8.41**)

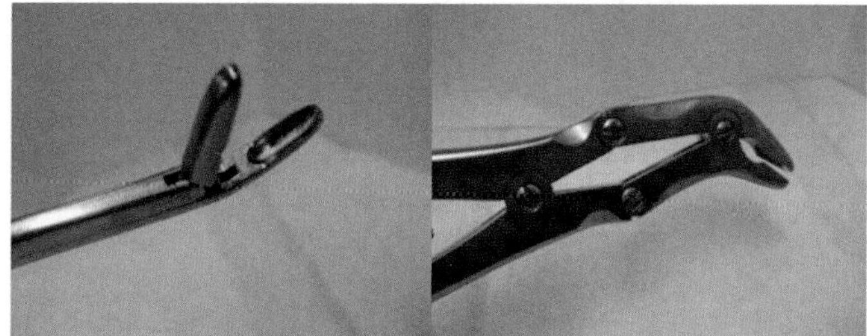

Figure 8.41 Tips and crevices are difficult to clean.

Instruments tagged for repair must still be cleaned and decontaminated. When instruments are returned from repair, they must be considered contaminated. Therefore, they must be cleaned, decontaminated and inspected before being returned to their respective sets.

Delicate instruments are a cleaning challenge; they must be separated from regular or heavy instruments during cleaning. Devices used for delicate surgical procedures are generally lightweight, with fine points and tips. Mixing them with heavy instruments or placing heavy devices on top of them can cause

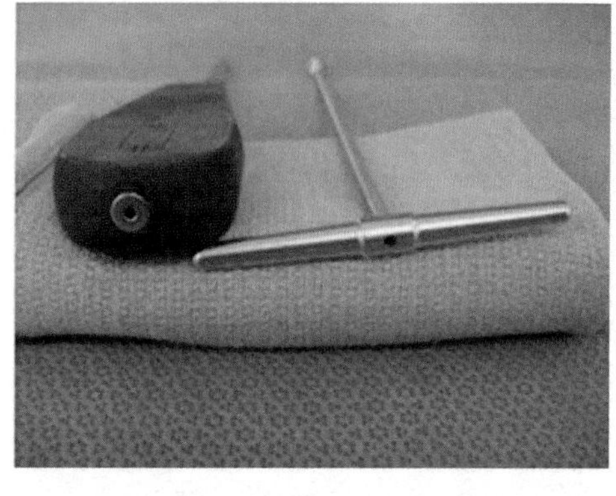

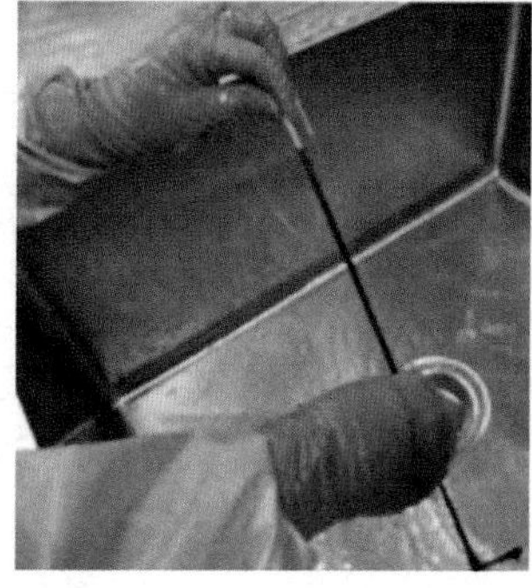

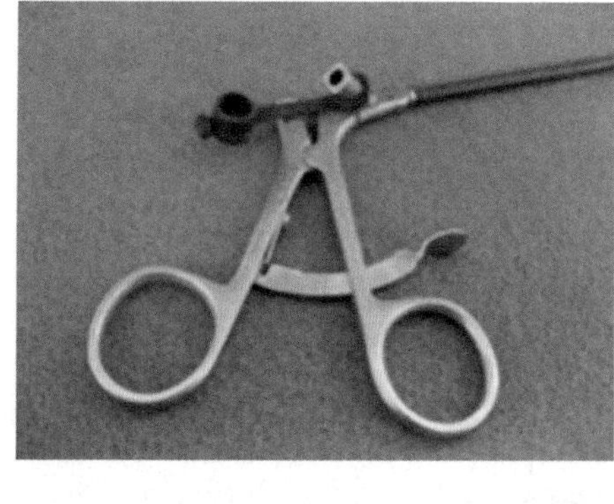

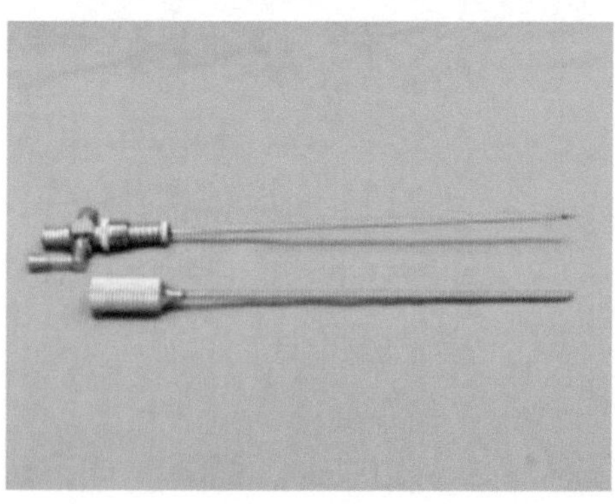

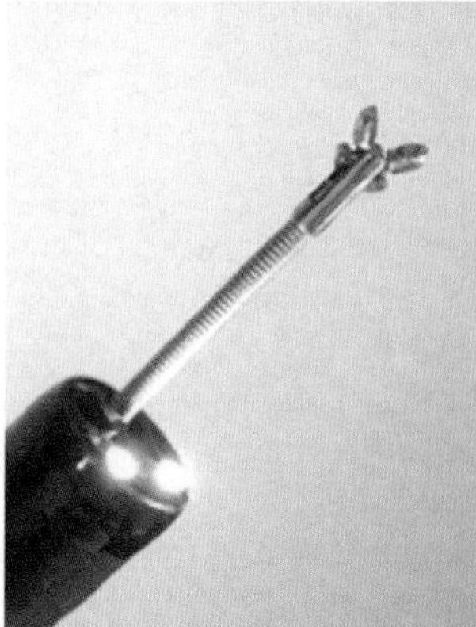

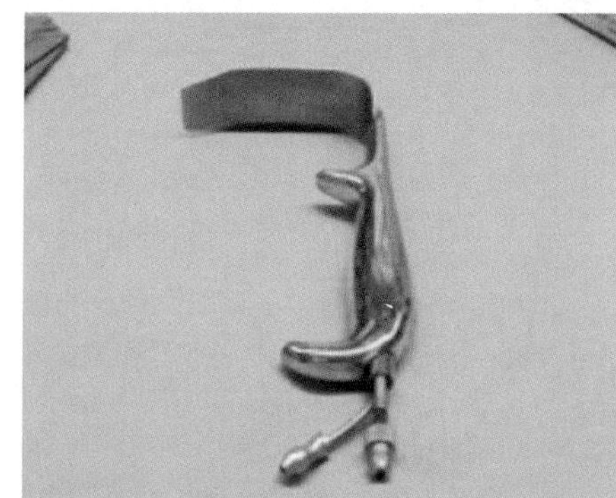

Figure 8.40 Check lumens carefully for cleanliness.

damage and misalignment. Delicate instruments, such as skin hooks, can slip through perforated baskets and become entangled. Also, check the IFU to ensure the proper cleaning chemical is being used. Unless otherwise stated by the manufacturer, clean these instruments as one would other surgical instruments, but with more care in handling. Always check the IFU to determine whether the instrument can be mechanically processed after manual cleaning. If processing in a washer-disinfector, a delicate cycle will likely need to be selected.

Ophthalmic instruments have special cleaning protocols because of the increasing incidents of **toxic anterior segment syndrome (TASS)**. Most instances of TASS appear to be related to instrument processing; therefore, the Instrument Cleaning Guideline in AORN's *Guidelines for PeriOperative Practice* recommends special precautions when processing intraocular ophthalmic instruments. The procedures for processing ophthalmic instruments are different from general instrumentation, which includes cleaning intraocular instruments separately from general surgical instruments. This separation can help prevent cross-contamination with bioburden from heavily soiled nonophthalmic surgical instruments. Manufacturer's cleaning instructions must be carefully followed. It is recommended that facilities have sufficient instrumentation to allow adequate time for processing between patients.

Toxic anterior segment syndrome (TASS)
Acute postoperative inflammatory reaction in which a noninfectious substance enters the anterior segment of the eye and induces toxic damage to the intraocular tissues.

There are thousands of instruments on the market and cleaning each one requires specific knowledge. Instruments that are designed to perform the same functions but are made by different manufacturers may need different cleaning processes. Consult the medical device manufacturer for special considerations and to determine whether these devices can withstand automated washers.

Orthopedic and neurologic surgeries have many instrument sets that require extended preparation and inspection prior to and during cleaning. Joint replacement cutting guides, rasps, reamers and broaches hide gross amounts of blood, bone and tissue. This can occur even with the best point-of-use treatment in the OR, and these instruments must be cleaned with brushes and extensive hand detailing. Presoaking with enzymatic detergents can help remove much of the bioburden from crevices. Some washer manufacturers have designed special washer racks to hold and flush out these devices.

Implants, such as orthopedic screws and plates, are not compatible with lubrication. When processing implants, use cycles that exclude the use of lubrication.

Laparoscopic and robotic instrumentation can be difficult and time consuming to clean. Instrument manufacturers provide extensive cleaning instructions that must be carefully followed to ensure the instruments are clean. Always use properly sized brushes in the lumened areas and carefully follow any flushing instructions provided by the manufacturer. For example, these instruments, especially robotic instruments, can be damaged if too much air and water pressure are used. Some types of mechanical cleaning equipment have special baskets, manifolds or connections to flush these items during mechanical cleaning. These items must still be manually cleaned and flushed, even when using a mechanical method.

Flexible and rigid endoscopes also pose special cleaning concerns. IFU for each specific model must be carefully followed.

TASS Precautions in the Decontamination Area

TASS occurs when contaminants enter the eye during eye surgery. Those contaminants can be the result of inadequate instrument processing. The risk of TASS can be reduced in the decontamination area by:

- Carefully following all manufacturers' IFU for cleaning
- Taking actions to prevent the formation of biofilm on instruments
- Using only enzymes and detergents recommended by the manufacturer
- Keeping cleaning tools, such as brushes and syringes, clean
- Flushing lumens
- Rinsing with copious amounts of the recommended rinse water
- Avoiding the use of lubrication
- Cleaning in a designated cleaning area, separately from general surgical instrument

New, repaired or loaned instruments received in the SPD must be cleaned prior to disinfection or sterilization. Although these instruments may look clean, their surfaces are covered in fine metal dust, oils and other debris from the manufacturing and repair processes. These instruments have also been handled and exposed to outside elements during shipping.

Instruments from back-up stock should be cleaned prior to use because they have been hanging on walls or stored in drawers for some time. These instruments could have been handled multiple times and most likely contain dust and other environmental contaminants. (See **Figure 8.42**)

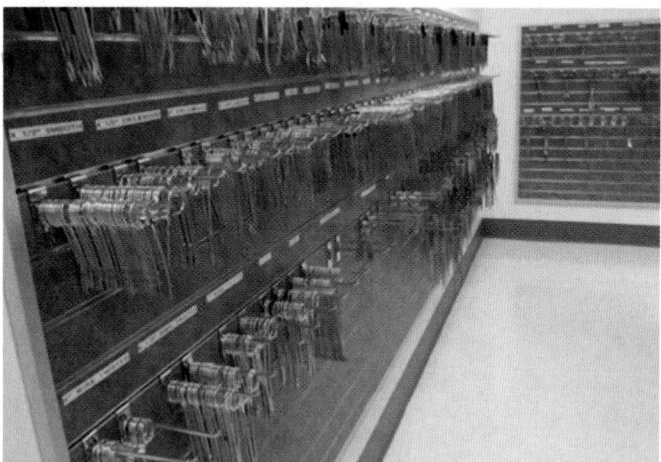

Figure 8.42

Cleaning Instruments That Cannot Be Immersed

Instruments, such as power equipment and cameras, cannot be immersed in water. The device manufacturer's IFU should be reviewed to ensure that proper cleaning chemistries and cleaning methods are used.

Hoses and cords should be carefully wiped down using the approved solution and a clean, soft, non-linting cloth. Special care should be taken at the ends of the hoses and cords because water will damage these items. Many of these types of instruments are a dark color, which makes it difficult to see dried blood; therefore, meticulous attention must be paid when cleaning these items. (See **Figure 8.43**) Unless approved by the manufacturer, do not rinse these items under running water. Carefully check these items to ensure there are no nicks, breaks or tears in the outer cover. If any damage is noted, mark the item for repair prior to sending it to the assembly area.

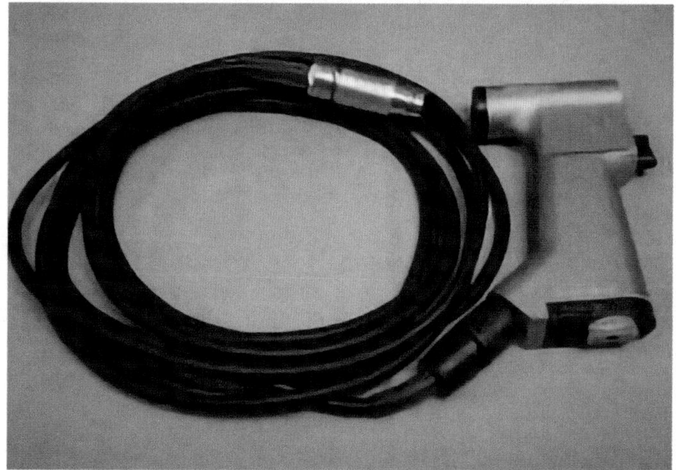

Figure 8.43

Power equipment presents challenges to SP technicians. These devices are powered by batteries, pneumatic air, or electricity. Care should be taken to prevent exposure of the connection points and battery contacts to moisture or chemicals. These connection areas can react with chemicals and cause damage and loss of electrical contact with the power source. The use of a battery, hose or cable designated for the decontamination area will help keep these connections dry. (See **Figure 8.44**)

Moisture can damage a powered surgical instrument (PSI)

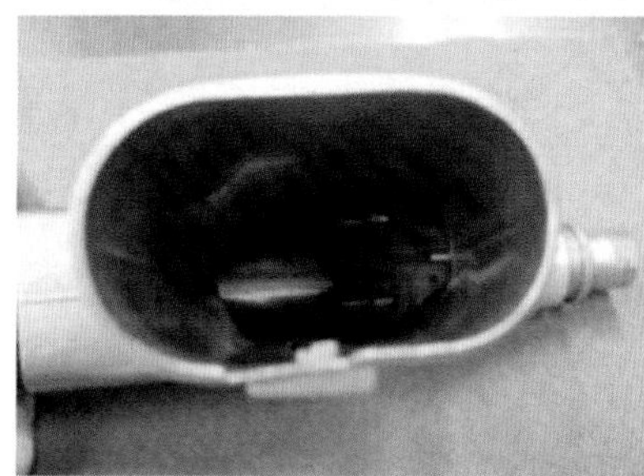

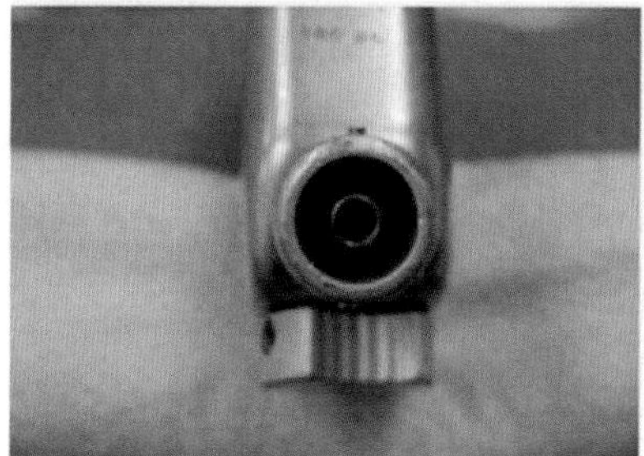

Prevent moisture from entering connection areas

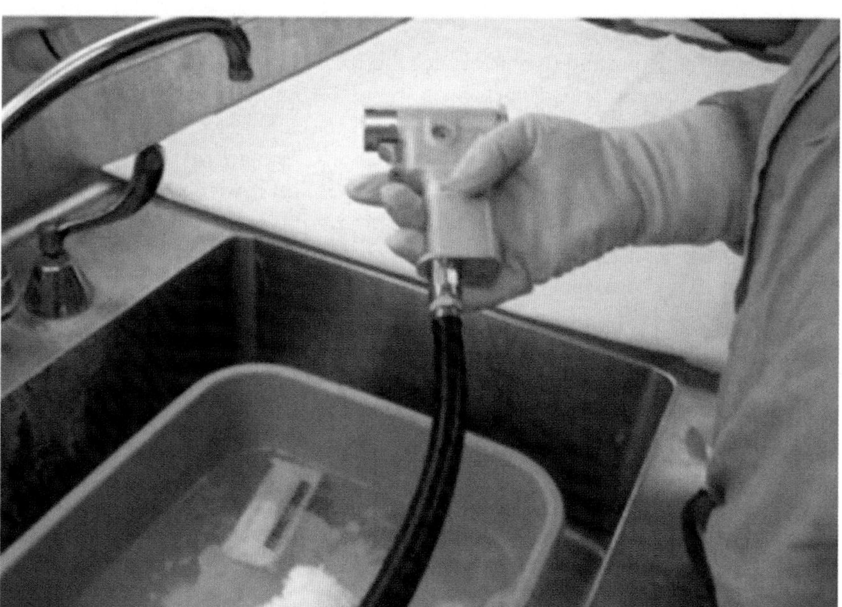

Figure 8.44 Powered surgical instrument (PSI) precautions

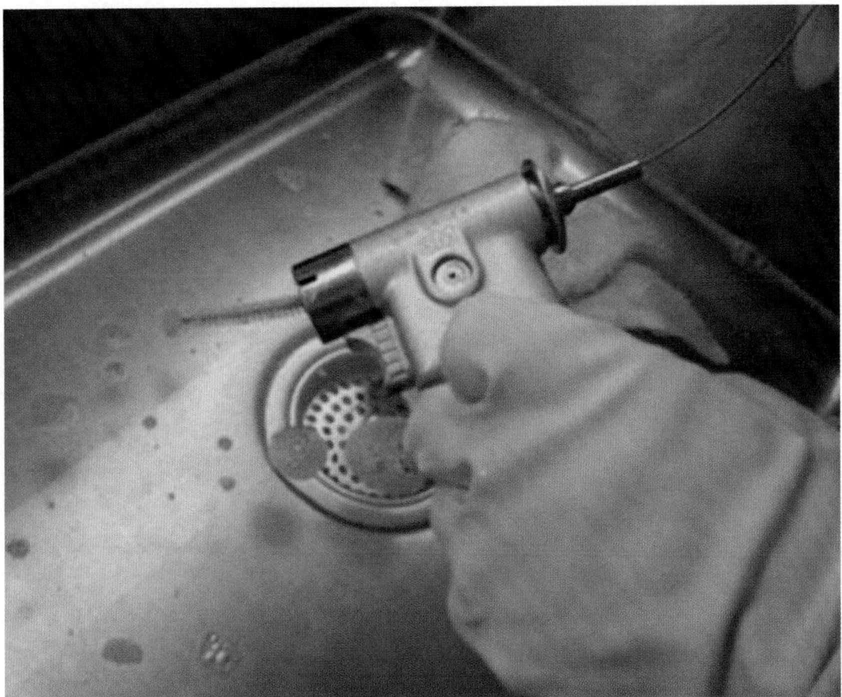

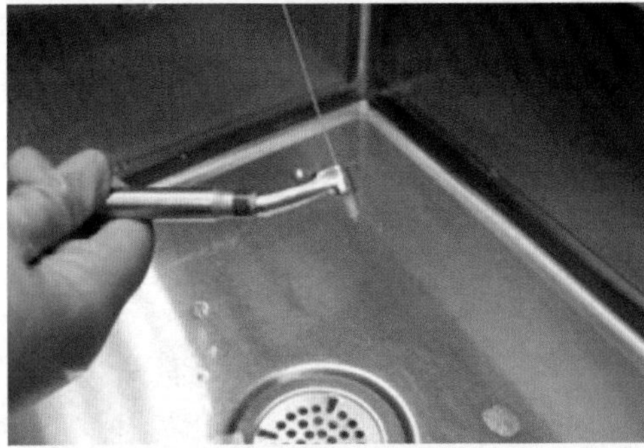

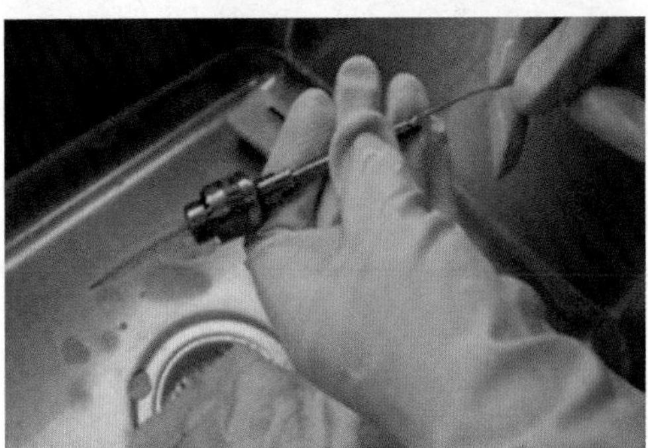

Figure 8.45 Cleaning PSI cannulas

Cannulated drills may have their lumens cleaned with running tap water, if approved by the manufacturer, and they should be brushed with a soft brush. (See **Figure 8.45**) A plastic syringe filled with water and enzymatic detergent can assist in delivering cleaning agents to hard-to-reach areas. If the instrument cannot be cleaned under running water, use a clean, soft cloth, appropriately sized brushes, and syringes filled with cleaning and rinsing solutions.

Frequently, orthopedic saws have residual bone chips and impacted bioburden in their working parts. They must be flushed and brushed clean under running water, if approved by the manufacturer.

Power accessories, such as chucks, can usually be immersed in the cleaning solution; however, some may need to be hand processed without immersion. Drill and saw attachments usually need non-immersion cleaning; consult and follow the manufacturer's IFU for the proper cleaning method.

Cleaning Instrument Containers and Basins

Cleaning rigid instrument containers and basins requires procedures that differ from those used for instruments. A neutral-pH detergent is typically recommended because acidic or alkaline pH detergents will damage aluminum and some composite materials. If processing manually, carefully clean all surface areas while the item is immersed in the cleaning solution, then rinse. If cleaning these items mechanically, place on the appropriate rack or manifold. When cleaning containers, the filter retention plate should be removed and not processed attached to the container or lid. Handles, locking mechanisms and container rims should be inspected for cracks and missing components. If basins are dented or bent or if containers are damaged, they should be marked for repair or removal from service prior to sending them to the assembly area.

Mobile Patient Care Equipment

Mobile patient care equipment has different processing needs than surgical instrumentation. In general, mild cleaning agents and disinfectants can be utilized to clean exterior components of patient care equipment. Use of an incorrect cleaning agent may affect product warranties and device functionality. Some chemicals may cause cosmetic changes in plastic and other materials.

Some devices have access doors and hatches that must be opened to clean intricate parts. (See **Figure 8.46**) Extreme care is needed to avoid damage to these critical parts. Soft materials and applicators may be used to clean these areas. Care must also be taken to thoroughly clean around switches and cords. It is important that the cleaning cloth is not overly wet (dripping), as water may damage the equipment.

SP technicians must clean many pieces of mobile equipment, including isolation and special procedure carts. Carts must be cleaned after each use. Do not empty the inside drawers of these carts while they are in the decontamination area because doing so will expose the supplies in the carts to the area's bioburden. Carts should also be emptied before transport. The empty cart should be transported to the decontamination area and all surfaces should be cleaned inside and out. The cart should then be transported to a clean room, and restocking tasks should be performed.

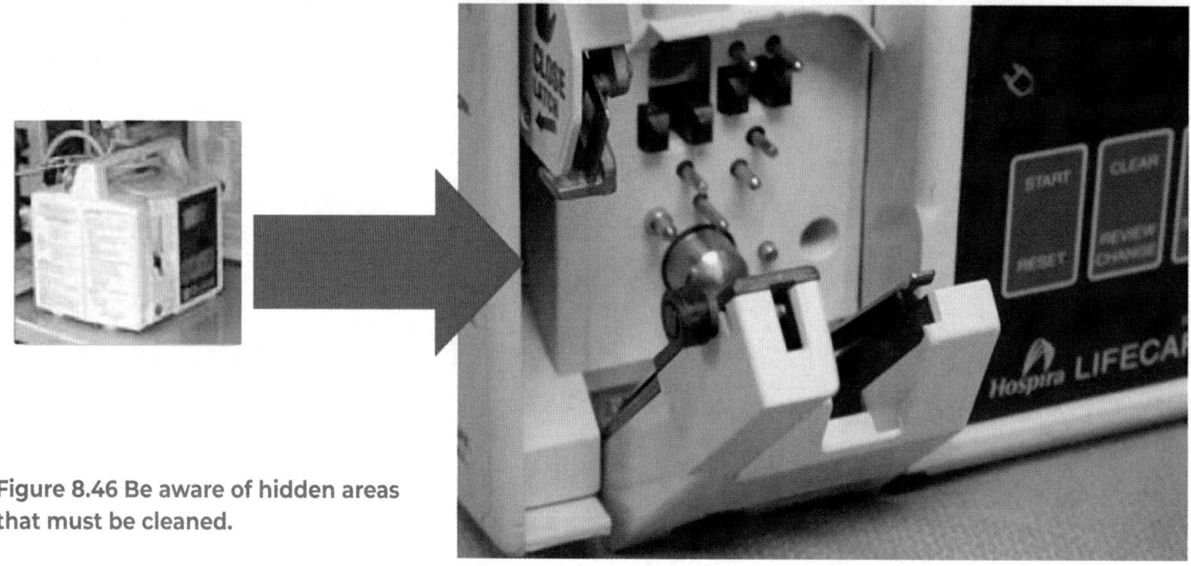

Figure 8.46 Be aware of hidden areas that must be cleaned.

Inspection

SP technicians play one of the most important roles in the next step of the decontamination process: inspection. Inspection is a crucial step in the process because it helps ensure the safety of the devices as well as employees and the patient. Each item cleaned must be carefully inspected for visible debris. If debris is detected, the item should be re-cleaned according to the manufacturer's IFU.

Quality Testing Cleaning Verification

Thorough cleaning is the foundation for disinfection and sterilization. Cleaning verification methods help demonstrate that the cleaning process is effective (see **Figure 8.47**) and are used for individual instrumentation and cleaning equipment.

Several devices, including lighted magnification, borescopes and cleaning verification tests, are available to inspect instruments for cleanliness.

Decontamination

The decontamination process involves the use of physical or chemical procedures to remove, inactivate or destroy bloodborne pathogens on an item's surface. The purpose of decontamination is to make devices safe for people who are not wearing gloves and to reduce the bioburden to make the next processing steps easier. Some instruments are safe for handling after they have been thoroughly cleaned; however, others require exposure to a microbiocidal process.

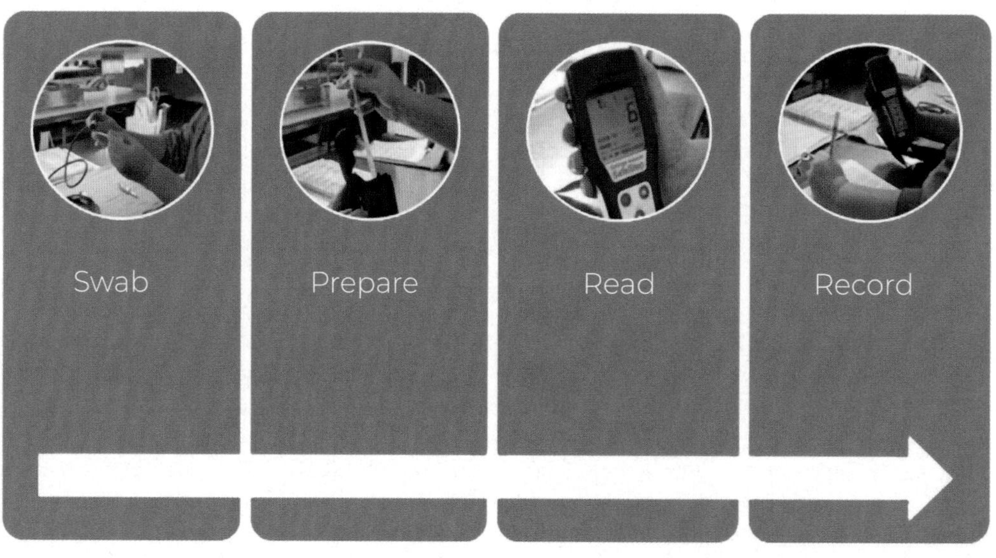

Figure 8.47 Example of cleaning verification using the adenosine triphosphate (ATP) method

CONCLUSION

Cleaning is a complex, multi-step process. The success of disinfection and sterilization processes depends on a successful cleaning process. SP technicians must understand the cleaning process for each medical device and perform it consistently to help ensure the safety of patients, visitors and healthcare personnel.

RESOURCES

Association for the Advancement of Medical Instrumentation. ANSI/AAMI ST79:2017 & 2020 Amendments A1, A2, A3, A4 (Consolidated Text) *Comprehensive guide to steam sterilization and sterility assurance in health care facilities.*

Occupational Safety and Health Administration. *Regulations Standards CFR 1910.1030, Bloodborne Pathogens.*

Association of periOperative Registered Nurses. *Guidelines for PeriOperative Practice: Instrument Cleaning.* Guidelines for PeriOperative Practice. 2022.

International Association of Healthcare Central Service Materiel Management. *Central Service Leadership Manual,* Chapter 20. 2020.

Ofstead CL, Hopkins KM, Smart AG, Brewer MK. "Droplet dispersal in decontamination areas of instrument reprocessing suites." *Am J Infect Control.* 2022;50(2):126-132. https://www.ajicjournal.org/article/S0196-6553(21)00689-1/fulltext [Open-access]

Ofstead CL, Hopkins KM, Daniels FE, Smart AG, Wetzler HP. "Splash generation and droplet dispersal in a well-designed, centralized high-level disinfection unit." *Am J Infect Control.* 2022;50(11):P1200-1207. https://www.ajicjournal.org/article/S0196-6553(22)00629-0/fulltext [Open-access]

STERILE PROCESSING TERMS

Decontamination area

Humidity

Negative pressure

Biohazardous waste

Utility water

Critical water

Biocide

Reverse osmosis (RO)

Deionized (DI) water

Distilled water

Cavitation

Electroplating

Impingement

Thermal disinfection

Emulsifier

Surfactant

Chelating agents

Toxic anterior segment syndrome (TASS)

Chapter 9

Disinfection

Learning Objectives

As a result of successfully completing this chapter, the reader will be able to:

1. Define the term disinfection and explain how it differs from sterilization
2. Explain disinfection levels as identified in the Spaulding Classification System
3. Provide basic information about the types of disinfectants commonly used in healthcare facilities
4. Identify good work practices for manual disinfection processes
5. Provide basic information about liquid chemical sterilants
6. Identify good work practices for automated disinfection processes
7. Explain disinfection quality assurance practices

INTRODUCTION

Once an item has been properly cleaned, there are some decisions to make. Is the item safe for its intended use or does it need further processing? If further processing is needed, what type of processing does it need and how can that be accomplished? (See **Figure 9.1**) Sterile Processing (SP) technicians must be able to identify the type of **bactericidal** process needed and select the method that will provide that process and perform it effectively. This chapter will provide basic information on disinfectants and disinfecting processes that are frequently used in Sterile Processing departments (SPDs).

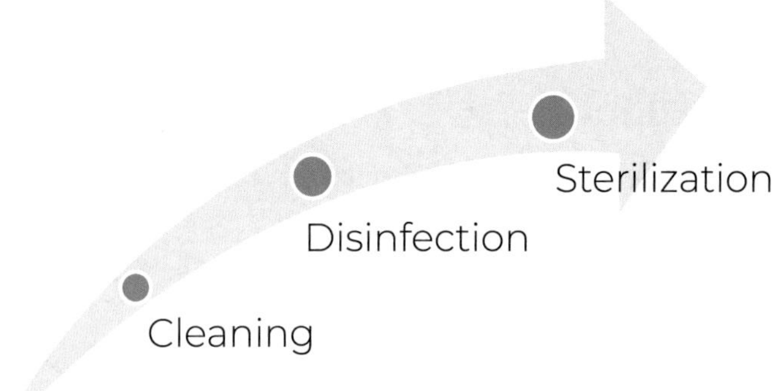

Figure 9.1 Which is needed?

INTRODUCTION TO DISINFECTANTS

The Spaulding Classification System

The selection of a **disinfectant** must be based, in part, upon the intended use of the device and the degree of **disinfection** required for that device. The **Spaulding Classification System** divides patient care items into three categories, each based on the degree of risk of infection when the items are used in patient care. The Centers for Disease Control and Prevention (CDC) and the Association for the Advancement of Medical Instrumentation (AAMI) use the Spaulding Classification System in their guidelines and standards. (See **Figure 9.2**) The three Spaulding categories are:

- Critical items – Instruments or devices introduced directly into the bloodstream or into other sterile areas of the body. Examples include surgical instruments, cardiac catheters, and implants. These items must be **sterilized** before use.

- Semi-critical items – These items come in contact with intact mucous membranes. They do not ordinarily penetrate body surfaces. Examples include non-invasive flexible fiberoptic endoscopes, endotracheal tubes, and anesthesia breathing circuits. Semi-critical items should be sterilized, if possible. However, if sterilization is not possible, the item, at a minimum, must undergo a **high-level disinfection (HLD)** process. HLD can be expected to destroy all microbial organisms, but not necessarily microbial spores.

- Non-critical items – These items usually come into direct contact with the patient's unbroken skin. Examples include crutches and countertops. These items require thorough cleaning and, in some cases, **low-level disinfection** to **intermediate-level disinfection.**

Bactericidal A substance that kills bacteria.

Disinfectant A chemical that kills most pathogenic organisms but does not kill all spores.

Disinfection The destruction of nearly all pathogenic microorganisms on an inanimate (non-living) surface.

Spaulding Classification System A system developed by Dr. E. H. Spaulding that divides medical devices into categories based on the risk of infection involved with their use.

Sterile/Sterilization Completely devoid of all living microorganisms.

High-level disinfection (HLD) The destruction of all vegetative microorganisms, but not bacterial spores.

Low-level disinfection The destruction of some vegetative forms of bacteria.

Intermediate-level disinfection The destruction of viruses, mycobacteria, fungi and vegetative bacteria (but not bacterial spores).

The Spaulding Classification System		
Device Classification	**Examples**	**Requires**
Critical – Enters sterile tissue or the vascular system	• Implants • Surgical instruments • Needles	Sterilization
Semi-critical – Touches mucous membranes, except dental	• Flexible endoscopes • Laryngoscopes • Endotracheal tubes	Sterilization, if possible; if not then high-level disinfection (HLD)
Non-critical – Touches intact skin	• Thermometers • Stethoscopes	Low-level disinfection

Figure 9.2 Spaulding Classification System

There is no single disinfectant that will work for all situations. That is why every SPD should have more than one disinfectant to choose from in the work area. SP technicians must be able to select the appropriate disinfectant for the job. To do so, a basic understanding of the different types of disinfectants is needed.

> **Caution!**
>
> Before using a chemical disinfectant, be sure to review the manufacturer's IFU. Using the correct chemical the wrong way is just as dangerous as using the wrong chemical.

SAFE WORK PRACTICES WHEN PERFORMING MANUAL DISINFECTION

No matter which disinfectant is chosen, failure to use a disinfectant properly, according to the manufacturer's instructions for use (IFU), can result in failure of the disinfection process, which puts both patients and staff at risk.

Work Area Setup

Disinfection processes should be performed only in designated areas that are separated from the area used for cleaning. The workflow should help ensure that the item(s) being processed are not recontaminated during or upon completion of the disinfection process.

Any accessories needed for the disinfection process, such as measuring devices, soaking bins and timers, should be collected prior to beginning the process. If cloths are used, they should be of clean, non-linting materials. Quality testing should be performed to ensure equipment is operating as intended. For example, automated dosing dispensers, suction irrigation devices, and automated reprocessors.

Labels

Since chemical disinfectants have different capabilities, it is important to read the product labels to ensure they are used appropriately. Check the IFU of the disinfectant and medical device(s) to be processed to ensure compatibility. (See **Figure 9.3**)

Disinfectants used in healthcare facilities are harsh chemicals. It is important to read and follow all safety precautions.

Preparation Instructions

In addition to choosing the appropriate disinfectant, there are various factors that are vital to the success of chemical disinfection. Cleaning and disinfecting chemicals cannot be mixed with other chemicals because the mixture may produce a lethal chemical. When preparing disinfectant solutions, check the label for essential preparation instructions, which include:

- The expiration date, if applicable
- Reuse-life date of the chemical, if applicable
- Appropriate concentration for use (diluted or full strength, depending on the IFU)
- Dilution or mixing requirements
- Correct temperature required for the disinfectant
- Water quality and pH requirements

Device Preparation

The device needs to be prepared for disinfection. It must be thoroughly cleaned to allow complete exposure to the disinfectant, and dried to prevent additional water from diluting

Read labels carefully

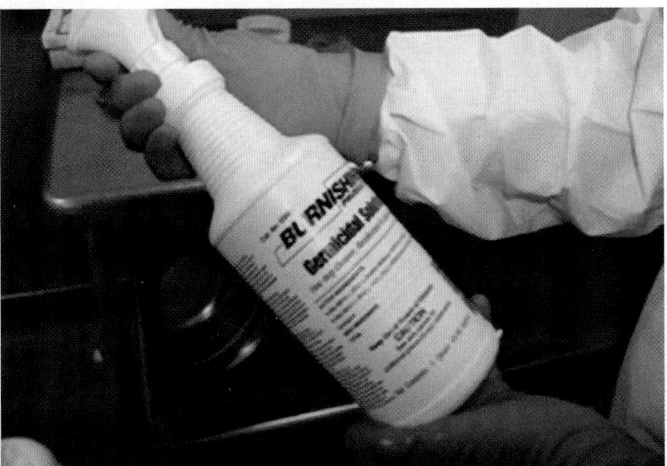

Measure for proper dilution

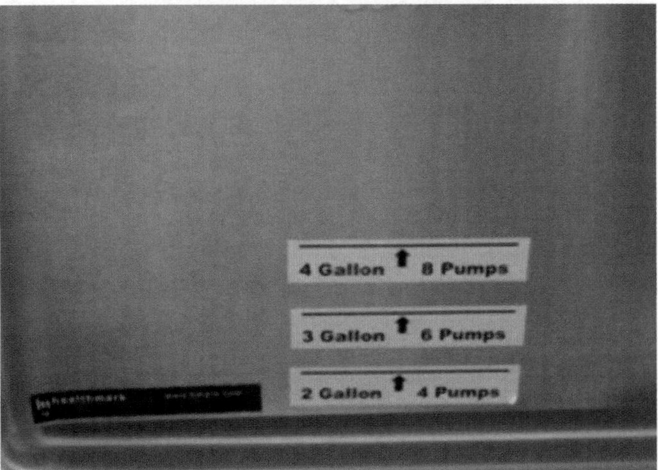

Figure 9.3 Follow IFU to achieve desired results.

the disinfectant. Multi-part devices should be disassembled to allow full contact of the disinfectant.

> **Important Safety Note**
>
> While manufacturers may combine chemicals to create a more effective disinfectant, SP technicians should never mix chemicals on their own. Some common chemicals can be lethal when combined.

Contact

Disinfectants are not effective unless they make direct contact with all surfaces of the device. Improper cleaning will leave organic matter, which prevents direct contact with the disinfectant. Lack of contact through improper application or because soil remains on a device will result in a failed disinfection process.

Direct contact may be impeded if items are not disassembled properly or if they are only partially submerged in a disinfectant soak solution. When disinfecting a lumen, care must be taken to ensure there are no air bubbles in the lumen that would prevent the disinfectant from contacting all interior surfaces of the lumen. (See **Figure 9.4**)

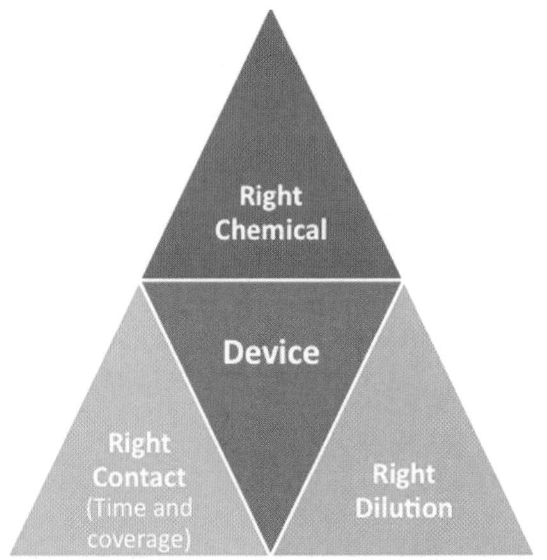

Figure 9.4 Chemical disinfection: Doing it right

Exposure Time

Exposure times vary by type and concentration of disinfectant. Many times, the term "wet contact" is stated in the IFU. This means the amount of time the device must remain wet with the disinfectant. Use a timer to ensure the proper exposure time is met.

> **What Is Wet Contact Time?**
>
> Wet contact time means that the item must remain wet with the disinfectant for the entire stated contact time. If the disinfectant evaporates or the item is allowed to dry before the total contact exposure time is met, the disinfectant must be reapplied, and the exposure time must begin again.

Rinsing

Disinfectants require a rinsing process. Critical water is preferred for non-critical items and is required for semi-critical and critical items unless sterile water is specified by the manufacturer's written IFU. Care should be taken to thoroughly rinse all surfaces according to the manufacturers' instructions.

Drying

After the cleaning and disinfection processes, items should be dried completely with clean, non-linting cloths. Lumened instruments should be dried with pressure-regulated, forced instrument air or high-efficiency particulate air (HEPA-filtered air), until no moisture is observed. Medical devices should never be stored wet because wet storage supports the growth of microorganisms and biofilms.

Storage and Transport

Following the disinfection process, items are placed into storage or transported for use. The storage area should be designated for patient-ready items and separated from the decontamination area/room. It should be clean, well-ventilated and free from dust, and devices should be stored in a manner that protects them from damage or contamination. They should be identified as being patient ready. These items should be transported in a manner that prevents contamination such as having a clean cover over them or placed in a clean container.

Containers

When using chemicals, it sometimes seems more efficient to pour chemicals from the larger, original container to a smaller, easier-to-handle container. Check with the department manager to determine if this practice is acceptable, and also check the department's procedure for labeling. All containers need to be properly labeled.

QUALITY ASSURANCE PRACTICES FOR DISINFECTION

In addition to reading and following the manufacturer's IFU when performing disinfection processes, other quality assurance practices should be in place. Those practices should help ensure that disinfection processes are performed correctly, safely and according to product-specific requirements.

Education

All technicians who perform disinfection activities should be trained and able to meet competencies for each disinfection process they perform. Each time a new product or process is introduced into the work area, training must be performed, and competencies must be completed.

Safety

Patient and employee safety is of concern when performing disinfection processes. Improperly disinfected medical devices pose a risk to patients. The harsh chemicals (and sometimes fumes) associated with chemical disinfection can pose a safety risk to SP technicians. It is important to understand the following recommendations for handling disinfectants:

- Personal protective equipment (PPE) requirements
- Environmental (ventilation) requirements
- Spill and leak procedures
- Storage requirements
- Disposal requirements

Spill Kit

When working with chemicals, safety precautions should be in place. It is a requirement of the Occupational Safety and Health Administration (OSHA) (Code of Federal Regulations OSHA, 29 CFR 1910.38) that a spill kit be available and that an emergency action plan be implemented in the event of a chemical spill. The spill plan should be for a worst-case scenario and provide instructions on how to handle a spill. The plan should also ensure employees are trained to respond appropriately. The reaction to a chemical spill depends upon the composition and volume of the chemical spilled, where the spill occurred, the resources needed and the personnel's level of training.

TYPES OF DISINFECTANTS

The term "disinfection" is a generic term used to describe a process. Within that process are products that perform at different levels. (See **Figure 9.5**)

The following is a review of common disinfectants used in SPDs and the level (type) of disinfection they are designed to provide.

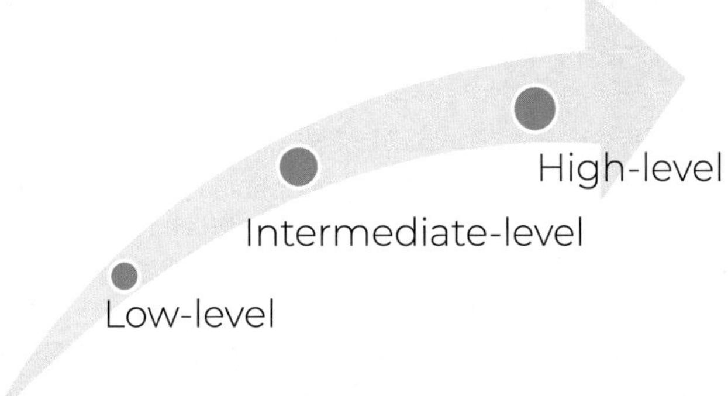

Figure 9.5 Which disinfection level is appropriate?

Low-Level and Intermediate-Level Disinfectants

Items requiring low-level or intermediate-level disinfection only come in contact with intact skin. These items usually only touch the outside of the body (this includes items like crutches and countertops). Low- and intermediate-level disinfectants may also be used on hard environmental surfaces and some mobile equipment. This group of disinfectants commonly includes quaternary ammonium compounds, alcohols, phenolics, chlorines and iodophors.

Low-level to intermediate-level disinfectants have one important thing in common: the germicidal action of each is reduced by the presence of **organic materials**. (See **Figure 9.6**)

> **Organic materials** Compounds containing oxygen, carbon and hydrogen; derived from living organisms. Organic matter in the form of serum, blood, pus, or fecal material can interfere with the activity of disinfectants.

No Soil!

The germicidal action of disinfectants is reduced by the presence of soil.

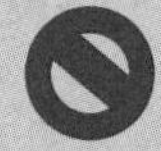

NO: Blood • Fluids • Feces • Tissue • Pus • Etc.

Figure 9.6

Quaternary Ammonium Compounds

Quaternary ammonium compounds (commonly called "quats") are low-level disinfectants. The most common chemical in most quats is benzalkonium chloride.

Quats are incompatible with soap. Soap is not recommended for use in the SP decontamination process because of the residue it leaves behind.

Some quats are absorbed by materials such as cotton and filter paper. A quat that is absorbed by cotton should not be used with cotton towels, cloths or mop heads. It is important to consult the specific quat's IFU to determine if cotton and/or paper can be used with them.

Summary of Quats
Advantages
• Bactericidal, fungicidal and virucidal against lipophilic viruses • Wetting agents with built-in detergent properties
Disadvantages
• Not sporicidal • Generally not tuberculocidal or virucidal against hydrophilic viruses unless multiple compounds are included • May be inactivated (absorbed or neutralized) by cotton or paper • Not compatible with soap • Not effective against some gram-negative organisms commonly found in hospitals • Deactivated by organic material
Uses
• Environmental sanitation of non-critical surfaces such as floors, walls and furniture • If multiple compounds are in the solution (super quat) may be used on instruments if properly rinsed • Must remain wet on surface to be disinfected six to 10 minutes (or according to the manufacturer's IFU)

Figure 9.7

Alcohol

Alcohol can be used as both an antiseptic and a disinfectant. Both ethyl and isopropyl (rubbing) alcohol have good disinfecting properties. One of the challenges when using alcohol as a disinfectant is that to achieve a reasonable level of disinfection the alcohol must remain in wet contact with the surface of the object being disinfected for a minimum of five minutes. Alcohol evaporates quickly, and maintaining wet contact for an extended period of time can be difficult. Alcohol can also act as a fixative for debris on surfaces, making the debris more difficult to remove.

Summary of Ethyl or Isopropyl Alcohol
Advantages
· Bactericidal agent against vegetative microorganisms · Relatively fast acting (five minutes or more) · No residue · Non-staining
Disadvantages
· Requires wet contact of at least five minutes to achieve a low level of disinfection · No residual activity · Volatile; flammable · Inactivated by organic material · Can dissolve lens mountings on certain optical instruments · Tends to harden and swell plastic tubing, including polyethylene · Non-sporicidal · Can be a fixative for debris on stainless steel
Uses
· To disinfect non-mobile equipment after cleaning and for patient care items such as stethoscopes · Can be used as a drying agent if approved by the device's IFU

Figure 9.8

Antiseptic or Disinfectant?

Antiseptics are used on living tissue (skin); for example, receiving an alcohol prep before an annual flu shot. Disinfectants are used on inanimate objects (for example, disinfecting a piece of equipment between uses).

Phenolics

Phenolics are intermediate-level to low-level disinfectants containing phenol. Phenolic compounds have long been the agent of choice for Environmental Services (EVS) departments. Because of the phenolic residue left after use, that residue can be reactivated later by damp mopping; however, this same residual film can become a problem when left on medical devices. For example, irritation of sensitive skin can occur after exposure to phenolic residues. Like all disinfectants, phenolics require a specific time for wet contact for maximum disinfectant effectiveness.

Stainless steel instruments should not be subjected to strong phenolics for a prolonged period of time because phenolics can be corrosive. Some plastics also react poorly to phenolics. Follow the device manufacturer's IFU for the types of materials that can withstand disinfection with phenolics.

Summary of Phenolics
Advantages
· Broad-spectrum of use: bactericidal for gram-negative and gram-positive bacteria, fungicidal and tuberculocidal; active against lipophilic viruses
· Residual activity. *Note: This can also be a disadvantage*
Disadvantages
· Not sporicidal
· Inactivated by organic material
· Corrosive to some plastics
· Copious rinsing is required to eliminate the potential for skin burns
Uses
· Environmental Services usage for walls, floors, countertops and furnishings
· Phenolics may be used in the decontamination area for disinfection of hard surfaces

Figure 9.9

Chlorine

Chlorine is an intermediate-level disinfectant that is commonly used for the treatment of water and sewage. Chlorine, a member of the halogen family, may be found in SPDs as a hypochlorite solution and is often recommended for biohazard clean-up procedures; however, chlorine is not considered a disinfectant of choice for SP due to its corrosive qualities. Metal instruments subjected to chlorine may have their finishes damaged by exposure to a chlorine solution.

Summary of Chlorine
Advantages
· Effective against gram-positive and gram-negative (vegetative) microorganisms; tuberculocidal, fungicidal and virucidal
· Fast acting
Disadvantages
· Inactivated by organic matter
· Corrosive to metals
· Non-sporicidal
· Stains fabrics, plastics and other synthetic materials
· Relatively unstable
Uses
· A 1:10 dilution of 5.25% sodium hypochloride has been recommended by the CDC for cleaning blood spills
· Must remain wet on items to be disinfected one to two-and-a-half minutes (check specific manufacturer's IFU)

Figure 9.10

Iodophors

Iodophors are buffered iodines that are also members of the halogen family. Like alcohol, iodophors are used both as antiseptics and disinfectants. The best-known and most widely used iodophor is povidone-iodine. Iodophors can stain both skin and patient equipment. Iodophors should not be used on surgical instruments.

Summary of Iodophors
Advantages
· Bactericidal, virucidal and tuberculocidal
· Rapid action against vegetative bacteria
Disadvantages
· Corrosive to metals unless combined with anti-corrosive agents when formulated
· Detrimental to some plastics
· Stains fabrics and other material
· May require long contact time to kill some fungi
Uses
· A 1:10 dilution used in skin preparations
· Disinfection of some equipment
· The corrosive nature of iodine on metals and some plastics limits its use as a primary disinfectant in Sterile Processing.
· Must remain wet on items to be disinfected for at least two minutes (check manufacturer's IFU). A dilution of 5.25% sodium hypochloride has been recommended by the CDC for cleaning blood spills
· Must remain wet on items to be disinfected one to two-and-a-half minutes (check specific manufacturer's IFU)

Figure 9.11

High-Level Disinfectants

High-level disinfectants are used to process semi-critical items that may come in contact with mucous membranes of the body. There are several types of disinfectants in this category. *Note: Manual HLD is no longer a method of choice for HLD processing. Manual HLD should only be used when an automated process is not available.*

The U.S. Food and Drug Administration (FDA) regulates high-level disinfectants and liquid chemical sterilants (LCS) used to process medical devices and surgical instruments. The FDA uses the term "liquid chemical sterilant," along with the term "high-level disinfectant" because, in some cases, the chemical can provide sterilization if the soak time is extended. This information is provided in the IFU.

Some HLD/LCS products are designed for single use, while others are designed for reuse. This information is provided in the IFU. Only HLD/LCS products labeled for reuse can be reused.

Add small activator bottle to solution

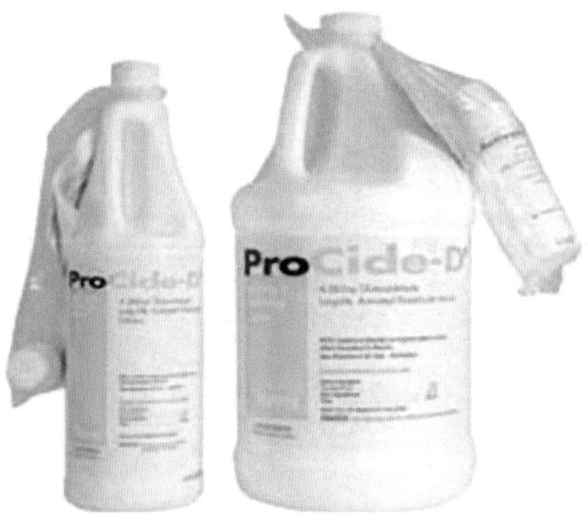

Solution changes color when activated

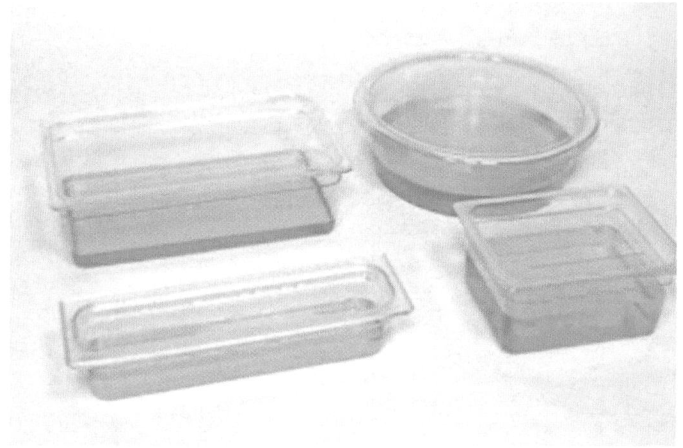

Figure 9.12 Glutaraldehyde requires activation.

Like their low-level and intermediate-level counterparts, high-level disinfectants are inactivated by organic materials; therefore, thorough cleaning is critical to successful outcomes. Medical devices should be thoroughly rinsed and flushed to remove residual debris and cleaning solutions. After rinsing, devices should be thoroughly dried using a clean, lint-free cloth or dried with instrument air or HEPA-filtered air in accordance with the device's IFU. Failing to follow the manufacturer's IFU can jeopardize the effectiveness of the disinfection process or the device's performance.

As with other disinfectants, SP technicians must understand the differences between high-level disinfectants and how to use them effectively. The following section provides some basic information about high-level disinfectants. As with all disinfectants, consult individual manufacturer's IFU before attempting to process items.

Glutaraldehyde

Glutaraldehyde is a high-level disinfectant used for semi-critical devices. Glutaraldehyde is compatible with materials used in many modern medical devices and can be used to process medical devices containing heat-sensitive materials. Glutaraldehyde is usually a clear liquid that turns color when **activated** (see **Figure 9.12**) and it has a sharp, pungent odor. It is a strong irritant to the skin, eyes and respiratory system. Nitrile or butyl gloves and face/eye protection should be used when working with glutaraldehyde.

> **Activated (activation)** Process by which a solution is combined with an activating chemical before use. Glutaraldehyde, for example, must be mixed with an activating solution before use.

Following immersion in a glutaraldehyde solution, instructions for rinsing items should be carefully followed to ensure the chemical is completely removed. Care must be taken to ensure that the item is not recontaminated.

Glutaraldehyde should be used in a separate, designated area, apart from the decontamination area. Any room where glutaraldehyde is used should be well-ventilated, with a minimum of 10 air exchanges per hour. When a dedicated area is not available, glutaraldehyde disinfection may be performed at an enclosed workstation. These self-contained workstations manage air flow and reduce exposure to fumes. **Figure 9.13** shows some examples of these stations.

Unused glutaraldehyde solution should be stored in a cool, secure location and in tightly closed, properly marked containers that contain the activation date.

Glutaraldehyde-based products can be used in automated or manual HLD processes. Most glutaraldehyde-based disinfectants are labeled for reuse for 14 to 28 days. During the recommended reuse period, the efficacy of the glutaraldehyde in the solution should be tested with test strips recommended by the manufacturer. If the solution falls below its **minimum effective concentration (MEC)** level, it should be discarded, regardless of how many days the solution has been in use.

Glutaraldehyde vapors increase whenever the solution is agitated such as when it is poured into or dumped out of a soaking bin. Exposure levels for SP technicians during disposal can be reduced by adding a glutaraldehyde neutralizing agent to the solution prior to disposal. Consult state and local requirements and the manufacturer's IFU for proper disposal measures, ventilation requirements and potential exposure monitoring.

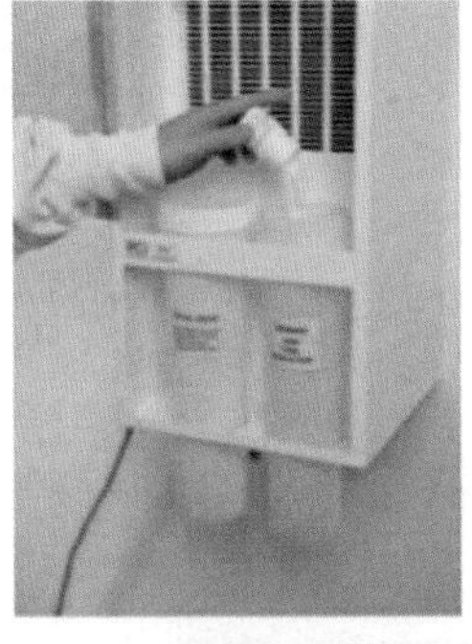
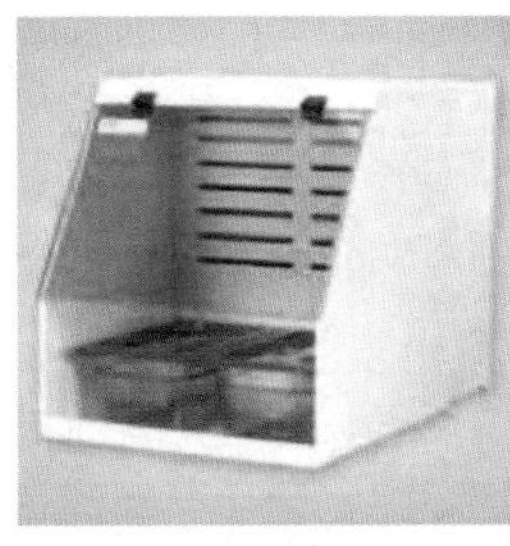
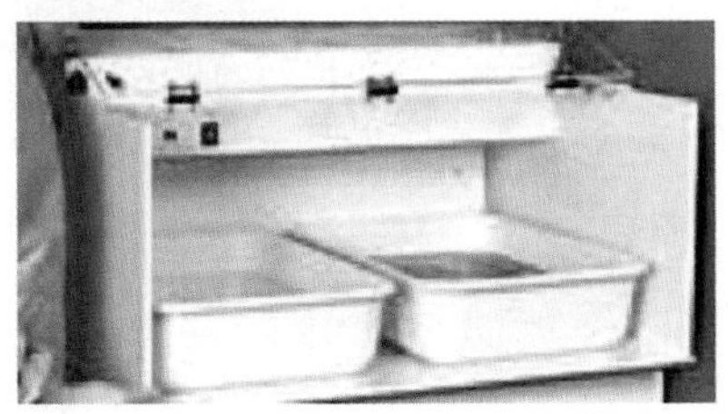
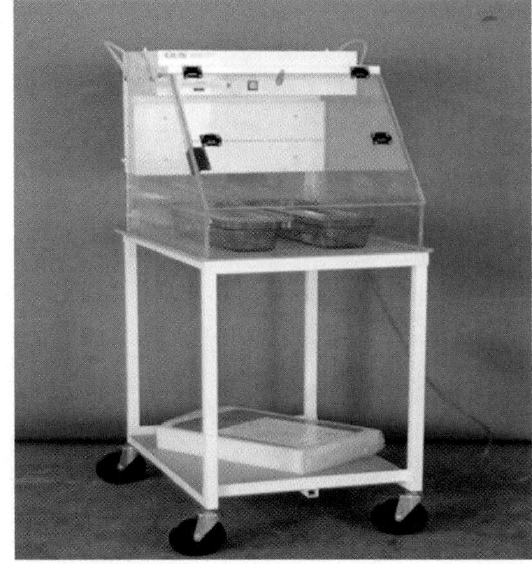

Figure 9.13 Examples of enclosed workstations for glutaraldehyde disinfection

Minimum effective concentration (MEC) The percentage concentration of the active ingredient in a disinfectant or chemical sterilant that is the minimum concentration at which the chemical meets all its label claims for activity against specific microorganisms.

Summary of Glutaraldehyde
Advantages
· Kills vegetative bacteria (within two minutes) · Bactericidal (gram-positive and gram-negative), tuberculocidal, fungicidal, virucidal and sporicidal. *[For sterilization (killing spores), the soak time is six to 10 hours. The manufacturer's recommendations should be consulted.]*
Disadvantages
· Noxious odors; good ventilation is required · Unstable (14- or 28-day product life) · Dilution of product reduces the activity necessary for high-level disinfection
Uses
· Semi-critical items such as laryngoscope blades, flexible endoscopes, etc.

Figure 9.14

Ortho-Phthalaldehyde

Ortho-phthalaldehyde (commonly called OPA) is a high-level disinfectant that provides a fast and effective way to disinfect a wide range of devices. Before processing any urological instrumentation, consult the IFU; OPA has been associated with anaphylactic-like reactions in bladder cancer patients.

The OPA solution may be used and reused within the limitations indicated by the manufacturer (for up to 14 days). The efficacy of the OPA solution should be tested with test strips recommended by the manufacturer before each use. If the solution falls below its MEC level, it should be discarded, regardless of how many days the solution has been in use.

Following immersion in OPA solution, instructions for rinsing items should be carefully followed to ensure the chemical is completely removed. Care must be taken to ensure that the item is not recontaminated.

Summary of OPA
Advantages
· Solution is compatible with a wide range of endoscopes and other medical devices · Requires no activation or mixing · 14-day reuse life · Can be discarded down facility drains in accordance with local regulations
Disadvantages
· Does not have a sterilant label claim
Uses
· Semi-critical item such as laryngoscope blades and flexible fiberoptic endoscopes

Figure 9.15

Hydrogen Peroxide

Hydrogen peroxide is a broad-spectrum high-level disinfectant that is available in different concentrations. As with other high-level disinfectants, hydrogen peroxide efficacy must be monitored by regularly testing the MEC. Follow the manufacturer's IFU for specific instructions.

Summary of Hydrogen Peroxide
Advantages
· Broad-spectrum HLD. Kills bacteria and viruses, including norovirus, rotavirus, RSV, MRSA and TB · Can be used as a sterilant at the right concentrations
Disadvantages
· Corrosive to some materials
Uses
· Disinfection of hard and soft surfaces

Figure 9.16

Peracetic Acid

This chemical achieves HLD in five minutes at room temperature. Some dilutions are designed to be used in a manufacturer-specific automated endoscope reprocessor (AER) as a sterilant only. Peracetic acid is compatible with many materials, it is also known to be corrosive, users must check with the device manufacturer to determine material compatibility. Follow the manufacturer's IFU for specific instructions.

Summary of Peracetic Acid
Advantages
· Broad spectrum HLD · May be used as a sterilant in the appropriate AER · Compatible with many materials
Disadvantages
· Corrosive to some materials
Uses
· HLD of laryngoscope blades, endoscopes

Figure 9.17

ACHIEVING DISINFECTION USING MECHANICAL PROCESSES

Mechanical HLD processes are the preferred method over manual processes because they are consistent and reduce errors related to human factors, while also reducing the risk for chemical exposure. Mechanical HLD involves placing the cleaned medical device into a mechanical system as specified by the manufacturer's written IFU and selecting the appropriate processing cycle. Mechanical processing equipment can be semi-automatic or fully automatic. They often provide documentation of the cycle, which should be maintained.

Washer-Disinfectors

The most common mechanical disinfection process is the one carried out in washer-disinfectors. These automated washers

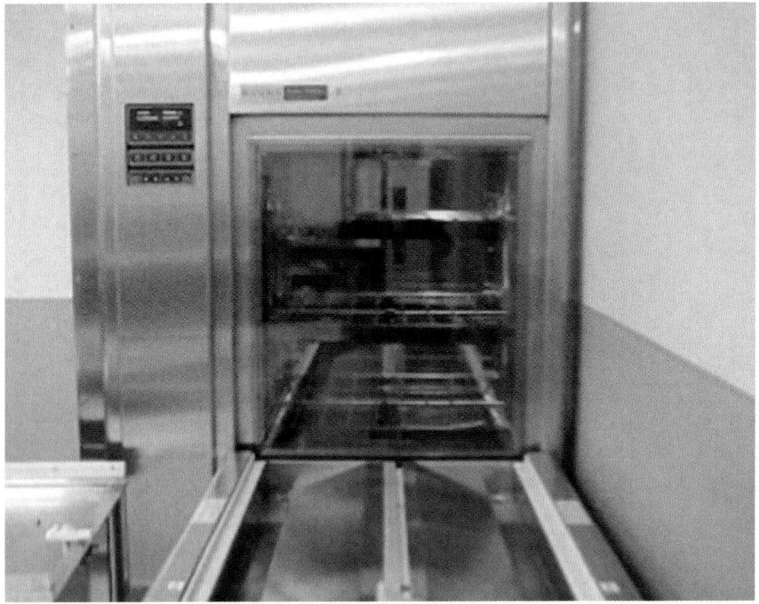

Figure 9.18 Terminal disinfection uses heat to disinfect medical devices.

provide a cleaning process followed by a thermal disinfection process. Thermal disinfection uses heat to reduce the number of microorganisms on items such as surgical instruments and utensils. (See **Figure 9.18**) Water temperature is the key source of disinfection in any automatic washer that claims to provide thermal disinfection. The exposure time and temperature used to achieve thermal disinfection differs by brand of washer. Check the manufacturer's IFU and the washer operator's manual for specific information.

Pasteurizers

Pasteurization equipment provides disinfection at water temperatures of 150°F to 170°F (65°C to 77°C). The temperature is maintained for a minimum of 30 minutes of exposure to the medical devices. Items must be able to withstand immersion in solution and be thoroughly cleaned prior to placing them in a pasteurizing unit. Water temperature and exposure time must be closely monitored. **Figure 9.19** is an example of a pasteurizer.

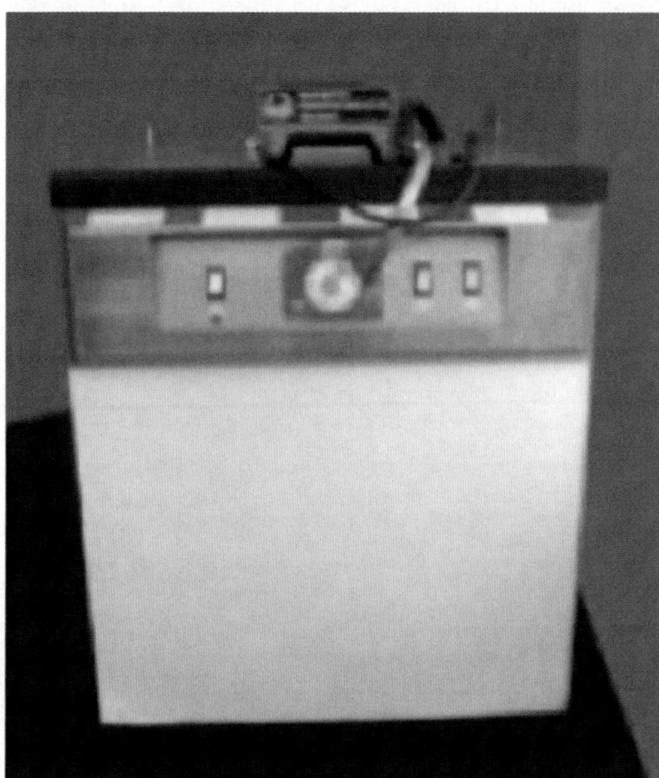

Figure 9.19 Pasturizers provide thermal disinfection using heated water.

Automated Endoscope Reprocessors

Automatic endoscope reprocessors (AERs) make the process of disinfecting flexible fiber optic endoscopes and some transesophageal echocardiography (TEE) probes simpler and safer. (See **Figure 9.20**)

AERs offer several advantages over manual processing. First, they reduce personnel exposure to the HLD disinfectant and its vapors. Their use may also increase quality assurance by providing consistent processes and documenting several cycle parameters.

Advantages of most AERs include:

- Consistent exposure to the cleaning agent
- Timed contact with the liquid chemical disinfectant
- Continuous movement of the high-level disinfectant
- Use of an air flush cycle to remove excess moisture
- Use of copious and consistent amounts of rinse water
- Documentation of the cycle parameters

Endoscope design limitations create the need for some manual reprocessing steps. Since most AERs do not completely dry endoscopes, additional drying is required after cycle completion. Refer to the AER's operating manual for information about limitations of automated cycles.

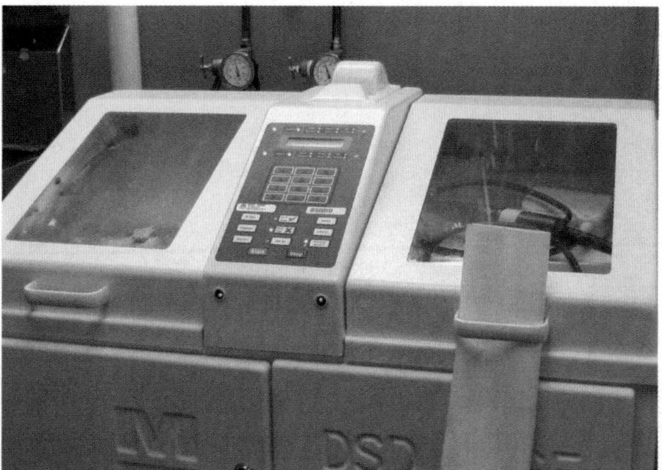

Figure 9.20

When using an AER:

- Follow the endoscope manufacturer's IFU for proper manual cleaning prior to placing the endoscope in an AER.
- Use the correct tubing and adapters and follow the manufacturer's instructions to connect the endoscope to the AER.
- Place valves and other removable parts in the AER, if possible.
- Follow the manufacturer's IFU for the types of disinfectants and their proper use.
- Set the AER for the recommended cycle time.

Liquid Chemical Sterilant Processing Systems

A liquid chemical sterilant (LCS) processing system utilizes a specific type of sterilant concentrate as recommended in the system's IFU. This type of processor provides a validated mechanical liquid sterilization system. Specialized tubing and adaptors are available to connect specific lumened items to the system so the required sterilant and rinse water reach all surfaces and angles of the device. Critical items, such as bronchoscopes, that undergo LCS are used immediately after processing. Critical devices that are not used immediately should be processed again when removed from storage before use.

Probe Processors

Probes are medical devices that are used in body cavities or that may have contact with non-intact skin. Some examples include transvaginal ultrasound probes, transrectal ultrasound probes and transesophageal echocardiography (TEE) probes. These probes are classified as intermediate-risk items because they come in contact with intact mucous membranes. Unlike flexible endoscopes, these probes are not usually fully immersible; however, as with flexible endoscopes, they can be processed either manually or mechanically.

The mechanical probe processors available are designed to perform HLD on probes. These systems use a high-level disinfectant where adequate concentrations can be monitored using an indicator, along with a printout or digital record to show the efficacy of the cycle.

Removing HLD Items from Processing Equipment

After items have undergone HLD/LCS, they should be handled in a manner that prevents contamination and damage. PPE should be removed, hand hygiene should be performed, and clean, non-latex gloves should be donned prior to handling the endoscope/probe. Carefully dry the device and place it in a transport device for immediate delivery or place the device into storage.

Storage

Proper storage of items after HLD/LCS is important to ensure the items are safe for patient use. Semi-critical devices like gastroscopes should be stored in an approved cabinet that is clean, well-ventilated and dust-free in order to keep them dry and prevent exposure to potentially hazardous microbial contamination. Endoscopes should be stored in a manner that protects them from damage or contamination, and disinfected items should be completely dry when placed into storage. Each endoscope should be identified as being patient-ready, as it distinguishes clean and disinfected items from non-processed items.

The storage time at each facility differs; therefore, the policy and procedure should specify the amount of time an HLD/LCS item can be in storage before reprocessing.

Transportation of HLD/LCS Devices

To protect the endoscope from contamination when removing HLD/LCS items from storage, the SP technician should perform hand hygiene and don (put on) new, clean, non-latex gloves. The processed item should be identified as clean and protected from contamination and damage.

QUALITY ASSURANCE TESTING FOR HIGH-LEVEL DISINFECTANTS

High-level disinfectants are much more complex chemicals than low- to intermediate-level disinfectants, and the items processed in these chemicals are used in semi-critical areas of the body. It is important to monitor these chemicals to ensure they are performing as expected and to document the results of that monitoring.

Minimum Effective Concentration Testing

To determine if the high-level disinfectant can be reused, it is important to test the solution with a chemical indicator. The disinfectants must be tested prior to each use, and the results must be clearly documented. Chemical indicators (CIs) are developed to be used for specific products. Be certain to use the correct indicator for the solution being tested. **Figure 9.21** provides an example of a chemical test strip. Follow specific manufacturer testing protocol and carefully document all MEC testing. **Figure 9.22** provides an example of an MEC testing log sheet.

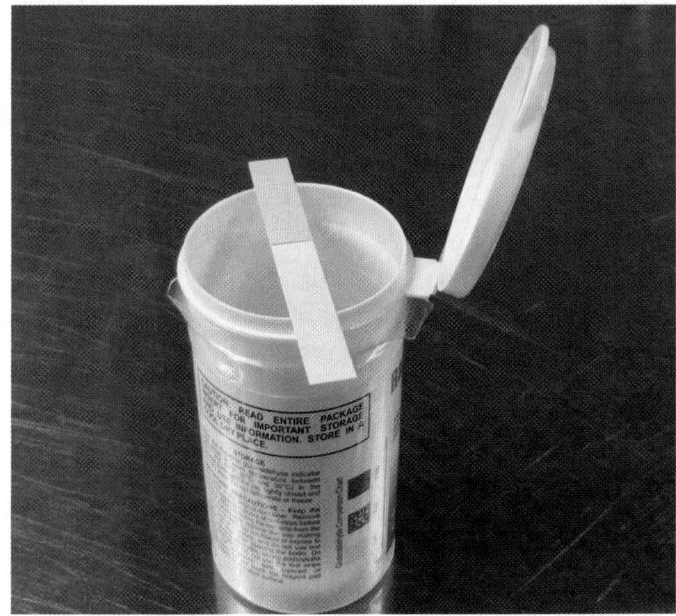

Figure 9.21

Location/Dept.		High-Level Disinfectant			Equipment		
Warning: Do not use solution beyond its stated reuse life or below the designated MEC							
Date solution opened	Date solution expires	Date test strips expire	Test date	Test time	Test results + = Pass - = Fail	Tested by (Initials)	Comments

Figure 9.22 Example of a high-level disinfectant MEC testing log sheet

Date/time of test	Patient ID	Physician/ procedure	Items processed (include serial numbers)	Technician who cleaned items	Technician performing HLD	HLD solution	Expiration date of high-level disinfectant	Test strip quality test results	MEC test results	HLD equipment used	Verification of rinsing (tech initials if manually disinfected)	Comments

Figure 9.23 HLD log sheet

Documentation

In addition to documenting the high-level disinfectant's MEC, concise documentation must be kept to enable tracking of the disinfected items to the patient receiving the items. A manual or computerized record should be maintained when using HLD. Documentation should at least contain:

- Lot number of the HLD process, including the AER or soak basin number
- Items being disinfected, including quantities and device serial numbers, if applicable
- Patient name or identifier
- Physician's name and procedure
- HLD solution information, including activation or dilution date and the last date the solution may be used (unless MEC efficacy testing fails before that date)
- Exposure time and temperature, if manually soaking
- Date and time of the process
- Technician identification
- MEC test strip results

Figure 9.23 provides an example of a HLD log sheet. *Note: It is not always necessary to have both an MEC and HLD log sheet. The documentation may be combined on a single document, as long as all required information is documented.*

CONCLUSION

Performing any successful disinfection process is much more difficult than it may appear. Careful attention to detail from the initial cleaning process through the completion of the disinfection process is critical to achieve desired results. SP technicians must select the appropriate disinfectant designed for the job they want to do, prepare the items properly and use the disinfectant as directed to ensure the safety of staff and patients. The success or failure of any disinfection process depends on the knowledge of the SP technician and their attention to detail. (See **Figure 9.24**)

Disinfectants:
• Are not all the same.
• Must be appropriate for the job.
• Are only effective when used accordingly to direction.

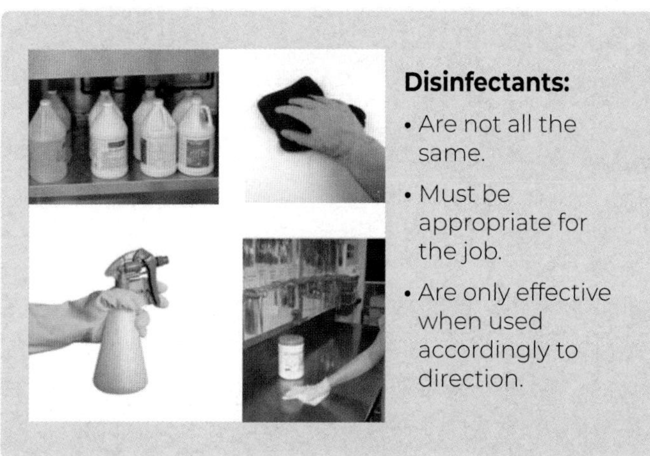

Figure 9.24

RESOURCES

Block S., McDonnell, G. *Disinfection, Sterilization and Preservation, 6th Ed.* 2020.

Society of Gastroenterology Nurses and Associates. *Guideline for Use of High-Level Disinfectants & Sterilants for Reprocessing Flexible Gastrointestinal Endoscopes.* 2017.

Centers for Disease Control and Prevention. *Guideline for Disinfection and Sterilization in Healthcare Facilities.* 2008.

Association of periOperative Registered Nurses (AORN). *Guidelines for PeriOperative Practice: Guideline for Manual Chemical High-Level Disinfection.* Guidelines for PeriOperative Practice. 2022.

AORN. Guidelines for PeriOperative Practice: *The Guideline for Environmental Cleaning.* Guidelines for PeriOperative Practice. 2022.

ANSI/AAMI ST58:2013 (R2018) *Chemical sterilization and high-level disinfection in health care facilities.*

ANSI/AAMI ST91:2021 *Flexible and semi-rigid endoscope processing in health care facilities.*

STERILE PROCESSING TERMS

Bactericidal

Disinfectant

Disinfection

Spaulding Classification System

Sterile/sterilization

High-level disinfection

Low-level disinfection

Intermediate-level disinfection

Organic materials

Activated (activation)

Minimum effective concentration (MEC)

Chapter 10

Surgical Instrumentation

Learning Objectives

As a result of successfully completing this chapter, the reader will be able to:

1. Discuss the importance of surgical instruments and the role of the Sterile Processing technician in instrument care and handling
2. Review basic steps in the surgical instrument manufacturing process
3. Define basic categories of surgical instruments based upon their functions and identify the points of inspection
4. Identify common chemical solutions that can damage stainless steel instruments
5. Explain procedures to test instruments for sharpness
6. Review instrument marking methods used for faster and easier device identification
7. Identify common errors when assembling instruments and how to avoid them

INTRODUCTION

Approximately 310 million major surgeries are performed each year, with 40 to 50 million of those procedure performed in the U.S. Ambulatory surgery centers and clinics significantly increase the total number of procedures performed in the U.S. Add in procedures from dental centers and other facilities, and it is easy to see that literally billions of surgical instruments are processed in the U.S. annually. Each of these devices has the potential to cause harm to a patient. (See **Figure 10.1**)

Sterile Processing (SP) technicians are responsible for helping ensure that instruments needed for each procedure are safe, functional and available when needed. To reach this critical goal, it is essential that SP technicians properly clean, decontaminate, package and sterilize instruments. It is also critical they understand how to identify, inspect and test these devices. SP technicians must also ensure that instrument sets and trays are complete and neatly organized to enable the end user to find instruments easily.

It is impossible for any technician to identify every instrument in existence; however, skilled technicians can identify the vast majority of instruments in their facility's inventory. This chapter provides some background information about common instruments and instrumentation-related processes applicable to most facilities.

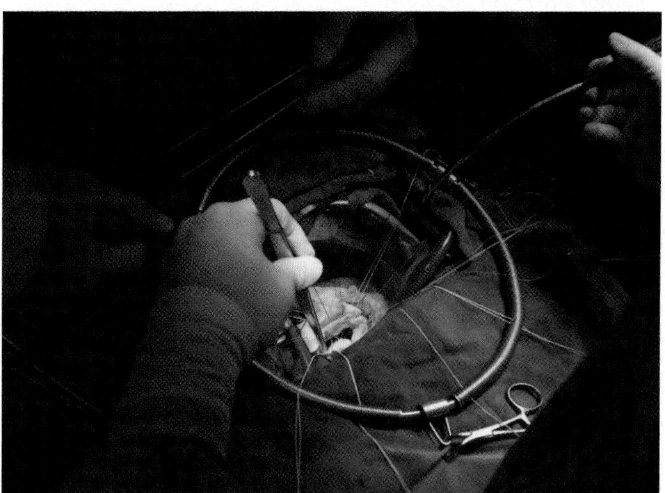

Figure 10.1

THE IMPORTANT ROLE OF INSTRUMENT SELECTION AND INSPECTION

Although many instruments may appear similar, they may have very different functions. Each is designed to perform in a specific situation. Placing the wrong instrument into a set can cause serious problems during a surgical procedure. Many instruments come in various sizes. Placing the wrong size instrument in a set may have the same effect as placing the wrong instrument in the set.

While identifying and selecting the correct instrument for each set is crucial, knowing how to inspect the instrument is just as important. Placing dull scissors or forceps with a missing tooth into a set, for example, can cause delays in the procedure and may also harm the patient. Loose or damaged parts can fall into a patient during a procedure, potentially causing injury to the patient. Each set must be functional, complete and neat. (See **Figure 10.2**)

Inspecting devices for cleanliness is also important. Instruments may appear clean on the outside, but careful inspection of the entire instrument may show that it was not properly cleaned. Instrument assembly is another vital role of the SP technician. When an instrument tray or set is completed by the SP technician, it will not be checked again until it reaches the point of use. At that point, errors—such as defective or missing instruments—can cause serious problems.

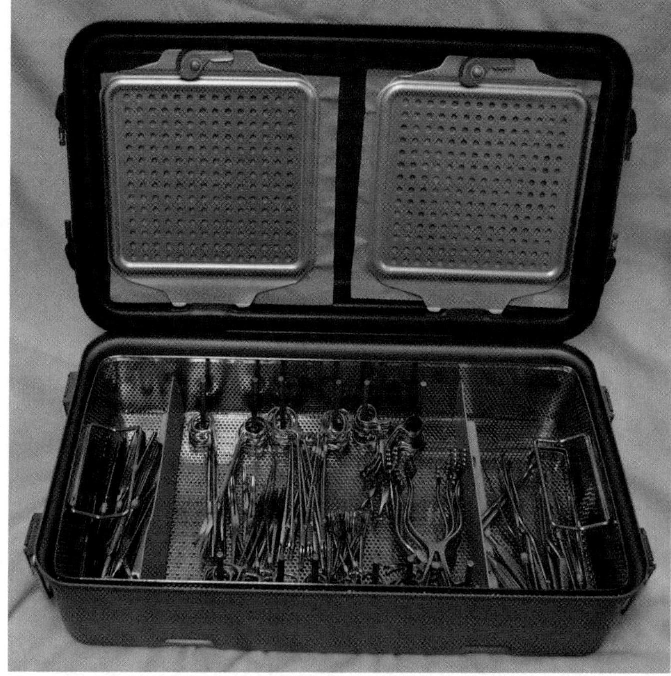

Figure 10.2 Proper instrument set assembly is critical for positive outcomes.

Some Basic Questions

Watching an experienced instrument assembly technician work may create the impression that the job is an easy one; however, that is not at all the case. Assembly technicians must know the instruments they handle. They must be able to identify them, identify quality issues, test them as necessary, correctly prepare them for the sterilization process and prioritize to ensure that instruments are ready when needed.

Those outcomes begin before the assembly process as technicians learn about the instruments they handle. There are several common questions that instrument assembly technicians ask when they begin working with instruments. Knowing the answers to those questions can help establish a good starting point for instrument care and handling. Some key questions may include:

Where do instruments come from?

Physicians identify the specific instruments needed to perform various procedures. Most instruments are purchased by the healthcare facility and maintained by SP. Some instruments are sent to the facility on loan for a specific surgery and must be returned to the vendor after use.

Why must all instrument requirements be so exacting?

The human body is very complex. Surgeons need exactly the right instrument to perform specific functions. Devices that appear similar can be used for very different procedures or purposes.

How do instruments get their names?

Many instruments get their names from the part of the anatomy where they were designed to be used. Instruments are sometimes named after the surgeon who invented them. The Bookwalter retractor, for example, is named after its inventor, Dr. John Bookwalter. Other common examples of instruments named after surgeons include Debakey and Mayo.

Do all healthcare facilities have the same instruments?

No. The type of instruments that a facility has will be determined by the types of procedures performed and by surgeon preference. Instruments also vary by manufacturer, so facilities may have instruments with the same names but different manufacturers.

How are instruments introduced into the facility?

Instruments usually enter the facility under three specific processes. Most instruments are purchased by the healthcare facility and maintained by SP. Some instruments are sent to the facility on loan for a specific surgery and must be returned to the vendor after use. Other instruments are owned by the vendor and left at the facility as consignment instruments.

Why are instruments so expensive?

Surgical instruments are precision tools. Manufacturing surgical instruments is very labor-intensive process. Most instruments are made using a combination of machine and hand labor. Fine details, such as sharpening, inspection and other steps, are performed by hand. The combination of materials used and labor costs makes instrument production expensive.

In this era of high technology, SP technicians may imagine that instruments are stamped out on a high-speed assembly line, packaged, and then shipped to the customer; however, this is not the case. The manufacturing process requires time-consuming, hands-on labor from highly skilled professionals.

THE INSTRUMENT MANUFACTURING PROCESS

Selecting Materials

The study of the surgical instrument manufacturing process begins by considering the raw materials used to create them. Most are produced from **stainless steel**; however, other materials, such as titanium, copper and silver, are also widely used.

Stainless steel can, in fact, stain, spot and rust; therefore, the more appropriate name is "stain-resistant." Proper care will ensure that a stainless instrument performs as it should and lasts a long time.

Several types of stainless steel are used to produce surgical instruments. One type (400 series stainless steel) is hard and used when sharp cutting edges are needed. Instruments produced with 400 series steel include **scissors**, **osteotomes**, **chisels**, **rongeurs**, **forceps**, **hemostatic forceps** and **needle holders**. This hardened steel is known as **martensitic stainless steel**.

Stainless steel An alloy of steel with chromium and sometimes another element, such as nickel or molybdenum, that is highly resistant to rusting and ordinary corrosion.

Scissors Surgical instruments used to cut, incise and/or dissect tissue.

Osteotomes Chisel-like instruments used to cut or shave bone.

Chisels Wedge-shaped instruments used to cut or shape bone.

Rongeurs Surgical instruments used to cut or bite away at bone and tissue.

Forceps Instruments used for grasping, holding firmly or exerting traction upon objects.

Hemostatic forceps Surgical instruments used to control the flow of blood.

Needle holders Surgical instruments designed to drive suture needles to close or rejoin a wound or surgical site. Also known as needle drivers.

Martensitic stainless steel This metal is also known as 400 series stainless steel. It is magnetic and may be heat-hardened.

The second most popular steel used to manufacture surgical instruments is 300 series stainless steel. While it offers high corrosion resistance, this material doesn't provide the hardness properties of its 400 series counterpart; therefore, it is more workable and malleable. Instruments produced with 300 series stainless steel include **retractors, cannulas, rib spreaders** and **suction devices**. This softer type of steel is called **austenitic stainless steel**.

Retractors Surgical instruments primarily used to move tissues and organs to keep the surgical site exposed throughout surgery.

Cannulas Surgical instruments with a hollow barrel (or lumen) through their center. Cannulas are often inserted for drainage.

Rib spreaders A retractor used to expose the chest.

Suction devices Surgical instruments used to extract blood and other fluids from a surgical site.

Austenitic stainless steel Also known as 300 series stainless steel. It is non-magnetic, cannot be heat-hardened and is more corrosion-resistant than martensitic stainless steel.

Manufacturing Steps

The next step in manufacturing a surgical instrument is forging the material to create a stamp of its rough outline from a heated bar of stainless steel. (See **Figure 10.3**) The heating and cooling process used to create an instrument is very important because good forging produces good instruments. Most high-quality forgings come from mills in Germany, but forgings also come from Japan, Pakistan, Malaysia, France and Sweden. After the forging is completed, the instrument must be ground and milled and have the excess steel removed. Some instruments require more than 20 milling operations to create the male and female halves and the cutting of **serrations** and **ratchets**.

Serrations Parallel grooves in the jaws of surgical instruments.

Ratchet The part of a surgical instrument that "locks" the handles in place.

In today's instrument manufacturing environment, there is more reliance on machines than in years past. Despite technical advances, however, there is still a significant amount of the milling process that must be done by hand. Instrument manufacturers perform hundreds of quality checks and finishing applications to every instrument during the manufacturing process to ensure quality.

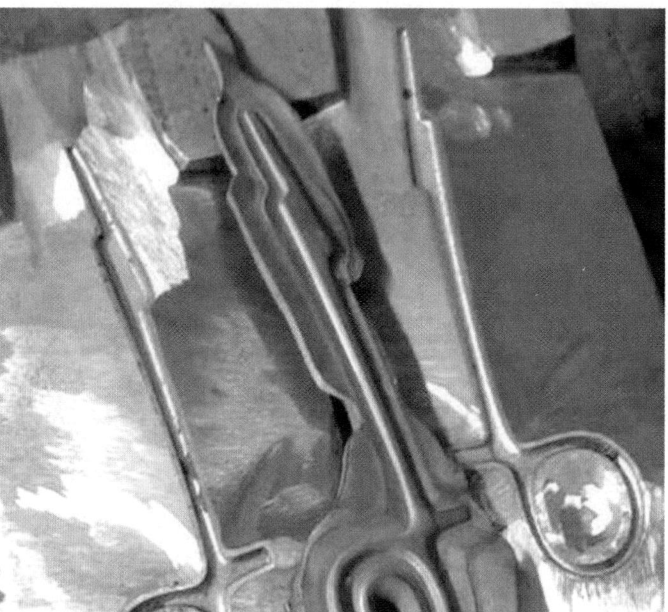

Figure 10.3

Upon completion of the assembly process, instruments undergo a final heating procedure, called tempering. After tempering, the instruments are polished. Polishing is necessary to achieve a smooth finish, which ultimately determines the final appearance or finish of the instrument. Surgical instruments may be shiny (mirror finish) or may have a matte or satin finish (gray-colored surface that does not reflect light). (See **Figure 10.4**) Both finishes are widely accepted and create a smooth surface; however, the mirror finish is smoother and tends to stain less frequently.

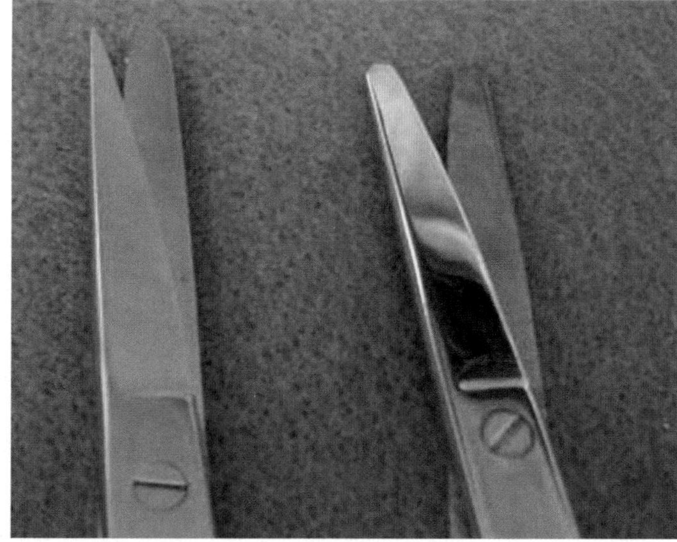

Figure 10.4

Next, the passivation layer is applied. **Passivation** uses nitric acid (HNO_3) to remove all of the iron content still found on the outside layer of the instrument. The removal of this iron helps build a protective outside layer of chromium oxide (Cr_2O_3). This layer is highly resistant to corrosion and continues to build up throughout the instrument's life. The passivation layer may become damaged when the instrument is abused by using abrasive cleaners, saline and chemicals not approved for use by the manufacturer. The instrument is then ready for final inspection where it will be carefully examined. Ratchets, tips, scissor blades, serrations, **box locks** and spot welds must be tested. Finally, the instrument is ready to be etched with the company name and catalog number. Acid chemical, stamping and lasers are some methods used for this purpose.

Passivation A chemical process applied during instrument manufacturing that provides a corrosion-resistant finish by forming a thin, transparent oxide film.

Box locks Point where the two jaws or blades of an instrument connect and pivot.

The surgical instrument manufacturing process is lengthy and detailed and requires a significant amount of experience, skill and craftsmanship. A typical manufacturing cycle—from forging to finished instrument—usually takes up to six weeks.

THE INSTRUMENT WORKSTATION

The first step in instrument inspection begins before the instruments are identified and inspected. Instrument technicians must have a workstation that includes the tools and supplies needed to properly identify, inspect, assemble and package instruments for sterilization. The area should be clean, well-lit, large enough to handle instruments comfortably and contain all the tools and supplies needed to carry out those functions, including:

Information – Each instrument must have instructions for identification, inspection, testing (if required) assembly, sterilization, packaging and any special instructions the assembly technician must be aware of when completing the specific set or tray. That information is contained in the instrument instructions for use (IFU) and may also be contained in the instrument computer system or manual count sheets. Technicians must always follow this information.

Inspection tools – Instruments require devices and/or supplies to carry out the inspection process. That may include lighted magnification devices, borescopes, specific testing supplies as specified in the instruments' IFU. For example, scissors testing materials, index cards, plastic dowels, etc.

Devices that facilitate sterilization and protect instruments – These devices can help ensure that the sterilant can reach all surfaces of the instruments and protect the instruments from damage. Stringers and tip protectors are examples of such items.

Workstations must be kept clean and free from contamination, dust and lint. This can be accomplished with routine cleaning and hand hygiene. *Note: Assembly technicians must take precautions to reduce the level of contamination in the area by keeping items, such as personal electronics, purses or bags, food and drink, and any personal items that can transmit bacteria, away from the workstation.*

Contamination must be kept to a minimum. Occasionally, when inspecting instruments for cleanliness, a soiled instrument will be identified. Those instruments must be returned to the decontamination area for cleaning. They should not be cleaned at the assembly workstation. After a soiled instrument is discovered, the instrument station should be cleaned to help reduce the risk of cross-contamination.

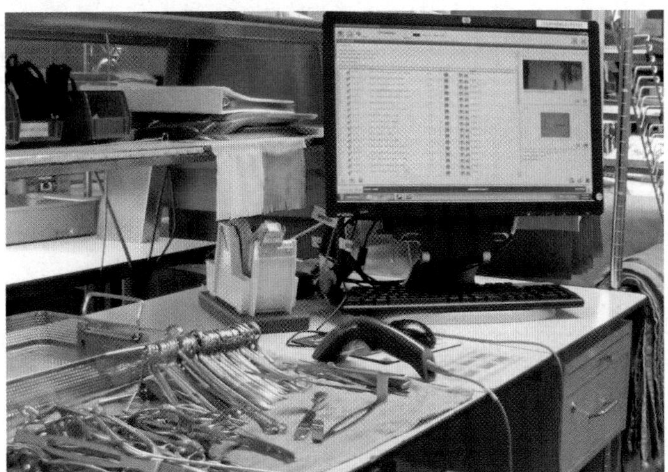

Figure 10.5 A clean and organized workstation sets the stage for an organized set.

CLASSIFICATION AND OVERVIEW OF SURGICAL INSTRUMENTS

Surgical instruments are designed for a specific surgical purpose. Injury to the patient and destruction of or damage to the instrument can occur when the incorrect instrument is used. For example, one might incorrectly pull a pin using a needle holder instead of a pin puller or a pair of pliars, which can damage the needle holder.

Hemostatic Forceps

The primary function of hemostatic forceps is to control the flow of blood. To properly inspect and test surgical instruments, SP technicians must know the anatomy and points of inspection of the devices and how to measure them. **Figures 10.6** and **10.7** show examples of how to measure hemostatic forceps. This will enable SP technicians to properly and efficiently assemble instrument sets.

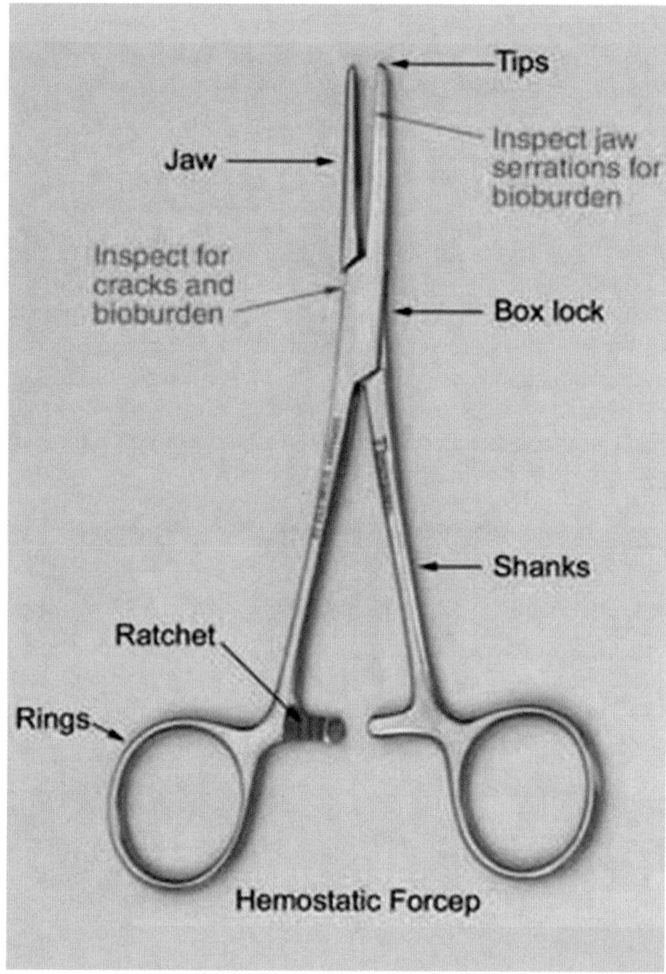

Figure 10.6

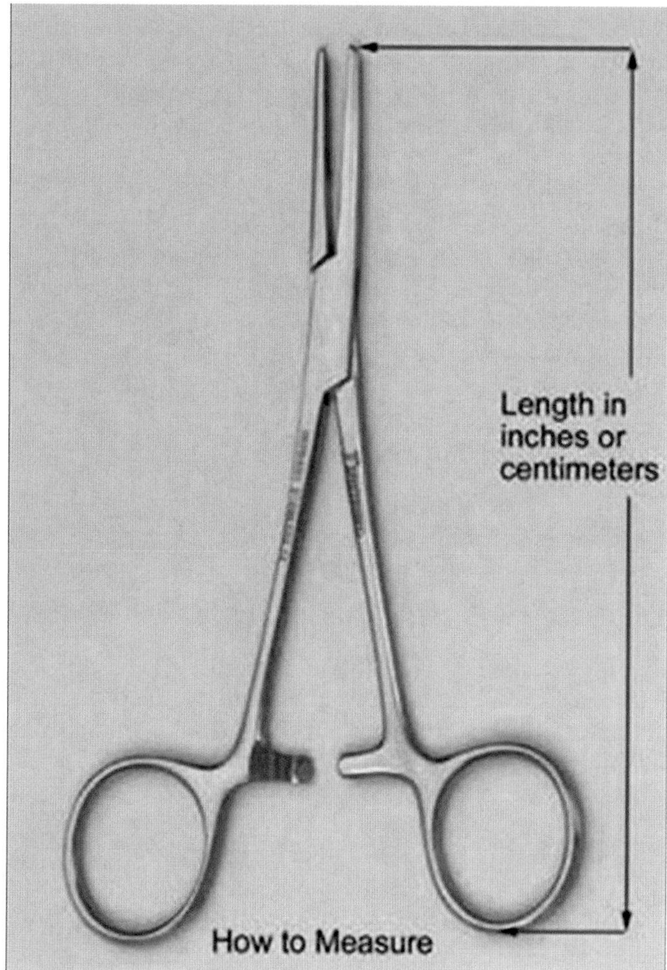

Figure 10.7

Basic instruments can also be identified by their size, serrations or blades. **Figure 10.8** provides an example of two different mosquito forceps. Instruments that look alike at first glance may be very different upon closer inspection. For example, **Figure 10.9** shows the difference in serrations between a Kelly and Crile forceps. The Crile has serrations the complete length of the jaw, while the Kelly only has serrations part of the way.

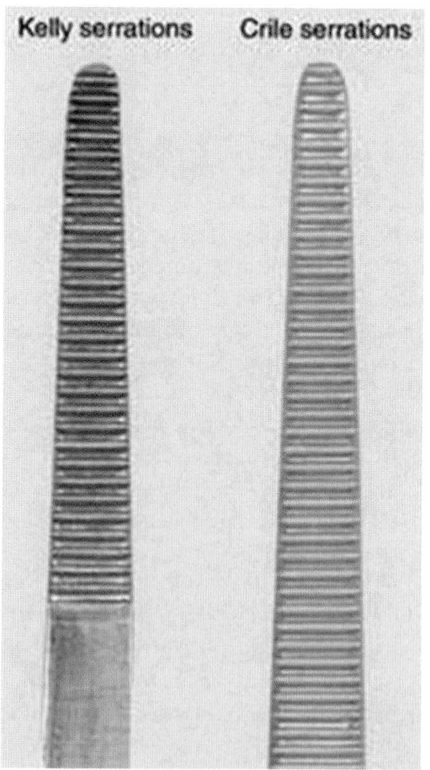

Figure 10.9

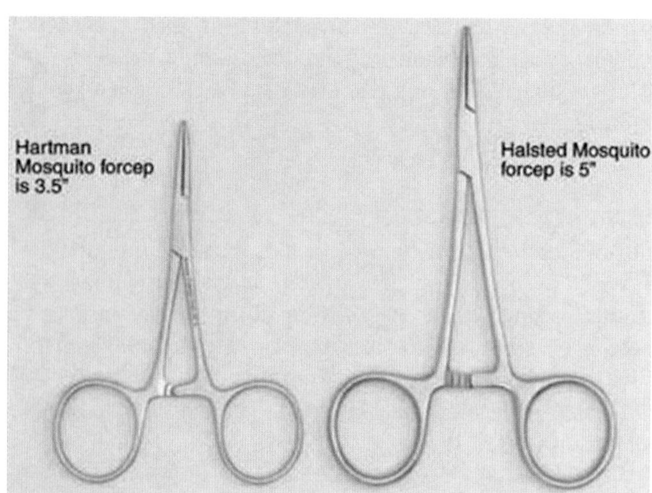

Figure 10.8

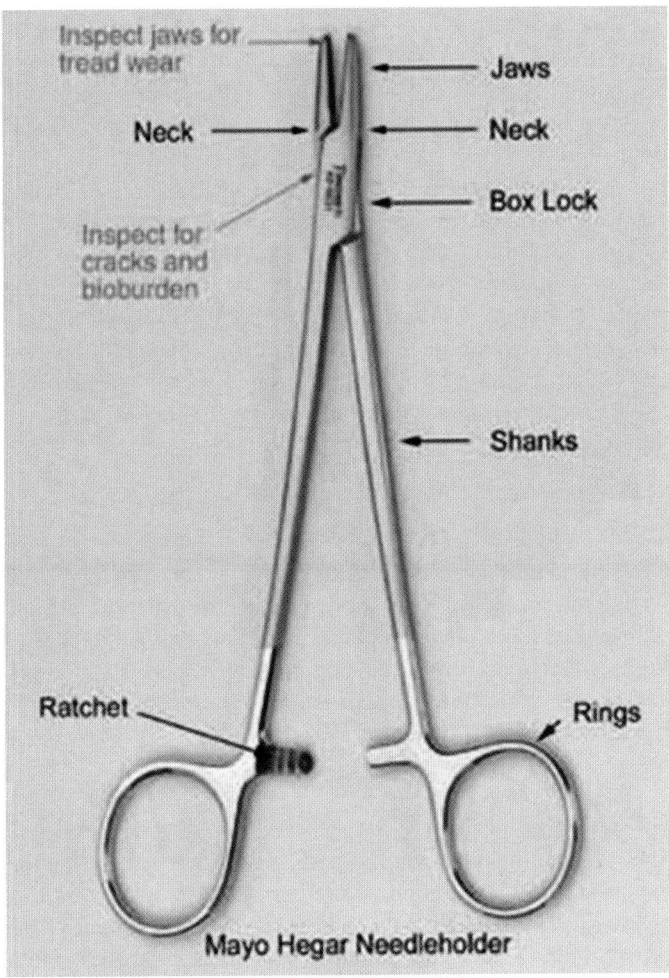

Figure 10.10

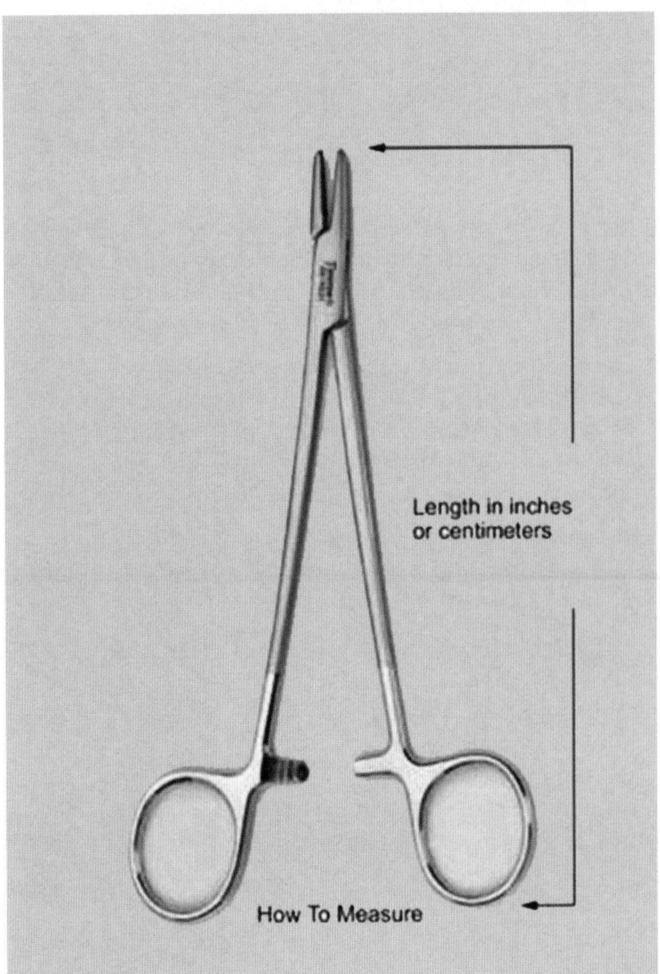

Figure 10.11

Needle Holders

These instruments are designed to drive suture needles to close surgical sites. **Figure 10.10** identifies the anatomy and points of inspection of a needle holder, and **Figure 10.11** shows the correct way to measure this instrument.

Needle holder **jaws**, the portion that holds the needle, can be manufactured with stainless steel or tungsten carbide:

- Stainless steel jaws – There are two patterns of jaw tread: smooth or serrated. Stainless steel jaw treads cannot be repaired, re-jawed, or have serrations replaced after they wear out. This can occur with one or two years of use, and then the needle holder must be replaced.

- Tungsten carbide jaws – The most popular needle holders used in surgical use have these jaws. The key visual factor is the bright gold rings on the handle. (See **Figure 10.12**) Gold placed on the instrument indicates that the working portion (jaw) is made of tungsten carbide. Jaws made from this metal are typically preferred because they are harder, last longer, grip the needle more firmly and can be replaced.

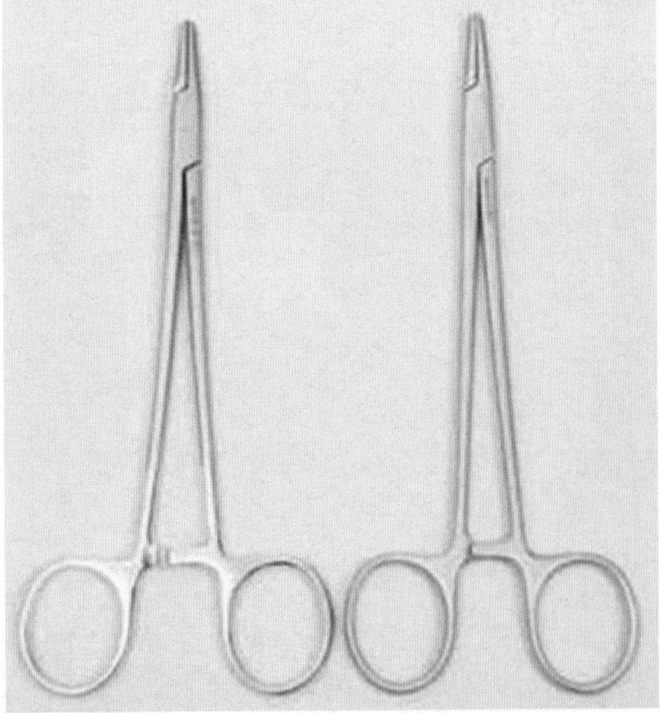

Figure 10.12

Jaws Two or more opposable parts that open and close; used for holding or crushing something between them.

Other names for needle holders are needle drivers, diamond jaws and gold handles. The two most common needle holder designs are Mayo-Hegar and Crile-Wood. (See **Figure 10.13**) *Note: The Crile-Wood is narrower than the Mayo-Hegar design.*

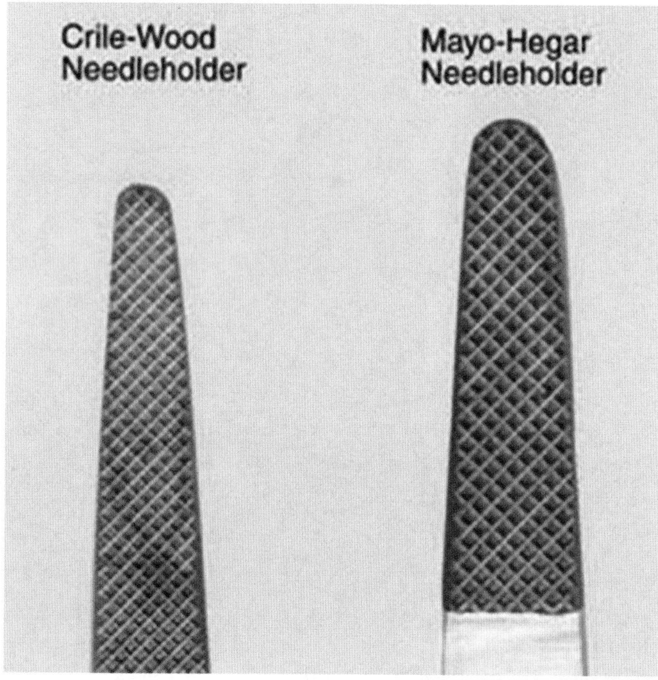

Figure 10.13

Tissue Forceps

The primary function of tissue forceps is to manipulate tissue. A design feature of this tweezer-like forceps is the multiple-teeth configuration at the distal tips. The teeth assist in grasping tissue and provide a more secure grip. **Figure 10.14** identifies the anatomy and points of inspection of a tissue forceps. **Figure 10.15** shows how to properly measure a tissue forceps.

The most common jaw or teeth configuration for tissue forceps is one tooth on one side and two teeth on the other. With this design, the teeth interlock and the configuration is indicated by 1x2. Other common teeth configurations are 2x3, 3x4, 5x6, 9x9 and 1x2 with serrations. Other names for tissue forceps are rat tooth, brown forceps and pickups.

Dressing Forceps

Dressing forceps are similar to tissue forceps, except they have serrations instead of teeth at the distal end. The primary function of this instrument is to manipulate tissue and pack surgical sites. **Figures 10.16** and **10.17** shows the anatomy of a dressing forceps and points of inspection. Other names for dressing forceps are smooth forceps and plain forceps.

Retractors

The primary function of a retractor is to move tissue aside for exposure and visualization of the surgical site. Retractors can be handheld, self-retaining or table mounted. Small finger-held retractors move and hold skin and subcutaneous tissues, while larger retractors are used to retract muscle tissue and organs.

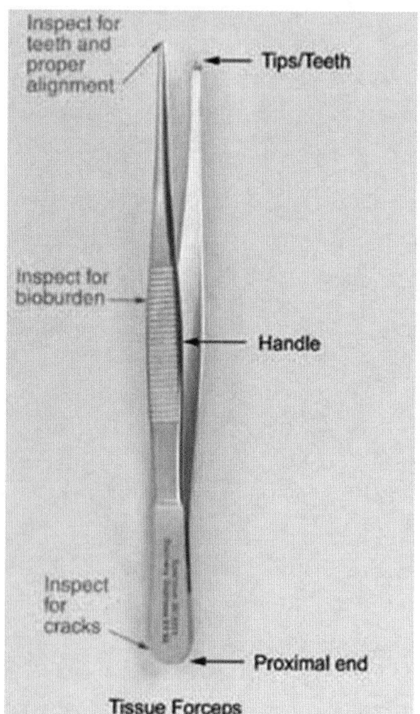

Figure 10.14

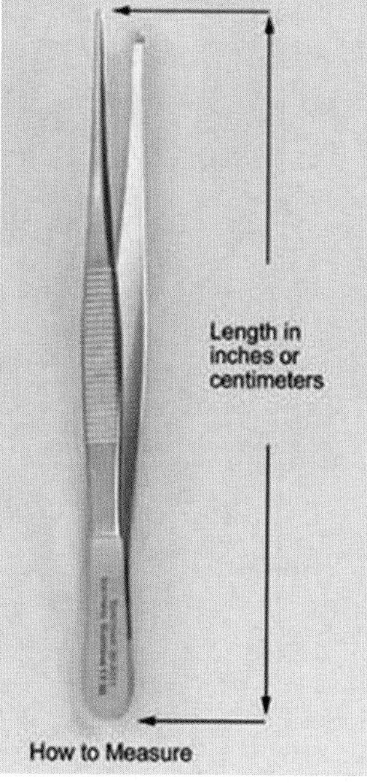

Figure 10.15

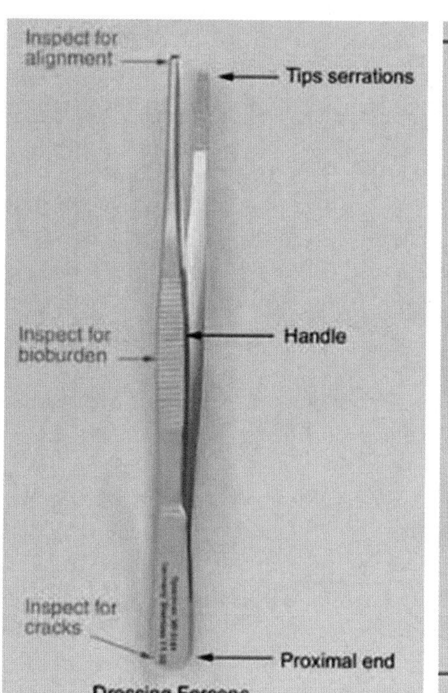

Figure 10.16

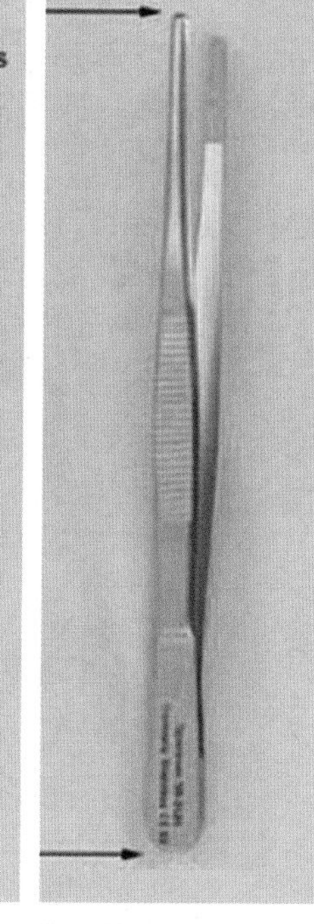

Figure 10.17

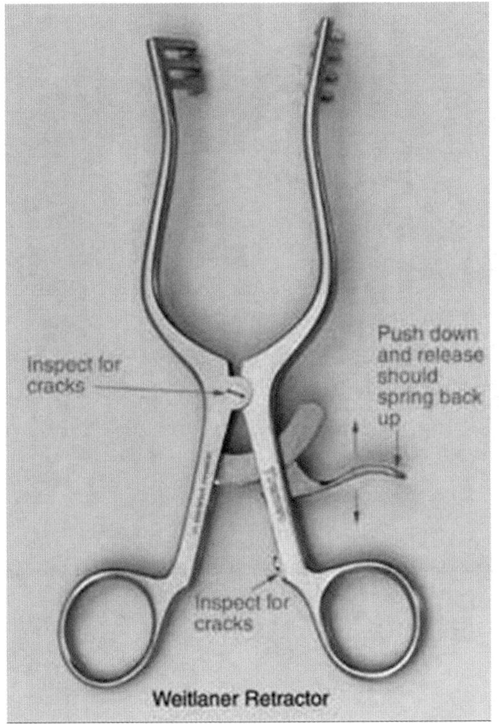

Figure 10.18

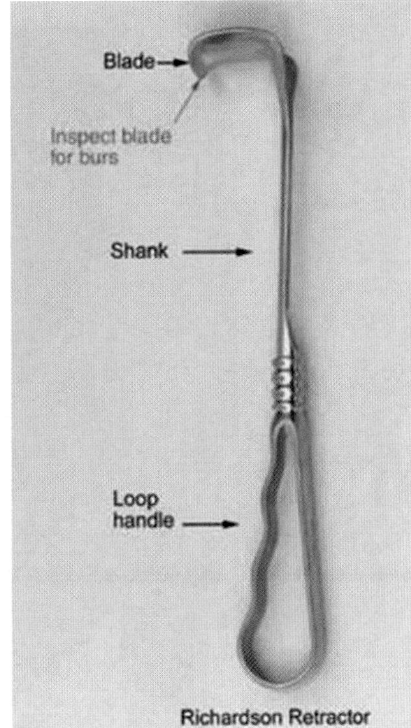

Figure 10.19

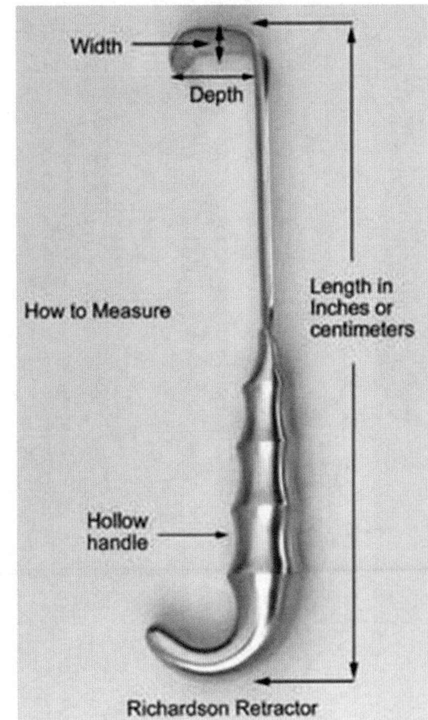

Figure 10.20

Self-retaining retractors are designed with a mechanical action that keeps them open to retract. (See **Figure 10.18**)

To test a self-retaining retractor, simply push down on the retractor lever and release. If the lever springs up, the instrument is working properly. If the lever remains in the down position, remove it from the instrument set and send the instrument to the repair vendor. Some common self-retaining retractors are Weitlaner, Gelpi, and Beckman-Adson.

Figure 10.19 shows the points of inspection of a loop-handle retractor. **Figure 10.20** shows the correct way to measure a hollow-handle retractor.

Scissors

The primary function of scissors is to cut tissue, suture and other material in the surgical field. For **dissection**, curved scissors are primarily used because their curve allows for better visualization. The opening action of the scissors also helps to dissect and spread tissue. **Figure 10.21** shows the anatomy and points of inspection for scissors.

Dissection The process of cutting apart or separating tissue.

Mayo scissors are one of the most popular scissors used and are identified by beveled blades. The second most popular Mayo design is the Mayo Noble. As seen in **Figure 10.22**, it does not have a beveled blade.

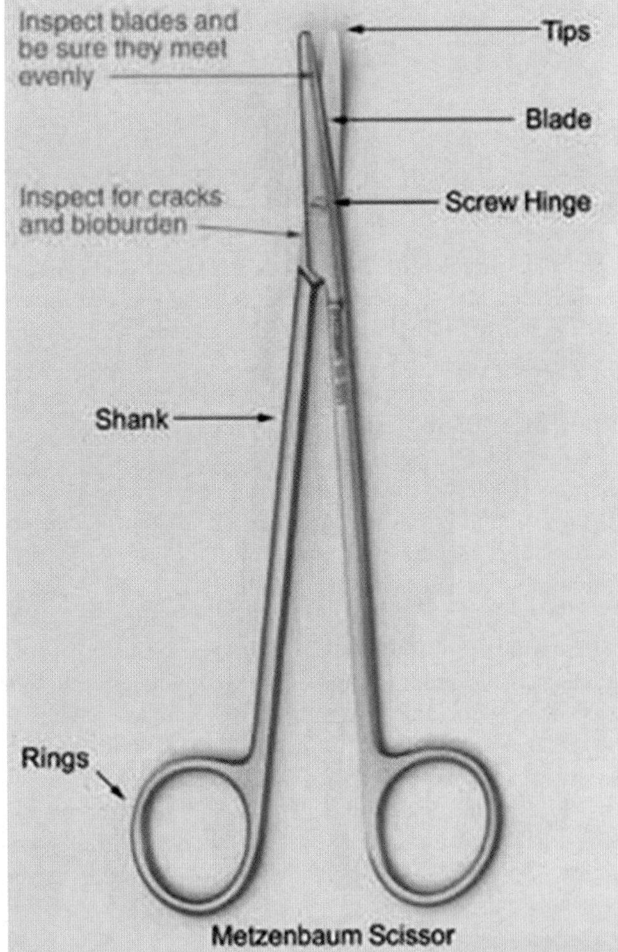

Figure 10.21

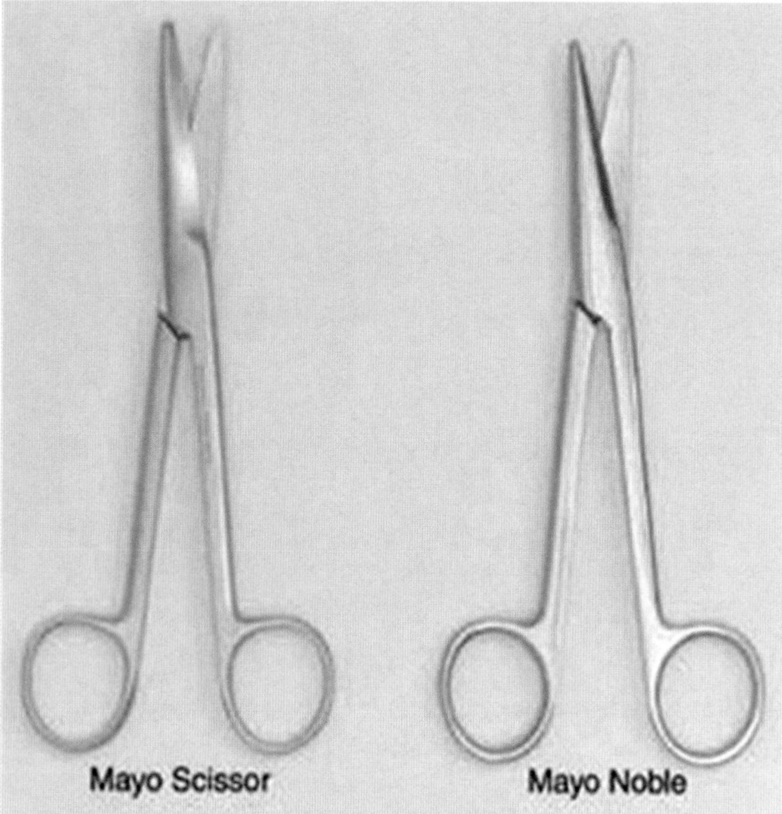

Figure 10.22

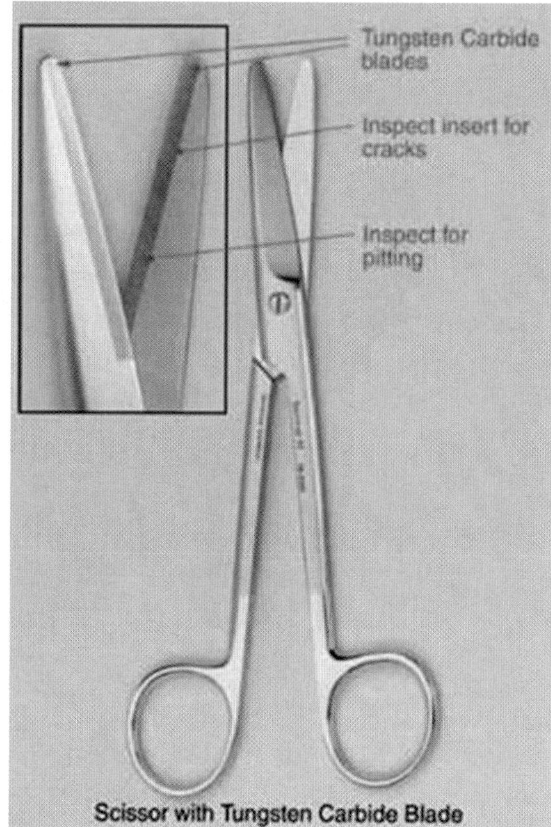

Figure 10.23

Surgical scissors have various blade features for specific surgical applications:

- Tungsten carbide blades – These scissors have gold rings on the handles and tungsten carbide blade edges. (See **Figure 10.23**) Scissors with these blades have a harder and stronger cutting edge and they allow the scissors to remain sharper for a longer time than other scissors. Their primary design function is tissue dissection.

- Serrated blades – The design feature of a serrated blade is the prevention of tissue slippage or escape during cutting. Serrations are generally found on one of the blades; however, there are some scissors with dual-blade serrations.

- Microgrind or supercut blades – Black rings visually identify these scissors from standard or gold-handled tungsten carbide scissors. The design of a black-handled scissors is to simulate a tissue lancing/slicing action. While all other scissors cut tissue with a crushing action, a black-handled scissors has one blade sharpened like a knife to slice tissue. The other blade is a standard design that causes a guillotine effect. (See **Figure 10.24**) Black-handled scissors must be specially sharpened.

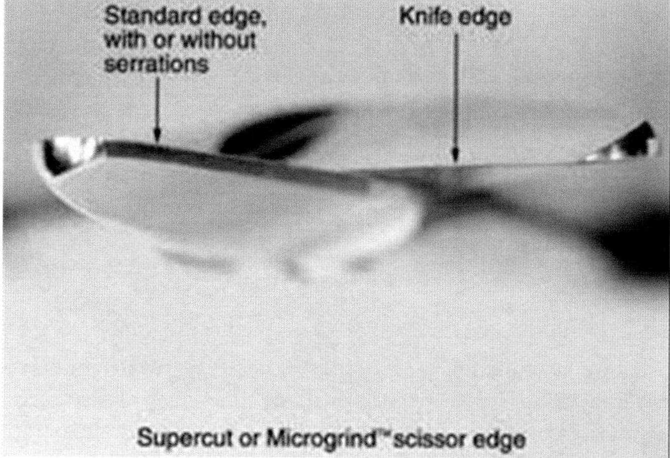

Figure 10.24

Suction Devices

The primary function of suction devices is to extract (suction) blood and fluids from the surgical site. **Figure 10.25** shows the anatomy and points of inspection for a suction device. The two most common suction devices are Baron and Frazier suction tubes. These suction devices include a metal stylet that is used during the surgical procedure to unclog the suction channel. A borescope can be used with lumened devices to help inspect and visualize cleanliness within the lumen. *Note: This stylet is not to be used for cleaning the device in SP. The only cleaning tool for a suction device is the proper cleaning brush or approved sponges designed to clean lumens.*

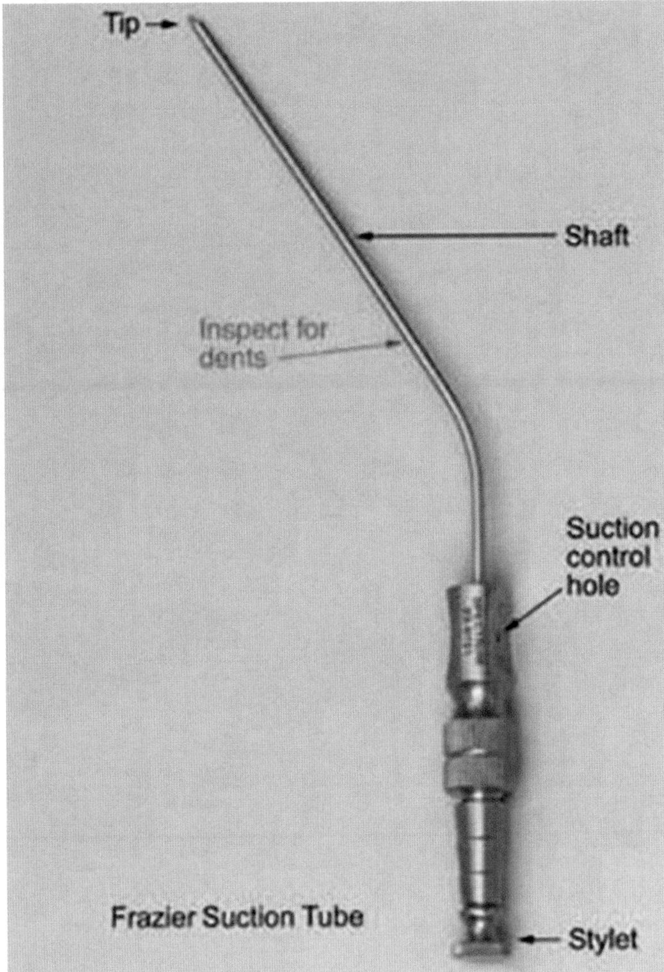

Figure 10.25

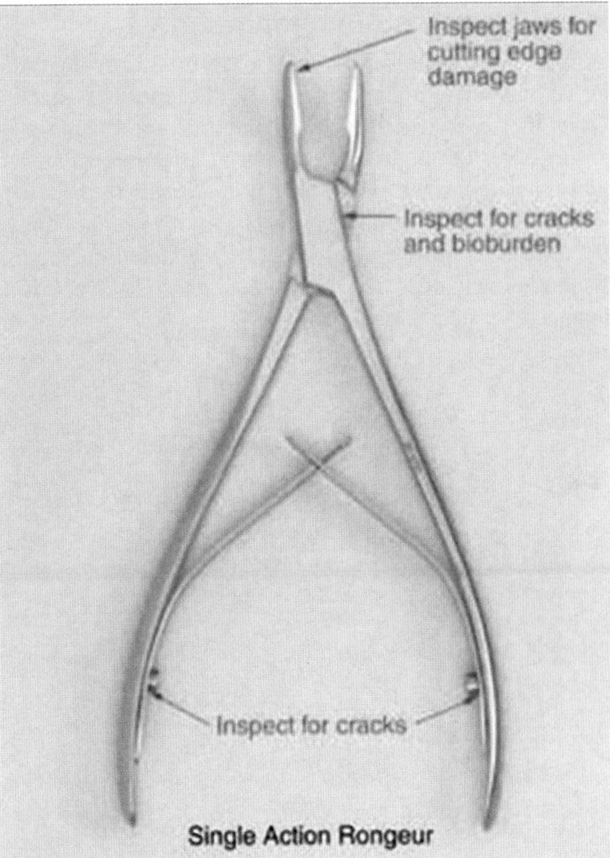

Figure 10.26

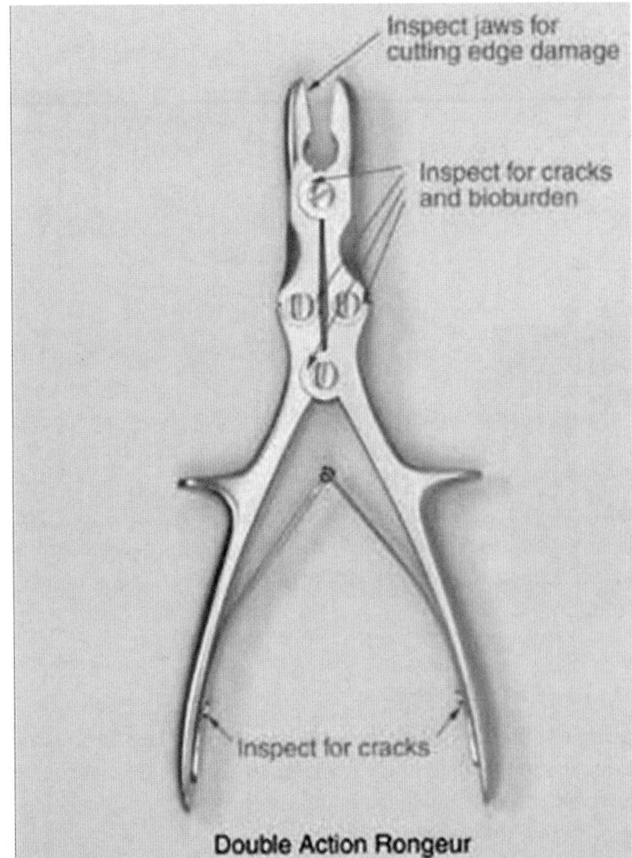

Figure 10.27

Single- and Double-Action Rongeurs

The primary function of a rongeur is to cut or bite away at bone and tissue. The difference between a single-action (**Figure 10.26**) and a double-action (**Figure 10.27**) rongeur is the design of how the jaws close. With a double-action instrument, the surgeon squeezes the handle, which creates two movements for the jaw to close. This double movement reduces the amount of hand strength needed, so the instrument bites more with less hand strength. The main inspection point on single- and double-action rongeurs is the jaws. Any dents or gouges of the jaws prevent the instrument from working properly.

Kerrison/Laminectomy Rongeurs

The primary function of this style of rongeur is to remove the disc or lamina during spine surgery. The distal portion must be inspected after each use to look for bioburden and damage to the cutting edge. (See **Figure 10.28**) When Kerrison rongeurs are being assembled in trays, it is important to identify the different bite designs (e.g., the 90-degree up bite, as shown in **Figure 10.29**). If a Kerrison rongeur is sticking in a closed position, a repair vendor will need to disassemble, polish, sharpen and reassemble the instrument.

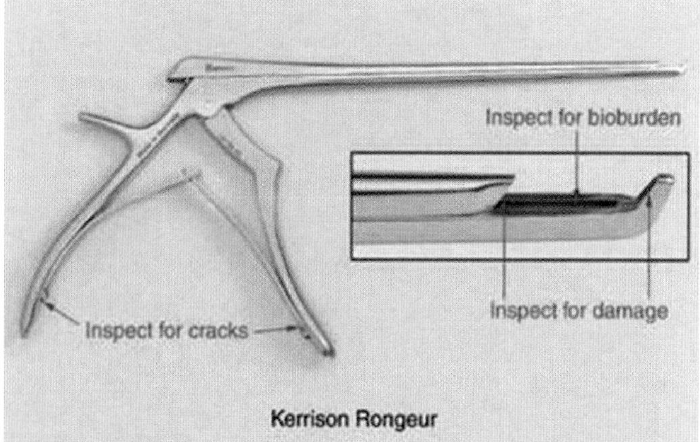

Figure 10.28

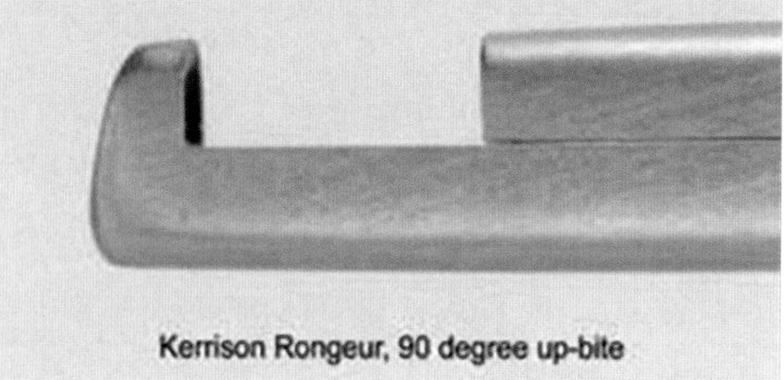

Figure 10.29

Graves and Pederson Vaginal Speculums

The primary use of these medical instruments is to expose the vaginal cavity. **Figure 10.30** shows the anatomy of a vaginal speculum. One important inspection point is to ensure that the thumb screws are present and functioning. It is also important to inspect all sides of the blades for damage. As noted in **Figure 10.31**, a Pederson blade is narrower than that on a Graves speculum.

Nail Nippers

The primary function of nail nippers (see **Figure 10.32**) is to cut toenails and fingernails and, occasionally, to trim small bone fragments. The cutting surface and edge should be inspected, along with the hinge area and spring.

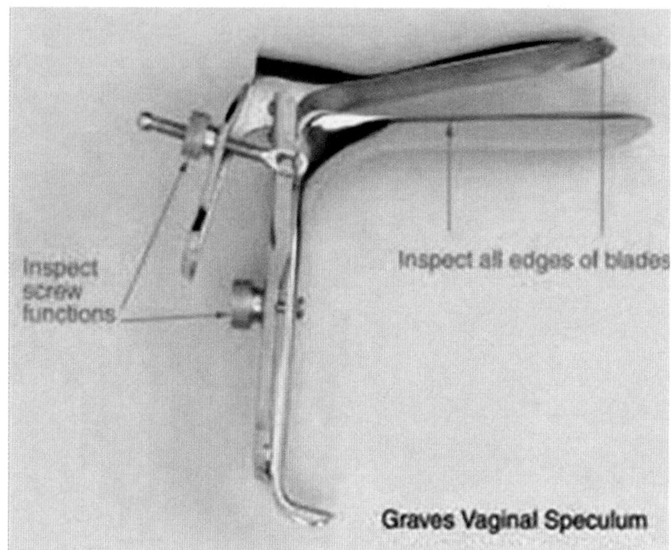

Figure 10.30

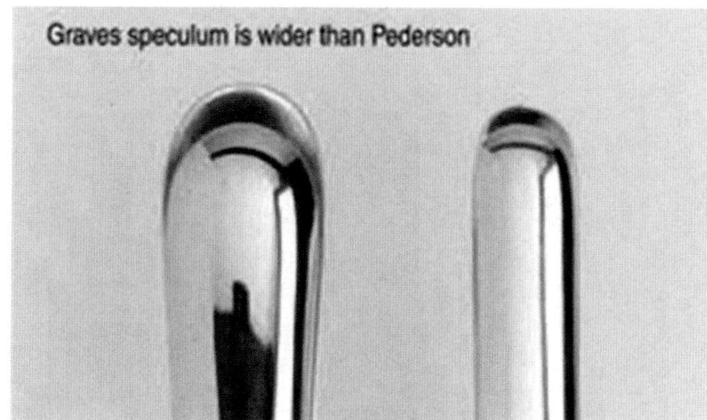

Figure 10.31

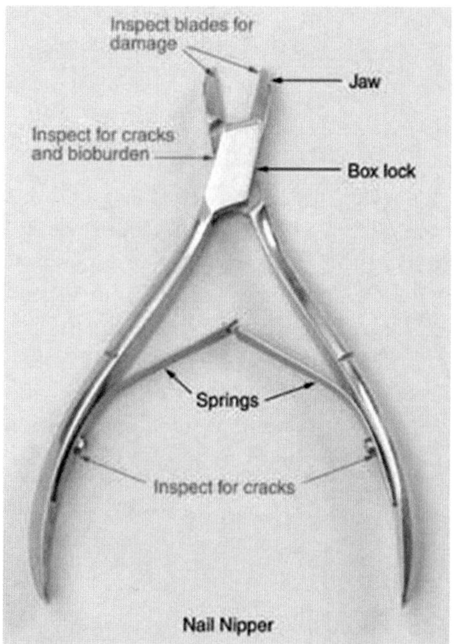

Figure 10.32

COMMON ABBREVIATIONS

When SP technicians assemble instrumentation, they may encounter several abbreviations listed on the assembly count sheet. Abbreviations can be used to identify the type of instrument and specific characteristics of the instrument. It is important for SP technicians to recognize and understand the abbreviations to ensure the correct instrument is placed in the proper set or tray. **Figure 10.33** list some abbreviations SP technicians may encounter. *Note: Only abbreviations that are approved by one's facility should be used on count sheets.*

MED	Medium
LG	Large
fr	French
"	Inches
mm	Millimeters
cm	Centimeters
oz	Ounces
L	Length
W	Width

Figure 10.33 Common abbreviations

SOLUTIONS THAT DAMAGE INSTRUMENTS

Numerous solutions, ranging from those typically used for housekeeping to kitchen-related cleaning purposes, can damage stainless steel instruments. If the solution's container does not specifically note that its intended purpose is for use on surgical instruments, the product should not be used to clean them. It is a good practice to follow the instrument IFU closely when using any chemicals or solutions. **Figure 10.34** identifies common solutions that can damage instruments.

Solutions That Damage Surgical Instruments
Betadine
Peroxide
Dish soaps
Soaking in water
Soaking in saline
Bleach
Iodine
Hand soaps
Saline
Long-term soaking in rust remover
Long-term soaking in stain remover
Porcelain cleaners
Household lubricants
Household powder cleansers
Surgeon's hand scrubs
Laundry detergents

Figure 10.34

The use of saline as a soaking or rinsing agent accelerates rusting and pitting of surgical instruments. (See **Figure 10.35**) In many cases, the use of saline may void instrument warranties; therefore, controlling instrument exposure to saline is very important. For clinical reasons, OR personnel cannot eliminate the exposure of stainless steel instruments to saline; however, after the surgical procedures are completed, saline must be removed as an early step in the cleaning process.

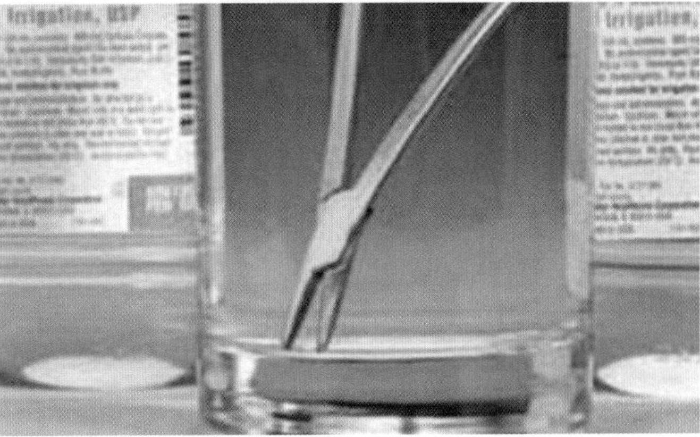

Figure 10.35

INSTRUMENT SHARPNESS TESTING AND IDENTIFICATION

Instrument sharpness testing is essential to monitor the sharpness of surgical instruments. **Figures 10.36** through **10.43** illustrate proper sharpness testing procedures for common surgical instruments.

Instrument: Scissors longer than 4.5"

Test material: Red test material (latex); orange material (latex free)

Test: Scissors must be able to cut through to the tip two to three times. The distal tips of scissors are the most crucial portion because this is where they first become dull. They must cut cleanly through the tips of the instrument.

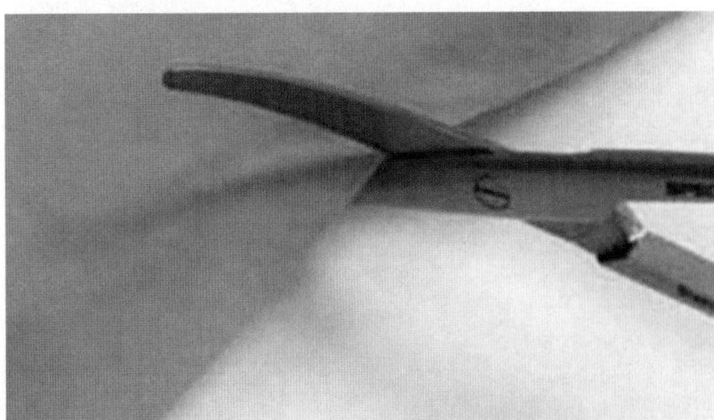

Figure 10.36 Scissor test material for scissors measuring longer than 4.5"

Instrument: Scissors 4.5" and shorter

Test material: Yellow test material (latex or latex free)

Test: Scissors must be able to cut through the tips two to three times. The distal tips of scissors are the most crucial portion; they must cut cleanly through the tips of the instrument.

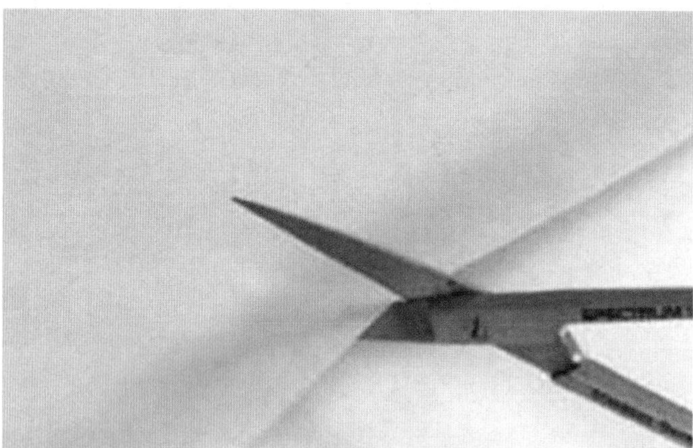

Figure 10.37 Scissor test material for scissors measuring 4.5" and shorter

Instrument: Kerrison rongeur

Test material: Index card

Test: Punch a clean hole through the card.

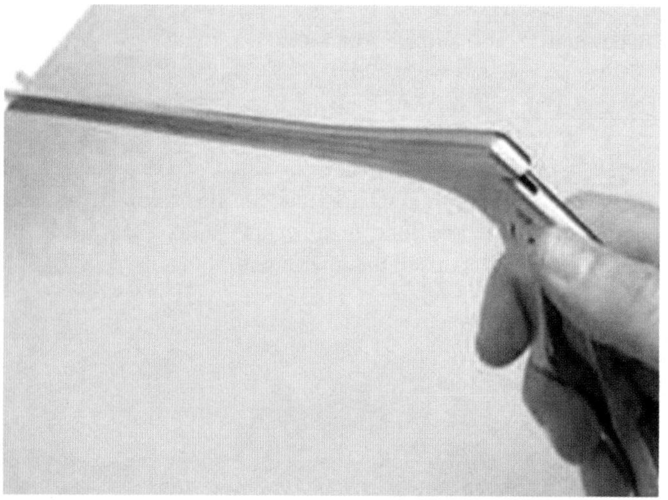

Figure 10.38 Sharpness test for Kerrison rongeurs

Instrument: Bone cutter

Test material: Index card

Test: Cut off a piece of the index card.

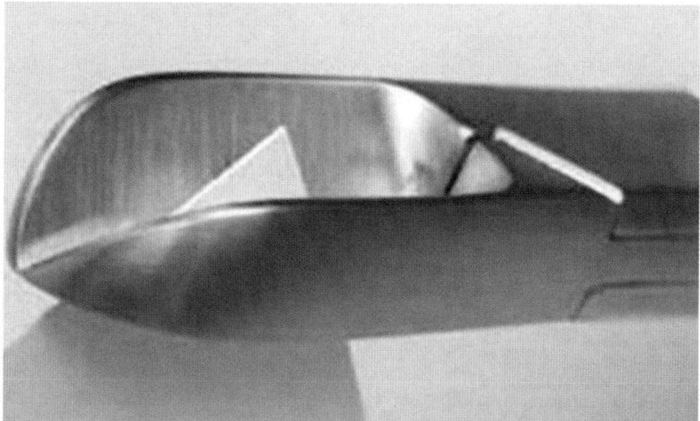

Figure 10.39 Sharpness test for bone cutters

Instrument: Laminectomy rongeur

Test material: Index card

Test: The rongeur should make a clean bite using half the jaw.

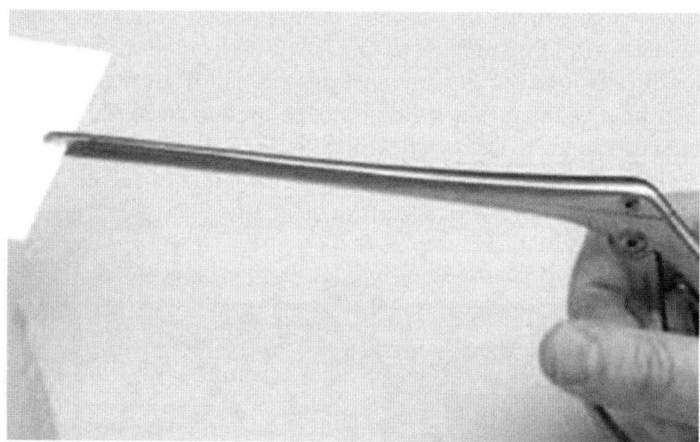

Figure 10.40 Sharpness test for laminectomy rongeurs

Instrument: Double-action rongeur

Test material: Index card

Test: The rongeur should make a clean bite through the card.

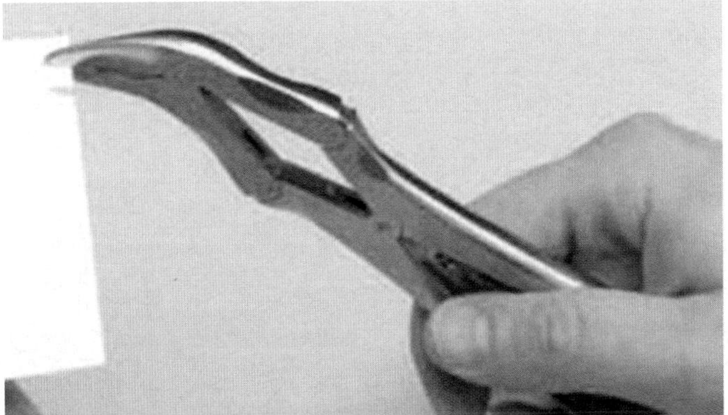

Figure 10.41 Sharpness test for double-action rongeurs

Instrument: Bone curette

Test material: Plastic dowel rod

Test: Shave off pieces of the dowel rod.

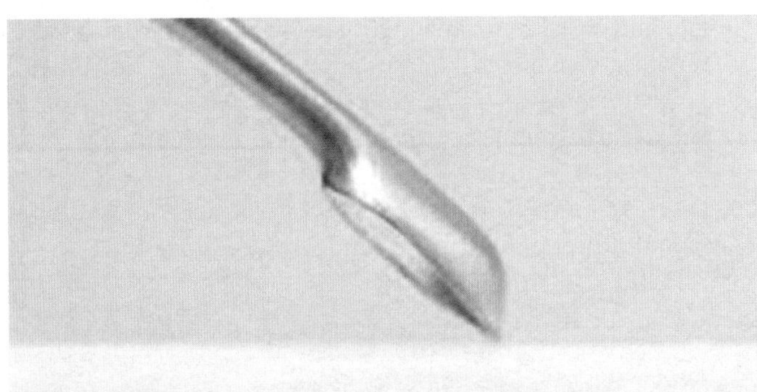

Figure 10.42 Sharpness test for bone curettes

Instrument: Chisels and osteotomes

Test material: Plastic dowel rod

Test: Shave off pieces of the dowel rod.

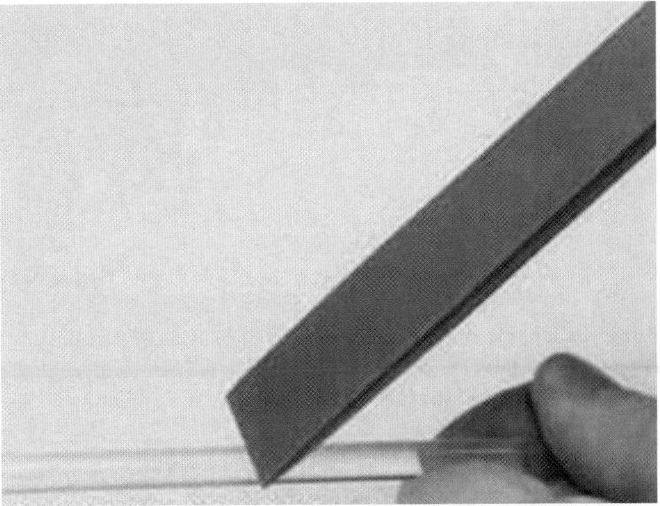

Figure 10.43 Sharpness test for osteotomes

Figure 10.44 provides a review of common instrument testing methods.

INSTRUMENT IDENTIFICATION METHODS

There are thousands of different surgical instruments and many may look quite similar. SP technicians must ensure that the correct instruments are placed into the proper trays. Many healthcare facilities use different instrument marking methods to mark instruments for faster and easier identification.

Marking surgical instruments for identification can be done several ways. The use of tape is one popular method for identifying instruments. (See **Figure 10.45**) Although this is a seemingly simple approach, it is important to follow the IFU of the tape manufacturer.

Sharpness Testing		
Instrument	**Test Material**	**Test**
Scissors longer than 4.5"	Red test material (latex) Orange text material (latex free)	Scissors must be able to cut through the tips two to three times. The distal tips of scissors are the most crucial portion; they must cut cleanly through the tips of the instrument.
Scissors 4.5" and shorter	Yellow test material	Same as above.
Kerrison rongeur	Index card	Punch a clean hole through the card.
Bone cutter	Index card	Cutter should cleanly cut off a piece of the index card.
Laminectomy rongeur	Index card	The rongeur should make a clean bite using half the jaw.
Double-action rongeur	Index card	The rongeur should make a clean bite through the card.
Bone curette	Plastic dowel	The curette should shave off pieces of the dowel rod.

Figure 10.44

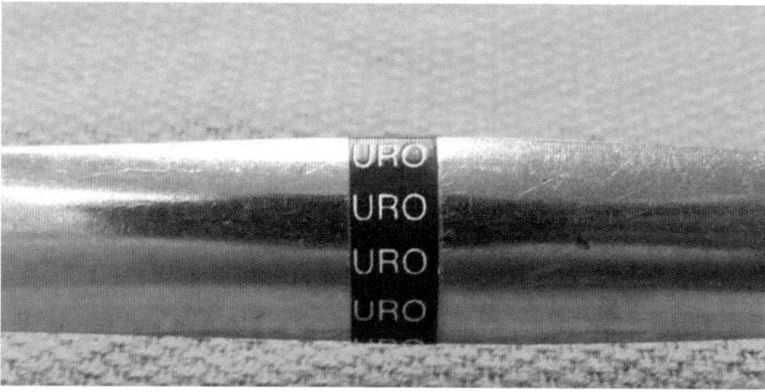

Figure 10.45

When using tape to identify instruments, inspection of the tape each time the device is processed is very important. Tape that is loose, damaged or peeling must be removed and replaced because microorganisms under the loose or damaged tape are very difficult to clean. Peeling and damaged tape can inadvertently fall into the patient, potentially causing an infection. (See **Figure 10.46**)

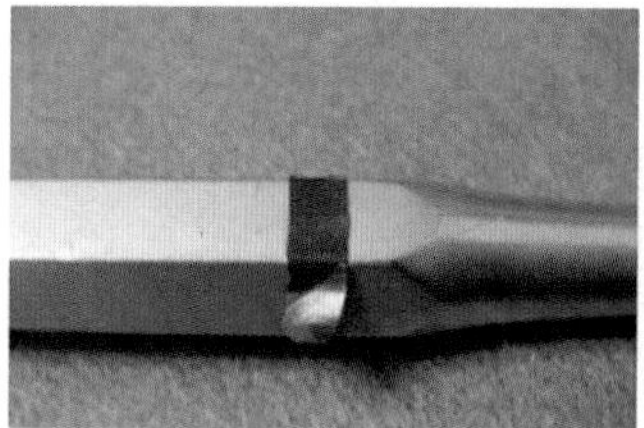
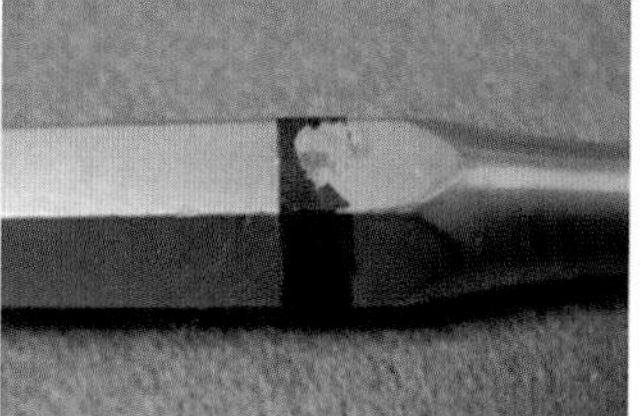

Figure 10.46 Tape that is peeling or flaking poses a threat to patients.

There are other methods of marking instruments. Before utilizing any of these methods, it is best to contact the instrument manufacturer for their advice.

- Acid-base etching – This process can be done by the instrument repair vendor, or a kit may be purchased so the etching process can be done at the facility. Acid-base etching uses a stencil, solutions and electricity to mark stainless steel. This process is semi-permanent and the etching can be buffed off during the instrument repair process. (See **Figure 10.47**)

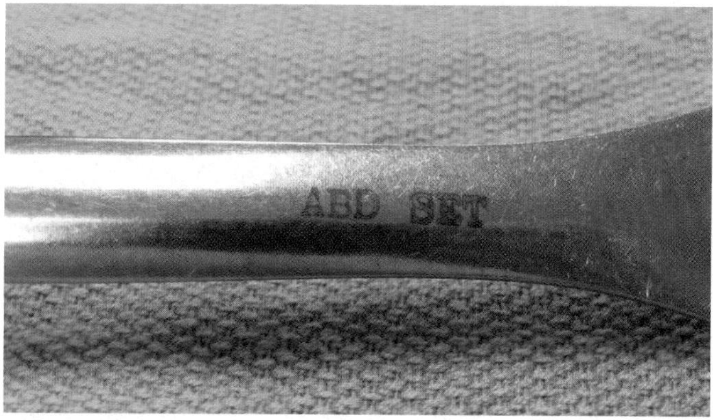

Figure 10.47

- Heat-fused nylon – This color coding is often referred to as "dipping" and is typically done in a repair facility. Heat-fused nylon is a liquid powder-coating process that leaves a thin layer of colored nylon on the instrument. Nylon coating can last years; however, once it begins to chip, all nylon must be removed from the instrument. (See **Figure 10.48**)

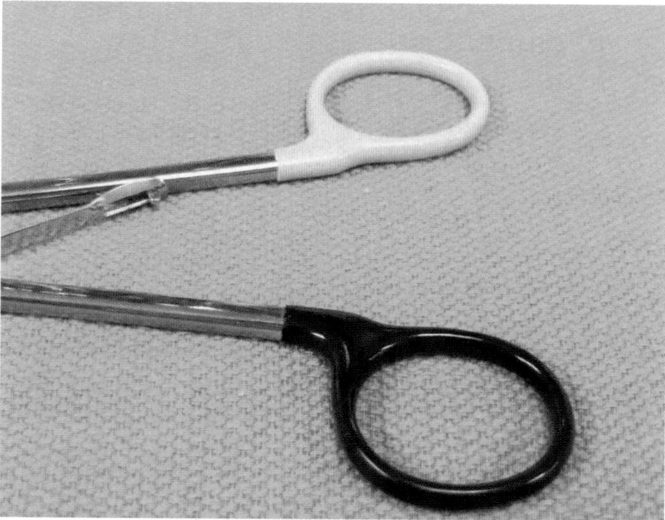

Figure 10.48

- Powder coating – This is a process that uses polymer resin combined with other additives to form a powder. The powder is then sprayed onto an instrument using an electrostatic spray gun and cured to form a high-density bond. Powder coating provides a durable, thin, smooth finish to the instrument. Powder-coated instruments are susceptible to cracks, nicks and damage from harsh cleaning chemicals over time.

- Laser etching – This durable process is usually done by the manufacturer or an outside vendor. (See **Figure 10.49**)

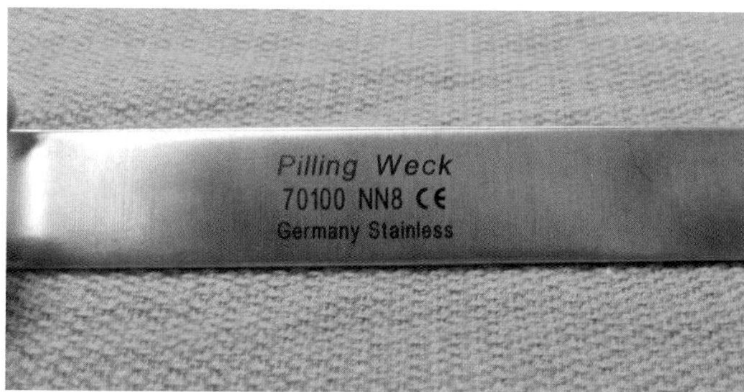

Figure 10.49

- Dot matrix – These systems are relatively inexpensive and can be applied by SP technicians. (See **Figure 10.50**) The two most popular types of dot systems are:
  - The dot marking system, where a small barcode containing the instrument information is applied with pressure-sensitive tape.

› The dot peen system, where a laser or tungsten stylet is used to implant the information onto an instrument.

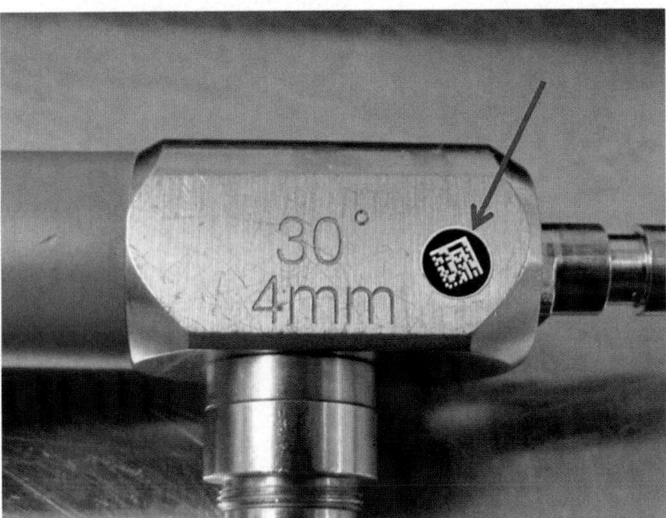

Figure 10.50

INSTRUMENT LUBRICATION

Many surgical instruments with moving parts must be lubricated after each use and in accordance with the manufacturer's recommendations. All lubricants must be approved for use as a surgical instrument lubricant and for the type of sterilization method that will be used on the instrument. The use of a neutral-pH lubricant extends the life of the instrument and makes the device easier for the surgeon to use. While most washer-disinfectors will lubricate instruments, some instruments may need to be lubricated again during assembly. Each SP workstation should have lubrication available for this purpose. Lubricants are available in spray bottle formulas. The point of application should be the instrument's hinged area or any working component such as a moving/sliding area. (See **Figure 10.51**)

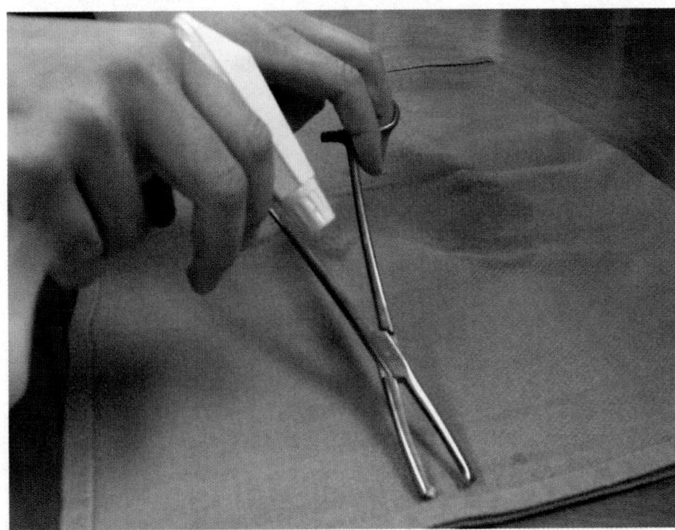

Figure 10.51

TIPS TO PROTECT INSTRUMENTS FROM DAMAGE

Instruments are an expensive asset for any facility. Protecting the instruments is a part of every SP technician's job. When handled properly, many instruments can remain in active service for many years. The following are some helpful tips:

- Always follow the manufacturer's instructions for cleaning, lubrication and sterilization. These instructions were developed by the instrument manufacturer to help ensure the instrument's longevity.
- Place heavy instruments on the bottom or side of the tray. This will help protect the smaller, more delicate instruments.
- Select an instrument tray that allows adequate space for weight distribution. Overcrowding instruments can cause damage.
- All curved instruments should be curved in the same direction to protect tips from damage.
- Tissue and dressing forceps should be softly nested together or placed close to each other in the tray or peel pack. Do not push the forceps together. Leave some space between each forceps so that the sterilant can reach all surfaces.
- Delicate instruments should be kept in approved micro cases or small protective cases within the surgical tray.
- The use of metal instrument holders, called stringers, can assist in faster sterile field assembly and safer handling of the instruments, especially sharps. Stringers also hold the instruments in the open position during sterilization. (See **Figure 10.52**)

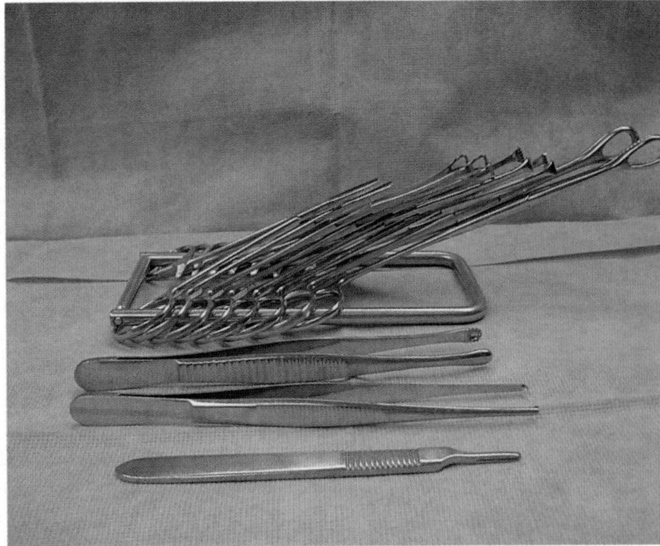

Figure 10.52

Error	Possible Result	Avoid By
Use nicknames/slang when describing or labeling instruments	Improper names/labels can cause confusion, communication delays and frustration.	Use proper names for all instruments.
Failure to follow instruments' IFU	Failure to follow specific IFU can result in defective instruments, sterilization failure or long-term damage to the instruments.	Be familiar with and follow each instrument's IFU.
Counting instruments instead of identifying each one (for example, Dr. Marsh's hand set has 11 instruments, so if 11 instruments are there, there is no need to identify each one)	Relying on a numeric count instead of identifying each instrument can result in incorrect instruments in the tray. Instruments that are not specifically identified are also more likely to go without inspection.	Identify and check each instrument as the tray is assembled.
Failure to test instruments as directed by the IFU	Failure to test instruments correctly increases the risk that defective instruments will make their way into surgical procedures. A defective instrument can pose a risk to a patient and can cause frustration for the surgeon and OR staff.	Test each instrument as directed.
Failure to assemble and then disassemble multi-part instruments	Multi-part instruments may be rendered unusable due to missing or defective parts.	Assembling a multi-part instrument as a part of the inspection process helps ensure that all parts are available and without damage that may impede the procedure.
Cutting corners due to time pressures	All instruments should receive through processing every time. Cutting corners may result in incorrect, unsafe or malfunctioning instruments being sent for use in a procedure.	Timelines can be tight in SP areas, and every effort should be made to meet them without compromising patient safety. Collaborate with colleagues to improve efficiencies and communicate with customers to establish realistic timelines.
Guessing about an instrument's identification or inspection protocol	Guessing about an instrument can lead to incorrect or unsafe instruments or malfunctioning instruments being sent for use in a procedure.	Become familiar with resources in the department and ask questions as needed.

Figure 10.53

COMMON INSTRUMENT ASSEMBLY ERRORS

When instrument errors happen, they can cause frustration, delay of treatment and, in some cases, physical harm to the patient. The goal should always be to eliminate errors in instrument inspection and assembly. That goal requires attention to detail, good education and information. Instrument assembly technicians also need the ability to adapt to changes. Technology is advancing, and needs continue to evolve. Assembly technicians must develop the ability to learn, unlearn and relearn as changes are implemented. **Figure 10.53** Provides some examples of common instrument errors and suggestions to prevent them from happening.

CONCLUSION

Properly identifying instruments and following the proper inspection protocols help ensure instrument trays are assembled correctly and all the instruments are clean and functional. Carefully following the manufacturers' IFU and paying meticulous attention to detail will help keep the instruments in good repair and extend the life of these expensive items.

SP technicians are the last individuals to touch instruments before they are received in a procedure area; therefore, their quality of work is critical to successful patient outcomes.

RESOURCES

Centers for Disease Control and Prevention. *FastStats.*

Dobson G. P. (2020). "Trauma of major surgery: A global problem that is not going away." *International journal of surgery (London, England), 81*, 47–54.

AST. (n.d.). *Standard Decontamination Surgical Instruments.*

ANSI/AAMI ST79:2017 & 2020 Amendments A1, A2, A3, A4 *Comprehensive guide to steam sterilization and sterility assurance in health care facilities.*

Schultz R. *Inspecting Surgical Instruments: An Illustrated Guide.* 2005.

Gregory B. *Orthopedic Surgery.* 1994.

Tighe S. *Instrumentation for the Operating Room.* 1994.

Glaser Z. "Surgical Instrument Quality." *Infection Control and Sterilization Technology.* 1997.

Storz Instruments. *The Care and Handling of Surgical Instruments.* 1991.

Reichert M. *Sterilization Technology for the Health Care Facility, Second Edition.* 1997.

STERILE PROCESSING TERMS

Stainless steel

Scissors

Osteotomes

Chisel

Rongeurs

Forceps

Hemostatic forceps

Needle holders

Martensitic stainless steel

Retractors

Cannulas

Rib spreaders

Suction devices

Austentitic stainless steel

Serrations

Ratchets

Passivation

Box Lock

Jaws

Dissection

Chapter 11

Complex Surgical Instruments

Learning Objectives

As a result of successfully completing this chapter, the reader will be able to:

1. Discuss procedures to care for powered surgical instruments
2. Explain critical protocols for processing endoscopic instruments
3. Discuss rigid and flexible endoscopes and their accessories
4. Discuss processes for loaned instrumentation

INTRODUCTION

Advances in many types of surgical procedures have improved patient outcomes and shortened hospital stays and recovery time. At the same time, the instruments used in these procedures have become more complex and difficult to process.

Surgical instruments have evolved from simple devices to the complex surgical devices used today. Forceps, scissors, needle holders and retractors, along with numerous other simple instruments, are still commonly used but are joined by powered surgical instruments, endoscopes, orthopedic, spinal, robotic, neurological and other highly sophisticated and delicate devices with complex components such as circuit boards and computer chips.

Many of the complex instruments that Sterile Processing (SP) technicians process require special handling and care. This instrumentation may range from a single instrument or a few sophisticated instruments in a small tray to those that comprise many trays and consist of hundreds of instruments.

The requirements for processing complex instruments are the same as for processing less-complex devices: thorough cleaning, detailed inspection, proper packaging, and disinfection or sterilization. One of the greatest challenges that SP technicians face is keeping abreast of new and evolving instruments and their specific processing requirements. Complex instruments are costly to purchase and repair and represent a large financial investment for the facility. Due to the associated expense, many facilities may not have backup instrumentation available, so careful handling of these instruments is essential.

This chapter addresses basic information about some of the complex instruments that may cause processing concerns for SP technicians.

POWERED SURGICAL INSTRUMENTS

The use of drills and saws by physicians dates as far back as 5,000 to 7,000 years ago. In the mid-1800s, the dental industry took the lead in powered instrumentation by developing powered dental drills. The fields of neurosurgery, orthopedics and otology have also played key roles in the development of powered surgical instruments now used in every specialty. These developments have revolutionized surgery, making procedures both safer and faster.

The size and design of powered surgical devices range from drills used on the tiniest ear bones to drills and saws used on the largest leg bones. Powered surgical instruments have greatly reduced the brute force and time required for orthopedic surgeries. This, in turn, has allowed surgeons to complete surgeries quicker and with more precision.

Materials used to construct powered surgical instruments are varied, so careful selection of cleaning and disinfection products is critical. Device manufacturer's instructions for use (IFU) must be followed to prevent damage. **Figure 11.1** shows some internal components of a motorized handpiece and demonstrates the complexity of powered surgical instrumentation.

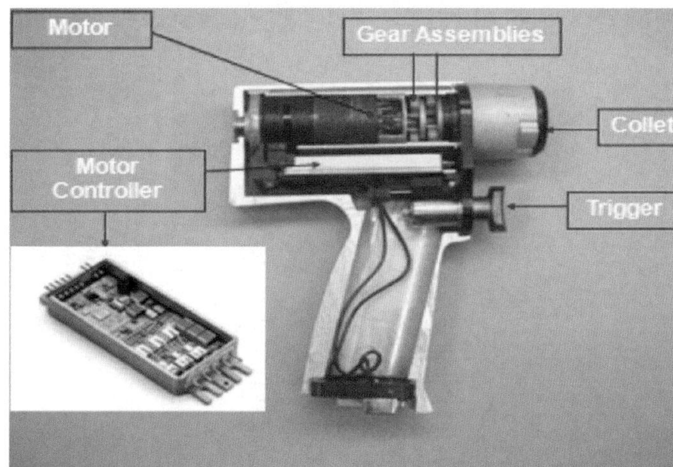

Figure 11.1

Powered surgical instruments contain several working components that will be damaged if fluid (such as water or a cleaning solution) is allowed to penetrate the device's interior. **Figures 11.2** and **11.3** illustrate the type of damage that occurs when powered surgical instruments and their accessories are invaded by fluid. SP technicians should be specifically trained to clean, process and handle powered surgical devices and ensure that fluid invasion does not occur.

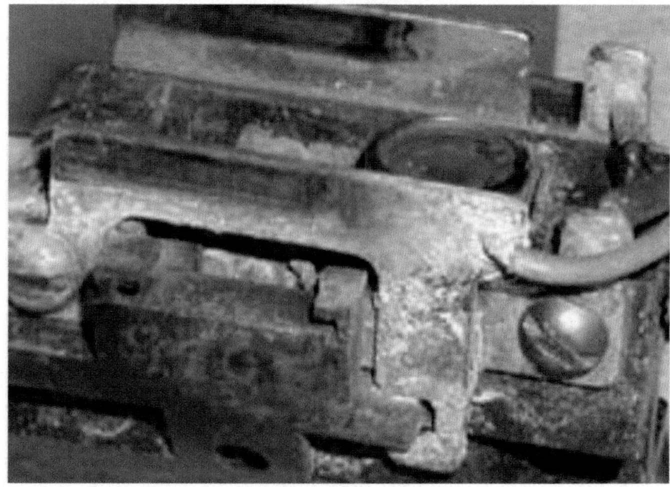

Figure 11.2 Fluid invasion damage on a powered surgical instrument

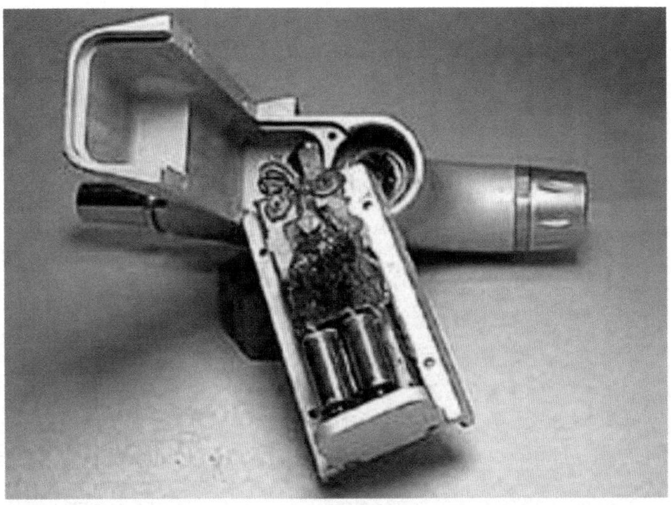

Figure 11.3

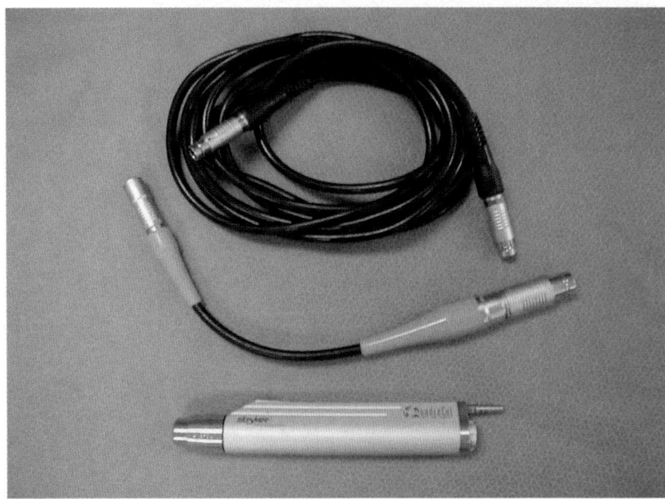

Figure 11.4

Power Sources

There are three main sources of power used for powered surgical instruments: electric, compressed gas (pneumatic), and battery.

Electric-Powered Surgical Instruments

Electric-powered instruments are used when physicians need a lightweight instrument for procedures where access is limited such as in maxillofacial, dental and small bone (e.g., hand) procedures. An arthroscopy shaver is an example of an electric-powered instrument. (See **Figure 11.4**)

Instruments powered by electricity require a power cable that can be sterilized. One end of the cable attaches to the motorized handpiece on the surgical field; the other end attaches to a power unit (motor/electrical adapter) that plugs into an outlet. These cables require routine maintenance that involves disassembly, cleaning, lubrication, and inspection to look for cuts, nicks and other damage. During cleaning, fluid must not enter the cable or handpiece. Many manufacturers recommend connecting the cable to the handpiece during the cleaning/decontamination process to help prevent fluid invasion. Care must also be taken not to bend the connector pins on the cable.

The most common problems associated with electric-powered equipment are:

- Damage to electrical parts during cleaning and disinfection/sterilization
- Condensation that enters the equipment when seals wear out
- Electrical contacts that become worn

The following are general guidelines for proper care and handling of electric-powered instruments and accessories:

- Do not immerse the equipment in any solution, including water, unless the manufacturer's IFU specifically states that the device can be submerged.
- Do not use solvents or lubricants, unless specified by the equipment manufacturer.
- Use a brush to clean the distal tip and lumens. Follow the IFU for the correct size and type of brush to use for each area.
- Carefully clean the accessory attachment area in the distal area of the handpiece.
- Dry the equipment with a clean, non-linting cloth.

Electric-powered devices usually have a control switch in the handpiece; however, some electric-powered equipment can be operated with a foot switch (foot-controlled pedal). **Figure 11.5** shows an operational foot pedal, and **Figure 11.6** shows a foot pedal damaged by fluid invasion.

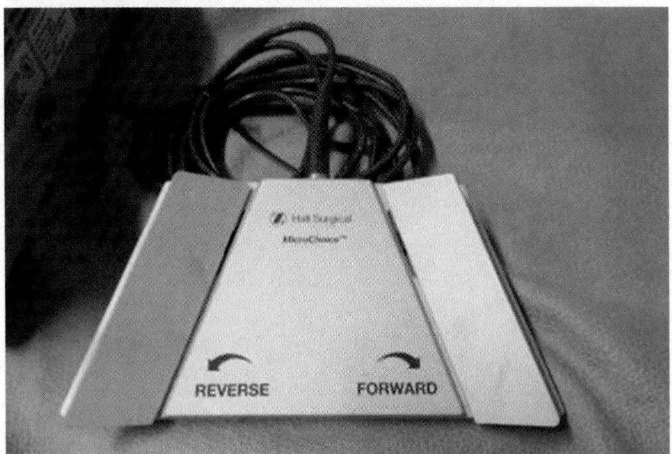

Figure 11.5

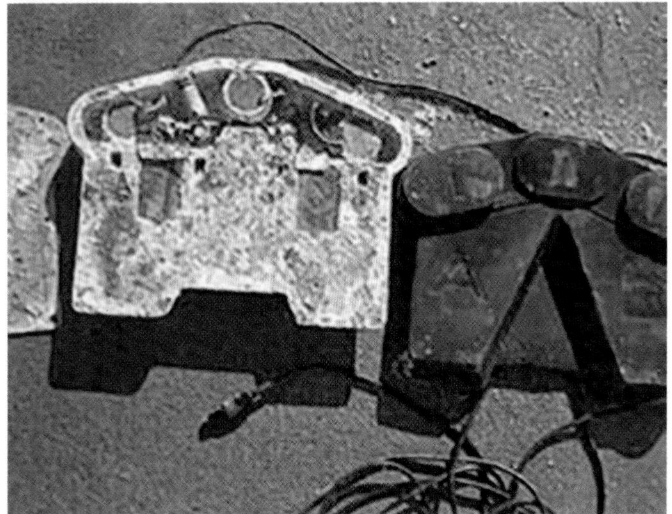

Figure 11.6

Foot switches may have a cable to attach to the instrument console, or they may be wireless. To clean foot switches, follow the manufacturer's instructions and avoid pulling on or kinking the power cord or damaging the sensors.

Pneumatic-Powered Surgical Instruments

Pneumatic (compressed air/gas-powered) instruments come in various sizes and allow the surgeon to work on small, medium and larger bones. Sternum saws, sagittal saws, and drills are popular pneumatic-powered instruments.

Pneumatic-powered instruments require a hose that can be sterilized. (See **Figure 11.7**) One end of the hose attaches to the motorized handpiece on the surgical field; the other end attaches to the source of compressed air/gas, which can come from a stand-alone cylinder (tank) with a pressure regulator (See **Figures 11.8** and **11.9**) or be "piped in" through a wall or column-mounted regulator panel. (See **Figure 11.10**)

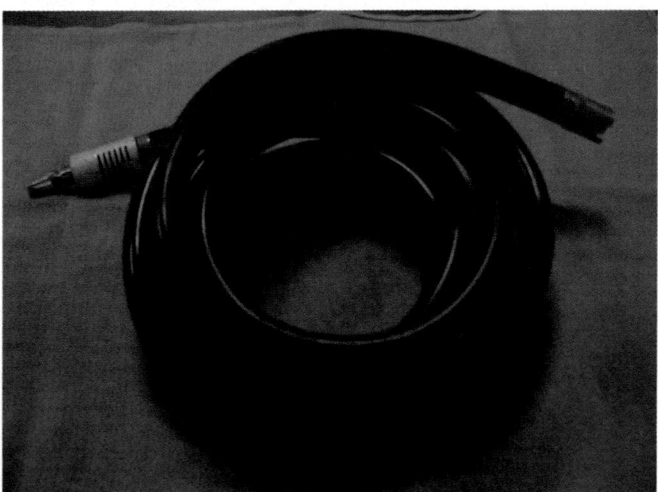

Figure 11.7

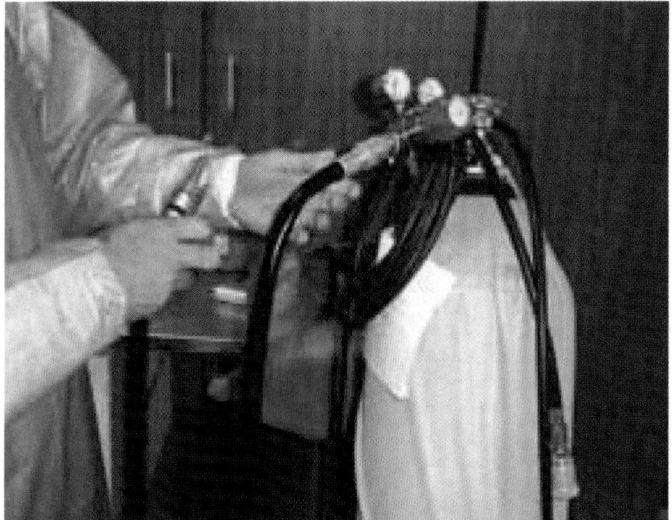

Figure 11.8

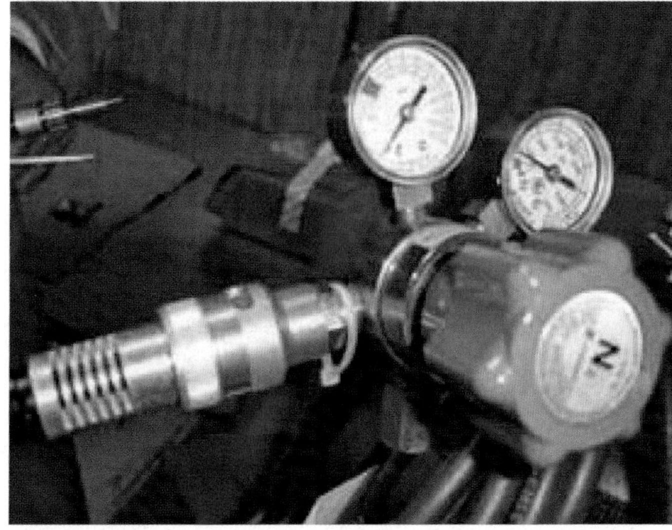

Figure 11.9

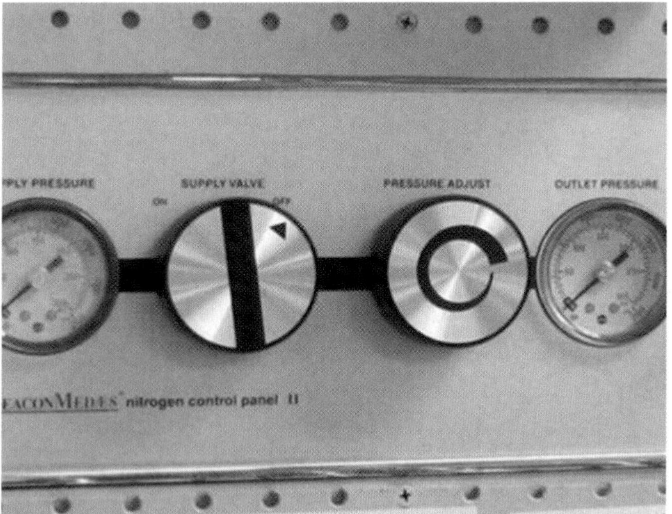

Figure 11.10

Instrument hoses must be carefully inspected for cleanliness. *Note: These hoses are typically black, so it is often difficult to see blood and debris.* Hoses must also be inspected for nicks and other possible damage. They must be pressurized for proper inspection; therefore, an air/gas source is required in the processing area.

If the hose casing becomes damaged (or "bubbled"), it must be removed from service. Fluid must not enter the hose or handpiece during processing. Many manufacturers recommend connecting the hose to the handpiece during cleaning to help prevent fluid invasion and related damage.

Different types of powered instruments require different operating pressures; a chart of these pressures should be available where the instruments are processed. SP technicians must follow the manufacturer's instructions and test instruments using the appropriate air/gas. Extreme care is required because testing instruments at an improper pressure can injure the operator and/or severely damage the instrument. **Figures 11.11** and **11.12** provide examples of pneumatic instruments.

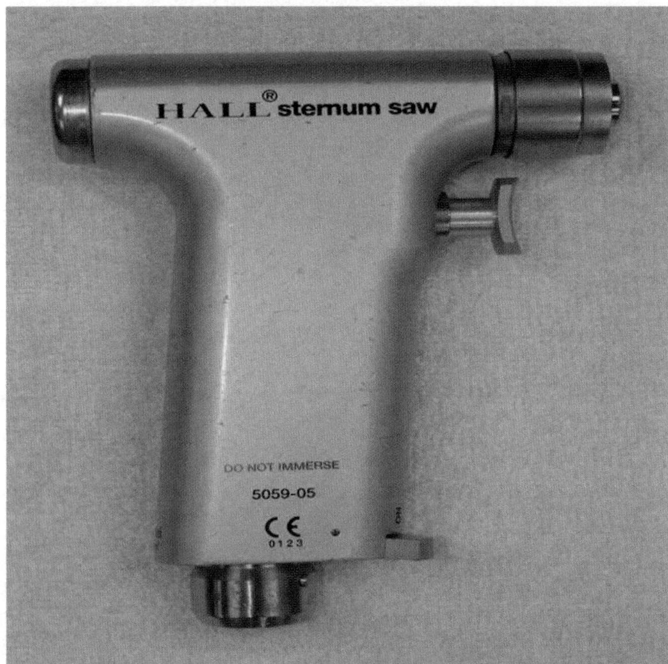

Figure 11.11 Pneumatic-powered sternum saw

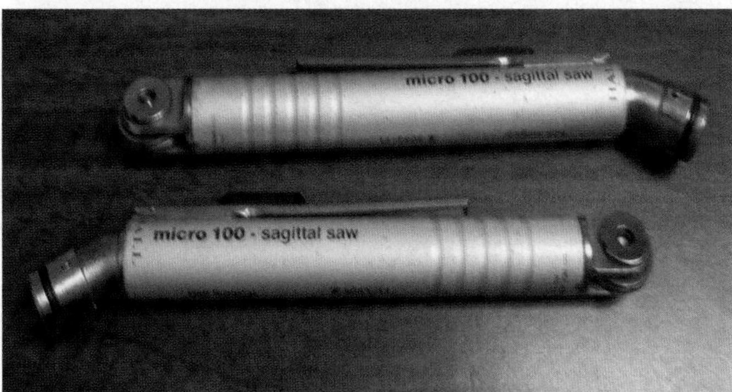

Figure 11.12 Pneumatic-powered sagittal saws

To properly care for and handle pneumatic equipment:

- Use a decontamination hose to protect inner components. (See **Figure 11.13**)

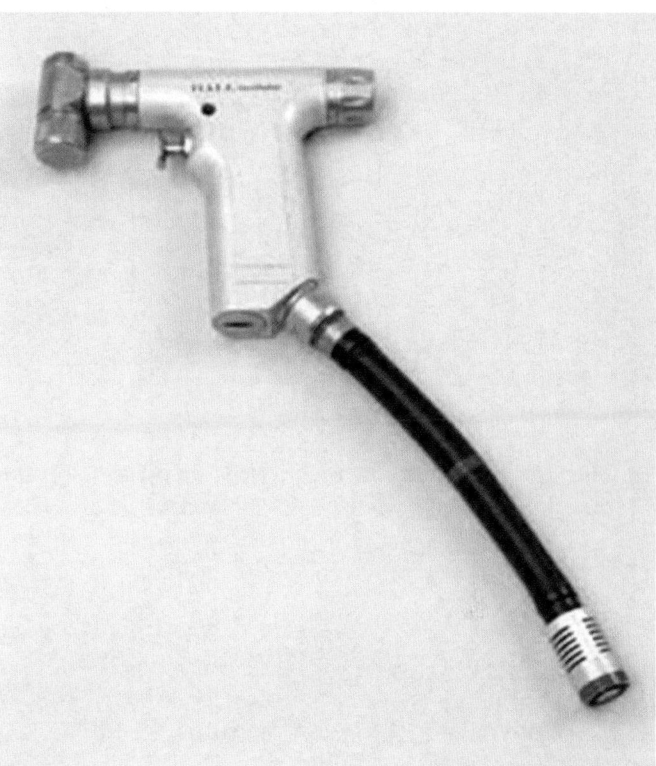

Figure 11.13

- Never immerse in any solution (including water), unless the manufacturer's IFU specifically states the device can be submerged.

- Carefully clean the outer casing of the handpiece using a damp, non-linting cloth. (See **Figure 11.14**)

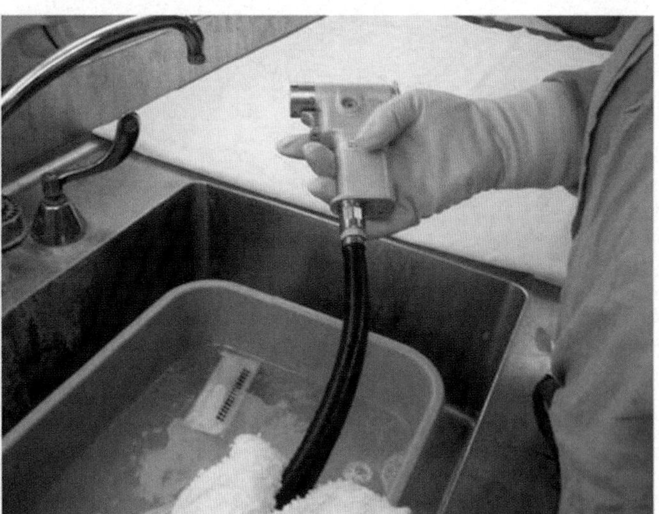

Figure 11.14

- To clean attachments, insert the appropriate manufacturer-recommended cleaning brush into attachments and burr guards. (See **Figure 11.15**)

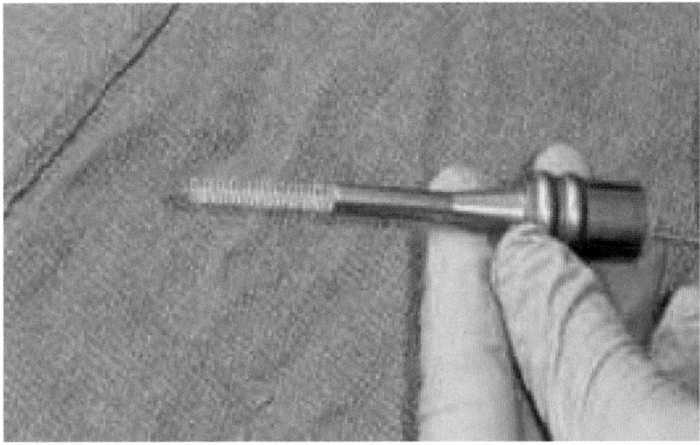

Figure 11.15

- Burr guards must be lubricated according to the manufacturer's instructions.
- Lubricate per the IFU.

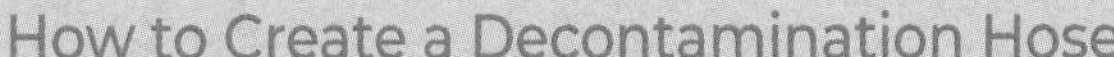

How to Create a Decontamination Hose

Decontamination hoses are made by cutting small pieces of a damaged pneumatic hose, placing both regulator ends on the hose, and marking the hose in some way to identify it as non-functional. A popular way of marking the hose is with red tape.

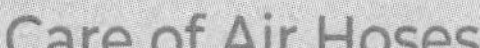

Care of Air Hoses

All pneumatic equipment must be attached to an air hose to operate. Sterilization issues are the primary reason hoses fail because heat from sterilization breaks down the rubber components and O-rings and causes air leakage. To clean the hose, use a mild detergent. Don't allow fluids to enter the hose and never use abrasives to wash the hose. Take care when coiling the hose during handling. Hoses should not be coiled tightly. Proper coil size for sterilization should be nine to 12 inches.

Battery-Powered Surgical Instruments

Battery-powered surgical instruments are cord free and work well with the procedures performed on larger, denser bones. Total hip and knee replacement surgeries are examples of such procedures. (See **Figure 11.16**) Batteries and chargers are specific to each system and are not interchangeable. (See **Figure 11.17**) **Figure 11.18** provides examples of battery-powered instruments.

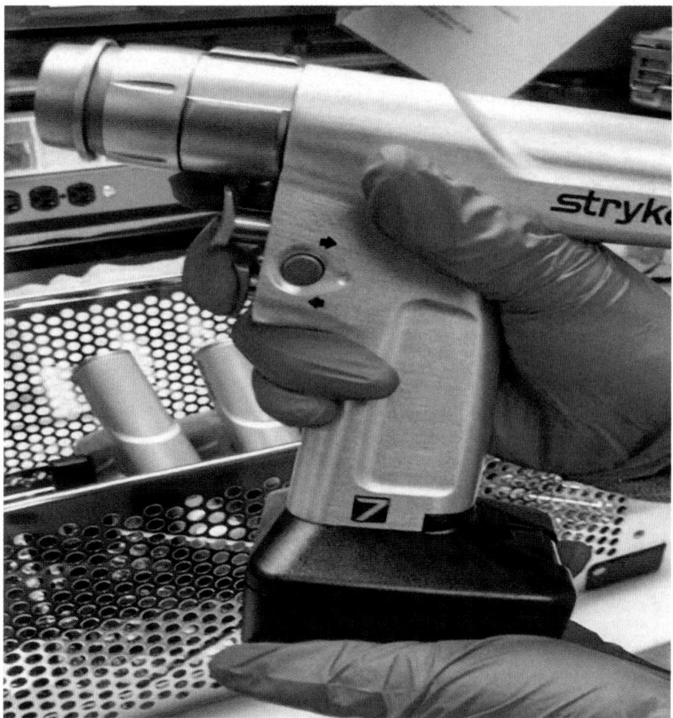

Figure 11.16

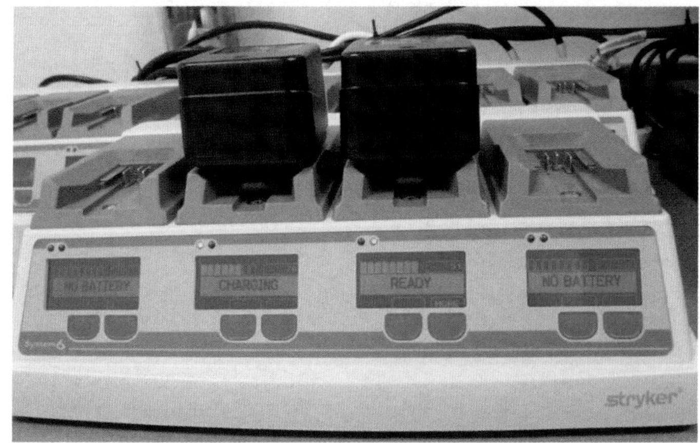

Figure 11.17

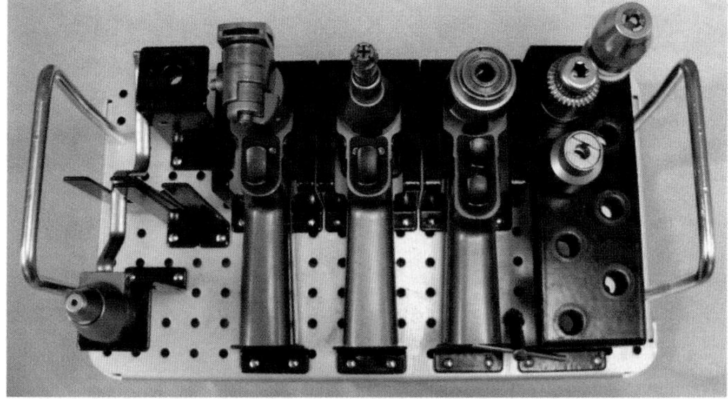

Figure 11.18

Common Powered Surgical Instruments

- Dermatome/dermabraders for harvesting skin grafts or reshaping skin surfaces
- Cebatomes for removing bone cement
- Sternal (sternum) saws to split the sternum and allow access for open heart surgery
- Dental drills for repair/reconstructive work on teeth and jawbones
- Micro drills for reshaping middle ear bones or driving very small wires through bones
- Wire drivers, drills and saws to work on the smallest facial bones to the largest bones (such as those in the leg)
- Saws designed to perform specific cutting actions

How to Create a Decontamination Battery

Locate an unrepairable battery for each style of powered surgical instrument. Use instrument marking tape to make a red "X" on the battery packs and keep these batteries in the decontamination area. When battery-powered equipment enters the Sterile Processing decontamination area, select and insert the appropriate battery pack to protect the electrical components from moisture. *Note: While this does help prevent moisture from entering the unit, care should still be taken to avoid contact with excess moisture.*

To properly care for battery-powered instruments:

- Never immerse handpieces, attachments or batteries in any solution, including water, unless approved by the manufacturer.
- Clean surgical debris from attachments, batteries and handpieces using brushes, a damp, non-linting cloth, and a manufacturer-recommended mild detergent. Carefully clean the attachment area of the handpiece.
- Rinse with water, while assuring that the water does not enter the battery contact area.

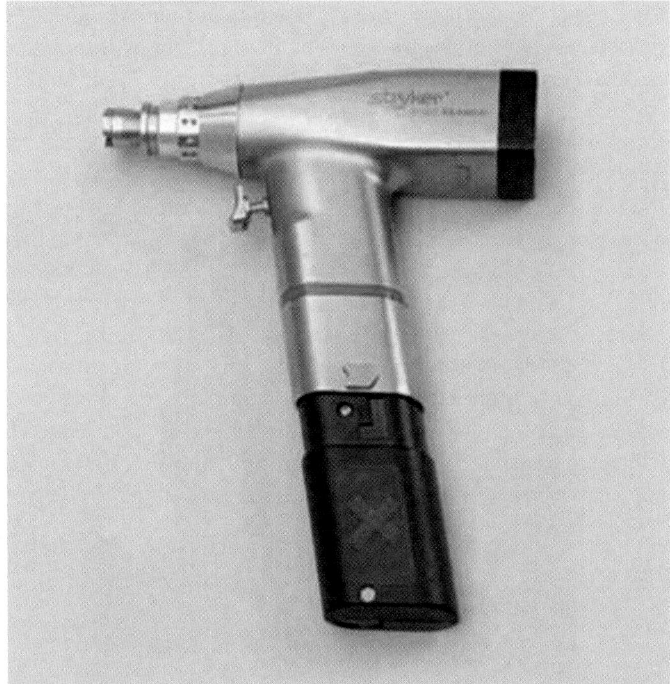

Figure 11.19

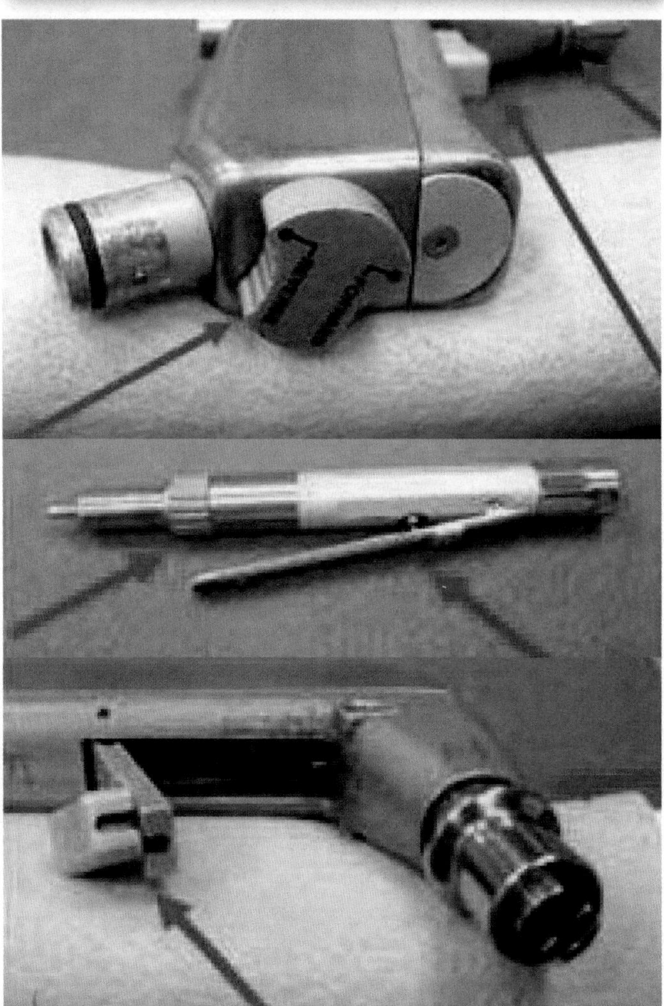

Figure 11.20 Check moving parts of powered surgical instruments.

- Use a decontamination battery to protect electrical components from moisture. (See **Figure 11.19**)
- Check all moving parts for cleanliness and function. (See **Figure 11.20**)

- Lubricate per the manufacturer's IFU. *Note: Not all powered instrumentation or accessories are lubricated. Refer to the device's IFU.*

- Some manufacturers recommend operating handpieces to ensure proper function and disperse lubrication (if added) prior to packaging for sterilization. (See **Figure 11.21**)

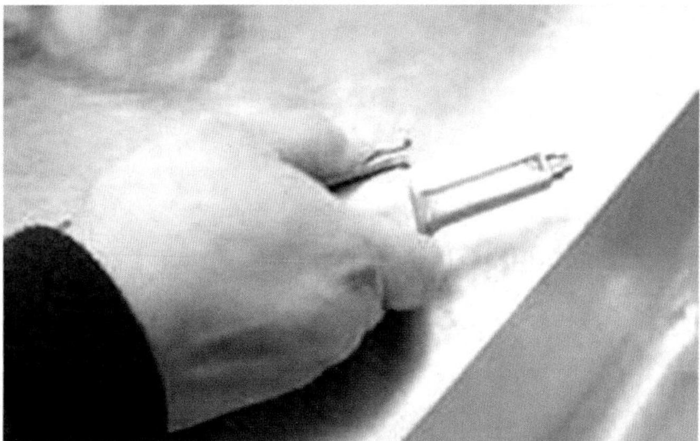

Figure 11.21

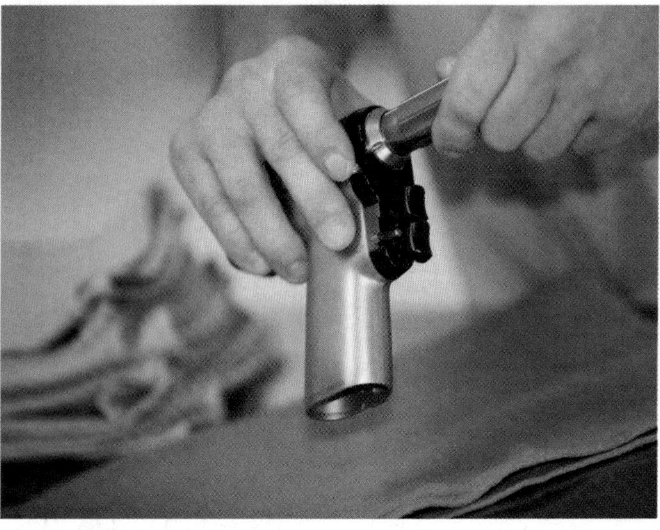

Figure 11.22

- Attach accessories, including batteries, to the handpieces to ensure they fit and function properly. (See **Figure 11.22**)

- Package and sterilize the device, per the manufacturer's recommendations. Special racks or positioning devices may be needed to ensure that all device surfaces are properly exposed to the sterilant and to ensure that condensation does not collect. Some types of packaging, such as peel packs, are not suitable for all types of powered instruments and accessories. Check the manufacturer's packaging recommendations.

- Charge, package and sterilize batteries per the IFU. Document the charging date on the outside of the package.

Common Reasons for Powered Equipment Repairs

Powered surgical equipment is expensive to purchase and repair. Common causes of damage include:

- Corrosion of internal components from condensation, steam, fluid invasion or improper cleaning.

- Physical damage due to mishandling. (See **Figure 11.23**)

- Lack of or improper preventive maintenance.

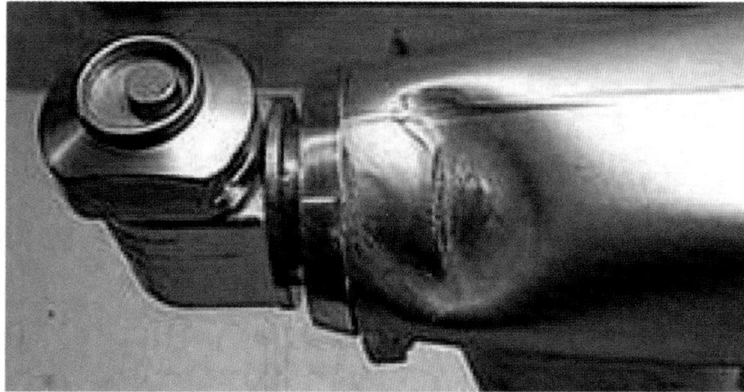

Figure 11.23

Motorized handpieces are very delicate and expensive and require special care. Proper use and handling, along with regular preventive maintenance and service, will help ensure that the devices are available for safe, effective use.

ENDOSCOPES

The term "endoscopy" means "looking inside." Endoscopic procedures allow a physician to look inside the body through an **endoscope**. Endoscopic procedures are considered minimally invasive because they do not involve a large incision. This minimally-invasive instrumentation allows the physician to perform procedures either through natural body openings like the mouth, nose or anus, or through small incisions that provide access for endoscopic instrumentation. This instrumentation may be used to view a specific area of the body or, with the addition of other instruments, perform multiple types of surgeries. The first endoscopes were developed in Germany in the 1800s; however, the use and development of endoscopes became more popular after World War II. In the 1950s, the flexible endoscope was introduced. Today, fiber optics [a technology that uses glass (or plastic) threads (fibers) to transmit data] and **light-emitting diodes (LED)** are the primary carriers/sources of light for endoscopic surgery.

> **Endoscope** An instrument used to examine the interior of a hollow organ or body cavity.
>
> **Light-emitting diode (LED)** Semiconductor diode that emits light when voltage is applied.

All endoscopes allow for light and image transmission. Some endoscopes also provide a working channel, allowing the surgeon to perform surgical procedures. LED serve as tiny light bulbs. Fiber optics do not produce light; instead, they act as wires to carry light generated from an external source. (See **Figure 11.24**)

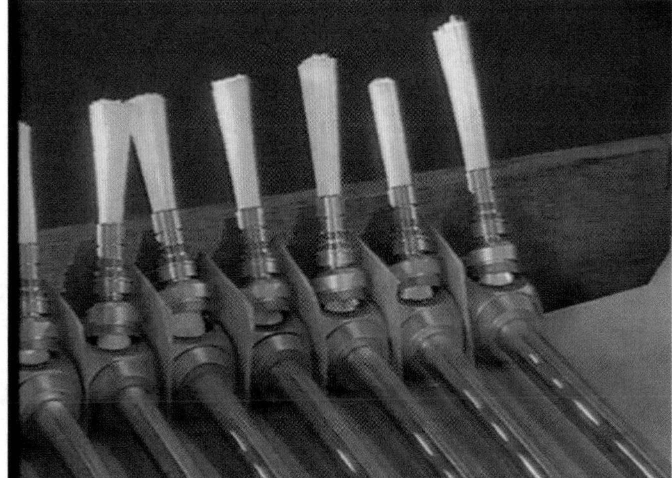

Figure 11.24 Light fibers before final assembly. Each strand of glass carries light from the light guide post to the distal end of the endoscope.

Light is a critical factor in endoscopic procedures, as the quality of the image or picture is largely dependent on light quality and quantity. It is important to check the endoscope, light source and carrier (fiber optic cord) to ensure they are in working order each time the endoscope is processed. The dark areas in **Figure 11.25** indicate damaged light fibers.

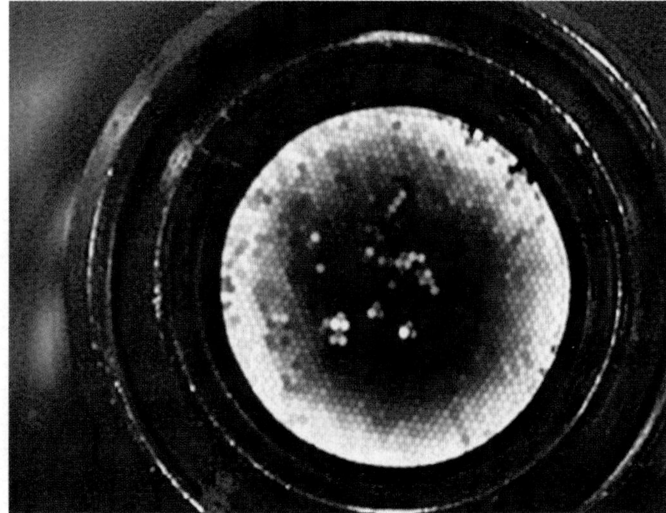

Figure 11.25 Badly damaged light fibers

The second function of endoscopes is to transmit the reflected image back to the surgeon's eye or to a video system. **Figure 11.26** shows endoscopy with the use of a video system. This can be accomplished through the use of fiber optic bundles or computer chips inside the endoscope.

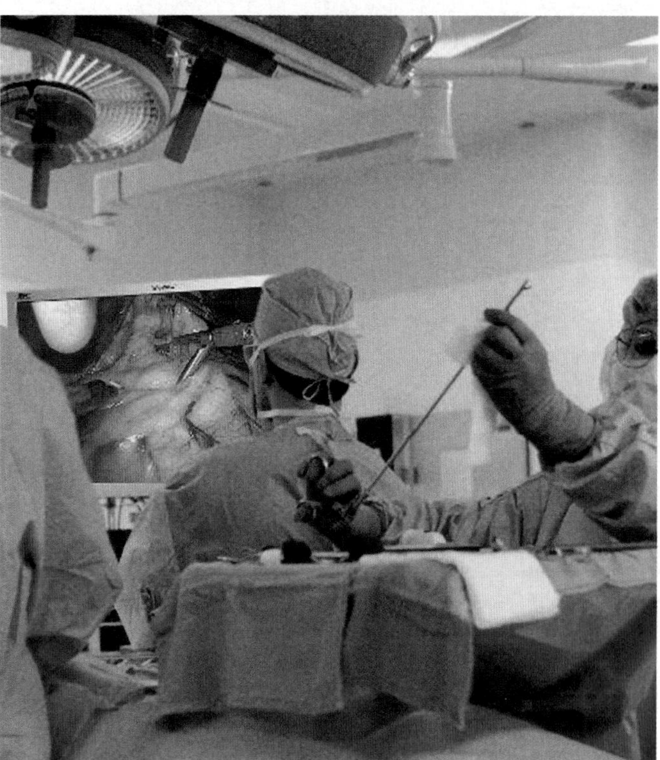

Figure 11.26

Endoscope Classification

The term "endoscope" describes all devices used to view inside a body cavity.

When discussing endoscopes, it is important to properly classify the type of endoscope in use because function, care and handling processes are different for each classification. This section will focus on rigid, semi-rigid and flexible endoscopes.

The classification of rigid, semi-rigid and flexible relates to an endoscope's ability to bend without damaging the device.

Operative and Non-Operative Endoscopes

The first endoscopes were non-operative, meaning the surgeon could view anatomy through the device but could not perform a surgical procedure such as a biopsy. Operative endoscope technology permitted surgeons to do much more than diagnose a condition; they could perform corrective surgeries with these new minimally-invasive instruments. Surgical procedures, such as laparoscopy and arthroscopy, came into demand as physicians and patients realized the benefit of shorter hospitalizations, less painful surgical procedures, lower healthcare-associated infection (HAI) risks, and faster recovery times.

An operative endoscope has a working channel (lumen) through which instruments or accessories can be passed to perform surgical procedures. (See **Figure 11.27**)

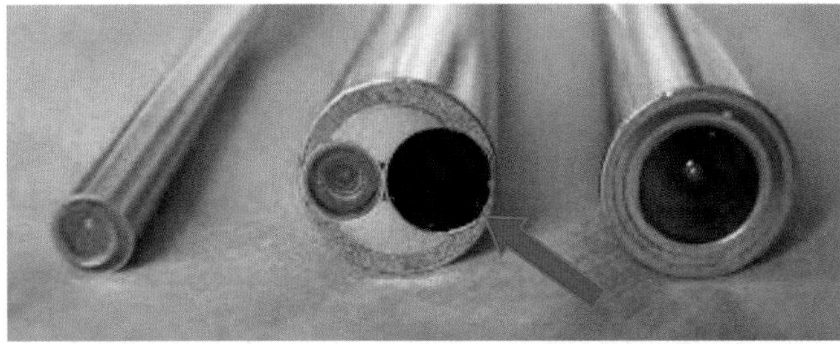

Figure 11.27 Operative and non-operative rigid endoscopes. Note the operative channel in the middle scope.

Technological advancements continue today across surgical specialties, much of which has been fueled by the development of smaller instruments and endoscopes. For example, surgeons can perform endoscopic abdominal, arthroscopic, urological, otolaryngeal, cardiac and neurosurgical procedures. Recent endoscopic developments permit heart conditions to be treated without opening the chest or cutting the ribs, pituitary surgery to be performed through the sinus cavity, and salivary gland stones to be removed endoscopically. Lesions in the gastrointestinal tract and lungs can be directly visualized, and diagnostic biopsies and therapeutic procedures can be performed without major surgery or general anesthesia.

Endoscope Use and Selection

Endoscopes are chosen by the physician based on the type of procedure they are performing. Rigid endoscopes are appropriate for viewing anatomy where there is straight-line access to the site. Semi-rigid endoscopes are useful where the line to the surgical site is relatively straight; however, some slight bending of the endoscope shaft may be needed to access the site such as in bladder surgery. Flexible endoscopes are used where straight-line access is not possible (such as when viewing the esophagus, lungs, kidneys or large intestine). Whether a rigid, semi-rigid or flexible endoscope is used, the device serves as the eye of the surgeon.

Due to these instruments' delicate construction as well as their size and frequent handling, endoscopes are at risk of being damaged every time they are handled. Damaged or poorly performing endoscopes result in costly procedure delays, staff and surgeon dissatisfaction and, possibly, patient harm.

RIGID AND SEMI-RIGID ENDOSCOPES

Rigid Endoscopes

Rigid endoscopes range in size from very tiny, 1.9mm endoscopes used for sialendoscopy (internal viewing of the salivary glands) to larger 15mm endoscopes used for robotic surgical procedures. Rigid endoscopes can be constructed using rigid rod lenses (non-video) or with a video chip mounted in the distal end (video). (See **Figure 11.28**)

Generally, all rigid endoscopes are manufactured using tubes of stainless steel. Rigid endoscopes are designed to allow for some minimal flexing of the shaft, but damage will occur beyond the flex limits.

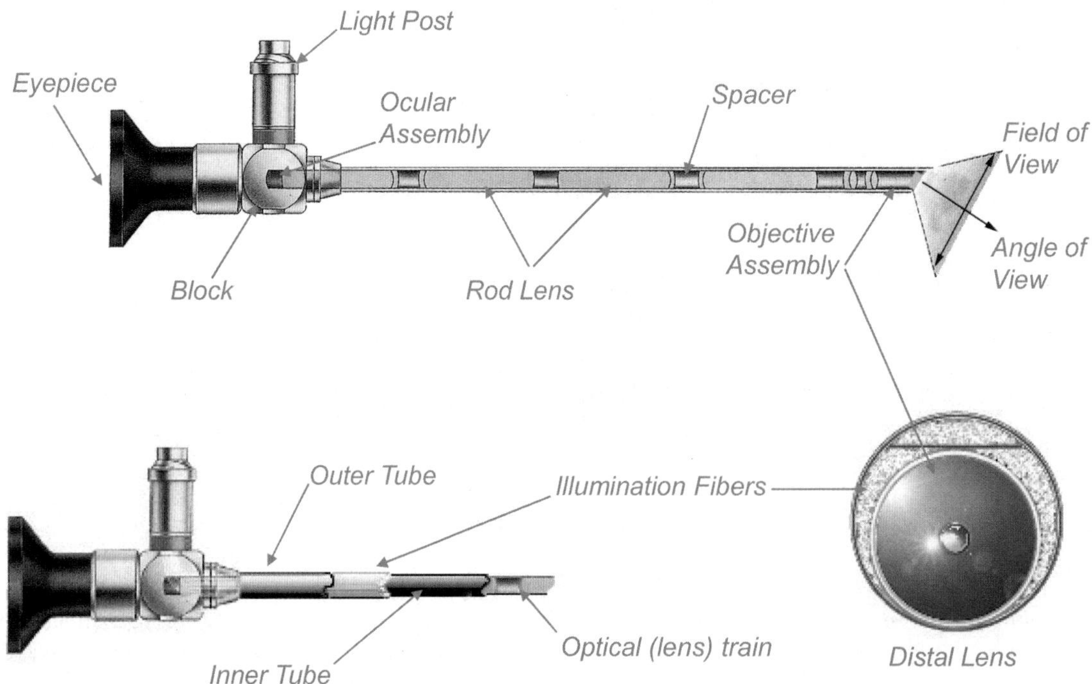

Figure 11.28

A general rule is that a rigid endoscope should not be bent. Fiber optics are housed between the inner and outer tubes and transmit light from the light guidepost to the distal end of the endoscope. (See **Figure 11.29**) Operative rigid endoscopes have a working channel that allows the surgeon to pass instruments to perform surgery.

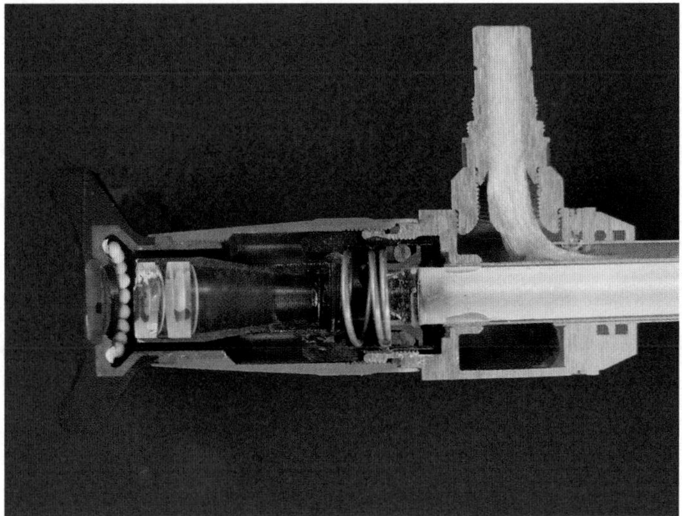

Figure 11.29 Cross-section view of a rigid endoscope

Specialty rigid endoscopes provide the ability to change the direction of view. The endoscope pictured in **Figure 11.30** allows the surgeon to change the direction of view by rotating a knob near the eyepiece. Other specialty endoscopes contain filters that help the surgeon identify diseased tissue when used in combination with pharmaceuticals and/or different spectrum light sources.

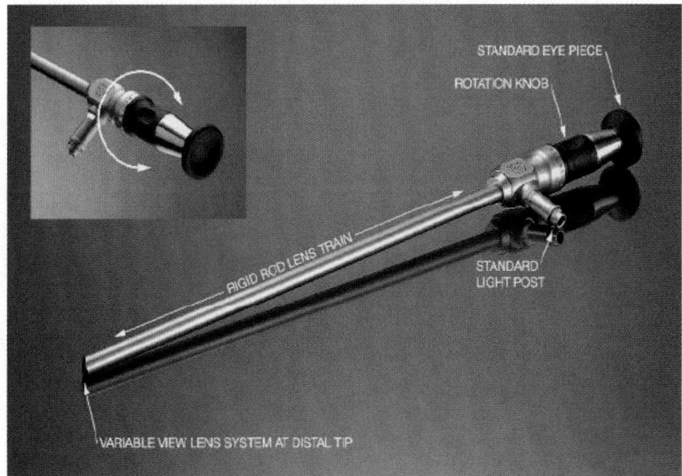

Figure 11.30 Variable direction of view

Semi-Rigid Endoscopes

Semi-rigid endoscopes are termed as such because the shaft is made of a very thin stainless steel, allowing it to bend slightly, without kinking the metal.

Semi-rigid endoscopes are primarily used in urology to view the bladder and the distal portion of the ureter. (See **Figure 11.31**) While they have the ability to bend slightly more than a rigid endoscope, they will be damaged if too much pressure is applied or if they are bent beyond their intended limits.

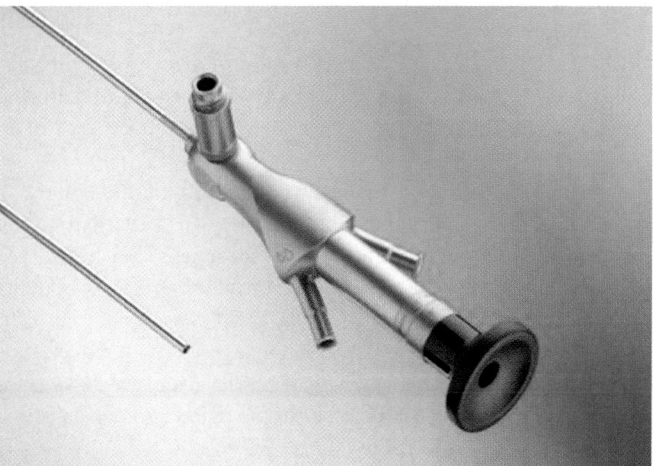

Figure 11.31

Rigid and Semi-Rigid Endoscope General Guidelines for Decontamination

The following are some general guidelines for cleaning rigid and semi-rigid endoscopes. Check with the individual endoscope manufacturer for specific instructions.

1. Remove the light source adapters from the light post. (See **Figure 11.32**)

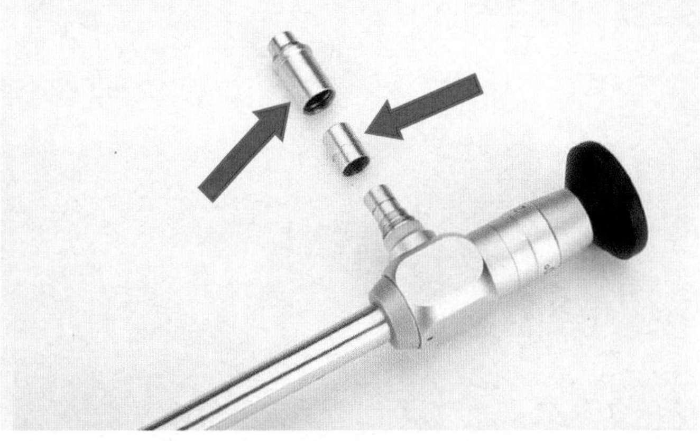

Figure 11.32 Rigid scope light source adaptors

2. Use the cleaning solution as identified in the manufacturer's IFU.

3. Hand wash the endoscope using a soft, non-linting cloth. Pay particular attention to the distal tip, as this is where debris collects and is most difficult to remove.

4. If the endoscope has a working channel, thoroughly brush the channel using the manufacturer's recommended brush type and size.

5. Thoroughly rinse the endoscope with critical water and flush the working channel to remove all traces of the cleaning solution.

6. Dry the outside of the endoscope with a clean, non-linting cloth. Dry the working channel per the manufacturer's IFU.

New technology allows for automated washing of non-operative rigid endoscopes. Check the manufacturer's IFU to verify that the tray and endoscope are approved for automated washing. (See **Figure 11.33**) Automated washing provides multiple benefits such as consistent quality of the wash process.

Note: Ultrasonic cleaning cycles must not be part of the automated washing because damage will occur to the rigid endoscope.

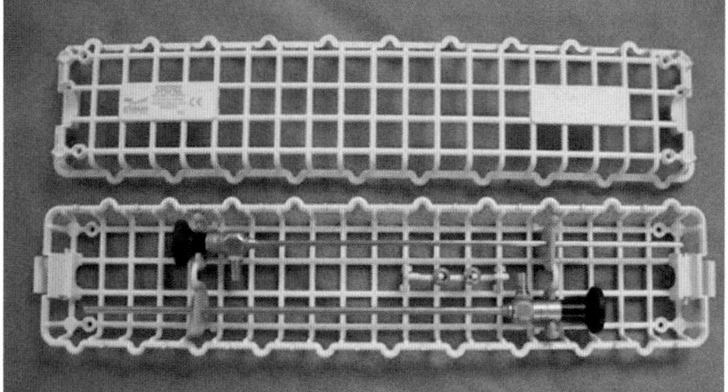

Figure 11.33 Basket and rigid endoscope approved for (non-sonic) automated cleaning

Rigid and Semi-Rigid Endoscope Inspection

The inspection process is very important for ensuring proper function of an endoscope. The technician must understand the proper procedure for inspection, and the manufacturer's IFU should be followed. The following are basic guidelines for addressing endoscope inspection:

- Closely inspect for damage and cleanliness.

- Functions, such as light output, image quality and angulations, should be examined (if applicable or possible).

- For rigid endoscopes used with bridges/sheaths, fit should be checked to ensure that the two devices go together with little to no force applied.

- For all endoscopes, the distal and proximal windows should be inspected for cleanliness and wiped off with an approved cleaner and a soft cloth, if necessary.

- For non-video rigid endoscopes, the image quality should be tested by viewing typewritten print through the endoscope from a distance of about one inch. (See **Figure 11.34**) The image should be closely examined in the center and for 360 degrees around the outside edge to ensure there are no blurry or dark areas. *Note: Most flexible fiber optic endoscopes have a focus-adjusting mechanism near the eyepiece.*

Rigid Endoscopic Instruments

Rigid endoscopic instruments come in hundreds of shapes and sizes, and many contain lumens that require special care to ensure that they are properly cleaned. Many instruments come

Check Rigid Endoscopes for Visual Clarity

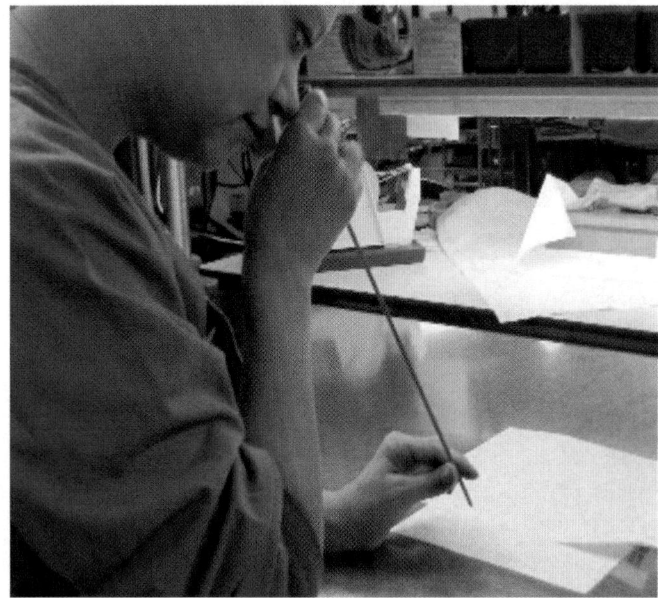

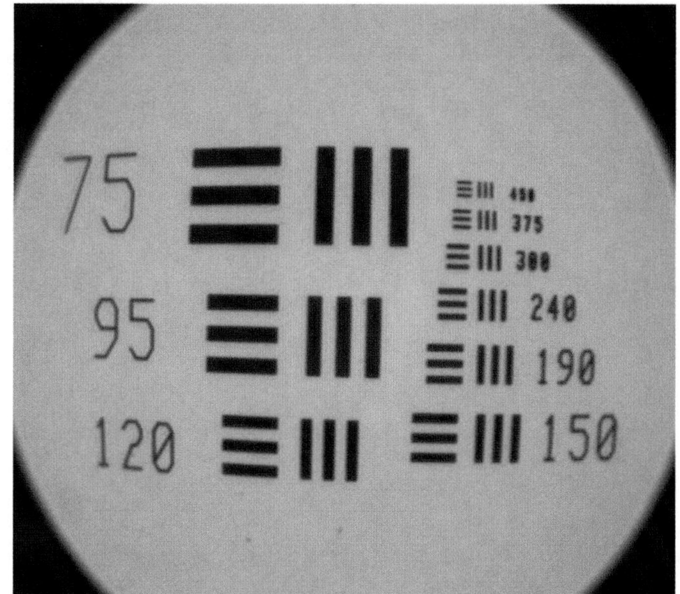

Figure 11.34 Rigid endoscope testing

with multiple parts such as a laparoscope with a handle, working insert and outer shaft. (See **Figure 11.35**)

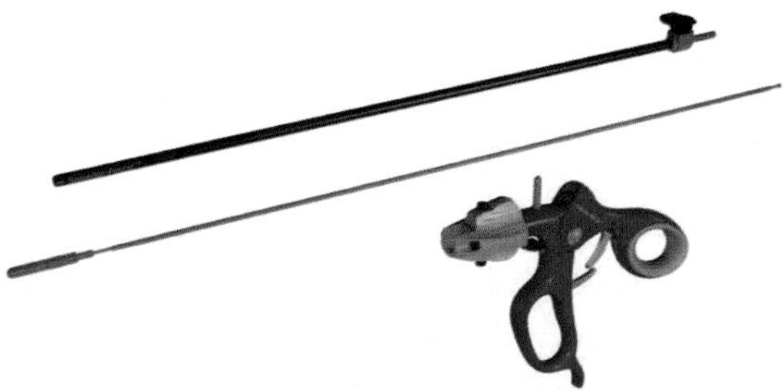

Figure 11.35 Disassembled laparoscopic instrument

Care and handling are often complicated due to some instrument designs. Hidden areas and moving parts can protect soil during the cleaning process. (See **Figure 11.36**) If the instrument cannot be easily disassembled into component parts, it may be impossible for a technician to determine that the lumens are clean.

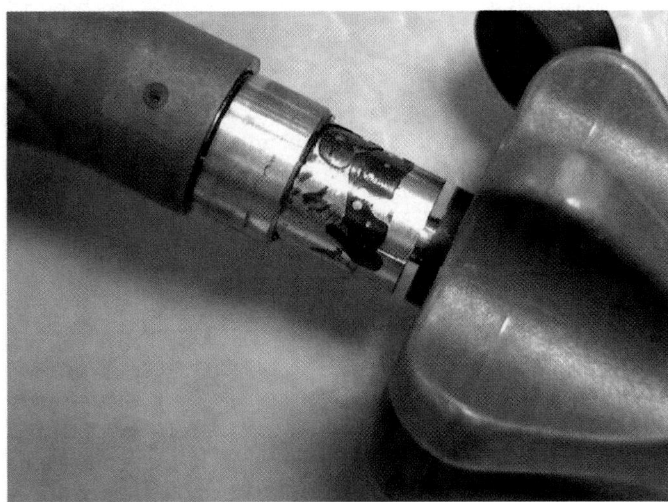

Figure 11.36 Debris under a rotating knob

Endoscopic and Robotic Instruments

Operative endoscopes require special instrumentation. The following section addresses common instruments used with rigid and semi-rigid operative endoscopes.

Laparoscopic Instruments

Most laparoscopic instruments can be easily identified because they are very slender (3mm to 10mm in width) and longer than other instruments. The shafts look like the shaft of pencils or small rods, and many of the tips have the same design as general instruments with the same name. The distal tip of a laparoscopic Allis forceps, for example, is the same design as the distal tip of a general surgery Allis forceps. (See **Figure 11.37**)

Some laparoscopic instruments are used to cut or cauterize during surgery. These instruments will have insulation covering the shaft, which protects the patient from electrical current that flows through the instruments. Laparoscopic insulation is susceptible to pin holes, cracks, tears and overall loosening. These defects must be identified as the instruments are tested and assembled. Failure to discover pin holes or other damage to the insulation can result in leaked electricity that can damage nearby tissue and organs. These burns can cause infection, extended patient recovery times and other complications.

To inspect the insulation, locate the metal collar at the distal tip. The insulation should fit tightly against the collar; this union should be snug, with no spaces visible. Next, grip the insulation and try to slide it back. If the insulation slides (moves), the instrument should be sent for repair. Finally, visually check the instrument shaft to look for cuts, cracks and nicks to the insulation, and inspect the insulated handle for chips or cracks.

Electronic testing devices (See **Figure 11.38**) can detect microscopic holes in the insulation of shafts and handles of laparoscopic instruments. Electronic testing with an approved testing device should be done prior to set assembly on the clean side of the Sterile Processing department (SPD). *Note: All insulated instruments (including non-laparoscopic devices) need to be tested for electrical leakage each time they are processed.*

Allis forceps

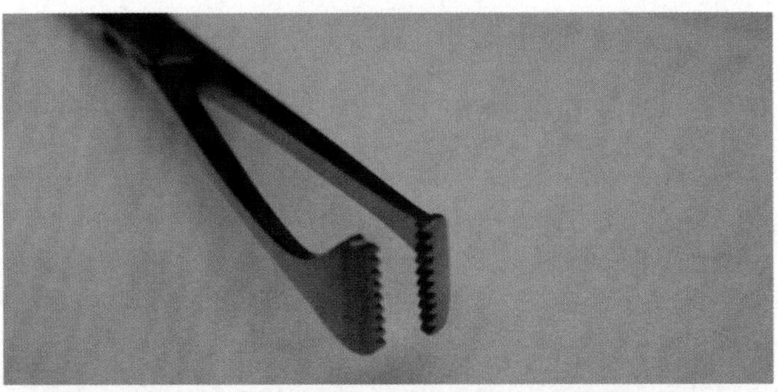

Laparoscopic Allis forceps

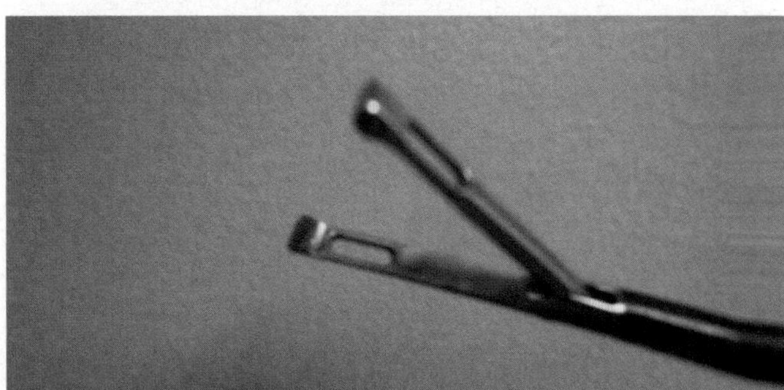

Figure 11.37 General and laparoscopic Allis forceps

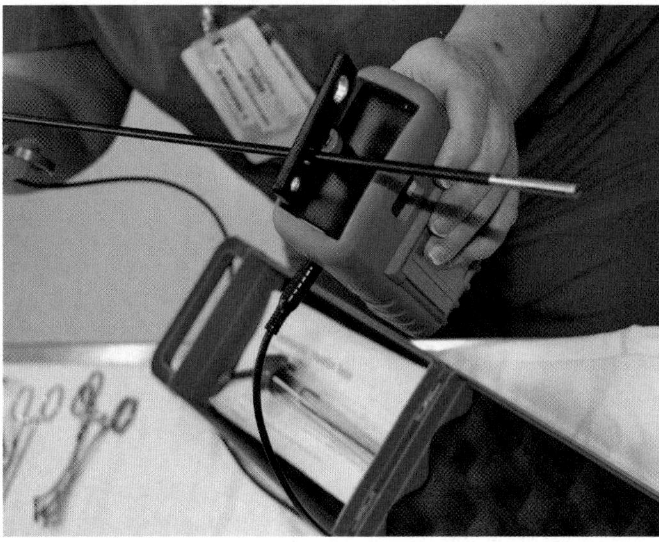

Figure 11.38

Laparoscopic hooks and spatulas are used to cut and/or cauterize. They must be inspected for insulation failure in the shaft and at the distal tip. (See **Figure 11.39**) Cannulated instruments require a brush for proper cleaning. Always use the brush type, size and length recommended by the manufacturer.

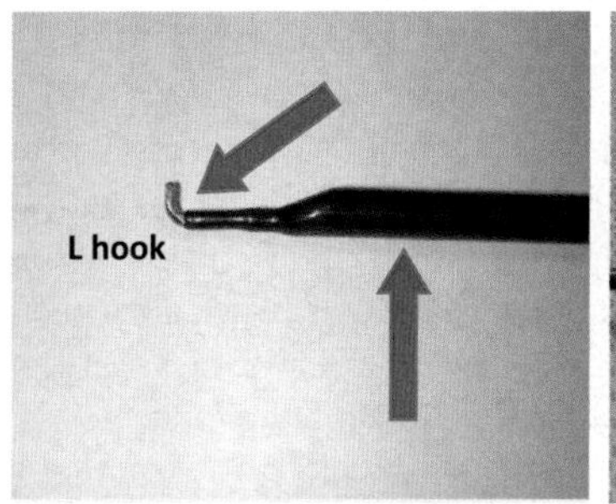

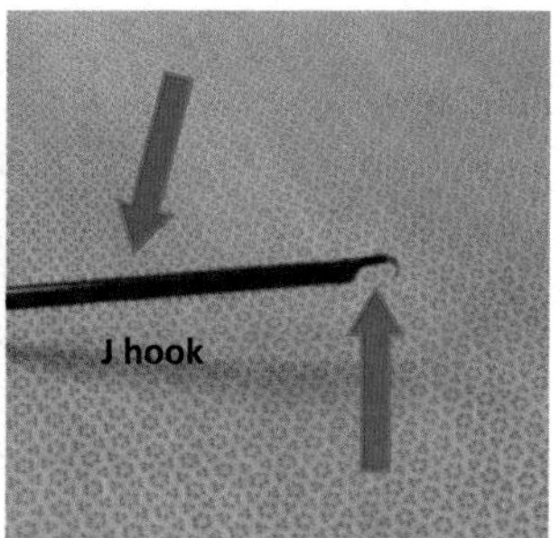

Figure 11.39 Laparoscopic hooks. Check tip for cleanliness and ensure insulation is intact.

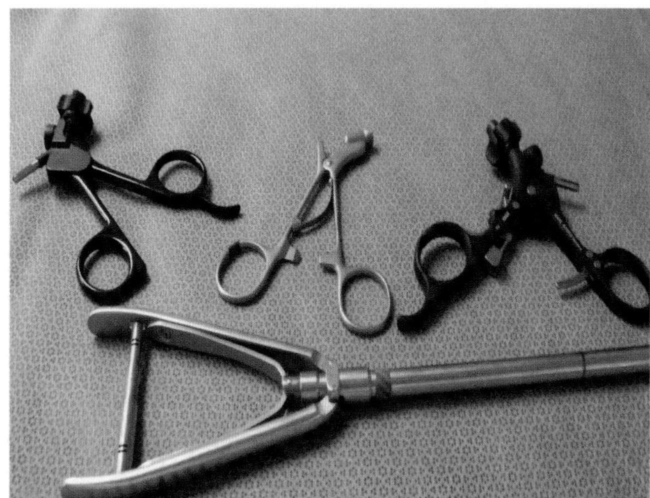

Figure 11.40

Laparoscopic ring handles are available in several styles (See **Figure 11.40**) such as:

- Free handle – No ratchet or spring finger, with an open-and-close action
- Spring handle – Opens under slight tension and closes by spring action
- Ratchet handle – Similar to hemostats, with various locking points on the ratchet

While most laparoscopic instrumentation can be mechanically cleaned, careful manual cleaning must take place first. Some laparoscopic instruments, such as scissors, can use disposable tips. Disposable tips should be removed and discarded prior to instrument cleaning. Manufacturers' cleaning instructions should be meticulously followed. All ports should be flushed, and lumens should be flushed and brushed. Instruments that come apart should be disassembled. Due to the dark-colored surface, insulated instruments must be carefully inspected for cleanliness. Spatulas and hook tips are very difficult to clean and must be carefully inspected for cleanliness.

During assembly, multi-part instruments should be assembled to ensure they are in working condition. Multi-part devices should then be disassembled for sterilization, unless otherwise stated by the instrument manufacturer. To protect these instruments from damage, care must be taken when placing them in a tray. If a tray designed for laparoscopic instruments is used, care should be taken not to bend the instrument shafts when placing or removing the instruments.

Electrosurgical cords connect instrumentation, such as laparoscopic instruments, to the electrical generator or power source. These cords carry electrical current from the generator to the instrumentation, where the surgical instrument focuses the electrical current to allow cutting and cauterization of tissue. Cords should not be dropped, kinked, twisted or coiled tightly during processing. Careful examination of the cord should be visually performed to inspect for cuts, nicks or any damage that could interrupt the electrical current.

Robotic Instruments

Over the past several years, robotic surgery has become very popular in many surgical specialties. While both laparoscopic and robotic surgery use small incisions to insert instruments and perform surgery, robotic surgery allows the surgeon to be remote from the patient (either across the room or even across a continent). As with laparoscopic surgery, robotic instruments are complex and require careful attention to ensure they are clean, sterile and functional when needed. (See **Figure 11.41**)

Robotic instruments are heavier than laparoscopic instruments. Mechanical and electrical components are located in the proximal

Robotic Instruments

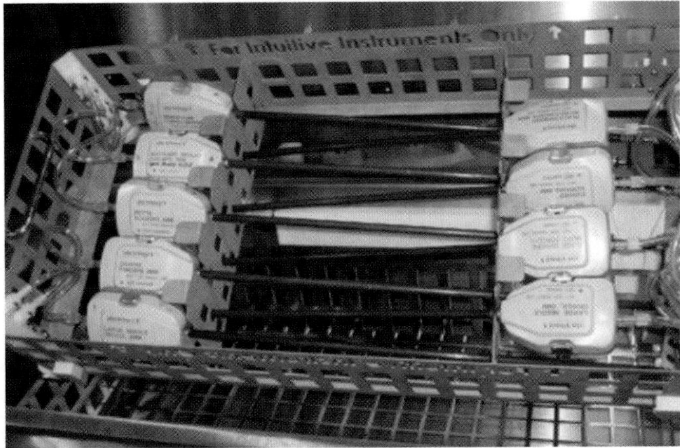

Figure 11.41

end of the instrument. Robotic instruments are more difficult to clean than standard laparoscopic instruments because:

- They do not come apart for cleaning.
- The distal end of the instrument rotates and may have open cabling that is difficult to clean.
- There may be multiple channels to flush in each instrument.

Robotic instrumentation is difficult and time consuming to process; carefully follow the manufacturer's cleaning instructions. Some IFU contain specific soak times and limit the number of sterilization cycles the instrument can undergo. Always flush and brush the lumens as instructed by the manufacturer. When connecting to an irrigating sonic, ensure the sonic is approved for cleaning robotic instruments and that the correct connectors are utilized. (See **Figure 11.42**)

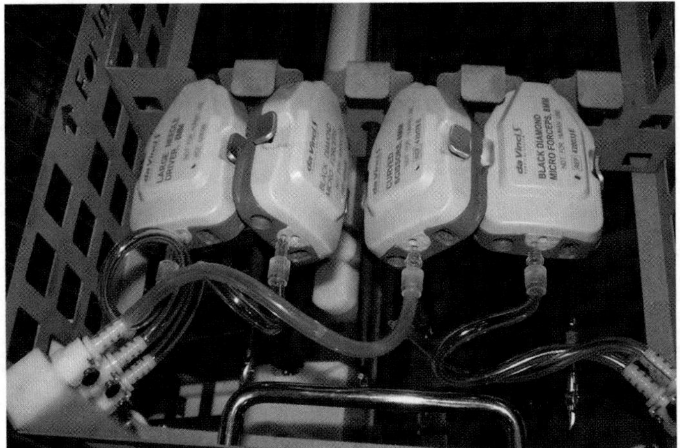

Figure 11.42

Robotic instrumentation is very delicate and complex. Careful attention to the manufacturer's IFU throughout the entire process is essential.

Laparoscopic Instruments

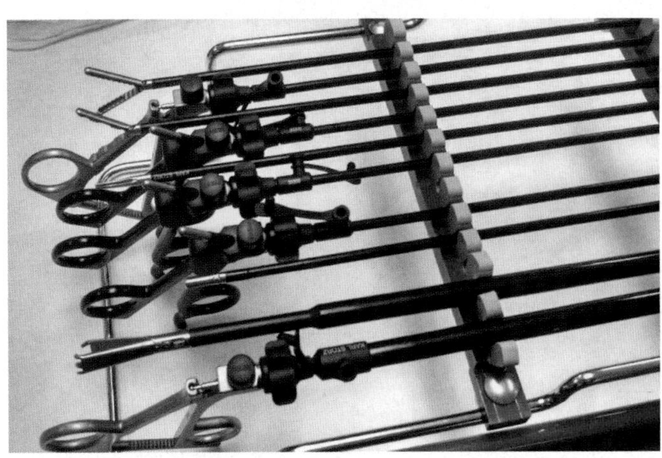

Arthroscopic Instruments

Arthroscopic surgery is a type of endoscopic procedure performed on joints. (See **Figure 11.43**) Because joints are small, enclosed areas, the instruments used for arthroscopic surgery are smaller than those used on other endoscopic procedures. Unlike laparoscopic instruments, most arthroscopy instrumentation does not look similar to general surgery instrumentation. (See **Figure 11.44**)

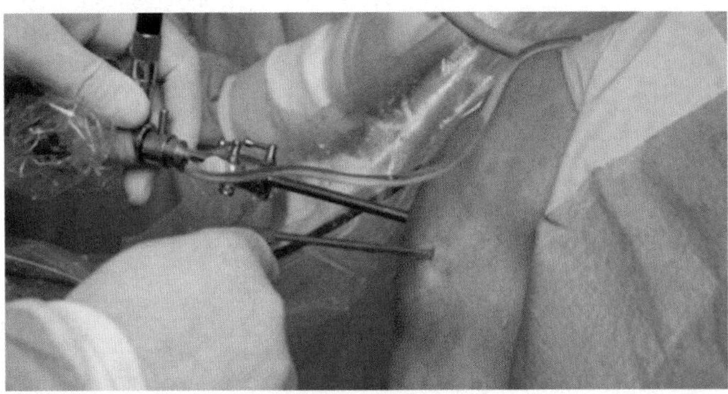

Figure 11.43 Knee arthroscopic surgery

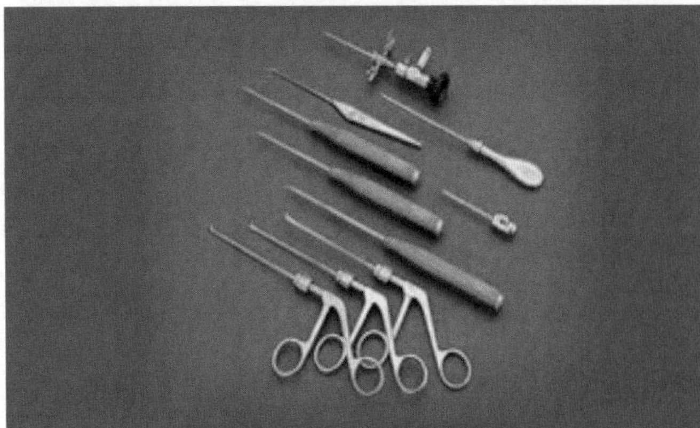

Figure 11.44 Arthroscopic instruments

Arthroscopic shavers can become clogged with debris during surgery, which can make them very difficult to clean. (See **Figure 11.45**) The use of a borescope is encouraged to check arthroscopic shavers for cleanliness.

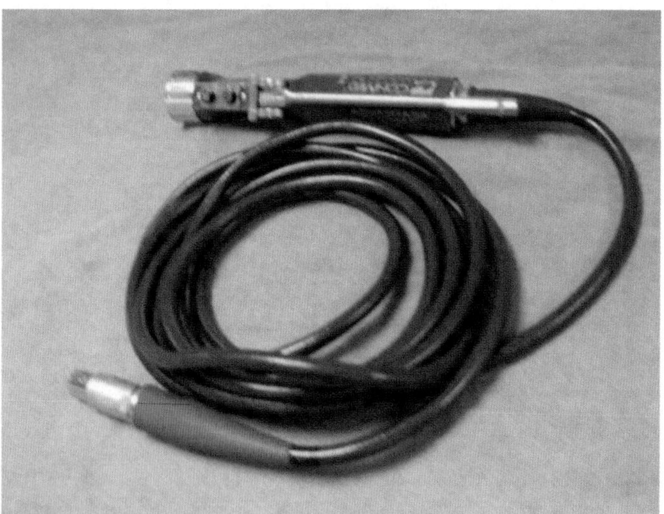

Figure 11.45

FLEXIBLE ENDOSCOPES

The term "flexible" means capable of bending and allows the physician to gain easier access to internal body organs. Flexible endoscopes are complex instruments used to visualize inside the body, perform diagnostic tests and surgical procedures, and/or obtain tissue specimens for biopsy.

Flexible endoscopes have revolutionized minimally-invasive surgical procedures because they give surgeons access to parts of the body without performing an open procedure. This minimizes tissue damage, patient discomfort and length of stay in the hospital. Like many sophisticated medical devices, the flexible endoscope is a complex instrument that requires processing between patients.

Flexible Endoscope Components

Flexible endoscopes are comprised of a body (handle assembly), universal cord (light cord) and an insertion tube (flexible shaft). The body features control knobs that, when actuated, cause the distal end of the endoscope shaft to move. Flexible endoscopes can be classified as either fiber optic or video. The difference between the two is how the image is captured and transmitted by the endoscope.

A fiber optic flexible endoscope gathers the image via a series of lenses at the distal end of the endoscope. (See **Figure 11.46**) The image is transmitted to the eyepiece via a fiber optic bundle. Video flexible endoscopes require a power source and a video system to view the image. The image is captured and transmitted as an electrical signal to the viewing monitor.

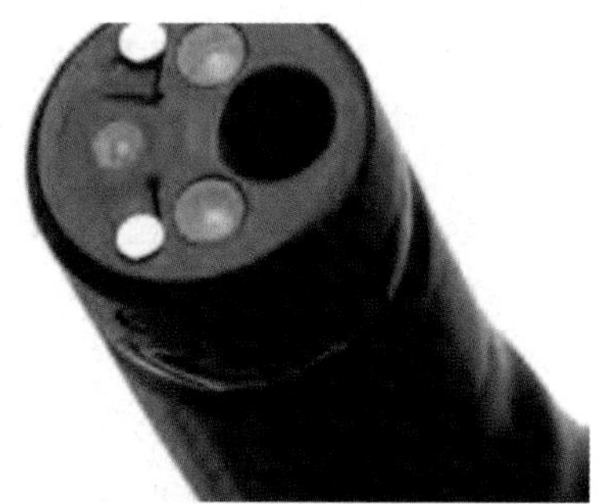

Figure 11.46 Distal end of a flexible scope

The internal components are contained and protected by an external sheath. The sheath is made of materials that can withstand exposure to bodily fluids and allows easy insertion and withdrawal. *Note: Care must always be taken when handling flexible endoscopes because sharp bends of the shaft or umbilical cable can cause damage.* Flexible endoscope lengths range from about 36" to 60" or longer. Like rigid endoscopes, flexible endoscopes can also be described as either diagnostic or operative. Operative flexible endoscopes have a working channel that allows the passage of a surgical instrument (i.e., biopsy forceps or diagnostic brushes for scrapings). These endoscopes may also have channel(s) for suction, irrigation, and insufflation to stretch the organ for better viewing.

Different caps are used to protect the endoscope from damage during various phases of reprocessing. If protective water caps are supplied, they must be in place whenever the endoscope is at risk of having water enter the endoscope. Flexible endoscopes may also come with a venting cap that opens the device to the outside environment. The venting cap is used to allow sterilants to enter and exit the endoscope channels. It is also used for shipping (particularly via air freight) to equalize pressure inside and outside the endoscope. *Note: A venting cap must never be used when the endoscope will be exposed to fluids, as it will allow fluid invasion and will likely result in damage.*

CLEANING AND PROCESSING FLEXIBLE ENDOSCOPES

Flexible endoscopes are difficult and time consuming to properly clean. The manufacturer's IFU, the Centers for Disease Control and Prevention's (CDC's) guidelines, the Association for the Advancement of Medical Instrumentation's standard, ANSI/AAMI ST91:2021 *Flexible and semi-rigid endoscope processing in health care facilities,* and facility protocols must be followed to help ensure the care, handling and processing of all endoscopes and accessory devices.

Technicians who process endoscopes should also follow standard precautions. They must wear personal protective equipment (PPE), including gloves, impervious gowns, face masks and shields (or goggles), shoe covers and hair coverings. (See **Figure 11.47**)

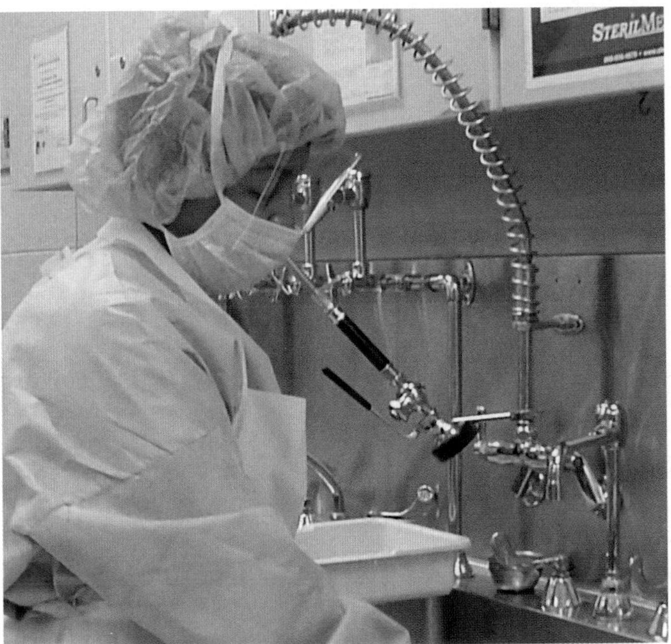

Figure 11.47

Endoscopes should be processed in an area large enough to allow for the safe handling of the instruments.

Be sure to follow the endoscope manufacturer's IFU to ensure that only approved cleaning chemicals are used. Cleaning should be performed with soft, clean, non-linting cloths or sponges and brushes specifically designed for use with each specific endoscope.

> **Not All Endoscopes Are Alike**
>
> Due to the significant difference in the processes required for video and non-video flexible endoscopes, it is important to follow the manufacturer's IFU for the model and brand of flexible endoscopes being cleaned.

Basic steps required to reprocess flexible endoscopes include:

1. Point-of-use treatment
2. Soiled transport
3. Leak testing
4. Cleaning
5. Rinsing
6. Drying
7. Cleaning verification and inspection
8. High-level disinfection (HLD)/sterilization
9. Rinsing
10. Drying
11. Storing

Note: ANSI/AAMI ST91:2021 Flexible and semi-rigid endoscope processing in health care facilities *now states endoscopes used in semi-critical applications should be sterilized prior to use. If sterilization is not possible, HLD is the minimum advised processing.*

Point-of-Use Treatment

Cleaning begins at the point of use to prevent blood or protein material from drying on the instrument. While performing point-of-use treatment, staff should wear the same type of PPE as is worn in the SPD's decontamination area. The IFU for point-of-use processes should be carefully followed to avoid damaging the endoscope. Suction channels should be rinsed with clean water to remove as much blood and tissue debris as possible. All disposable items should be removed and discarded. Endoscopes should be treated and transported to the SPD decontamination area as soon as possible following point-of-use treatment.

> **Delayed Processing**
>
> If endoscopes are not promptly transported to the decontamination area following the procedure, bioburden can harden on the devices and become more difficult to remove. Because of this drying process, some manufactures have developed **delayed processing** cleaning protocols. Delayed processing usually involves an extended presoak in the decontamination area, when the time from the end of point-of-use treatment until the start of manual cleaning exceeds 60 minutes. Even endoscopes that underwent point-of-use treatment can result in hardened, difficult-to-clean soil remaining if the device is not cleaned within one hour after the procedure. It is important to follow each manufacturer's protocol for their specific delayed endoscope processing procedures.

> **Delayed processing** Cleaning instructions for endoscopes that have not been processed within an hour after the completion of point-of-use treatment.

Transporting Soiled Endoscopes

Preparing flexible endoscopes is important to prevent damage to the endoscope and cross-contamination. Treated endoscopes should be placed in a leakproof, puncture-proof transport container. Again, the endoscope should be loosely coiled because tightly coiling flexible endoscopes will damage the device. Accessories, such as water bottles and biopsy forceps, should always be placed in a separate container. The container should then be sealed for transport. Containers should be properly labeled as a biohazard so others will know there are soiled items within the container.

Label the container with hand-off information to include:

- Patient identifier
- Procedure date
- Time point-of-use treatment was completed
- Any other pertinent information

Note: Remember to transport the endoscope to the decontamination area as soon as possible, ideally within 60 minutes after point-of-use treatment is completed. If transporting the soiled endoscopes offsite for cleaning, the devices should be transported per facility policy and regulatory requirements. The 60-minute limit for post-point-of-use treatment remains in effect.

Leak Testing

The majority of flexible endoscopes require a leak test be performed prior to submerging the device during cleaning and prior to HLD or sterilization. A leak test is necessary to ensure that the endoscope is watertight. A leaky endoscope should not be used on any patient, as the endoscope cannot be properly disinfected or sterilized, and chemicals or body fluids from the previous patient can potentially leak into the next patient. Fluid invasion will also damage the endoscope. (See **Figure 11.48**) Follow the IFU for each specific type and model of endoscope to ensure the proper type of leak testing is performed. *Note: Most endoscope manufacturers require the use of specific leak testers. Ensure the test is performed using the correct tool.*

Endoscopes that require leak testing must be tested each time the endoscope is used or processed. Be sure each leak tester is tested for proper function at least daily. Leak testers should undergo pressure verification each day that endoscopes are used.

Any endoscope that fails a leak test should be removed from service. Follow the IFU for further processing and send the endoscope to the manufacturer or an authorized repair company for service. Report the leak test failure according to facility policies and procedures and include the endoscope product identification and traceability information.

Note: The Occupational Safety and Health Administration (OSHA) requires that medical equipment be decontaminated to the maximum extent possible before transport.

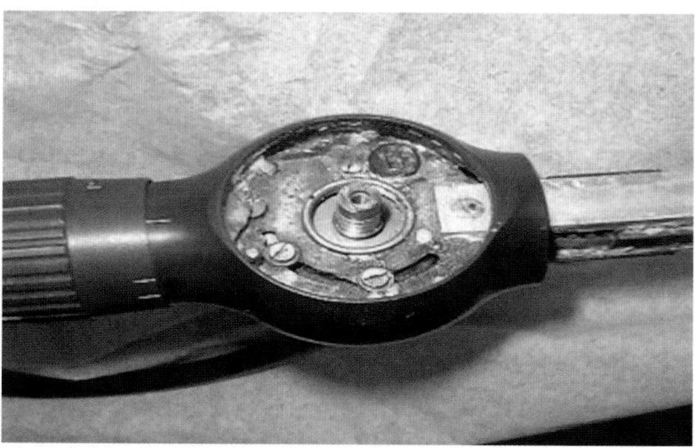

Figure 11.48 Inside of a scope with leak damage

Cleaning Steps for Flexible Endoscopes

The following are general recommendations for cleaning a flexible endoscope. Always consult the endoscope manufacturer's IFU for specific information pertaining to each endoscope's make and model.

- Thoroughly rinse the endoscope with water to remove all gross debris.
- Detach all removable parts (valves) and completely immerse the endoscope and valves in a solution recommended by the manufacturer. (See **Figure 11.49**)

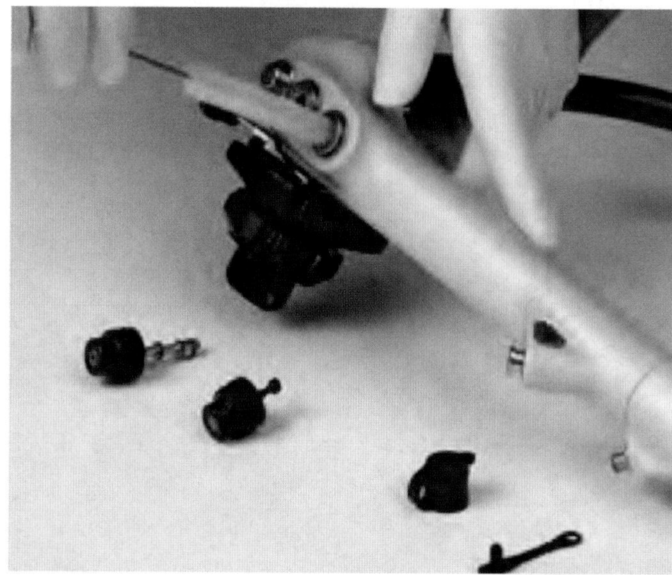

Figure 11.49 Remove detachable parts for cleaning

- Using a syringe or the manufacturer's supplied irrigation tubes, fill channels with cleaning solution.
- Keep the endoscope immersed for the time recommended by the manufacturer.

- While immersed, use a soft, clean, non-linting cloth or approved sponge to wipe the exterior of the endoscope. Use a soft-bristle brush to clean the valves and any crevices of the endoscope. Be sure to use the correctly-sized brush for the lumen's opening.

- Insert a long, flexible brush into the channel at the proximal end of the endoscope. Be sure it is the correct diameter to clean the channel. (See **Figure 11.50**)

- Carefully push the brush through until it exits the distal end. Rinse the brush bristles to remove debris and fully pull the brush back through the channel.

- Rinse the brush again and repeat until the brush remains clean after passing through the channel. Consult the IFU for any special brushing instructions.

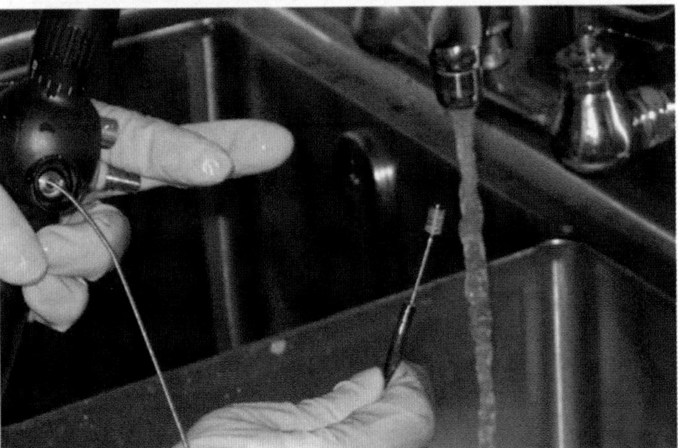

Figure 11.50

- After the immersion period, remove the endoscope and valves from the cleaning solution and completely immerse them in fresh water per the IFU. Be sure to flush all of the channels with water to remove the cleaning solution. Repeat the rinsing process using fresh water as recommended by the device manufacturer.

Alcohol and Endoscope Drying

In the past, alcohol was used as a drying agent. This process is no longer recommended because alcohol can act as a **fixative** if the endoscope is not completely clean. It is recommended to use pressure-regulated, forced instrument air [or, at minimum, high efficiency partial air (HEPA)-filtered air].

Fixative A substance used to keep things in position or stick them together. A chemical substance used to preserve or stabilize biological material for examination.

Endoscopes must be dried thoroughly to prevent the growth of microorganisms. External components can be dried with a clean, soft, non-linting cloth. Consult the device manufacturer's IFU for specific internal drying instructions.

Cleaning Verification and Inspection

An endoscope that appears clean can still harbor debris. Cleaning verification is used to detect whether residual organic soil and microbial contamination were removed. Cleaning verification is performed after endoscope cleaning and before disinfection or sterilization. Visual inspection involves examining the internal and external components of the endoscope to ensure all areas of the endoscope have been cleaned. Helpful tools used in visual inspection include lighted magnification for external components and borescope examination of internal structures and lumens. Cleaning verification tests include protein, carbohydrate, hemoglobin (blood), and adenosine triphosphate (ATP). Inspection using a borescope allows for visualization of the internal working channels to identify damage and residual soil and contaminants. An endoscope that has failed a cleaning verification test should be recleaned and retested. If an endoscope is suspected of having damage, it should be removed from service and sent to an appropriate repair service for evaluation.

High-Level Disinfection

HLD is the minimum biocidal requirement for endoscopes. ANSI/AAMI ST91:2021 now states that flexible endoscopes should be sterilized when possible. Always refer to the specific endoscope manufacturer's IFU for the proper HLD information for each make and model.

Sterilization of Flexible Endoscopes

Package and sterilize the endoscope following the manufacturer's IFU. Some flexible endoscopes that are sterilized using low-temperature sterilants may require a venting cap during sterilization. (See **Figure 11.51**) *Note: Always be sure to use the appropriate sterilization method and cycle.*

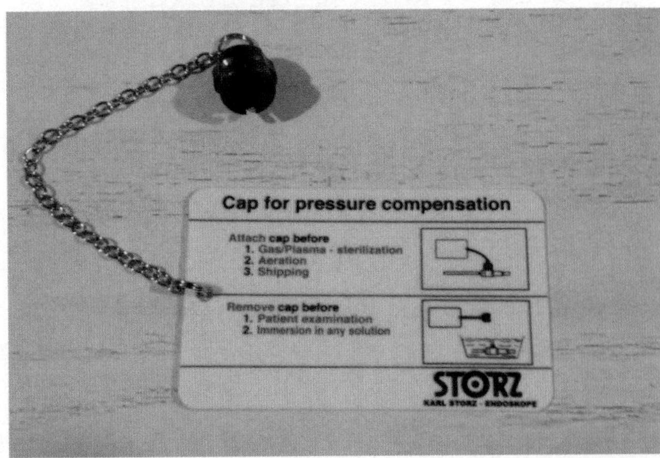

Figure 11.51 Venting cap

Storing Endoscopes

Proper storage of endoscopes is an important part of endoscope processing to ensure the devices are safe for patient use. Before being placed into storage, endoscopes should be identified as patient-ready to distinguish processed endoscopes from non-processed endoscopes. The patient-ready label or tag is attached to the patient ready endoscope with information that includes:

- Processing date
- Name(s) of the person(s) who performed the processing (as specified by facility policy)
- Expiration date, based on the facility's established risk assessment, if applicable.

Two types of endoscope storage cabinets are recommended for processed endoscopes:

- Drying cabinets – Closed cabinets designed for storage of flexible endoscopes that circulate HEPA-filtered or instrument air through the cabinet and each endoscope channel at continuous positive pressure.
- Conventional cabinets – Those that circulate HEPA-filtered or instrument air through the cabinet at continuous positive pressure, but do not include forced air through endoscope channels.

There are specific requirements for storing endoscopes, depending on the type of storage cabinet used. Refer to the facility's policy and the manufacturer's IFU for proper storage information.

Sterilized endoscopes are stored like all other sterilized trays.

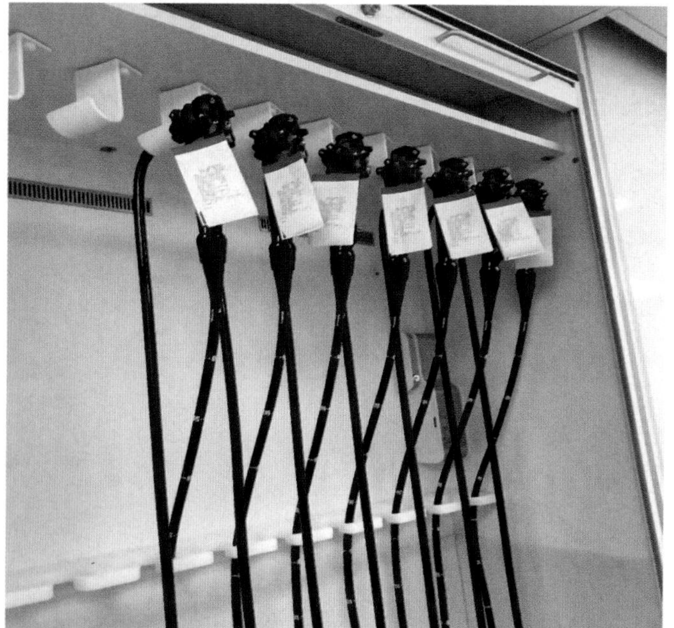

Figure 11.52

Transporting Processed Endoscopes

When removing endoscopes from storage, they must be protected from contamination and damage. Before removing endoscopes from the storage cabinet, hand hygiene must be performed and new, clean, non-latex gloves must be worn. The patient-ready label stays attached to communicate to the patient care team that the endoscope is safe for use. During transport to the point of use, the endoscope should be protected from contamination and damage. The endoscope should be loosely coiled and placed in a clean container that is large enough to accommodate a single endoscope.

Carrying Cases

The carrying case used to transport endoscopes outside the healthcare environment should not be used to store an endoscope or transport the instrument within the facility. The use of disposable carrying cases may be a better practice than using a reusable case.

Flexible Endoscope Accessories

Water Bottle Precautions

The water in an endoscope's water bottle (See **Figure 11.53**) is sprayed through the water channel to the patient's internal organs. For this reason, the bottle must be cared for properly. The water bottle should be sterilized at least once a day (ideally, after each use). Only sterile water should be used to fill the bottle, and water should never be stored in the water bottle overnight. Clean and sterilize the water bottle per the manufacturer's IFU.

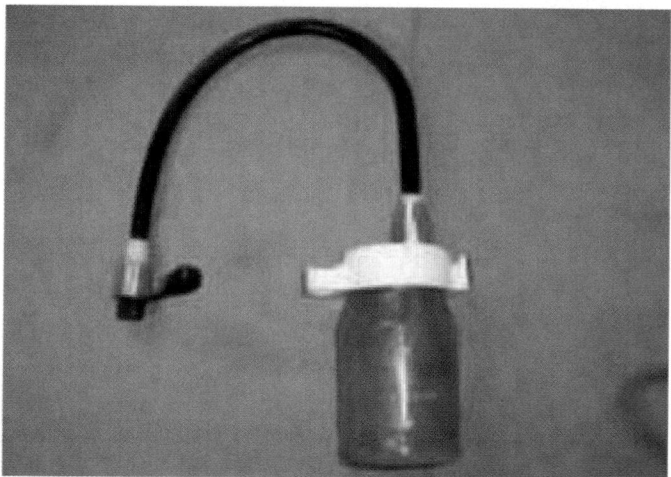

Figure 11.53

Flexible Endoscope Instruments

All reusable flexible endoscope instruments should be carefully cleaned following the manufacturer's IFU. These items usually come in contact with sterile membranes, so they must be sterilized prior to use.

ENDOSCOPE-RELATED INFECTION PREVENTION

Effective infection prevention policies and practices are critical for minimizing or eliminating endoscope-related cross-contamination. Flexible endoscopes are particularly challenging for infection control. Their long, dark and narrow lumens pose a processing concern because they are not directly accessible and are extremely difficult to clean. In addition, if channels are not thoroughly dried after processing and are stored wet, they become a dark and damp environment that is suitable for bacterial growth.

ENDOSCOPE CAMERA CARE AND HANDLING

Endoscope cameras are complex and delicate devices. **Figure 11.54** shows one type of endoscopic camera.

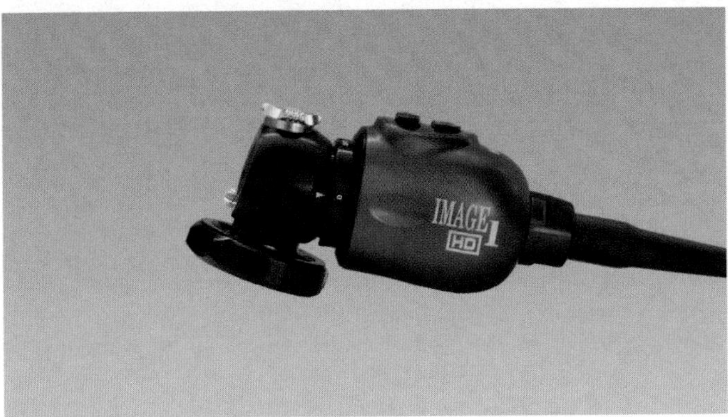

Figure 11.54 Endoscopic camera

Camera Cleaning

The manufacturer's IFU should be followed to help ensure proper care and handling of the camera, including cleaning. The use of improper chemicals is a major contributor to premature failure of external components. In general, cameras should be precleaned in the operating/procedure room to remove gross debris and then transported to the decontamination area as quickly as possible to prevent drying of debris (again, ideally within 60 minutes of the end of the procedure). An inspection of the camera should be performed to closely examine the camera cable for any cuts, nicks or other damage. *Note: A damaged camera should not be used in any procedure. It should be removed from service and sent for repair.*

Cleaning is performed using a soft, non-linting cloth and solution recommended in the IFU. Particular attention must be paid to the camera window.

Camera Inspection

Every manufacturer's cameras are unique to the company; therefore, inspection of each camera make and model must be done by carefully following the camera's specific IFU. Disinfection and/or sterilization processes must always be performed with strict adherence to the manufacturer's IFU.

STAFF EDUCATION

SP technicians working with complex medical instrumentation, such as endoscopes, must be thoroughly trained in proper processing protocols. Competency should be performed annually.

IMPLANTABLE DEVICES

Implantable devices (implants) are used in many types of surgeries. Implants can be a simple k-wire, a breast implant, total joint, spacers or plates, and screws. While there is a movement toward receiving implants that are already sterile, many implants are still received unsterile and need to be carefully processed. (See **Figure 11.55**) IFU must be reviewed for each type of implant because there are different processing instructions for many implantable devices. Most implants cannot be run through an automated process with a lubrication cycle as lubricants may interfere with the patient's recovery.

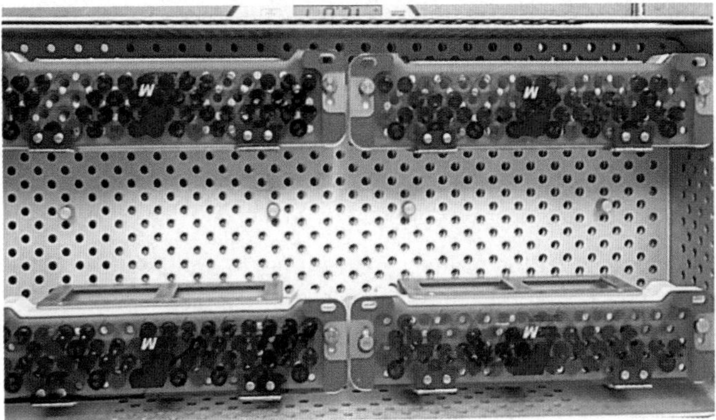

Figure 11.55 Yukon posterior cervical implants

When sterilizing an implant, the load must contain a biological indicator (BI) and should not be released prior to reading the BI results after incubation.

Implants removed from patients are called explants. The facility should have a policy on whether or not an explant can be returned to the patient because a damaged explant often needs to be returned to the manufacturer. As with all other surgical devices, explants should be properly cleaned and decontaminated prior to returning these items to a patient. Many times, due to the difficulty of properly cleaning these devices, there will be no manufacturer's IFU for the proper cleaning protocols.

THREE-DIMENSIONAL DEVICES

One of the newest types of devices being used today are three-dimensional (3D) devices. These devices can be created and customized for specific sets or even a specific patient. Because these are custom-made devices and may be created from different materials, it is very important to follow the manufacturer's IFU for each processing step. Sterilization is also varied with these devices based on the materials used to create the specific device. (See **Figure 11.56**)

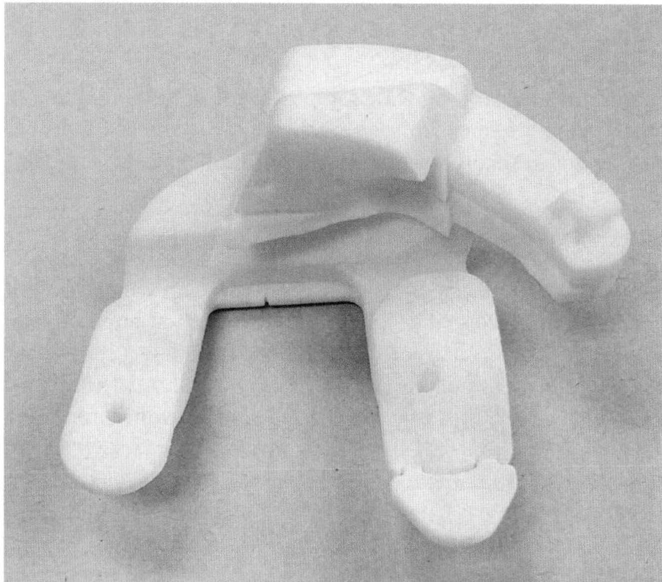

Figure 11.56 Three-dimensional device

LOANED INSTRUMENTATION

As the name implies, **loaned instrumentation** is instrumentation loaned from a vendor for a specific case or procedure. Loaned instrumentation comes for many specialties, and each represents different challenges pertaining to ordering, receiving, decontamination, assembly, sterilization, storage and return of the borrowed items. Loaned instrumentation, once primarily used in orthopedic and neurosurgical specialties, is now used in almost all surgical and procedural specialties. Facilities borrow instrumentation from manufacturers, distributing vendors and even other healthcare organizations because:

- The cost of the instrumentation to perform relatively few procedures can be prohibitive.
- More specialty cases are being performed than what the facility's instrument inventory can support.
- A physician or surgical specialty wants to trial the new instrument(s) or technology.

Loaned instrumentation Instruments or sets borrowed from a vendor or other facility for emergency or scheduled surgical procedures that will be returned following use.

Loaned instrumentation may be received as one instrument or as numerous trays for a specific procedure. (See **Figure 11.57**) Each instrument requires special attention during processing. As the concept of borrowing instruments continues to grow, departments may receive several hundred trays in one day. Many of these instruments require special disassembly, cleaning and assembly protocols, which makes them a challenge for most SPDs. It is important to have loaned instruments delivered with enough time to properly process them for scheduled procedures. After the procedure, enough time must be allocated to properly clean and decontaminate the instruments prior to returning them to the loaning vendor or facility.

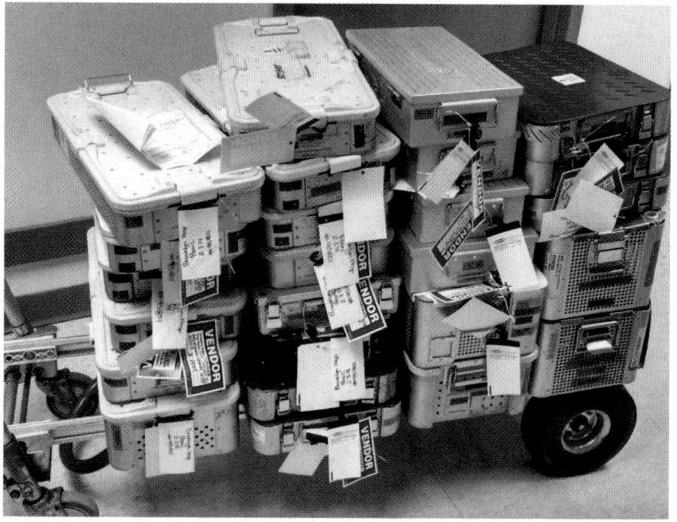

Figure 11.57

Loaned Receipt and Inventory Procedures

Loaned instruments may be received at the facility in several different ways. Company representatives may personally deliver the instruments, or they may also arrive by next-day carriers, U.S. mail and local courier services. This makes managing the process difficult. Policies and procedures need to be in place, so standard practices are followed when receiving, handling and returning these expensive instruments.

SP technicians should log the receipt of loaned instrumentation and implants per facility policy. As soon as possible after receipt, loaned instruments should be inspected. This process should be done with the vendor representative present, whenever possible. Damaged and missing instruments should be documented, the user area should be notified, and the representative should arrange for immediate replacement. Because the quality of the previous cleaning is unknown, gloves should be worn during the inspection process.

When completed properly, an inventory control sheet provides valuable information to protect the facility and the vendor. (See **Figure 11.58**) Many times, the inventory control sheet is a preprinted inventory list provided by the vendor, or it may be a custom sheet designed by the facility.

Responsibility for the instruments should not be taken until the above procedures are completed, as the facility will be responsible for lost or damaged instruments.

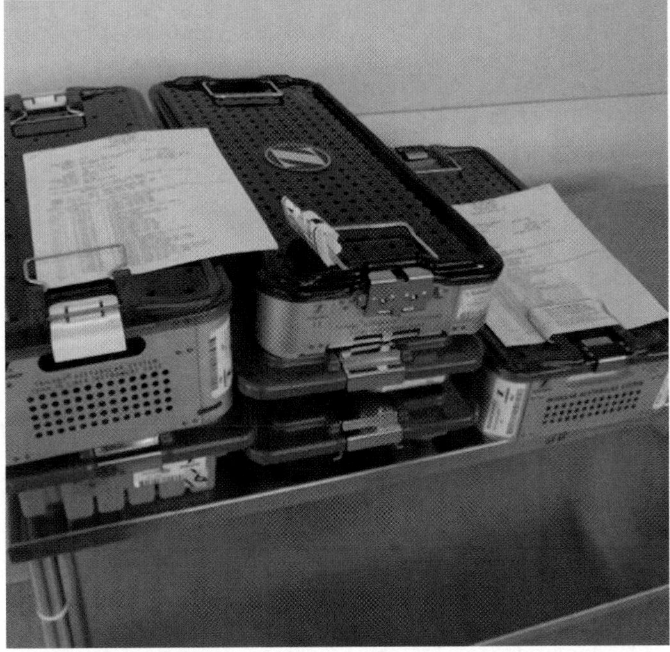

Figure 11.58 Loaned instrument trays with inventory sheets

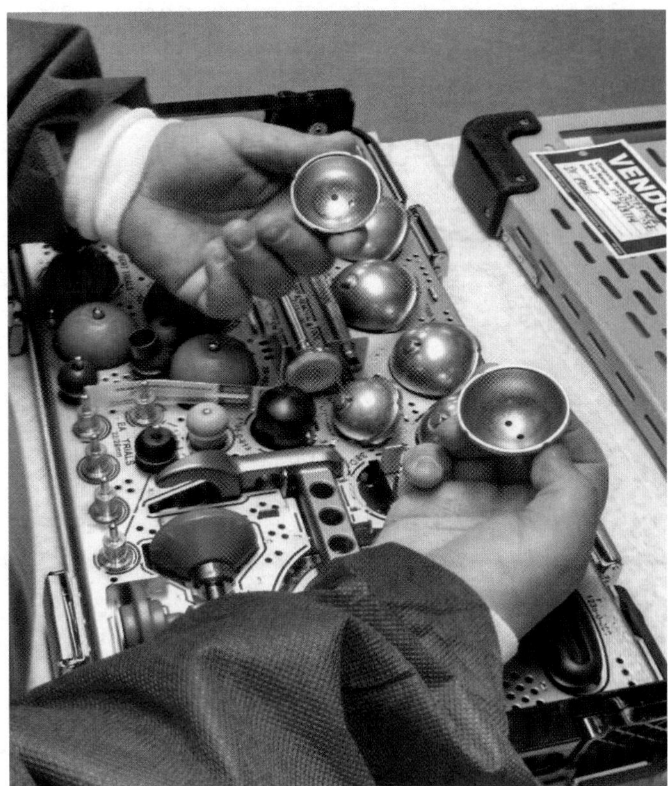

Figure 11.59 SP technician checking loaned instrumentation

Decontamination of Loaned Instrumentation

All loaned instruments should be cleaned and decontaminated upon their receipt and after use. Instruments that appear clean (even those received in sterilized containers or wrap) should be considered contaminated and must be properly processed. Each manufacturer has specific instructions about the type of solutions, temperature, and mechanical cleaning method to be used.

Loaned Instrument Inspection and Assembly

After cleaning and decontamination, SP technicians must inspect each device for cleanliness and functionality and then assemble and prepare the loaned instrumentation for sterilization. Each instrument should be examined for residual bioburden and for any defects that might cause the device to malfunction. (See **Figure 11.59**) Defective instruments should be documented and reported to the appropriate supervisor to prevent delays in scheduled procedures. Loaned instruments should be packaged according to the manufacturer's IFU.

Each manufacturer establishes instructions for the sterilization of their instruments and sets. These instructions are based, in part, on the tray configuration and the complexity of the instrumentation. Facilities must follow the sterilization times and temperatures established by the manufacturer to help ensure sterilization of the loaned instruments.

Loaned Instrument Handling and Storage

After the loaned instruments have been sterilized, they should be moved to a department area with low traffic and allowed to cool away from the direct airflow of cooling vents. *Note: Trays should not be handled until properly cooled, which could take several hours.* After cooling, trays should be handled as little as possible to prevent contamination or damage to the wrap. Care should be used when handling and moving the trays after they have cooled. These trays are often heavy, and their packaging may be easily compromised (torn) if not handled properly. Never slide these trays across a surface; always lift the trays and set them on storage shelves or case carts for use in the OR.

Sometimes, instruments are loaned to a facility for an extended period. These instruments should be stored in a protected area to decrease the potential of instrument loss or damage.

Loaned Instrument Return

After the loaned instrument trays have been used in the procedure, they must be processed. Each instrument should be carefully cleaned and decontaminated according to manufacturer's instructions prior to releasing them to the vendor representative or before sending the trays back via courier or shipping company. Vendor representatives may be in a hurry to take the instruments to another facility. Regardless, all instruments must be thoroughly cleaned and decontaminated prior to their release.

An exit inventory of all loaned instruments is recommended to help ensure that any missing or damaged instrumentation is identified in a timely manner.

CONCLUSION

As technology advances, surgical instruments and equipment will become more complex, and this has been evident within many surgical specialties. SP technicians will continue to be challenged with staying current with new technologies.

RESOURCES

Centers for Disease Control and Prevention. *Guideline for Disinfection and Sterilization in Healthcare Facilities.* 2008.

ANSI/AAMI ST58:2013/(R)2018 *Chemical sterilization and high-level disinfection in health care facilities.*

ANSI/AAMI ST79:2017 & 2020 Amendments, A3 2012, A4 2013, section 6, *Comprehensive guide to steam sterilization and sterility assurance in health care facilities.*

AAMI TIR12:2020 *Designing, testing, and labeling medical devices intended for processing by health care facilities: A guide for device manufacturers.*

ANSI/AAMI ST91:2021 *Flexible and semi-rigid endoscope processing in health care facilities.*

STERILE PROCESSING TERMS

Endoscope

Light-emitting diode (LED)

Delayed processing

Fixative

Loaned instrumentation

Chapter 12

Preparation and Packaging

Learning Objectives

As a result of successfully completing this chapter, the reader will be able to:

1. Explain the setup and function of the assembly area
2. Review basic procedures to prepare pack contents for packaging
3. Explain the basic objectives of the packaging process
4. Provide an overview of reusable packaging materials
5. Provide an overview of disposable packaging materials
6. Discuss basic package closure methods

INTRODUCTION

When instruments have been cleaned, they are transferred to the **preparation and packaging** area of the Sterile Processing department (SPD). This area is also known as the prep and pack or assembly area and is where instruments are inspected to ensure they are clean and in good working order before they are packaged for sterilization. This is a critical step because it is the final time the instruments will be handled before being dispensed to the Operating Room (OR) or other user areas. Potentially serious problems can arise if a defective or unclean instrument arrives in the user department. When these incidents are detected, delays occur. When they are not detected, risks to the patient increase; therefore, it is imperative that protocols for inspection, assembly and packaging are followed at all times. Like other areas of the SPD, attention to detail is critical in the assembly area. SP technicians working in this part of the department must understand the configuration of their work area and the specific requirements that must be followed to work safely and effectively in that area.

Preparation and packaging A clean area of the SPD where instrument inspection, assembly and packaging are performed. The preparation and packing area is sometimes called the prep and pack or assembly area.

PREPARATION AND PACKAGING AREA

Physical Environment

The preparation and packaging area is a designated clean area, and meticulous care must be taken to maintain that cleanliness. Airflow plays a critical role in keeping the prep and pack area clean and free of contaminants. Air pressure in the prep and pack area should be positive. The purpose of this positive airflow is to ensure that when the doors to the prep and pack area are opened, air flows outward instead of into the work area. Positive airflow reduces the risk of airborne bacteria being introduced into the area.

Maintaining proper temperature is also critical. The healthcare organization monitors the prep and pack room temperature and humidity based on ANSI/ASHRAE/ASHE 170 when the heating, ventilation and air conditioning (HVAC) system was initially installed or last upgraded.

Environmental Services (EVS) standards for the assembly area should be the same as those for delivery rooms and the OR. To reduce the number of bacteria in the area, all fixtures, worktables and furniture should be constructed of non-porous, easy-to-clean materials. In addition to routinely cleaning surfaces, care must be taken to minimize dust and lint in the area. Dust and lint may settle on pack contents and be introduced into the patient's body during a procedure. Workstations should be cleaned at least once each shift and as they become soiled.

The Danger of Lint

Lint is comprised of fine fibers that separate from items such as wraps, textiles, paper and more. Lint can be carried on air currents and deposited anywhere. Microorganisms often adhere to lint. When lint is introduced into the sterile field, it can settle into a wound and cause infection.

SPDs should make every effort to minimize lint. Good cleaning practices and compliance with attire and EVS protocols can reduce lint and the chance of it entering the OR.

To further maintain environmental cleanliness, hand hygiene stations should be conveniently located and readily accessible to all SP staff. Hand hygiene should be performed frequently in this area.

Dress Code and Personal Behaviors

Personal cleanliness and adherence to dress code is essential for preventing microorganisms and contaminants from entering the work area. The cleaner the environment, the less chance there is of contaminants entering a pack.

Nail polish and artificial nails should not be worn in the prep and pack area because there is a potential for nail polish to chip and artificial nails to fall off. Natural fingernails should be clean and kept at a length that does not extend beyond the fingertips. Long nails harbor bacteria that may hinder effective handwashing. **Figure 12.1** shows clean natural fingernails.

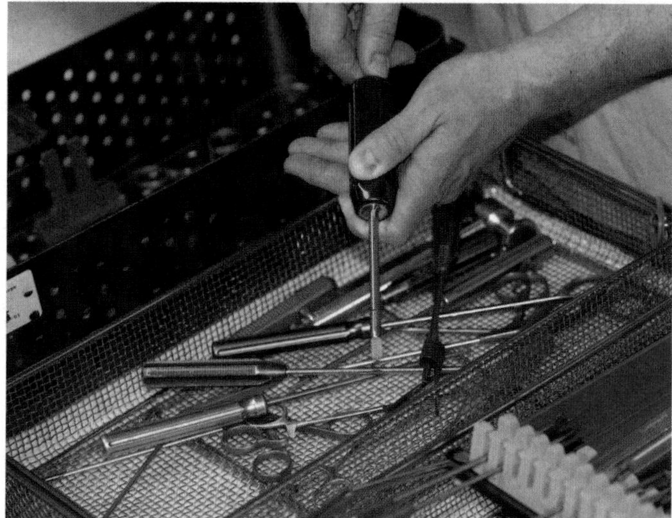

Figure 12.1

According to ANSI/AAMI ST79:2017 & 2020 Amendments A1, A2, A3, A4 (Consolidated Text) *Comprehensive guide to steam sterilization and sterility assurance in health care facilities*, all head and facial hair (except for eyebrows and eyelashes) should be completely covered with a surgical-type hair covering. *Note: Beards and mustaches must be covered using an approved beard cover.* Jewelry (all types, including wedding bands) and wristwatches should not be worn in the area because they can harbor microorganisms.

All staff members in the area must monitor their cleanliness and change scrub attire if it becomes soiled. SP technicians should not bring items into the area that may contaminate hands (e.g., money, personal items and personal electronics). *Note: SP personnel should consult their facility's policy about the use of personal electronics and how it relates to infection prevention. Studies have shown that personal items contain a high microbial load.*

Traffic Control and Environmental Management

Everyone assigned to the preparation and packaging areas should be mindful and protective of that clean environment. Traffic should be restricted, and traffic control requirements must be followed. Care must be taken to ensure that items that may serve as vehicles for microorganisms are not allowed into the area. (See **Figure 12.2**)

ATTENTION:
Entering
Semi-Restricted
Surgical Area.
Surgical Scrubs, Hair
Covering REQUIRED.
NO Food or Beverage
Beyond This Point.

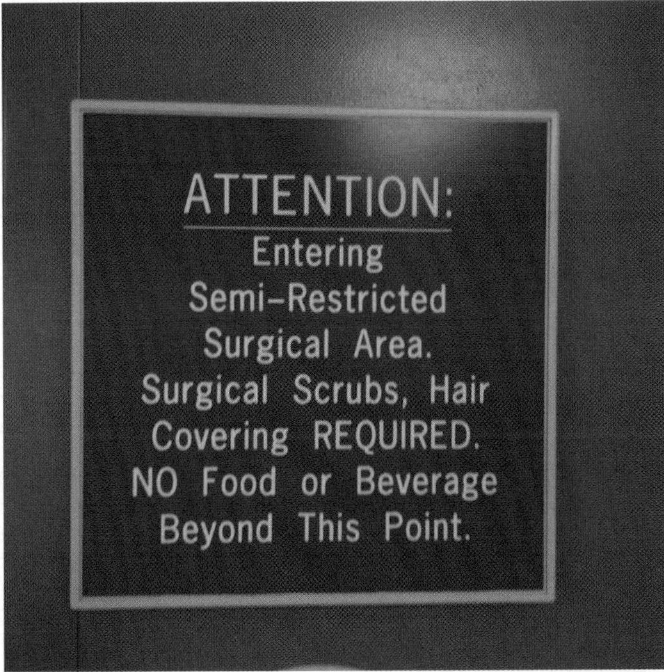

Figure 12.2

Food and beverages are not allowed in the preparation and packaging area. Food and drinks may attract insects and rodents, and residues left on hands after eating may transfer to instruments and impede the sterilization process. Personal behaviors, such as following dress code, performing proper hand hygiene and avoiding situations that pose a threat of contamination, all help protect the patient.

Personal items, such as electronics, cell phones and tablets, are discouraged from being used in the SPD. There are circumstances, however, when facility-issued electronics are brought into the department; these devices should be cleaned according to the device manufacturer's instructions for use (IFU) and facility policy before these items are brought into the SPD. Cleaning these devices and implementing hand hygiene reduces the numbers of microorganisms present on the devices, thus protecting the SP environment.

Work Area Requirements

The work area in preparation and packaging should be adequately sized to perform inspection, testing and assembly duties. Supplies needed for those processes should be readily available. Equipment, such as computers, printers and specialized instrument testing devices, should also be readily available. (See **Figure 12.3**) The work area should be routinely cleaned to reduce bacteria and lint. (See **Figure 12.4**)

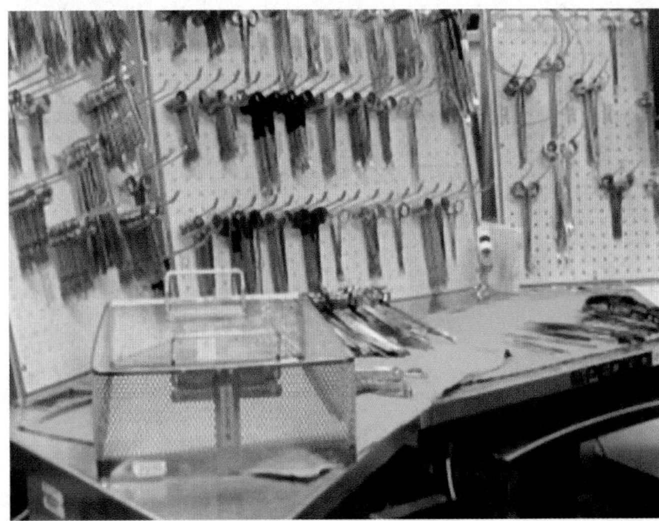

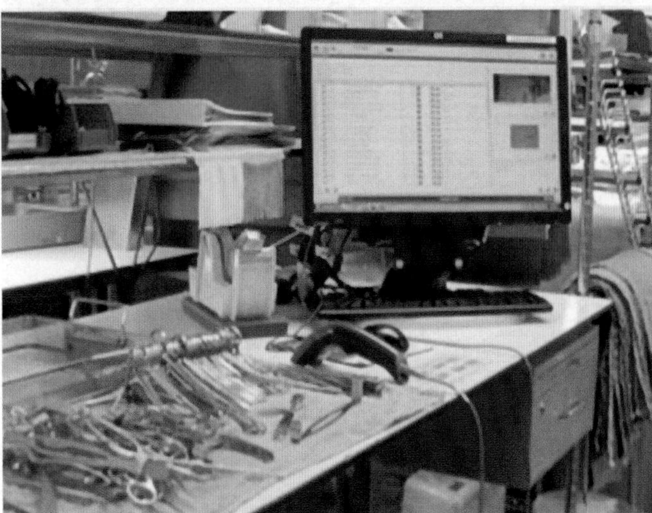

Figure 12.3 Pack assembly workstations

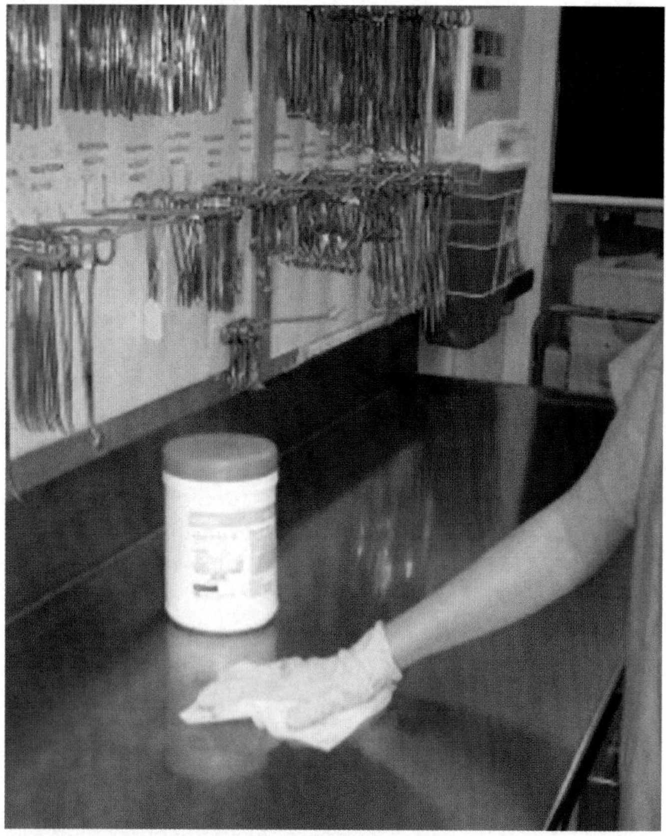

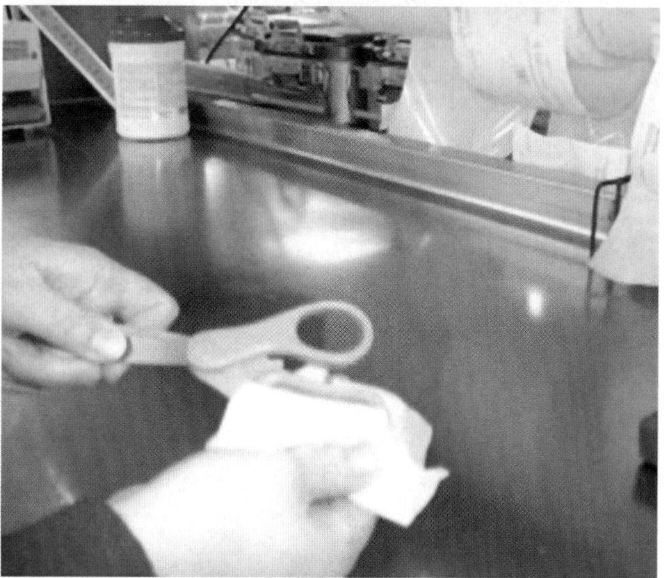

Figure 12.4 Keep work areas clean.

PRIMARY GOALS OF PACK PREPARATION

SP technicians assigned to the preparation and packaging area must understand the primary goals of creating an instrument pack. The first goal is to create a pack that meets users' needs. The acronym "FAN," which stands for functional, accurate and neat, can help reinforce that goal.

- Functional – Each item in the pack must function as it was designed. This means that scissors must be sharp, clamps must hold securely, and multi-part items must be complete and functional when assembled. Technicians reach that goal by understanding how instruments operate and by relying on specific test methods to ensure they work properly.

- Accurate – Instruments must be correct, and quantities must be exact. Technicians meet this goal by learning to identify specific instruments, working from an up-to-date pack count sheet and verifying that all specifications for the pack, including quantities and configuration, are correct.

- Neat – Pack contents must be organized, and instruments must be easy to locate. Disorganized packs may waste time or delay treatment and care.

The FAN Principle

When assembling any pack for sterilization, remember the "**FAN**" principle. All items must be **f**unctional, **a**ccurate and **n**eat.

In addition to creating organized packs that contain correct and functional instruments, SP technicians must also arrange pack contents in a manner that facilitates the appropriate sterilization process. As technicians arrange pack contents, they must also take precautions to protect instruments from possible damage or content shifting that may occur during handling and transport.

Technicians must then adhere to the packaging method recommended by the instrument manufacturers—one that is appropriate for the sterilization method that will be used for the items being packaged. Finally, technicians must use the proper packaging technique, as instructed by the manufacturer.

GENERAL GUIDELINES FOR PREPARATION OF PACK CONTENTS

Most instruments are prepared in groups called packs, sets, trays or kits. *Note: The specific name (kit, tray, set or pack) is determined by the healthcare facility.* Smaller groups of instruments used for minor procedures in areas outside of the OR are often called procedure trays (also known as floor trays). No matter which type of tray is being assembled, and regardless of its size, preparation of pack contents begins with planning.

Clearly written, illustrated and standardized count sheets should be readily available and used by all personnel. Count sheets provide specific information that help ensure all packs are assembled, packaged and sterilized according to exact specifications. Pack standardization helps ensure packs are organized and uniform so users can quickly locate contents.

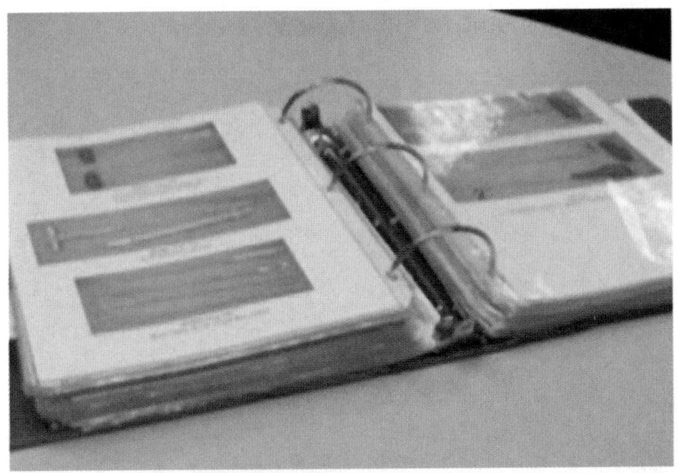

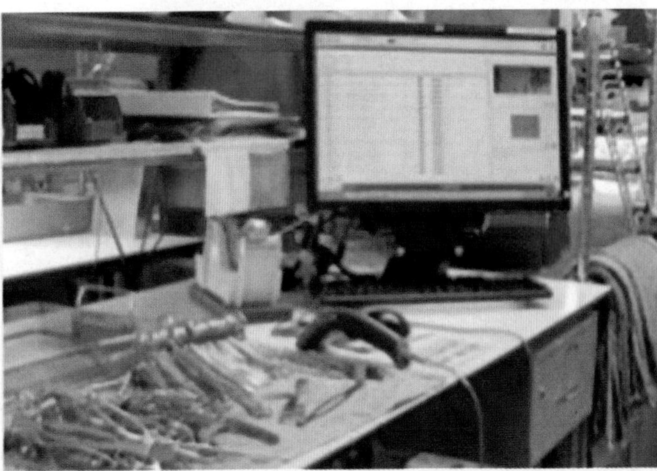

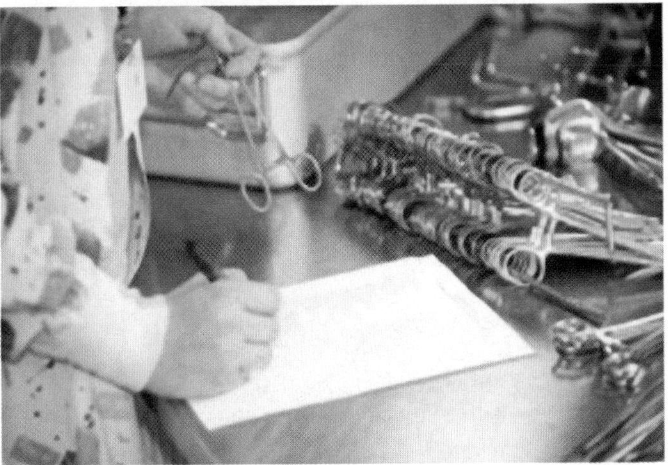

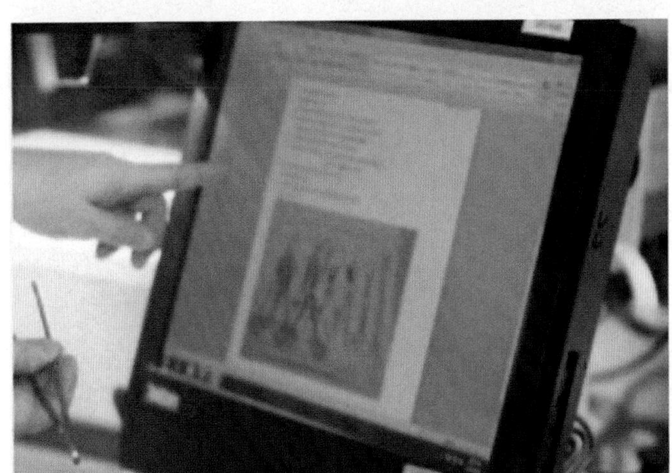

Figure 12.5 Pack preparation

Item requirements for tray contents are usually identified by users. For example, a surgeon and OR staff would determine the contents of specific surgical trays. Pack content information may be collected and maintained in a manual or computerized system. (See **Figure 12.5**) Whichever method is used, the same basic information is provided to the assembler. This includes:

- Correct and complete name of the tray
- A detailed list of tray contents, including item quantities, sizes and catalog or reference numbers
- Essential steps for preparation and inspection, including assembly and disassembly of device(s) according to the manufacturer's written directions and/or specifications.
- Specific instructions for correct placement of items in the tray
- Sterilization method and required cycle used for processing the tray
- Type(s) and size(s) of packaging to be used
- Type and placement of internal and/or external chemical process indicator(s)
- Destination or storage location of the tray

Pack Assembly

Before items can be assembled into trays, sets or packs for sterilization, they must be inspected—and in some cases, tested—to ensure that they are clean, dry, correct and functional.

Inspection Guidelines

It is imperative to inspect for cleanliness. Even though instruments have been cleaned, there may still be instances where some soil was not removed. (See **Figure 12.6**) Organic material, such as blood or other contaminants, will interfere with sterilization and optimal functioning. Inspecting instruments for cleanliness adds a safeguard to the process by reducing the chance that a soiled instrument will be delivered to a user area.

Soiled box locks on scissors

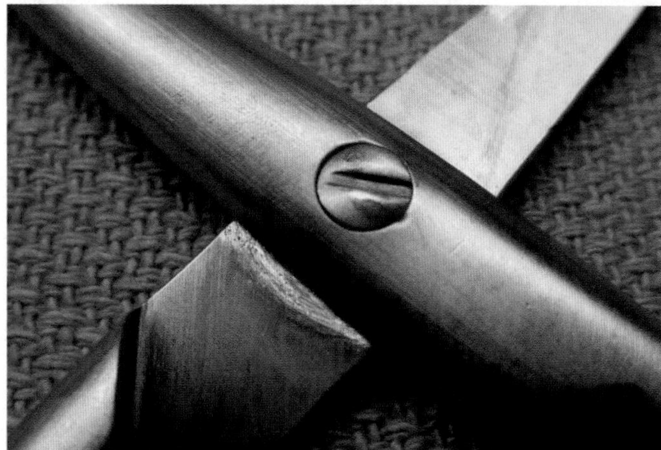

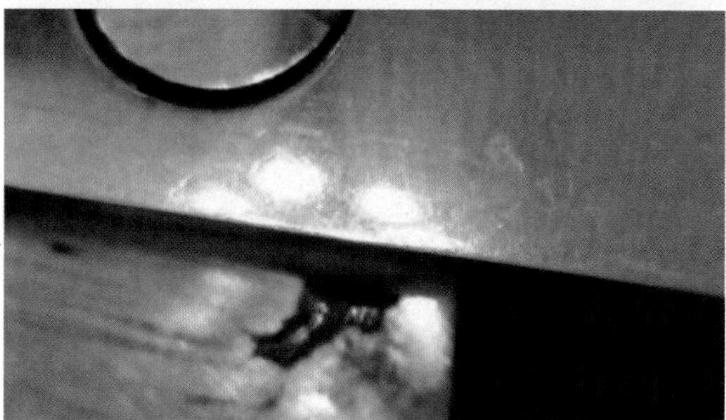

Magnified view of soil on a shaver

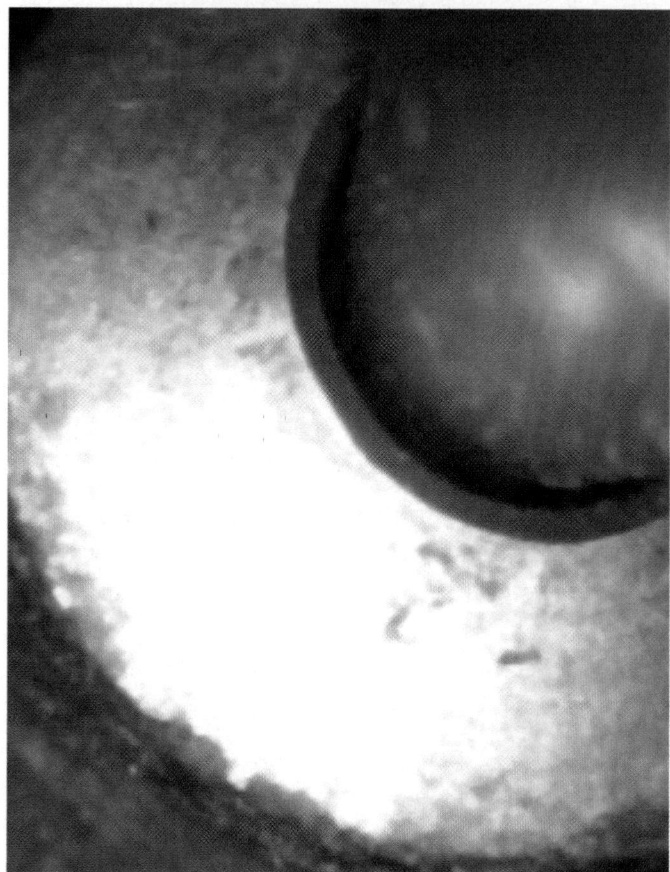

Figure 12.6 Inspecting for cleanliness is important.

If a soiled instrument is detected during the inspection process, it should be sent back to the decontamination area for proper cleaning. The tray in which the soiled instrument was located should also be sent back to the decontamination area because other instruments may have also been contaminated through contact with the unclean instrument. *Note: Do not attempt to clean the instrument in the assembly area. Doing so may contaminate the immediate area and may cross-contaminate other areas of the department.*

Ensure all instruments are dry unless otherwise indicated in the IFU.

Inspect for damage. Instruments may become damaged through use, misuse, transport and processing. Look for cracks, breaks, bent tips, misalignment and other signs of damage.

Inspect for signs of wear. Even with the best of care, instruments eventually begin to show signs of wear. Scissors and other sharp instruments become dull, surfaces break down, springs may weaken, screws may loosen, and moving parts may begin to stick.

Damaged and worn instruments should be removed and sent for repair or discarded as necessary. The continued use of broken or excessively worn instruments could put patients and facility personnel at risk. (See **Figure 12.7**)

Multi-part instruments also must be checked carefully. Instruments that have been dissembled for cleaning should be reassembled and tested for functionality, then disassembled again for sterilization. (See **Figure 12.8**) *Note: Small parts, such as wing nuts, should be placed in an approved containment device.* (See **Figure 12.9**) When placing disassembled instruments inside the tray, keep all parts near one another, so they can be readily accessible for the user.

Assembly technicians should also ensure that the following information is available and followed:

- Specific instructions for correct placement of items in the tray
- Sterilization method and required cycle used for processing the tray
- Type(s) and size(s) of packaging to be used
- Type and placement of internal and/or external chemical process indicator(s)
- Destination or storage location of the tray

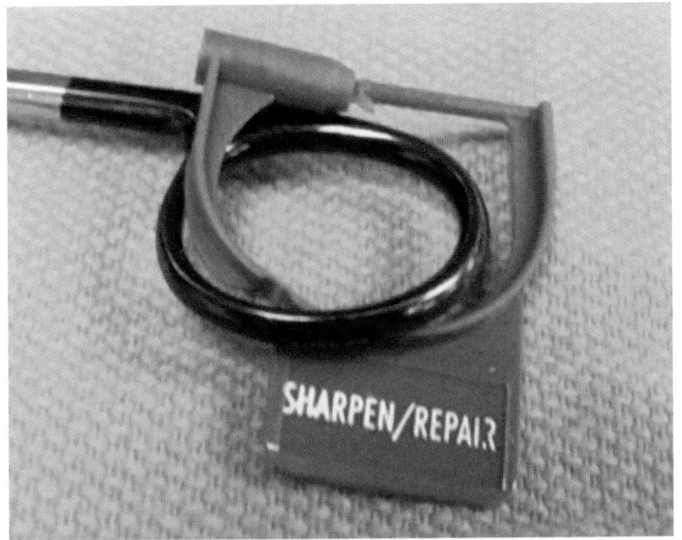

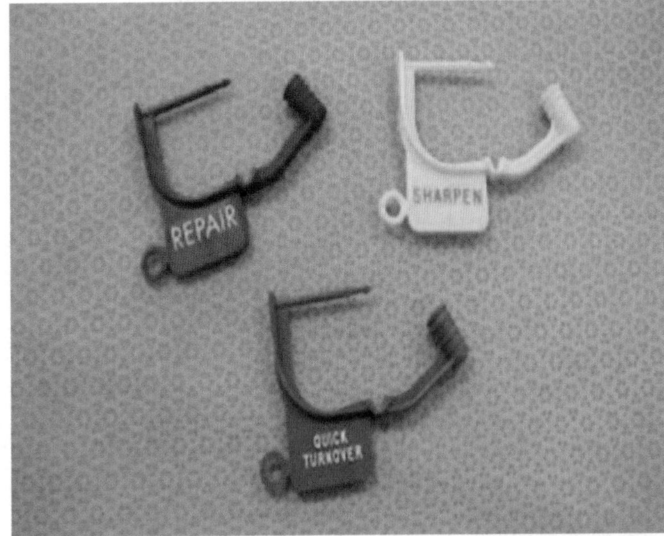

Figure 12.7 Examples of sharpen and repair tags

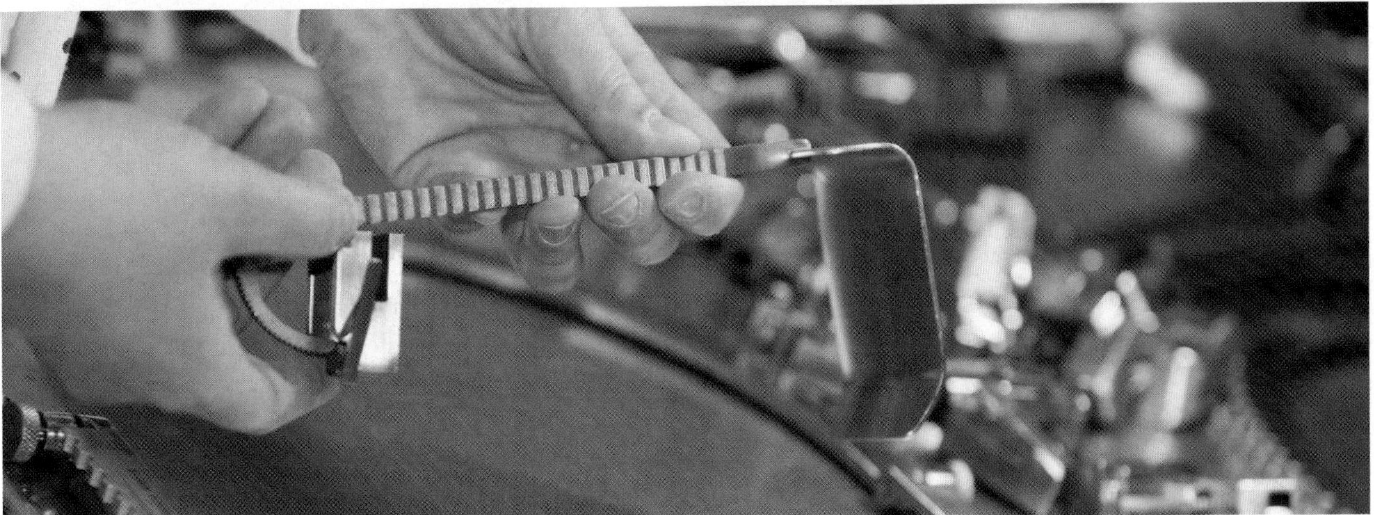

Figure 12.8 A technician checks a retractor by assembling and disassembling it.

Paper sterilization pouches

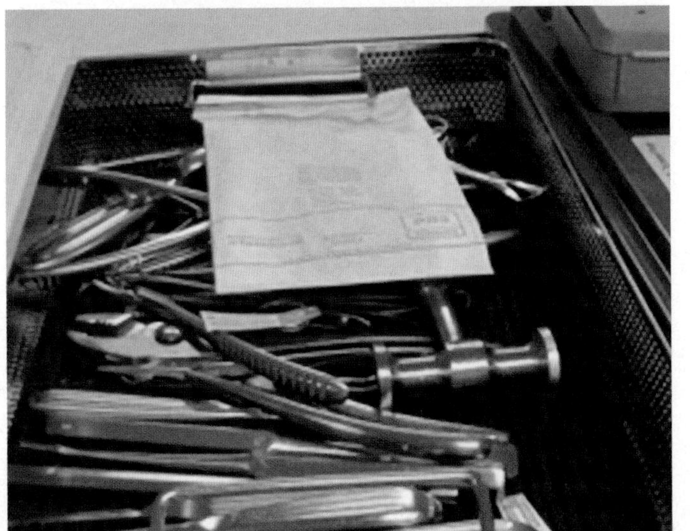

Metal holders

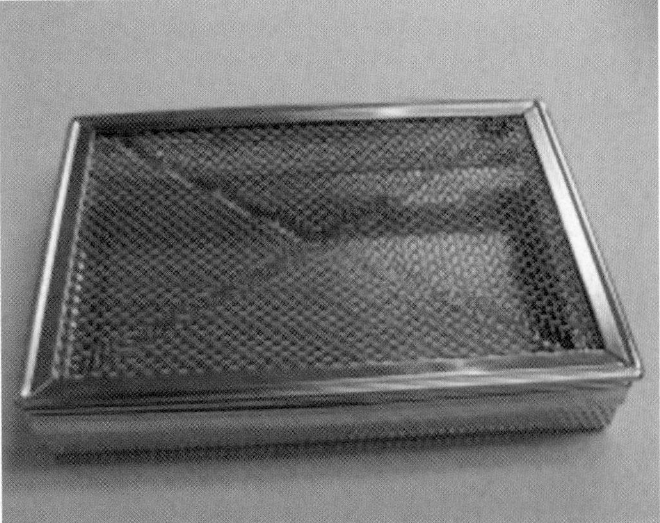

Figure 12.9 Examples of devices designed to hold small parts within packs

Testing

All instruments must be inspected before assembly. Some instruments must also be tested. For example, scissors should be tested for sharpness (See **Figure 12.10**), and the insulation of electrosurgical instruments must be tested for integrity between uses. (See **Figure 12.11**) The instrument shaft should be inspected for cuts, cracks and nicks. The handle should be inspected for chips or cracks. The insulation should fit tightly against the metal collar at the distal end of the instrument.

Demagnetizers – Occasionally, instruments may become magnetized. This is a source of frustration for the surgeon, especially with needle holders, as magnetization may make working with suture needles very difficult. Demagnetizers work by reversing the magnetic field away from the instrument. **Figure 12.12** provides examples of demagnetizers.

Tools for inspection – There are many tools available to help with instrument inspection. Lightened magnification, computer magnifiers, and borescopes can enlarge areas to help detect residual soil, wear and damage. (See **Figure 12.13**)

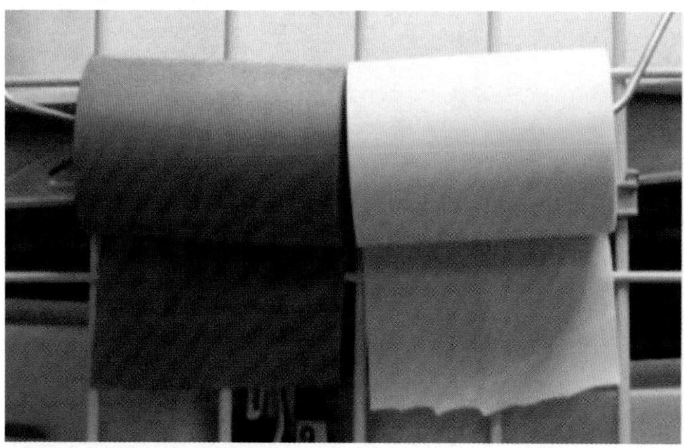

Figure 12.10 Scissors sharpness testing

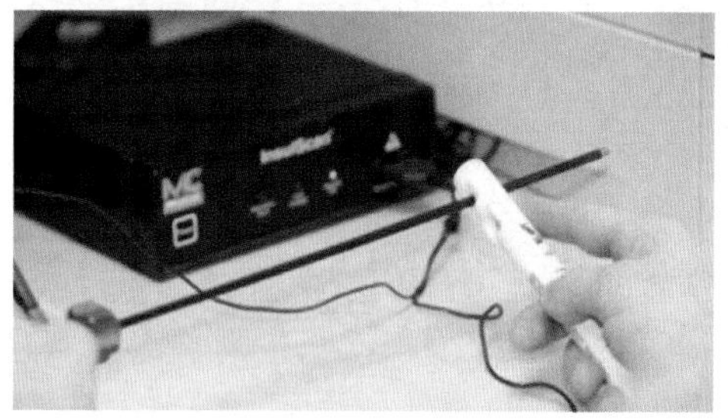

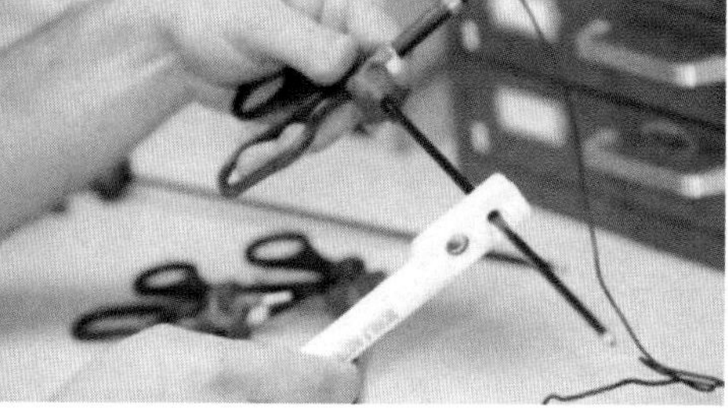

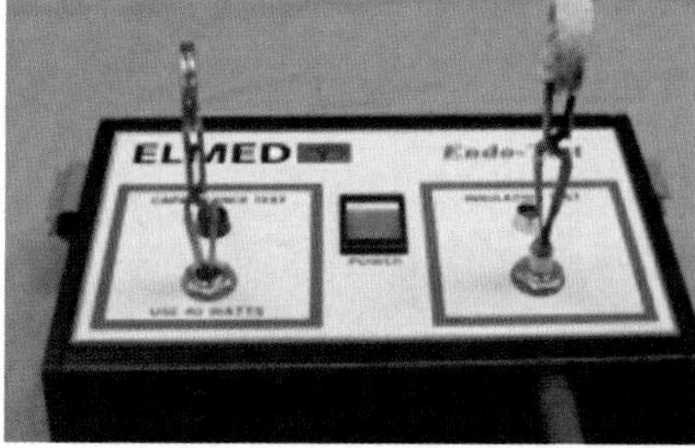

Figure 12.11 Insulation testing

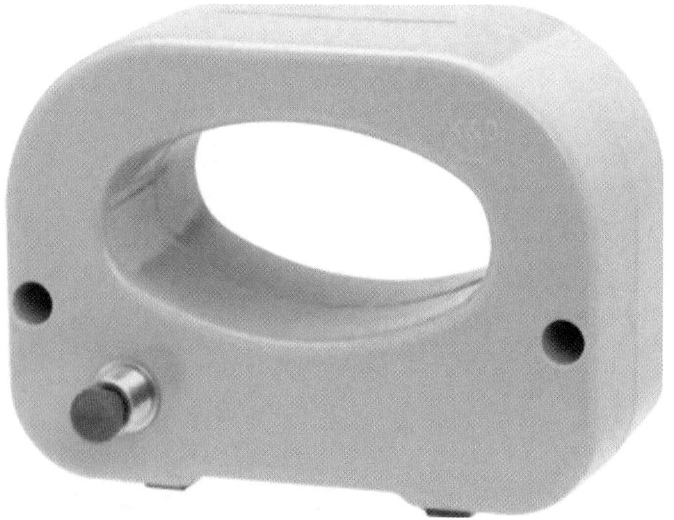

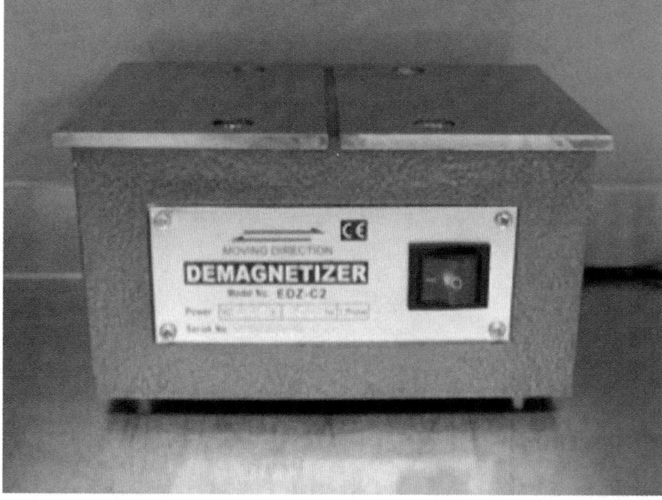

Figure 12.12 Examples of demagnetizers

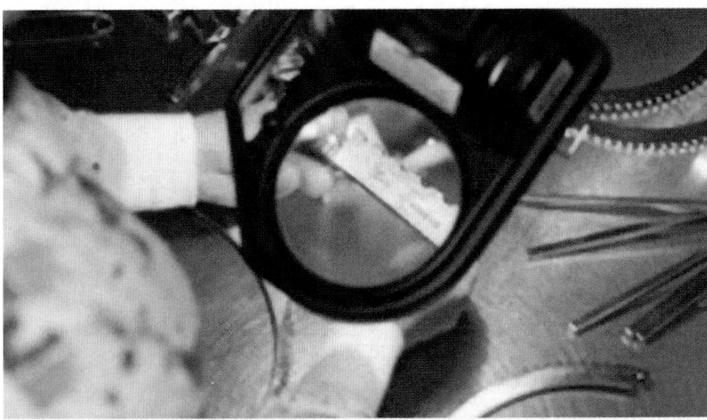

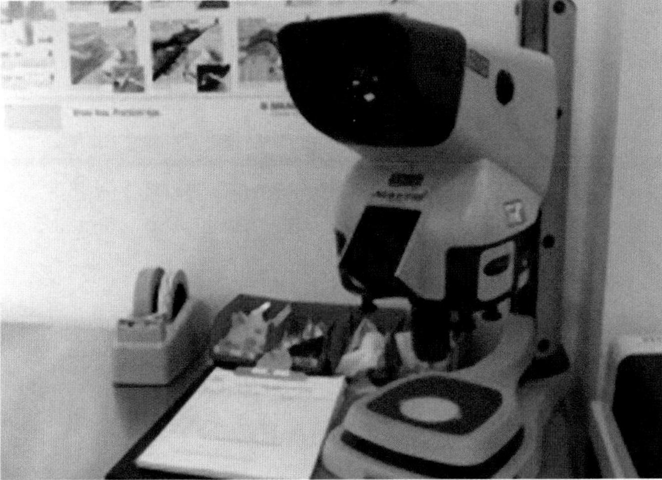

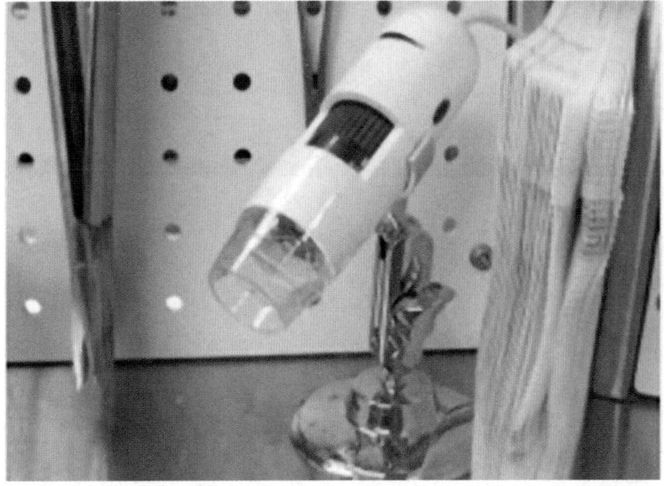

Figure 12.13 Magnification devices

Scannable codes

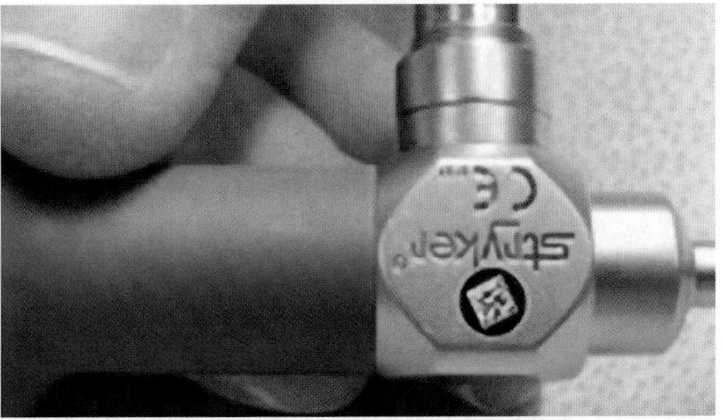

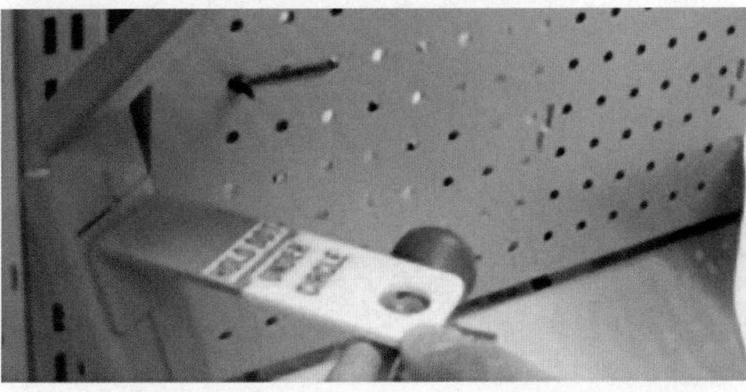

Etching and tape

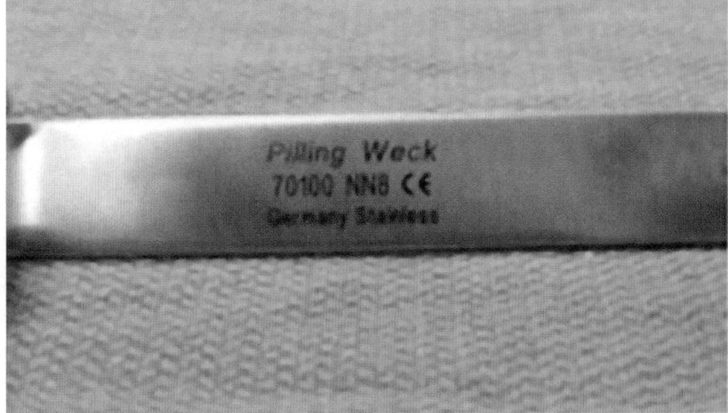

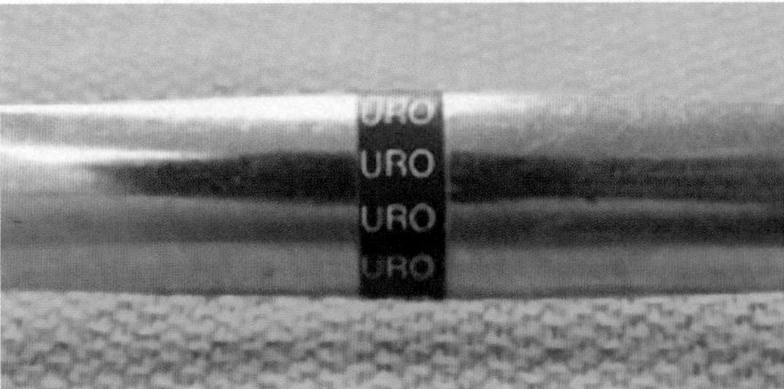

Figure 12.14 Examples of instrument identification systems

Photographs – Photos of instruments and instrument configuration can help ensure that items are assembled correctly.

Instrument identification – Instrument scanning systems, approved instrument marking systems and instrument tape can help SP technicians identify devices and assist with pack assembly. (See **Figure 12.14**)

Instrument holding trays – Groups of instruments for a specific procedure or specialty are contained together in trays specifically designed to protect the devices and facilitate the sterilization process. (See **Figure 12.15**) Other instrument groups are contained in trays that can be adapted to several configurations. (See **Figure 12.16**) In most cases, the container is selected when the instrument tray is put into the surgical instrument system.

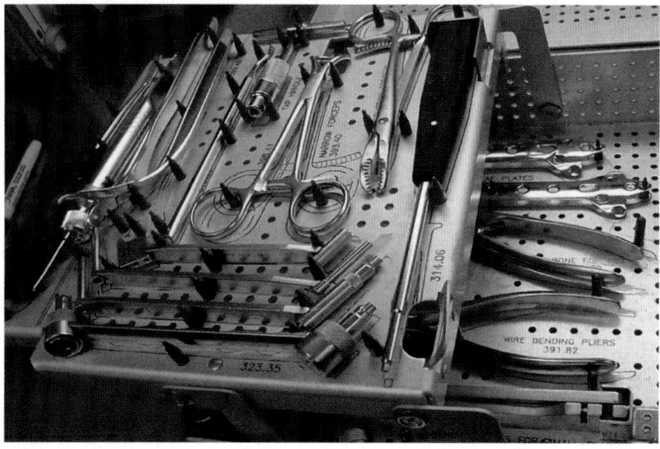

Figure 12.15

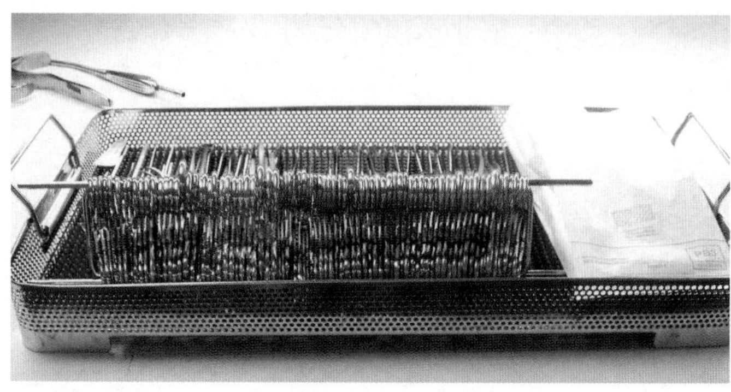

Figure 12.16

The following are points to consider when using instrument holding trays:

- Use the holding tray correctly. Read the manufacturer's IFU and use the tray as instructed. Failure to do so can damage instruments or cause the sterilization process to fail. For example, trays with silicone finger mats must be aligned with drainage holes to help ensure air and water removal.

- Do not overcrowd the holding tray. Overcrowding often occurs when instruments are added to an existing tray. Over time, physicians' needs may change, and instruments may be added to trays, creating a situation where the holding tray is too small for its contents. When this happens, there is a greater risk of instruments becoming damaged. In some cases, severe overcrowding may negatively affect sterilization and drying.

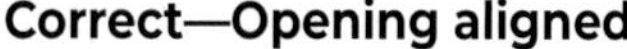

Incorrect—Opening offset and closed. No path for air removal and water drainage.

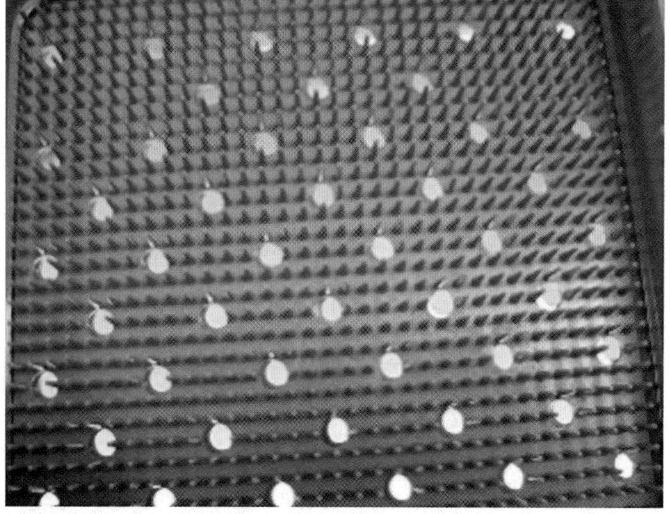

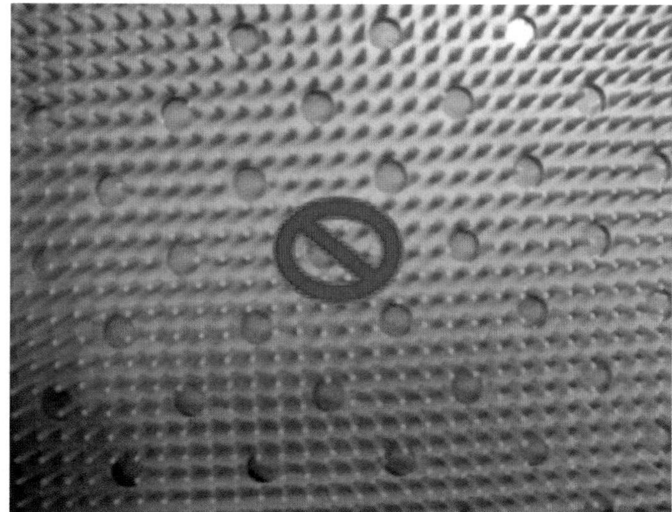

Figure 12.17 Using silicone finger mats

- Don't create overweight trays. Be aware of tray weight and density recommendations from the manufacturers of sterilizers, instruments and packaging systems. In addition to possible issues associated with heat-up and drying, excessive tray weight can present ergonomic challenges for those who must lift the trays. ANSI/AAMI ST77 *Containment devices for reusable medical device sterilization* and ANSI/AAMI ST79 2017 & 2020 Amendments A1, A2, A3, A4 (Consolidated Text) *Comprehensive guide to steam sterilization and sterility assurance in health care facilities* recommend a maximum weight of 25 pounds for containerized trays; this includes both the weight of the instruments and the instrument container. (See **Figure 12.18**)

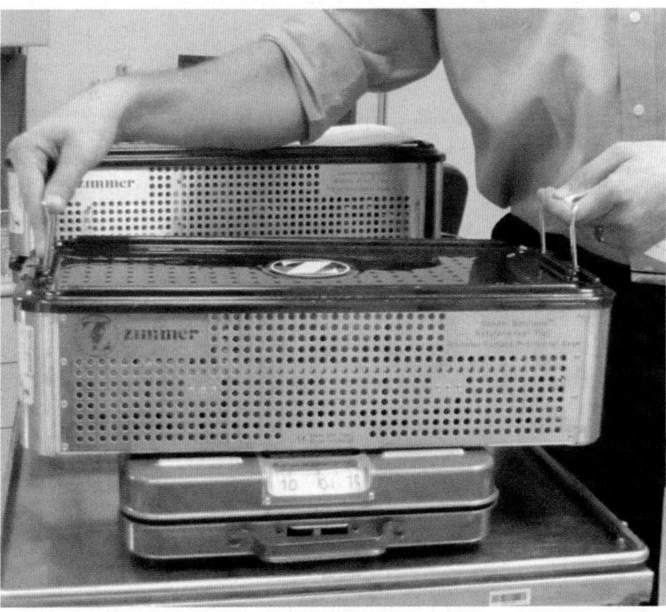

Figure 12.18 Instrument trays being weighed upon receipt in an SPD

- Protect instruments from damage. All instruments should be protected from damage when handled. Delicate and sharp instruments are of special concern. Sharp points may be protected with special holders, commercially available tip guards, silicone mats, holding brackets, posts or foam sleeves. **Figures 12.19** and **12.20** provide examples of methods to protect instruments. Suppliers of protective devices should be consulted to ensure that the devices are permeable to the sterilant being used. For example, latex tubing should not be used to protect instrument tips, as it may prevent the sterilant from making direct contact with the instruments.

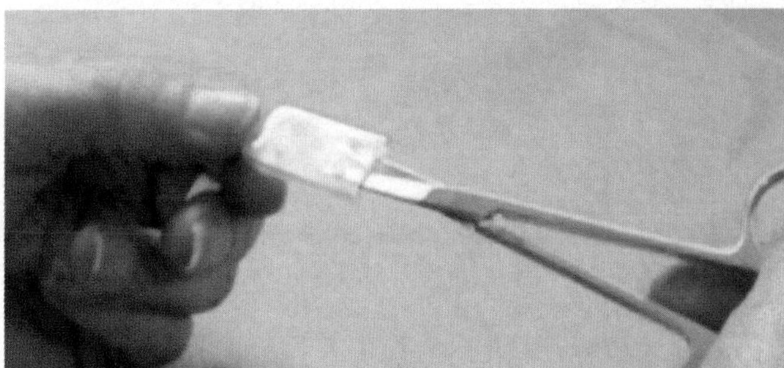

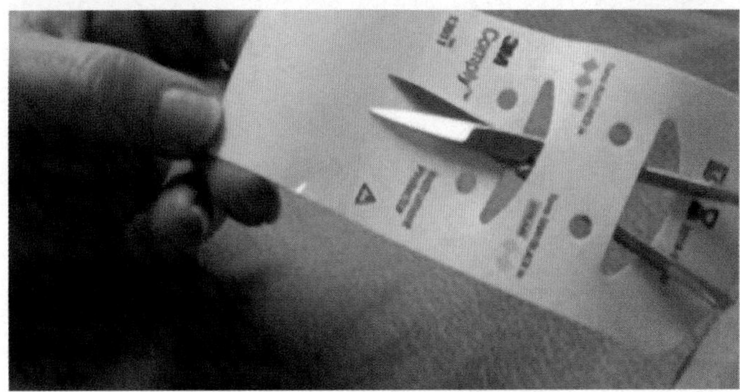

Figure 12.19 Examples of tip protectors

Silicone finger mats

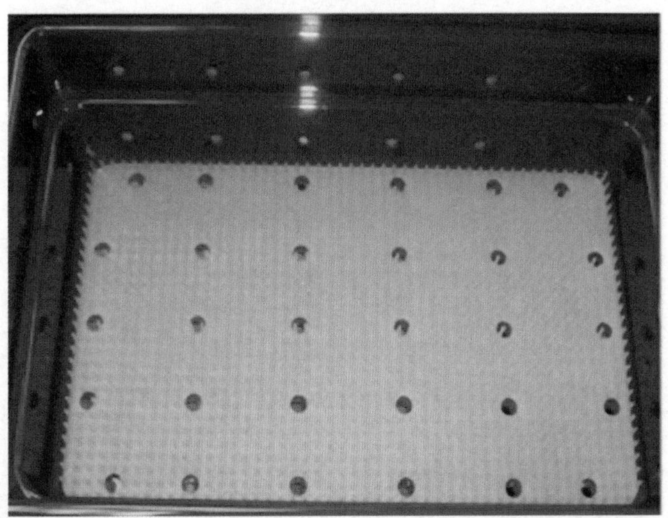

Foam protectors

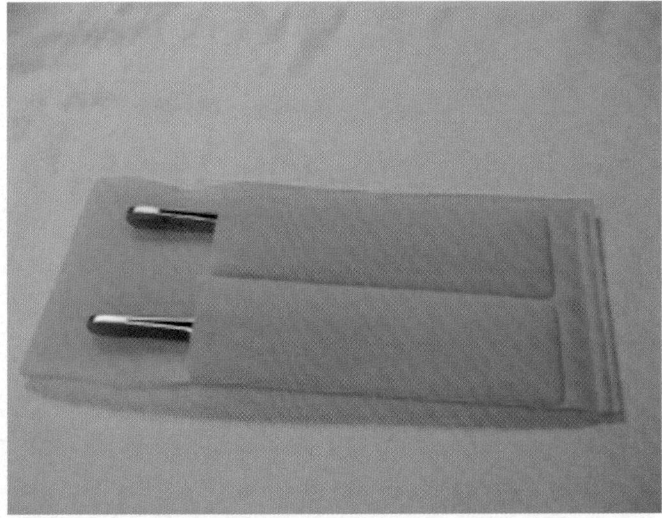

Figure 12.20 Examples of instrument protectors

Instruments that open, such as scissors and hemostats, should be kept in an unlocked or unlatched and opened position to enable the sterilant to reach all parts. Devices, such as stringers and racks, can be purchased to keep hinged instruments open. (See **Figure 12.21**) Always follow the manufacturer's IFU for specific requirements.

Protect the alignment of forceps tips by placing all tips in the same direction. (See **Figure 12.22**) Forceps tips can also be protected by using an approved containment device.

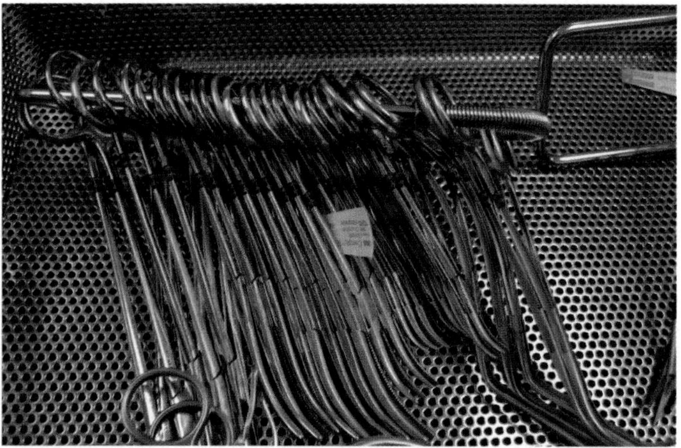

Figure 12.21

The most important thing to remember with all pack preparation is that all items must be functional, accurate and organized because the next time the pack is accessed, it will be used for patient care.

Assembly Procedures

Pack contents and pack configurations are unique. SP technicians must apply basic principles to pack assembly to create packs that can be successfully sterilized and meet the users' needs. The following section provides an overview of general assembly guidelines.

Procedure Trays

Procedure trays are used in patient care settings, such as nursing units, and in procedure areas like Radiology and Emergency Departments. Procedure trays are often designed to include all or most of the items needed for a minor procedure. It is important to disassemble multi-part items and place all items in trays in a manner that prevents air entrapment and pooling of condensate during the sterilization process.

In the past, the inclusion of disposable (single-use) items, such as needles, scalpel blades and suture, in trays was common; however, today, this practice is not recommended. To sterilize single-use items, the manufacturer's IFU (including resterilization instructions) must be kept on file and carefully followed. If the manufacturer's instructions for resterilization of a single-use item cannot be obtained, the item should not be included inside an in-house sterilized procedure tray. If approved single-use items are sterilized in the healthcare facility, they must not be resterilized if they are returned unused.

Gauze sponges and surgical (huck) towels were also commonly used in procedure trays in the past. Now, many studies show that lint from these items can be transferred to a patient wound—even in minor procedures—causing complications such as blood clots or infection. Prepackaged sterile towels purchased from an outside vendor or processed in house should not be opened and used on trays because they may **super heat** within the sterilization cycle. If super heating occurs, the tray they are in (and other trays within the load) will potentially be unsterile. Towels should be laundered after sterilization to rehydrate the fibers prior to sterilization. Prepackaged sterile towels from an outside vendor should not be laundered unless the IFU have been obtained from the towel manufacturer. These towels are usually made of lower-

Correct

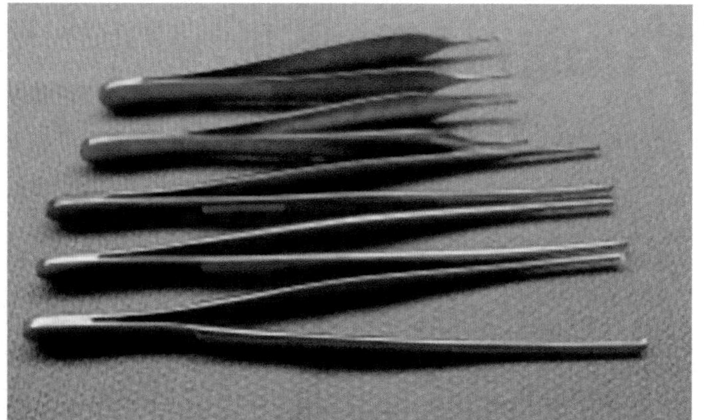

Incorrect

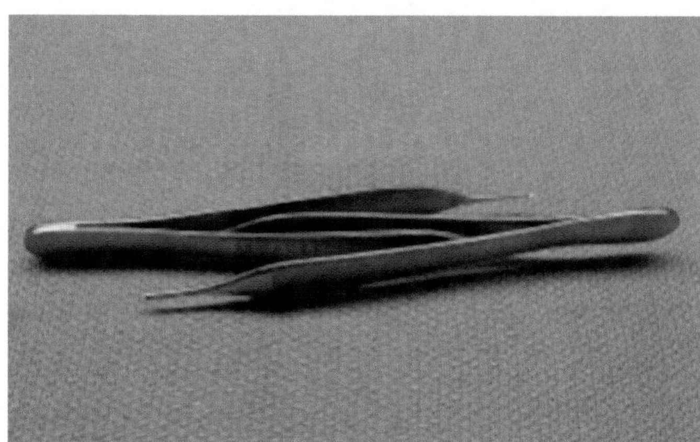

Figure 12.22 Protect forceps tips

quality material, which makes them single use and not meant for re-laundering.

Super-heated steam Occurs when dry steam becomes too hot compared to saturated steam; dry steam rises to a temperature higher than the boiling point of saturated steam. This commonly occurs when dehydrated linen is processed in a steam sterilizer. Due to the lack of moisture, dry steam is not an effective sterilant and will often char or burn items in the sterilizer.

Instrument Trays

As with procedure trays, each instrument tray should have a detailed count sheet available during instrument assembly. Technicians should never try to assemble an instrument tray from memory because contents may change and items could easily be forgotten. Technicians should avoid counting total tray contents as a method of assembling instrument trays (e.g., counting a total of 100 instruments instead of verifying each type of instrument needed). Each instrument should be identified, inspected, verified against the count sheet and placed properly in the tray.

Standardization of the instrument arrangement within each tray is important. Instrument trays should look the same, regardless of which technician assembled them. This saves time and reduces stress for the user. The order or arrangement in the tray should be determined by the SP manager and user department personnel.

It is important to note that SP technicians must place the required number of instruments in the tray. Placing too few or too many in the tray will disrupt the instrument count and may delay a surgical procedure while the needed instruments are located. Instrument substitutions should not occur, unless approved by the user department. If packaging an incomplete instrument tray is unavoidable, the users should be notified, and the tray should be clearly marked to indicate what is missing. (See **Figure 12.23**)

Instruments of the same type should be arranged together to facilitate their location during an emergency. Hinged instruments may be grouped together on racks, tray pins or stringers to ensure that instruments with locks or ratchets are maintained in the open position. Heavier items must be placed at the bottom of the tray to avoid damage to more delicate instruments. Delicate instruments should be protected using items such as approved foam pouches, tip protectors, silicon mats, holding brackets, or posts. Instrument protectors should be approved by the manufacturer for the type of sterilization method to be used. Instruments that could hold condensate should be placed in a way that allows the condensate to run out during the sterilization process.

The use of approved towels or tray liners for cushioning instruments or wicking should be determined based on the metal mass in the tray and the external package manufacturer's IFU.

Gauze sponges should never be used as additional packaging (wicking) material in trays or packs. Surgical staff count gauze sponges during procedures, and their counts must be exact. Introducing additional sponges into the OR as packaging material may cause confusion and affect sponge counts, or they may be inadvertently inserted into the patient's operative site and accidentally retained. Retained surgical items can cause damage to surrounding tissue, lead to infections, and cause irreputable damage to the patient.

Sterilant penetration or weight distribution concerns may prevent the "perfect tray" arrangement requested by the user department. SP managers should inform user department personnel about sterilization limitations. The ultimate goal must always be to create a tray that can be successfully sterilized.

Powered Surgical Instruments

Manufacturer instructions should always be followed when preparing powered surgical instruments for sterilization. This includes the use of the correct disassembly and lubrication

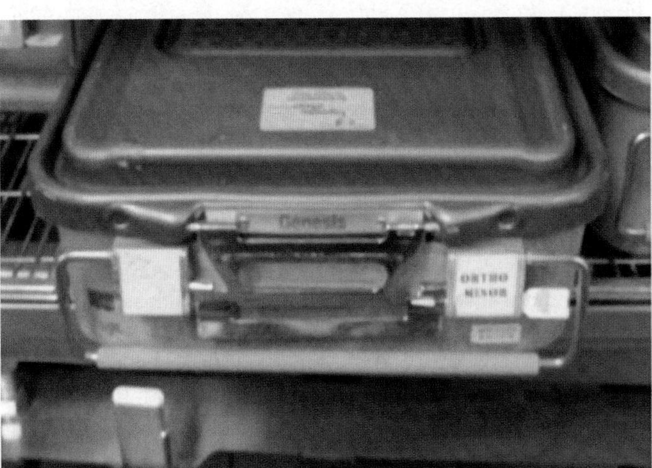

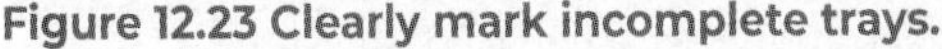
Figure 12.23 Clearly mark incomplete trays.

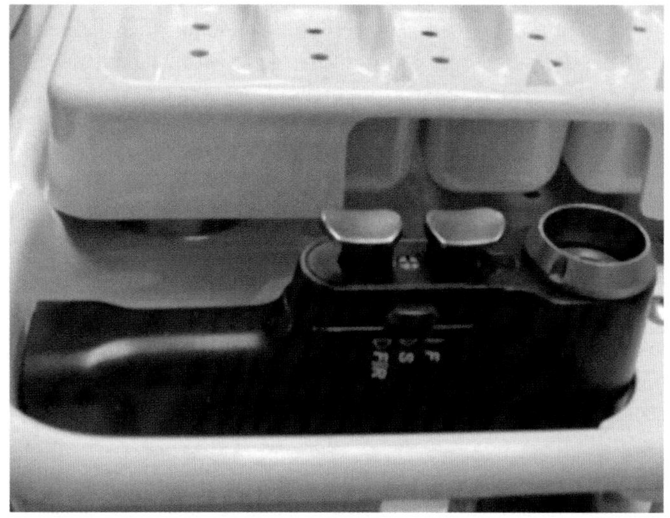

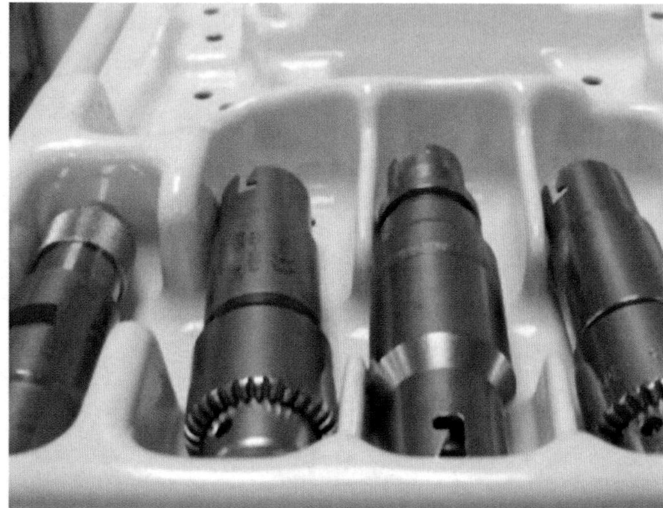

Figure 12.24 Powered surgical instruments in manufacturer's tray

procedures. Trigger handles should be placed in the safety position, and power switches should be turned off before placing the instruments in the tray.

Powered surgical instruments often use a sterilization container supplied by the manufacturer. (See **Figure 12.24**) After items are inspected, disassembled (if necessary) and placed in a container according to the manufacturer's instructions, the tray is ready to be packaged for sterilization.

Specialty Instruments

Specialty instruments, such as laparoscopic instruments, robotics, endoscopes and cameras, are of special concern for SP technicians. Manufacturers' IFU must be carefully followed to ensure that proper disassembly, assembly and sterilization procedures are completed. Some instrument IFU state the specific number of times the item can undergo sterilization.

Single Instruments

The term "single instrument" is used to describe instruments that are to be packaged alone; it can also refer to like instruments packaged together (e.g., a single Mayo scissors or a package of two Kelly clamps). These instruments should be assembled according to the department's established protocols for the size and number of instruments.

Surgical Supplies

Numerous non-instrument surgical supplies, such as cotton balls and dressings, may be required by users. Most of these items are available as commercially sterilized products, and it is often more cost effective to purchase them pre-sterilized. If the facility chooses to process them internally, these and similar items should be wrapped individually or in usable quantities based on the product manufacturer's IFU and the user's need. These items should not be sterilized without the manufacturer's IFU on file within the department. Due to the linting factor, most surgical supplies should not be sterilized inside trays or packs.

Quality Assurance Measures

Part of the assembly process for every pack includes a quality assurance test designed to measure sterilant penetration. Incorrect placement of pack contents, incorrect packaging methods or improper loading can impede the sterilization process by creating air pockets or barriers that can prevent the sterilant from penetrating the pack and making direct contact with the items inside. Internal **chemical indicators (CIs)** are designed to identify those issues before a pack is used.

> **Chemical indicators (CIs)** Devices used to monitor the presence or attainment of one or more of the parameters required for a satisfactory sterilization process.

A CI is a small, disposable test that helps the user verify that the pack contents were exposed to a sterilant. (See **Figure 12.25**) A CI's color changes when exposed to the specific sterilant it is designed to detect; this provides a visual indication of the presence of sterilant in the pack. When the pack is opened at the point of use, it is checked by the user. Users will not use a pack that has a failed internal CI and will also not use a pack that does not contain a CI.

When used properly, the CI becomes a very important early warning that something may be wrong with some aspect of the sterilization process. CIs should be placed inside each pack in the area considered the least accessible by the sterilant being used. The location may or may not be in the center of the pack's contents. In some cases, multiple CIs may need to be used if multiple areas could pose a challenge for sterilant penetration. Multi-level trays should have a CI placed in the most difficult area for sterilant penetration on each level of the tray.

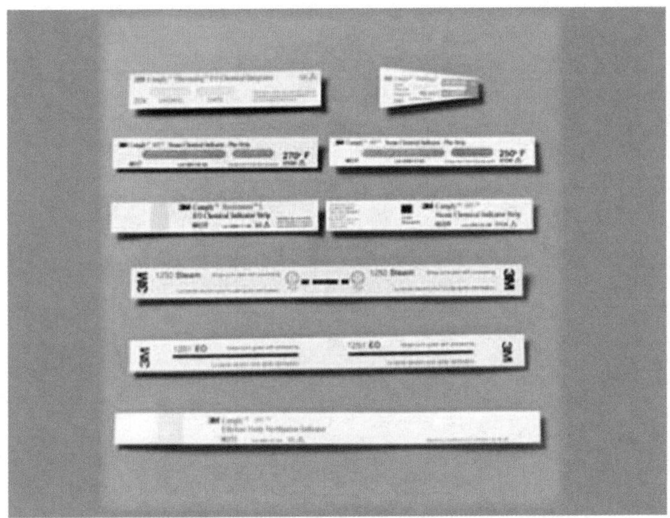

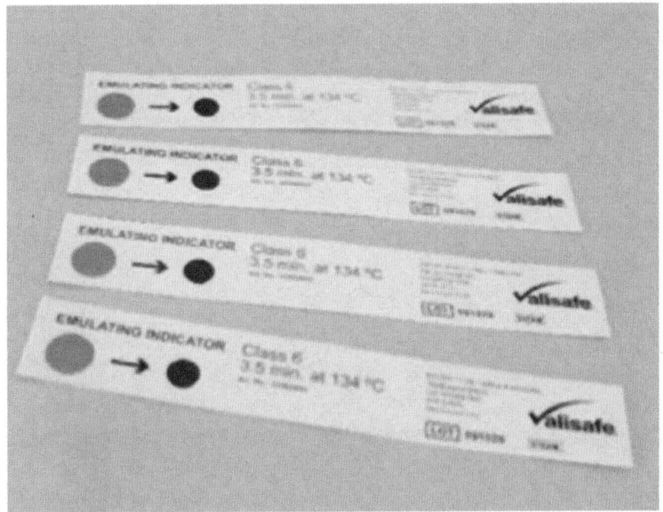

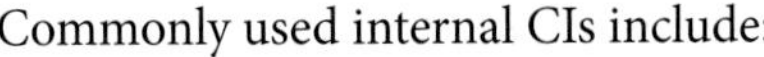
Figure 12.25 Examples of internal chemical indicators

Commonly used internal CIs include:

- Type 4 multi-critical process variable indicators – Designed to react to two or more of the critical process variables and are intended to indicate exposure to a sterilization process at stated values of the chosen critical process variables.

- Type 5 integrating indicators – Designed to react to all critical parameters and be equivalent to or exceed performance requirements over a specified range of sterilization cycles. When used inside a **process challenge device (PCD)**, non-implant loads may be released with the appropriate results indicated on the CI.

- Type 6 emulating indicators, also called verification indicators or cycle-specific indicators – Designed to react to all critical parameters of a sterilization cycle. Class 6 indicators are designed to be run within one specific cycle (e.g., 270°F, four-minute exposure). This is the *only* cycle in which this specific indicator may be used. If a 275°F, three-minute exposure cycle is to be run, an emulator specifically made for that cycle must be used.

Note: It is important to use the appropriate indicator for the intended method of sterilization and cycle.

Process challenge device (PCD) Object that simulates a predetermined set of conditions when used to test sterilizing agent(s).

BASIC PACKAGING PROCEDURES

Once items have been cleaned, dried, inspected and assembled, they are ready to be sterilized. In order to maintain their sterility, items must be packaged before they are sterilized. The packaging allows the sterilant to enter and helps maintain the integrity (sterility) of the sterile items until they are opened and used.

The following sections address packaging selection and application.

Overview of the Sterile Packaging Process

SP technicians must select the appropriate packaging material and apply it correctly to create a pack that can be sterilized successfully and maintain sterility until opened.

One can draw some comparisons between food packaging and sterile packaging. Both types of packaging must protect items and keep them from becoming contaminated before they are used. Both can be compromised in a way that affects the package's contents and makes them unsafe for use.

Some sterile packaging is designed with **tamper-evident seals**, so users can tell if the package has been opened. (See **Figure 12.26**) Many food products use these tamper-evident seals on their packaging for the same reason. There are several packaging options for food products and sterile items, and not all types of packaging are appropriate for all items and processes. For example, soup could not be packaged in aluminum foil, carried to work and heated in a microwave oven. Sterile item packaging must also consider the sterilization process that will be used.

Tamper-evident seals Sealing method that allows users to determine if sterile packages have been opened (contaminated) and helps users identify packages that are unsafe for patient use.

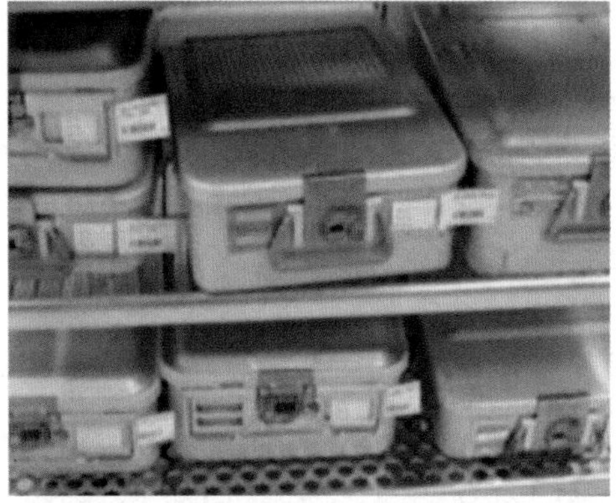

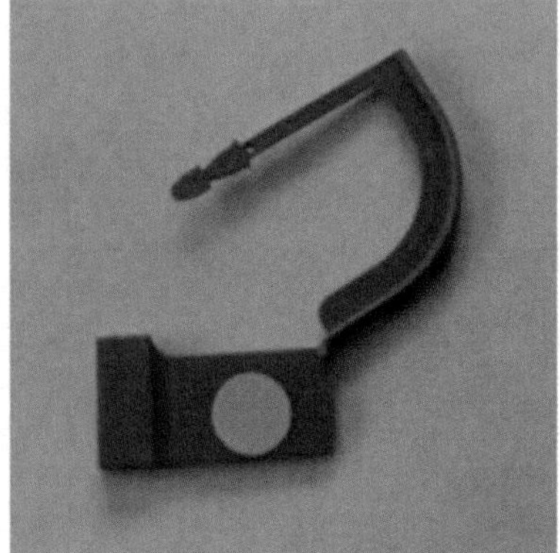

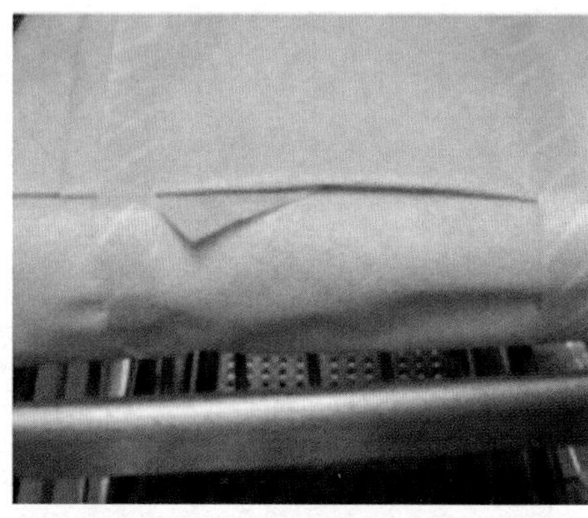

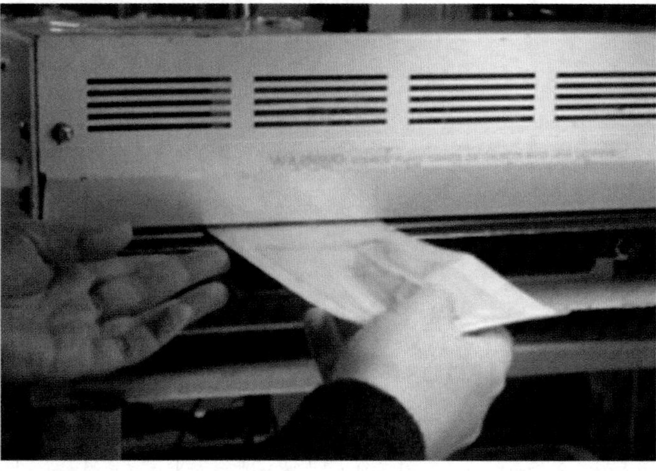

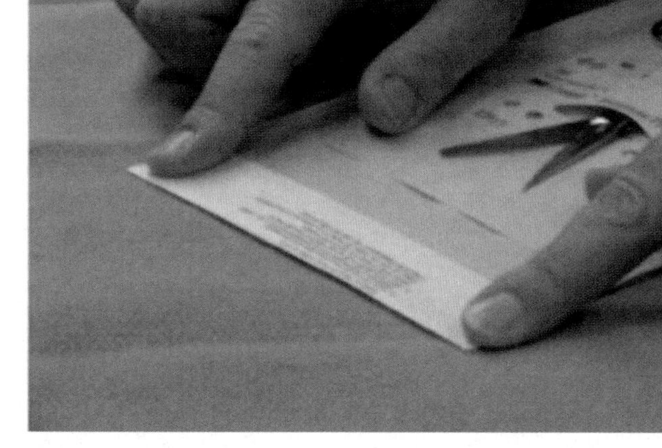

Figure 12.26 Examples of tamper-resistant seals

Objectives of the Packaging Process

There are three primary objectives for any sterilization packaging system. It must:

- Allow penetration of the chosen sterilant and be compatible with any other requirements of the specific sterilization process such as drying
- Maintain the sterility of the package contents until the package is opened
- Create a package that can be opened aseptically (without contaminating the contents)

Packaging systems must also:

- Have a sealing method that is tamper evident
- Be non-toxic
- Be non-linting
- Be easy to use
- Be cost effective

The U.S. Food and Drug Administration (FDA) classifies sterilization packaging as a Class II medical device (a device that presents a potential risk). The consequences of using a nonsterile item during a surgical procedure can be life-threatening. In addition to selecting and applying the appropriate packaging material, SP technicians must also be able to construct packages that allow the sterilization process to be successful and protect the package contents from contamination.

Selecting the Appropriate Packaging Material

The first step in the packaging process is selecting the appropriate packaging material and method. Different types of packaging are needed for alternative sterilization methods, and styles of packaging may vary based on package contents.

SP technicians must make good packaging choices. Only materials specifically designed for sterilization packaging and cleared by the FDA are acceptable.

In addition to selecting the appropriate packaging material, SP technicians must understand how to use sterilization packaging properly to achieve the desired results, sterilant penetration, barrier effectiveness and aseptic opening.

Packaging systems used in healthcare facility-based sterilization are generally classified into reusable packaging and disposable (single-use) packaging materials. Each packaging system has advantages and limitations. The following sections provide some basic information about common packaging systems and their application.

REUSABLE PACKAGING MATERIALS

There are two basic types of reusable packaging material: woven fabric and rigid containers.

Woven Fabric Materials

Muslin, Type 140 cotton, calico, and barrier cloth are common names for fabric made of 100% unbleached, loosely woven cotton fibers. Muslin wrappers are generally made of two-ply (double thickness) fabric fastened together as one wrap. (See **Figure 12.27**).

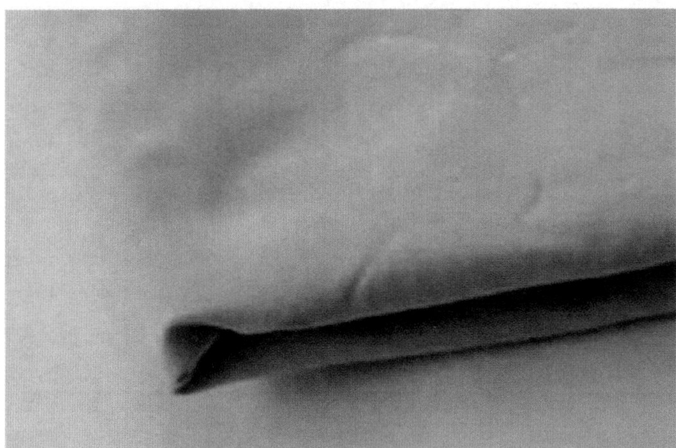

Figure 12.27 Muslin wrap

Other woven fabrics used in sterilization are:

- Duck cloth
- Twill
- Treated barrier fabrics

Note: Canvas is not recommended as a packaging material because its tight weave impedes steam penetration and drying.

Textile packaging is still the packaging method of choice for some healthcare facilities. The selection of reusable textiles is often impacted by costs and/or environmental sustainability concerns (the desire to reduce waste generated by disposable packaging materials).

Textile packaging requires more labor because it must be laundered and inspected to ensure that there are no tears, punctures, worn spots, or stains from previous use. That inspection is performed using a light table that has a light source built into the tabletop to identify small holes and punctures. As the wrap is passed over the lighted table top, light shines through small holes and punctures, making them easier to identify.

If holes, punctures or worn spots are discovered, the linen wrap must be repaired using a heat-sealed patch designed to cover the hole. The size of the surface area covered by heat-sealed patches on reusable fabrics should be considered before the fabric is reused. (See **Figure 12.28**)

If stains are discovered, the wrap should be re-laundered. If stains cannot be removed, the wrap should be removed from service.

Textiles must also be de-linted as needed to minimize the risk of lint entering the sterile pack and, ultimately, the sterile field. (See

Light table

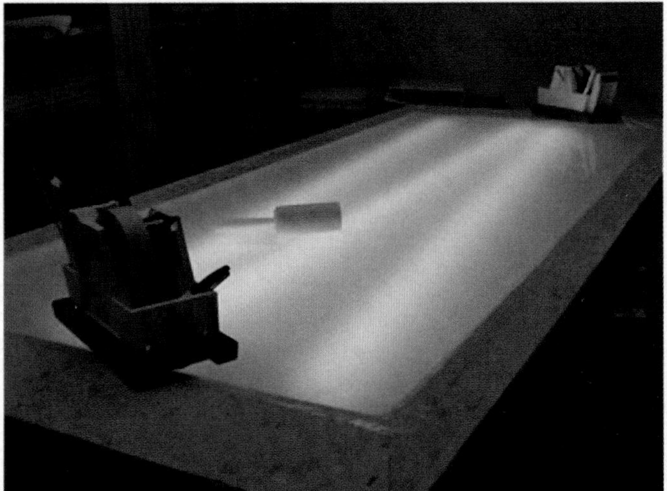

Textile patch

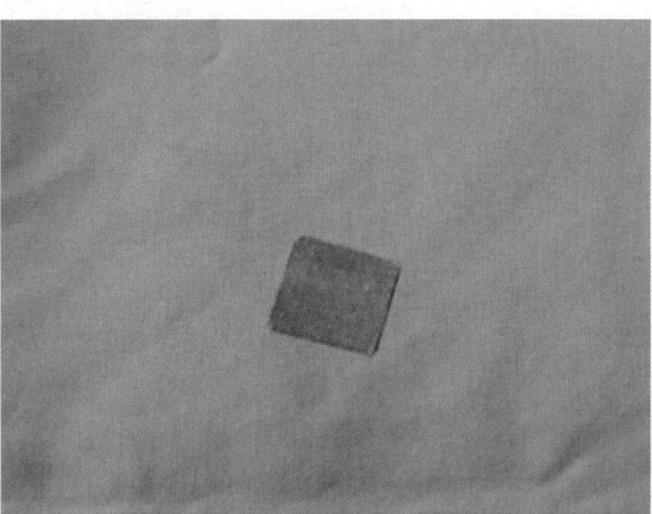

Figure 12.28 Reusable textile inspection and repair

Figure 12.29) Reusable textiles can be a significant source of lint. If lint enters a patient's incision, it may cause negative effects.

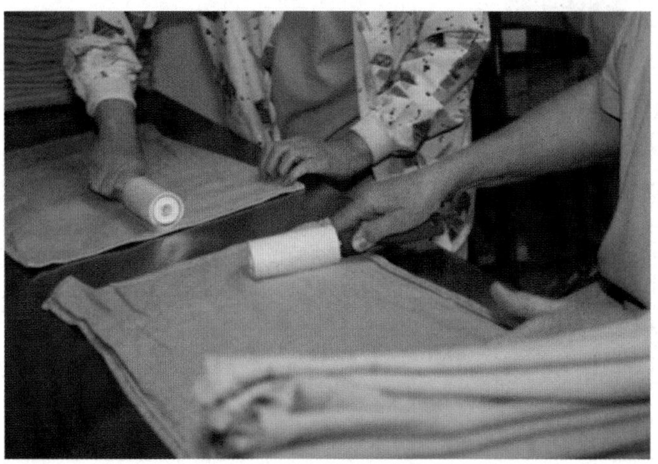

Figure 12.29 De-linting reusable textiles

When assembling linen packs using textiles, refer to the textile and sterilizer IFU for size and weight restrictions, as these restrictions may differ from their single-use counterparts.

Linen wrappers should be securely applied without compressing package contents. Contents must be packaged with sufficient spacing to allow the sterilant to reach all surfaces.

Tight packaging will not allow for fiber swelling (expansion); when expansion occurs, the sterilant will not penetrate the material. It is possible to wrap even a small pack so tightly that its density will be too great for adequate sterilant penetration.

Rigid Container Systems

Rigid container systems are box-like structures with sealable and removable lids. They are made of anodized aluminum, stainless steel, plastic or a combination of these materials. Rigid containers have lids and filters that allow sterilant penetration, while providing a microbial barrier. Filters may be disposable (a synthetic spunbond product) or reusable (with ceramic filters or a valve system). Rigid containers consist of an inner basket to hold the instruments and an outer container that acts as a protective barrier. Instruments should only be inside the basket, not outside the basket or resting on the container. Both the inner basket and outer container have handles for easier carrying. After placing the lid on the container, tamper-evident locks must be applied.

Rigid container system Instrument containers that hold medical devices during sterilization and also protect devices from contamination during storage and transport.

Figure 12.30 identifies the common components of a rigid sterilization container system's outer container.

Some manufacturers of rigid container systems recommend that times for instrument sterilization, drying and aeration be extended when using their containers. It is important to consult the specific container manufacturer's IFU before using a rigid container system. The IFU specifies the type of sterilization modality to use and cycle type such as dynamic air removal and gravity. Rigid containers are regulated by the FDA.

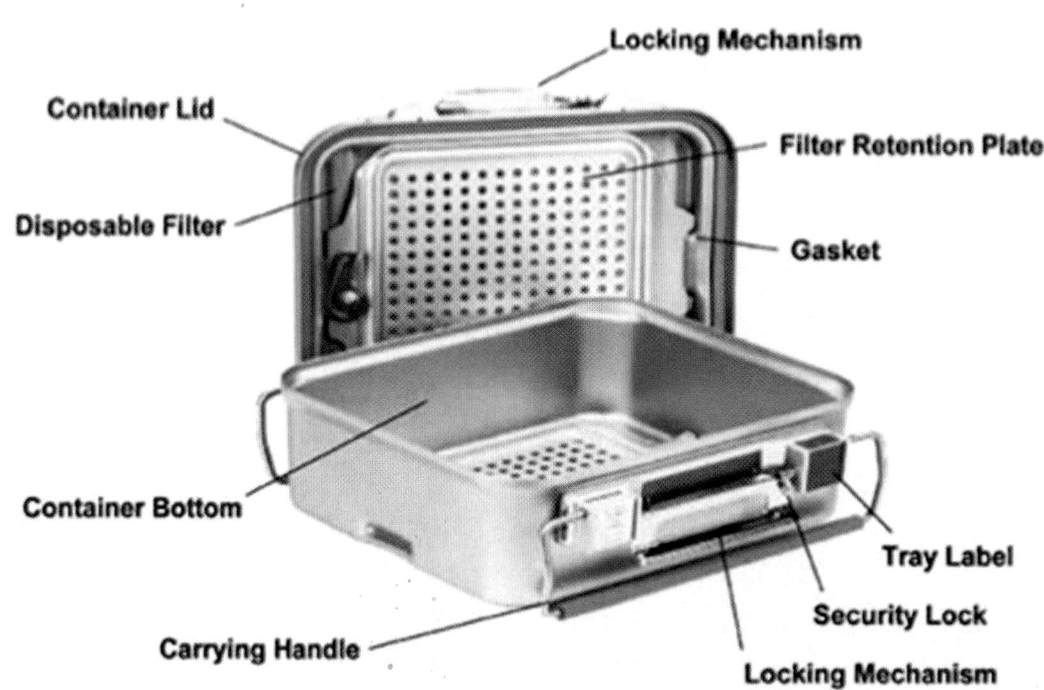

Figure 12.30 Example of a rigid container system

When using sterilization containers, it is imperative to review and follow the IFU carefully. Not all sterilization containers can sterilize all medical devices; there may be restrictions related to density of materials, weight and distribution of contents. Other sterilization container restrictions include:

- Lumen size
- Number of lumened devices
- Types of material used
- Stacking
- Weight

Advantages and Disadvantages

There are several advantages of rigid sterilization containers. They:

- Provide an excellent barrier to microorganisms
- Are easy to use
- Eliminate torn wrappers
- Help protect instruments from damage during processing, storage and transport

There are also potential disadvantages to the use of rigid sterilization containers, including:

- Safety concerns linked to ergonomics – Some large, empty containers weigh approximately seven to nine pounds. This requires SP technicians to use good body mechanics when lifting and moving containers.
- Additional cycle time may be required to thoroughly dry the container – Sterilization efficacy is also impacted as a container's weight increases because of excess condensation. While it is difficult to generalize about specific causes of **wet packs**, it is known that heavier sets and those with greater metal mass are more likely to experience this problem, especially when instruments are not properly disbursed in the container.
- Plastic containers may require longer dry times because they lack metal, which produces heat by conduction to help drying.

Wet pack Package or container that contains moisture after the sterilization process is completed.

- Additional space may be needed to store those containers that are larger than traditional wrapped containers. (See **Figure 12.31**)

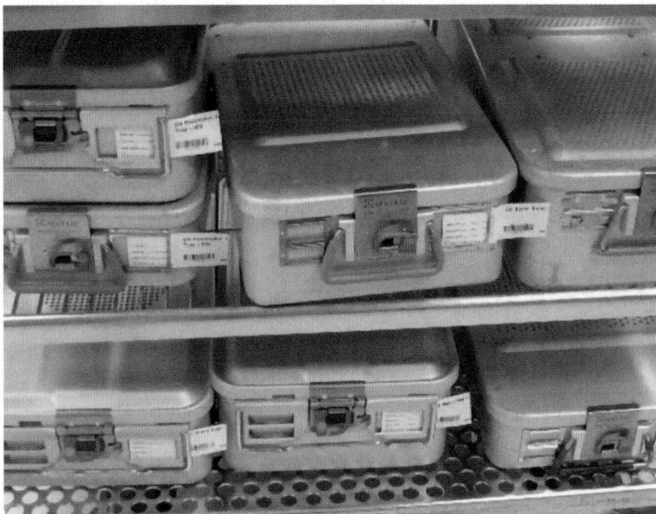

Figure 12.31

- Additional labor may be required since the containers must be cleaned between uses. This may also affect washer loads if a mechanical washer is used. (See **Figure 12.32**)
- Latching mechanisms on containers create potential problems. When latches and welds break, the containers cannot be used. Also, sharp edges can injure employees.
- Filter retention plates may become dislodged and contaminate instruments.

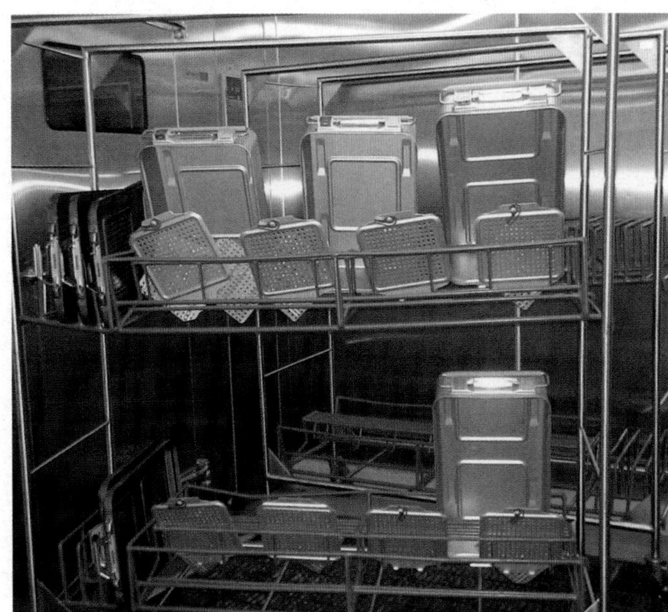

Figure 12.32 Rigid sterilization containers should be cleaned between uses.

Cleaning and Inspection Procedures for Rigid Containers

To clean a rigid sterilization container, first remove its disposable filters or release its filter protector/holder. Valve-type closures must be cleaned according to the manufacturer's written instructions. Interior baskets must be removed and cleaned. Dividers and pins may need to be removed if they interfere with the cleaning process.

Cleaning and rinsing instructions provided by the container manufacturer should be followed. Particular attention should be given to the type of detergent used. For example, some containers cannot be exposed to certain chemicals such as high-alkaline solutions.

Inspection of rigid sterilization containers is necessary to detect flaws and wear that may interfere with the sterilization process or sterility maintenance. Inspection should also focus on the top and bottom valve or filter mechanism and the latching mechanism. For example:

- The filter retention plate should be intact and not bent; the retention plate should seat over the filter and securely lock into place.
- The surfaces and edges of the container and lid should be free of dents and chips.
- The retention post should be secure and not move.
- If using disposable filters, they should be checked for holes prior to placing them in the container. (See **Figure 12.33**) Filters should fit the space allotted, with no folding or crimping of edges. Filter material must be approved for the type of sterilization to be used.

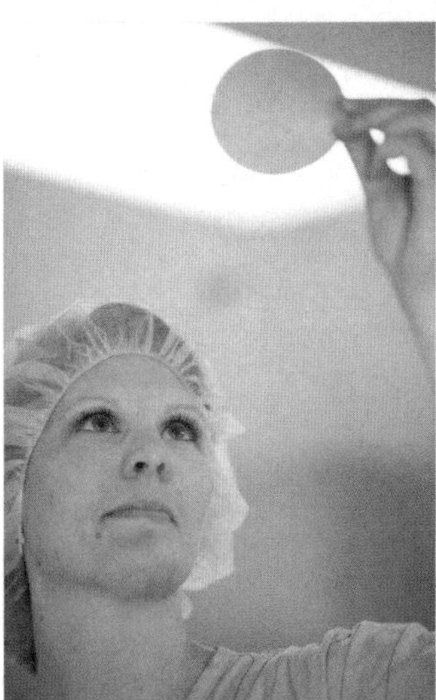

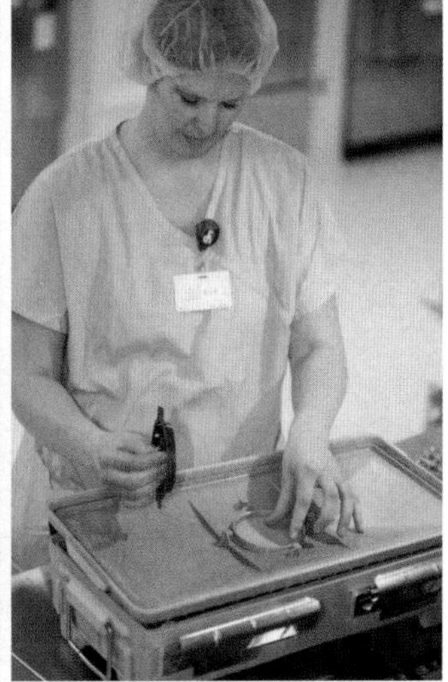

Figure 12.33 Check filters before use.

- Only filters recommended by the container manufacturer should be used; filters cannot be altered or made from other materials.
- If using reusable valves, they should be clean and free of debris, with no breaks or chips in the valve mechanism. (See **Figure 12.34**)

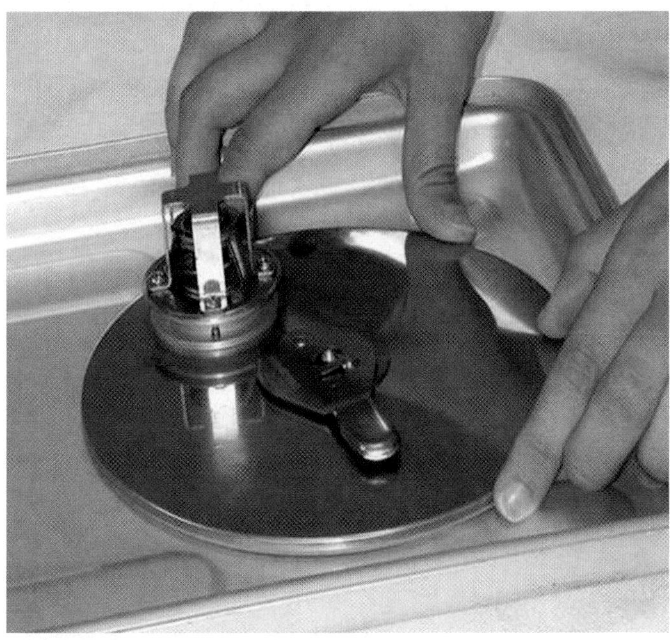

Figure 12.34

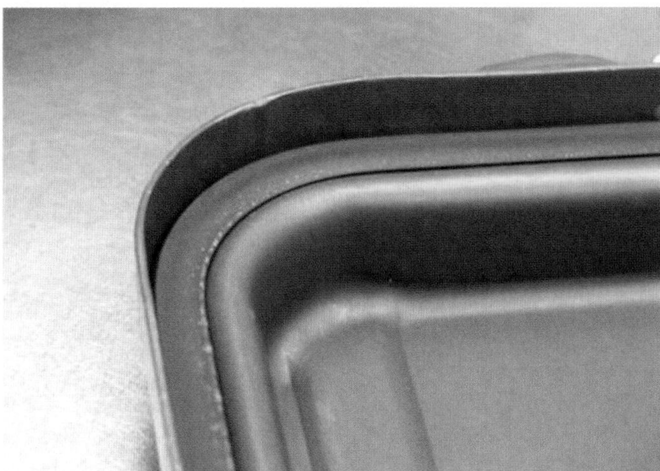

Figure 12.35 Check gaskets for cleanliness, damage and signs of wear.

- The lid gasket should be pliable, clean and free of cracks and nicks. There should be no ridges on the gasket. *Note: Ridges are caused by a tight fit between the top and bottom of the container.* (See **Figure 12.35**)
- Rivets in the handle area should be checked to ensure that they are secured and not separating from the container. If loosened, they can become a safety hazard and a pathway for entry of bacteria.

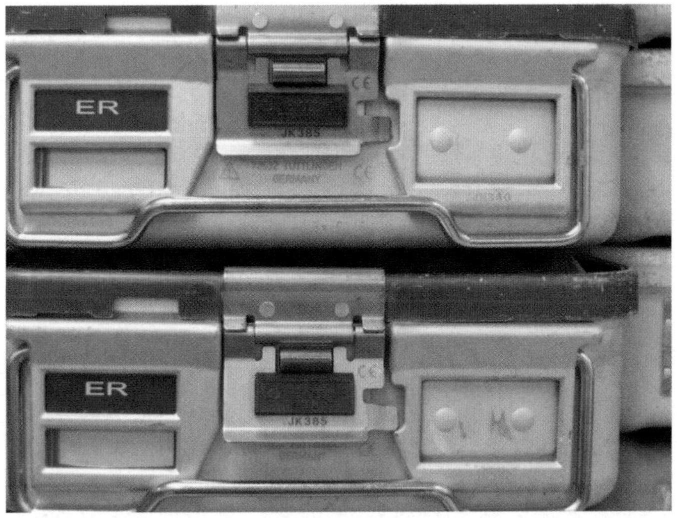

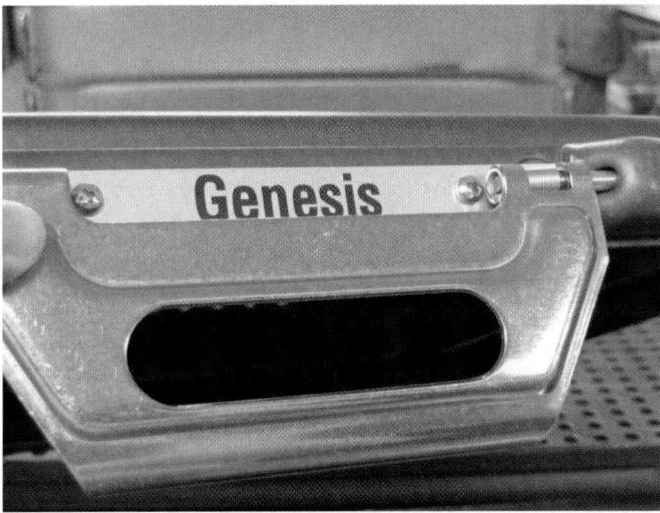

Figure 12.36 Check handles for cleanliness and signs of wear.

- Handles should move up and down easily. Ensure the latch springs are in place and once locked, checked to ensure the latching mechanisms are functioning to maintain the seal. (See **Figure 12.36**)

As noted previously, the weight of instruments placed in the container is an important concern. The number of instruments placed in the tray must not exceed the quantity that can be effectively sterilized and dried.

Rigid containers should be carried by both of their handles (not by the lid) to avoid breaking the container's seal or damaging the instruments inside.

DISPOSABLE PACKAGING MATERIALS

Disposable (non-woven) materials were introduced as "engineered fabrics" in the 1940s and have made their way into everyday life. Coffee filters, teabags, vacuum cleaner bags and disposable diapers are all examples of engineered fabrics (also referred to as disposable non-woven materials). These materials are used in both disposable flat wrap and rigid container filters. (See **Figure 12.37**) Before using, both disposable flat wrap and rigid container filters should be inspected for tears or holes that may have occurred during transport and handling. Disposable/ non-woven materials are a popular choice for sterilization packaging because they have excellent barrier effectiveness and can be discarded after use. There are three types of disposable packaging materials in common use: paper, polyolefin plastic and disposable non-woven wrap.

Important Note: Be Aware of Packaging Expiration Dates

Some disposable packaging materials contain expiration dates from the manufacturer. It is important to check for an expiration date prior to using any disposable packaging material. The expiration date usually indicates a decrease in the packaging's ability to perform at optimal standards, including the packaging material's microbial barrier properties.

Flat wrap

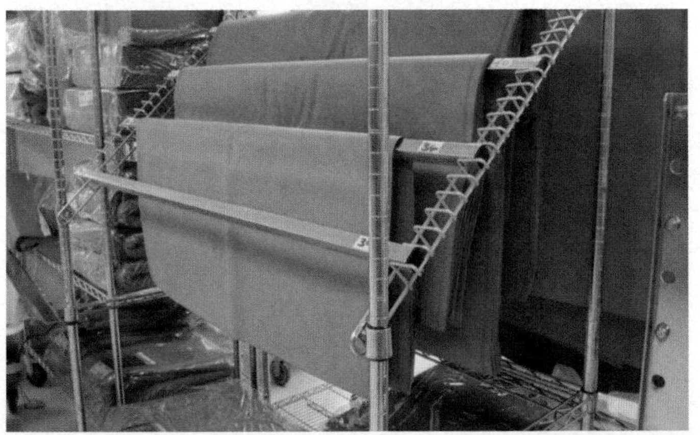

Rigid container filters

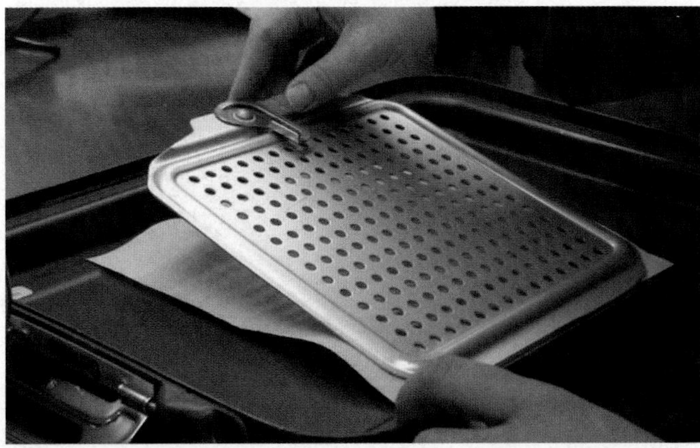

Figure 12.37 Disposable non-woven materials play a significant role in sterilization packaging.

Paper is commonly used as sterilization packaging materials. It is important to ensure that the paper packaging is intended for use as sterilization packaging, and that it has been cleared by the FDA. *Note: Paper containing cellulose cannot be used in hydrogen peroxide sterilizers because cellulose absorbs the sterilant and reduces penetration. As this occurs, the contents being sterilized may not be exposed to the proper amount of sterilant.*

Kraft-type paper (medical grade) is generally smooth surfaced and is available in sizes to accommodate many medical devices and porous or soft-good items. Pouches of medical-grade paper specially formulated for sterilization are also available. Pouches with both sides consisting of Kraft-type paper can be used to hold small parts and instruments inside the instrument sets. (See **Figure 12.38**)

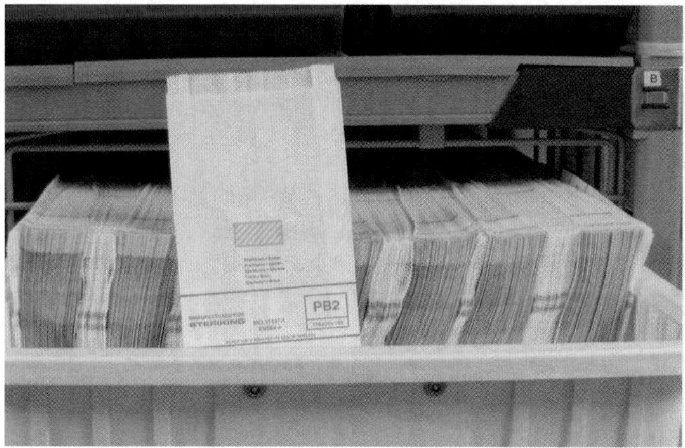

Figure 12.38 Examples of Kraft-type paper pouches

Kraft-type paper (also known as crepe paper) can also be purchased as flat wrap. These products may be utilized in steam and ethylene oxide (EO) sterilization but cannot be used with hydrogen peroxide.

Paper/plastic and spunbond polyolefin-plastic combinations (called peel packs or peel pouches) are the most commonly used packaging materials for small instruments and lightweight items. (See **Figure 12.39**) They are called peel pouches because after they are sealed, they must be peeled open for aseptic presentation.

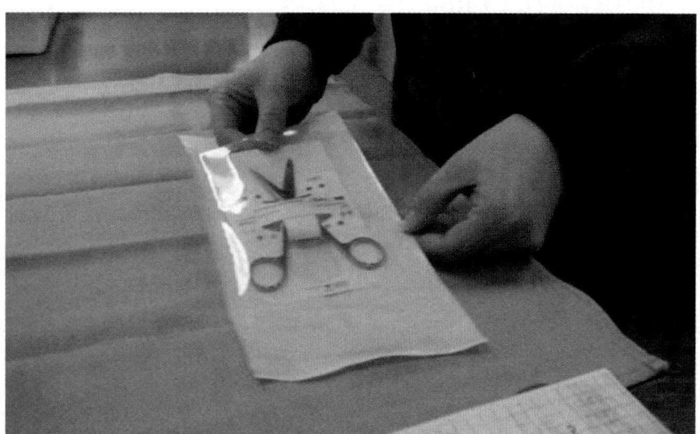

Figure 12.39 Example of a peel pouch

There are two basic types of combination peel pouches:

- Paper/plastic combinations – These are typically acceptable for use with steam and EO sterilization processes. They are not compatible with hydrogen peroxide. As suggested by their name, they have a paper side and a plastic side. The plastic side allows visibility of the package contents, and the paper side allows sterilant penetration. *Note: Sterilant cannot enter through the plastic side, so proper positioning is important to achieve sterilization.*

- Spun bonded high-density polyethylene (HDPE) combinations (sometimes referred to as Tyvek® pouches) – These are used for low-temperature hydrogen peroxide sterilization. Like paper/plastic combinations, they have a plastic side so package contents are visible. The other side is composed of polyolefin that contains no cellulosic materials and is, therefore, compatible with hydrogen peroxide sterilization processes.

Important Note: Use Caution When Selecting Peel Pouches

Paper/plastic and spunbond-polyolefin packages look alike. Paper/plastic combinations are not compatible with hydrogen peroxide sterilization, and spunbond-polyolefin combinations will melt in high-temperature processes such as steam sterilization.

Flat wrap is another commonly used packaging material. Instead of inserting objects into a ready-made pouch and sealing it, flat wrap requires the user to "create" a barrier package using specific folding techniques. (See **Figure 12.40)**

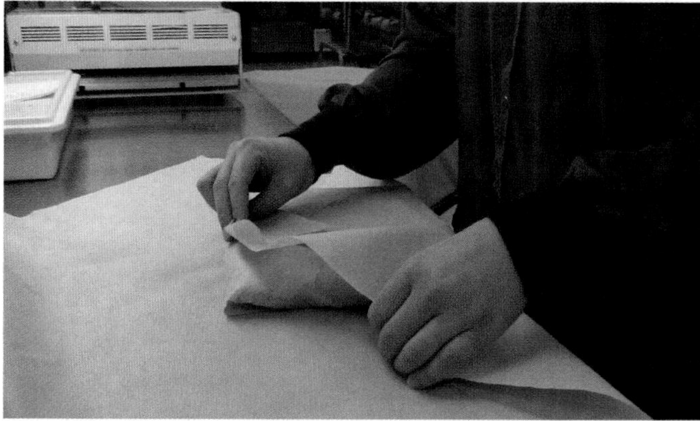

Figure 12.40

One non-woven packaging material, spunbond-meltblown-spunbond (SMS), is a popular flat wrap. It is made by a process in which polyolefin layers (synthetic materials softened by heat and hardened by cooling) are exposed to high heat and are pressure-bonded together to form sheets. Flat wrapping products constructed of non-woven SMS fabrics for sterilization wrapping are designed as single-use disposable products and must never be reused. These materials are available in a range of weights and a wide variety of sizes. Flat wrap is also available as single- or double-sheet wraps that are bonded together.

The use of each packaging material has advantages and disadvantages. SP technicians must ensure that they select the type of packaging most suitable for the item(s) being packaged and the type of sterilization selected. SP technicians can then begin preparing the package contents for packaging and the sterilization process to follow.

WRAPPING TECHNIQUES

Peel Pouching Techniques

Peel pouches are usually used for smaller, lightweight items and are useful when it is important to see inside the package. Peel pouches are available on rolls that allow SP technicians to cut off the length desired for each package; they are also available in precut sizes. Inserts or tip protectors help to protect a pouch's contents from damage and prevent the tips from penetrating the package. If inserts or tip protectors are used, ensure that the material is appropriate for the type of sterilization method to be used, and that it is nontoxic and free of non-fast dyes. (See **Figure 12.41**)

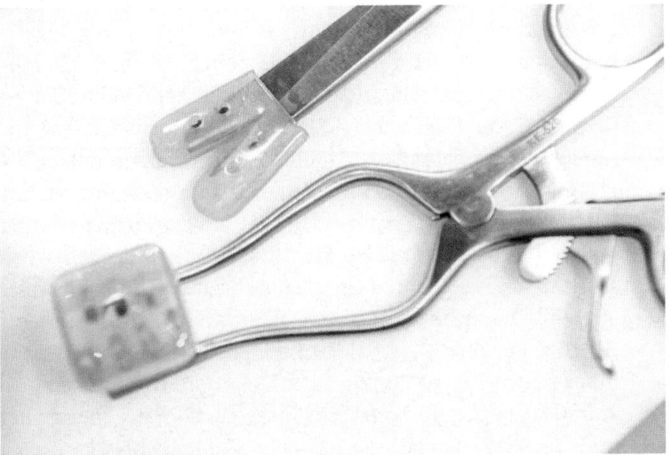

Figure 12.41

Before placing items in the peel pouch, carefully inspect the pouch to ensure there are no tears or holes. Items should be placed in the pouch so the end of the item to be grasped during presentation (i.e., finger rings of an instrument) will be presented first when the package is opened at the point of use. *Note: This is the chevron end for pre-made pouches.* **Figure 12.42** illustrates the chevron end of a pre-made pouch. It is designed in a manner that makes it easier to open. This reduces the risk of product contamination during aseptic opening.

Instrument tips should always face the plastic side of the package to avoid penetrating the paper side and contaminating the contents.

Hinged instruments must be packaged in a manner that keep the instrument open for sterilization. This can be accomplished by using commercially purchased products.

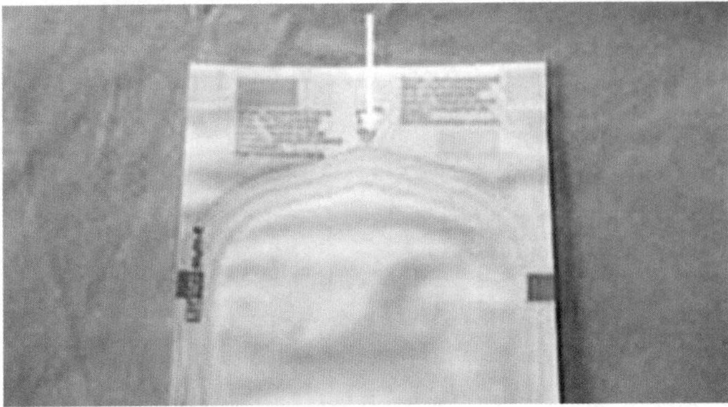

Figure 12.42 Chevron end of a peel pouch

Pouches must be sized and applied properly to allow for adequate air removal, sterilant penetration and drying.

To allow space for package contraction and proper circulation, leave about one inch (1/4" per side of the package) of space between the items in the pouch and the sealed edges. When packaging is too small, the packaged instruments cause stress on the sides of the pouch. (See **Figure 12.43**) Stress compromises the package's barrier and will likely rupture the side seams of the package during the harsh air removal and heat-up phases of the steam sterilization process or the high vacuum phase of the hydrogen peroxide sterilization process. Items placed in packages that are too small can also rupture the seams during normal handling and transport. Pouches should not be too large because movement of the items inside the pouch may result in the contents sliding from end to end or side to side. The excessive movement of contents could break seals or puncture the pouch's paper. (See **Figure 12.44**) Pouches should not be overfilled because this can cause the paper to tear, or the seals to rupture during sterilization or handling. (See **Figure 12.45**)

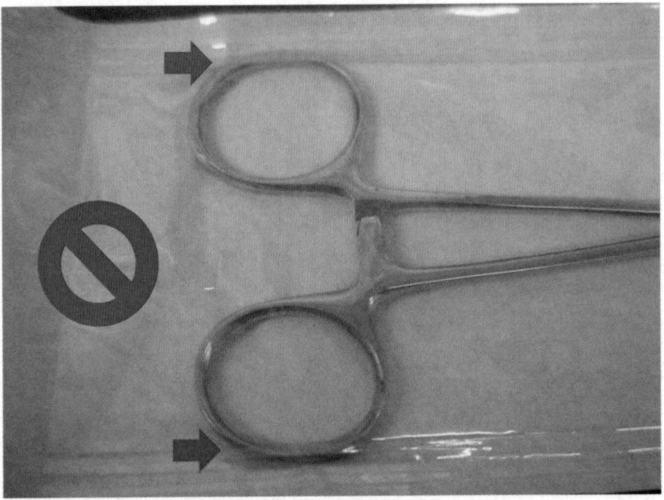

Figure 12.43 An instrument placed in a too-small peel pouch can stress the edges of the package.

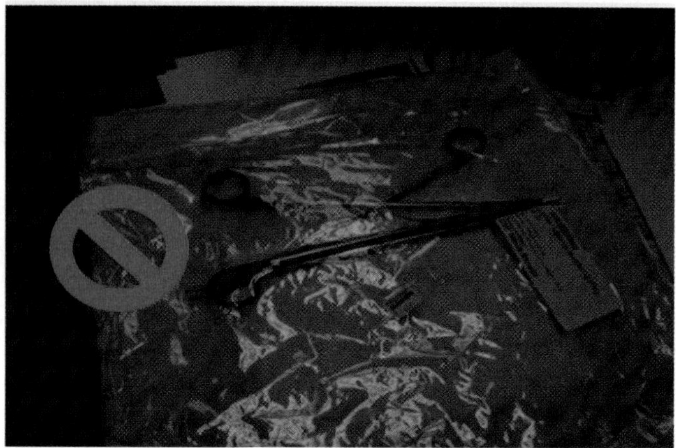

Figure 12.44 Packs that are too large are vulnerable to seal breaks when contents move excessively.

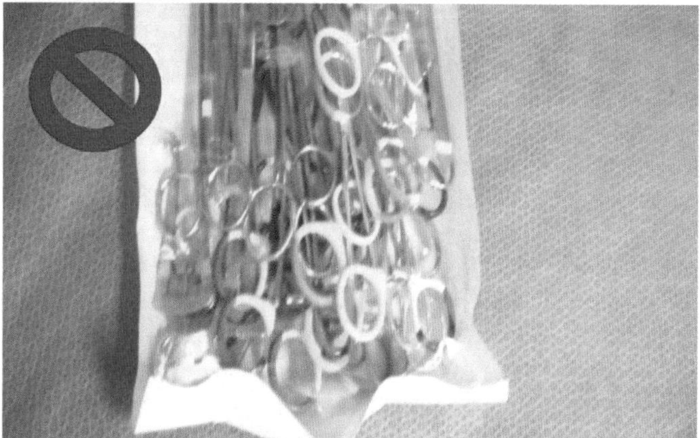

Figure 12.45 Over-filled pouches may stress seals and tear the paper side of the pouch.

Trapped air acts as a barrier to heat, moisture and sterilant penetration, so it is important to remove as much air as possible before sealing. To remove trapped air, gently push the pouch's top and bottom layers together, just prior to sealing. *Note: Applying too much pressure can damage the pouch.*

Paper/plastic pouches must only be labeled on the plastic side or on areas specifically provided by the manufacturer (e.g., on fold-over paper flap seals). Writing on the paper side of the pouch will damage the package, which may not be noticeable but can compromise the barrier protection. Use only felt-tipped pens approved for writing on the plastic surface and for the sterilization method to be used. Using the wrong type of pen, such as a ballpoint pen, can damage packaging.

Pouches must be closed with a tamper-evident seal so there is no danger of packages being opened and resealed for later use. Package seals should be either a self-seal or heat seal. Sterilization tape should not be used because tape hinders aseptic removal. After a sterile package is opened, it is contaminated and may not be resealed and reused.

Most heat sealers have a temperature control. The temperature of the heat sealer is dependent on the type of packaging used, which is included in the packaging IFU. Paper/plastic heat sealers function at a higher temperature than plastic Tyvek® pouches.

There are two types of heat sealers available: lift sealers and continuous-feed heat sealers. Whichever is used, it must be kept in proper working condition to prevent the heat sealer from burning the package or from not thoroughly sealing the package. The heat sealer's IFU provides information regarding its care and maintenance. Verification testing devices are available to verify that the peel pouch seals are holding.

Common ways that paper/plastic and polyolefin-plastic packages can be used to meet specific packaging needs include:

- Wrap within a pouch – Sometimes, usually to accommodate unique sterile presentation issues, it is desirable to place a single-wrapped package into a pouch. The initial wrap is done using the flat wrap packaging and wrapping method. It is not necessary to seal the wrapped item. The wrapped item is then inserted into the appropriately sized pouch. The pouch should be sealed and labeled. *Note: The manufacturer's IFU for both the peel pouch and the flat wrap must be reviewed to see if this process is approved. Using this method if not approved by both manufacturers could result in an unsterile product.*

- Double pouches – While double pouching is not necessary for sterility maintenance, it may be required for aseptic presentation of multiple items or for instruments having more than one part. Before double pouching, the packaging manufacturer IFU should be reviewed for approval to double package. Double packaging should be performed using the same type of packaging. Double pouches are prepared by placing the item(s) into one paper/plastic pouch and sealing it. This pouch is then placed inside another slightly larger pouch and sealed. (See **Figure 12.46**) Care is needed when selecting the appropriate sequential sizing. The same rules apply for the inside peel pouch as for pouching instruments (leave about one ¼" per side of the package). Never fold the inner pouch because doing so can interfere with air removal and sterilant penetration. (See **Figure 12.47**) Place the smaller inner package paper side to paper side and plastic side to plastic side to help ensure sterilant penetration, drying, and content visibility.

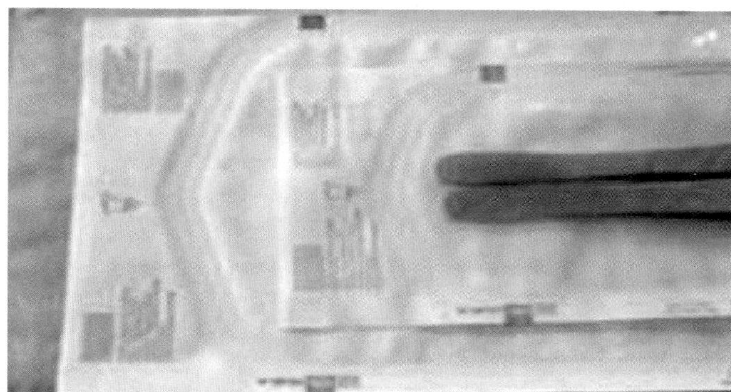

Figure 12.46 Double peel pouch

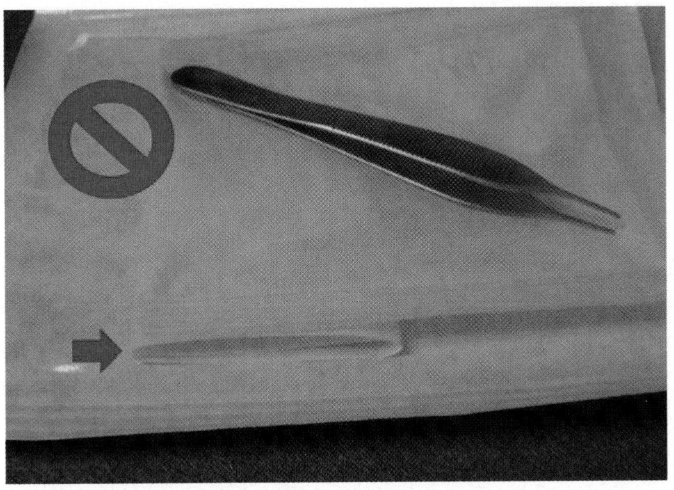

Figure 12.47 A folded-over inner pouch can cause penetration and drying issues.

Flat-Wrapping Techniques

Flat-wrapping procedures are primarily used for large packages but may also be used for smaller items. These procedures involve using either reusable woven textiles (linens) or disposable non-woven wraps.

There are two methods of using flat wrap packs:

- Sequential – The package is wrapped twice and is "a package within a package." The term "sequential" indicates that the contents have been wrapped in sequence (one after the other). This method is used for muslin, Kraft-type paper and single layers of SMS wraps.
- Simultaneous – The package is only wrapped once but requires a special, double-layered synthetic nonwoven material bound on two or four sides.

The advantage of sequential wrap is that it affords a "second chance" for sterile presentation. The disadvantages: sequential wrap requires more time for wrapping and unwrapping. The advantage of simultaneous wrap is reduced labor costs and increased output in the SPD and OR.

There are also two techniques for wrapping packages, and both are used with the sequential and simultaneous wrap methods:

- Square fold – This is also called the in-line or parallel fold; it is most frequently used for larger packs and instrument trays.
- Envelope fold – This is more commonly used for individual items, small packs and most instrument sets.

Regardless of the packaging system used, flat wrap should be inspected for holes and tears prior to use. Wrap must be free from holes, tears, abrasions or any other deviations that could allow bacteria to enter the package.

SP technicians are responsible for creating a package that will protect the contents and allow for sterilization and aseptic opening from flat sheets of wrapping material. This requires that every package be created according to specific protocols. The following photos illustrate the proper techniques for sequential and simultaneous wrapping in both the envelope and square styles.

Figures 12.48 through **12.58** illustrate sequential wrapping techniques using the envelope style. In this method, flat wrap is applied one after the other (in sequence).

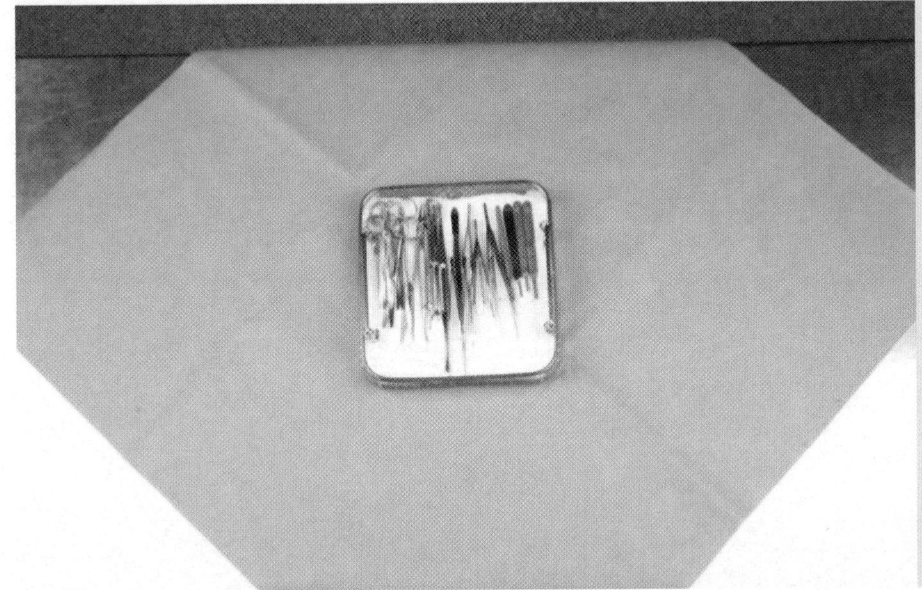

Figure 12.48

Sequential Envelope: Step 1

With the sequential envelope technique, the wrap is placed on the table to form a diamond shape. The item to be wrapped is placed in the center of the wrap, parallel with the edge of the table.

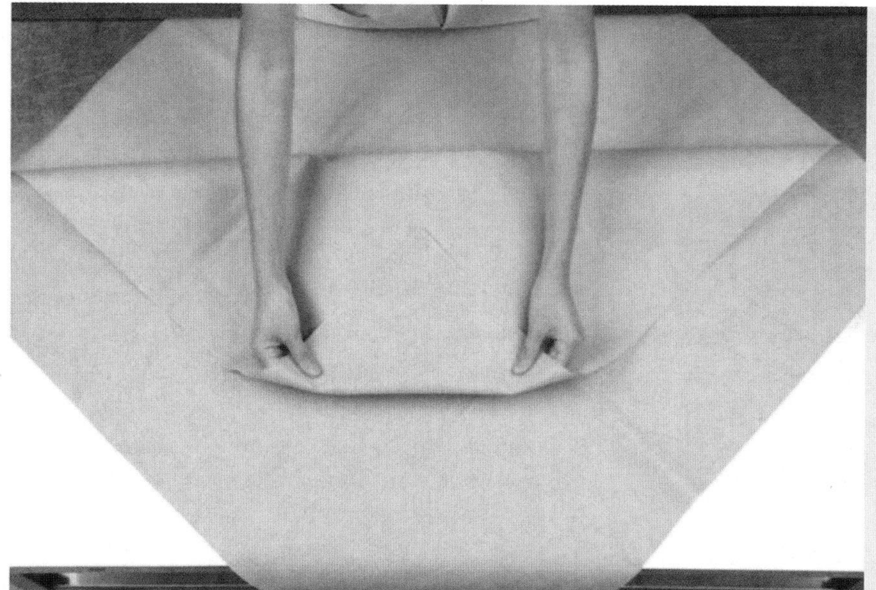

Figure 12.49

Sequential Envelope: Step 2

The lower corner is brought up to completely cover the contents, and the tip is folded back onto itself to form a flap. This flap may be used later to assist with opening the pack aseptically.

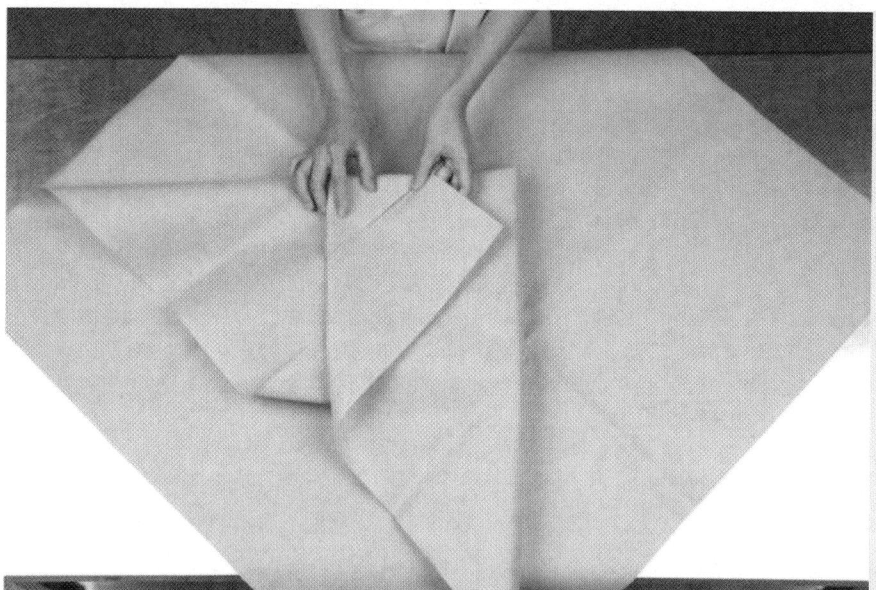

Figure 12.50

Sequential Envelope: Step 3

Fold the left corner over the contents and fold the tip back to form a flap. Ensure the entire tray/ pack is covered with this fold.

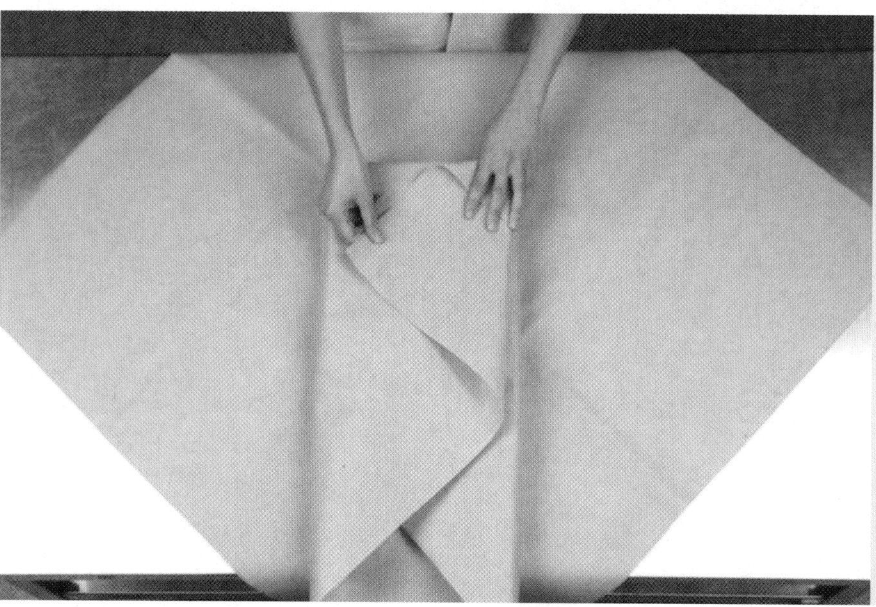

Figure 12.51

Sequential Envelope: Step 4

Fold the right corner over the left fold and fold the tip back onto itself to form a flap. Ensure the entire tray/pack is covered with this fold.

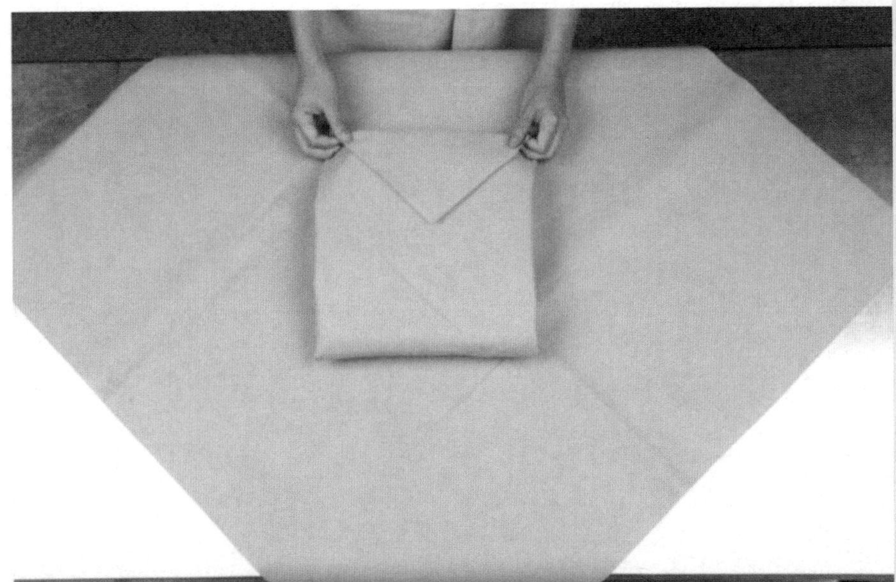

Figure 12.52

Sequential Envelope: Step 5

Bring the top corner down over the contents and tuck the corner under the right and left folds, leaving a small tab visible for easy opening.

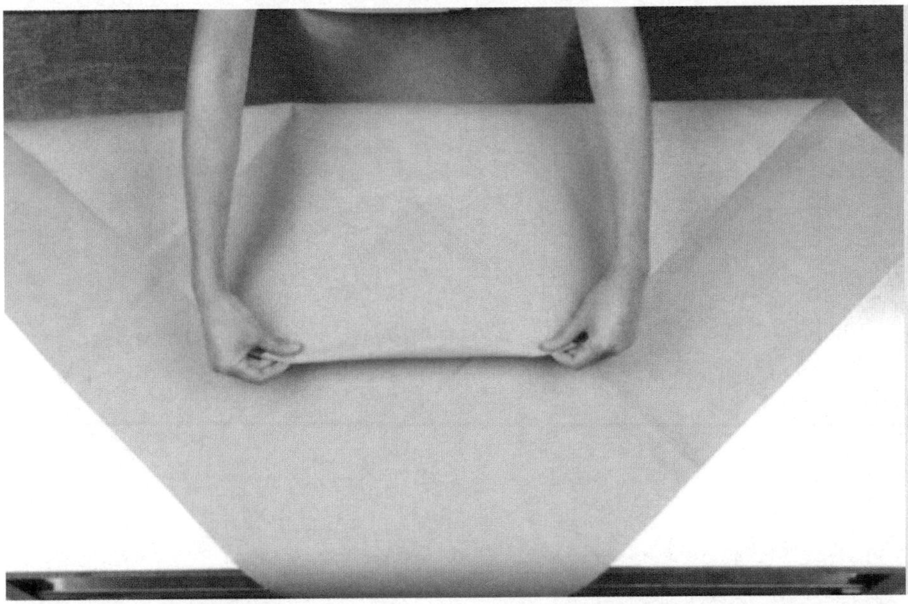

Figure 12.53

Sequential Envelope: Step 6

The second wrap is applied by placing the single-wrapped item into the center of the remaining wrap and then repeating the wrap sequence to form a package within a package.

The lower corner is brought up to cover the single-wrapped item, and the tip is folded back onto itself to form a flap.

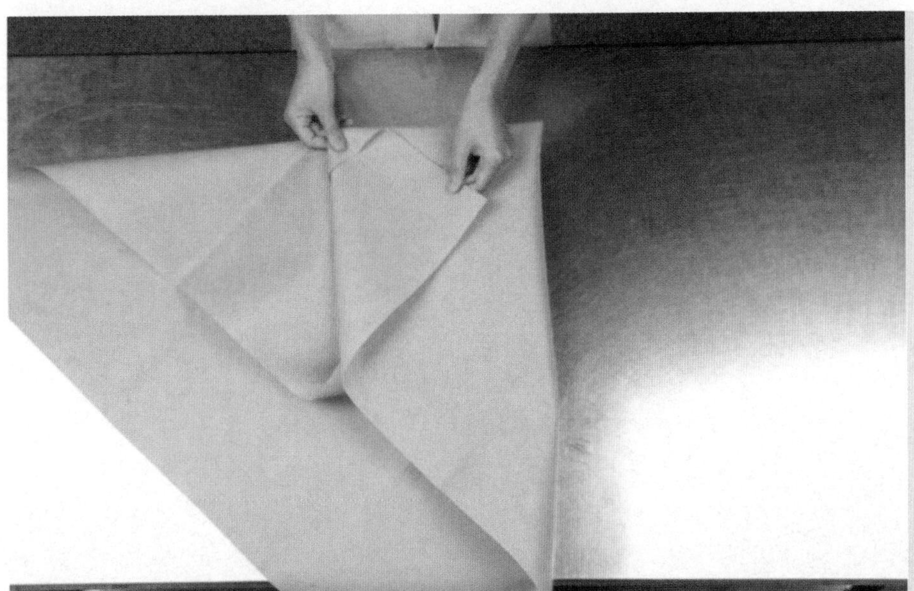

Figure 12.54

Sequential Envelope: Step 7

Fold the left corner over the single-wrapped item and fold the tip back to form a flap. Ensure the entire tray/pack is covered with this fold.

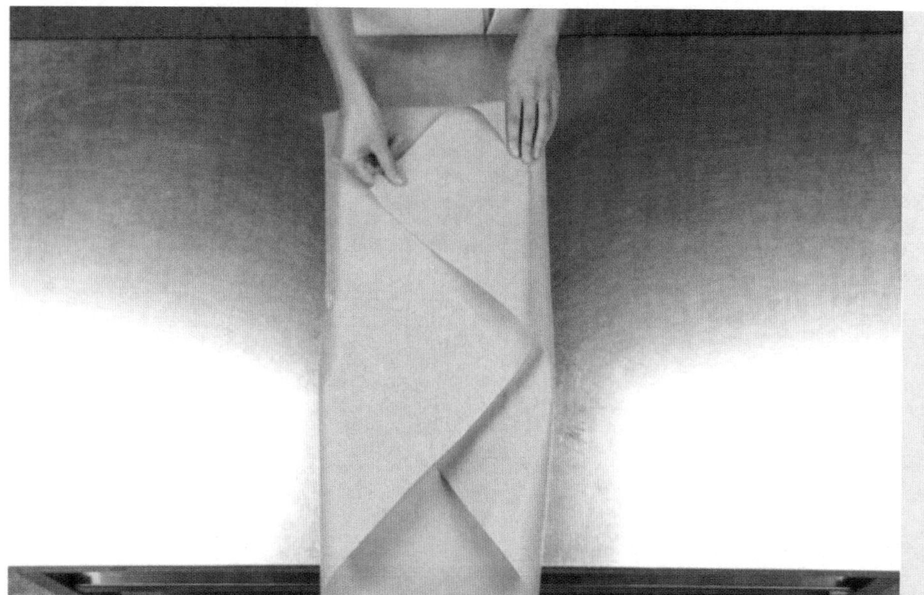

Figure 12.55

Sequential Envelope: Step 8

Fold the right corner over the left fold and fold the tip back onto itself to form a flap. Ensure the entire tray/pack is covered with this fold.

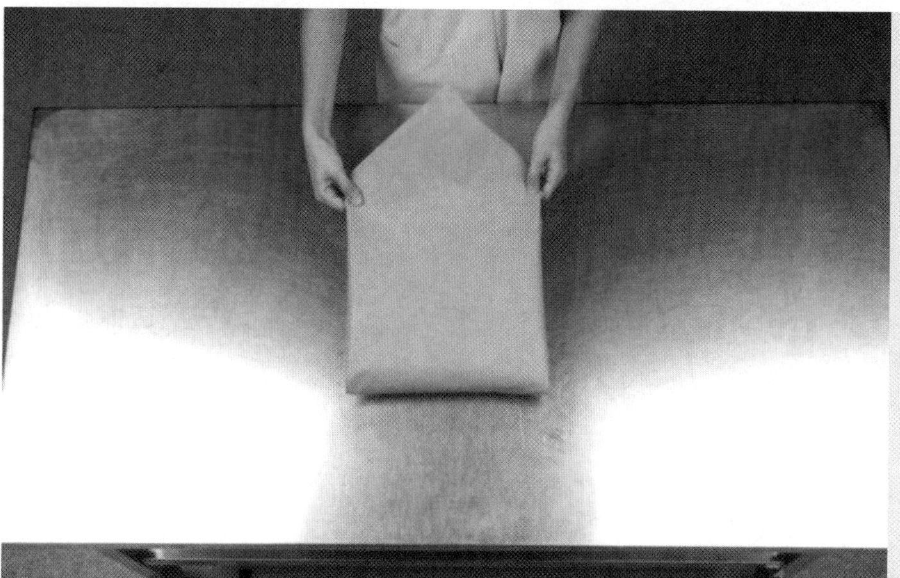

Figure 12.56

Sequential Envelope: Step 9

Bring the top corner down over the single-wrapped item.

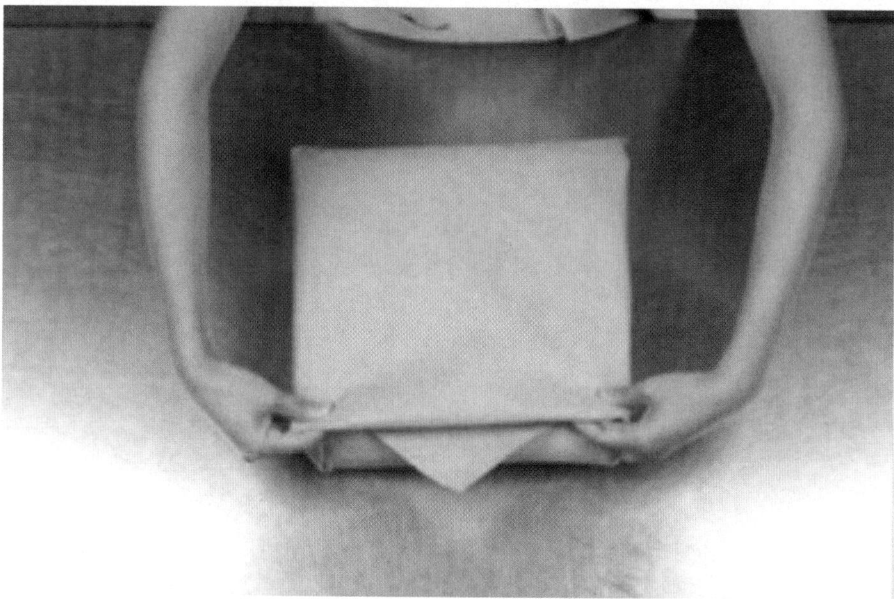

Figure 12.57

Sequential Envelope: Step 10

Tuck the corner under the right and left folds, leaving a small tab visible for easy opening.

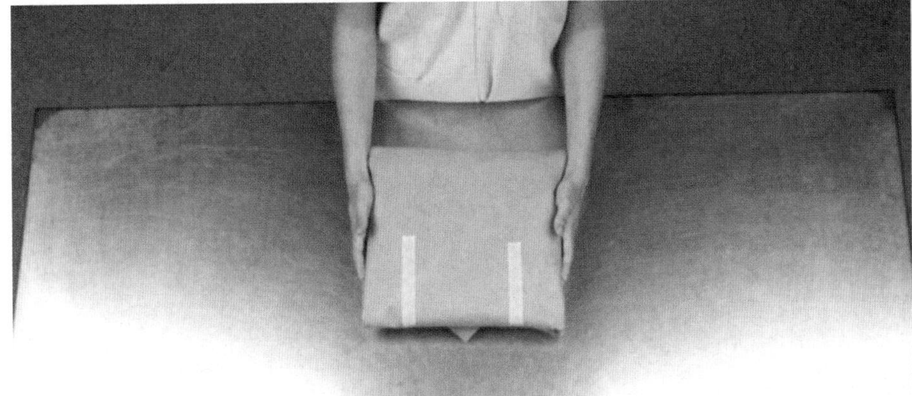

Figure 12.58

Sequential Envelope: Completed

The package is then secured with indicator tape to complete the wrap process.

Note: ANSI/AAMI ST79 states to secure the wrap with two pieces of tape (one piece for smaller packs). Using excess tape will interfere with the sterilization process and make aseptic presentation of the pack very difficult.

Figures 12.59 through **12.68** illustrate sequential wrapping techniques using the square style. This method is primarily used for large packs.

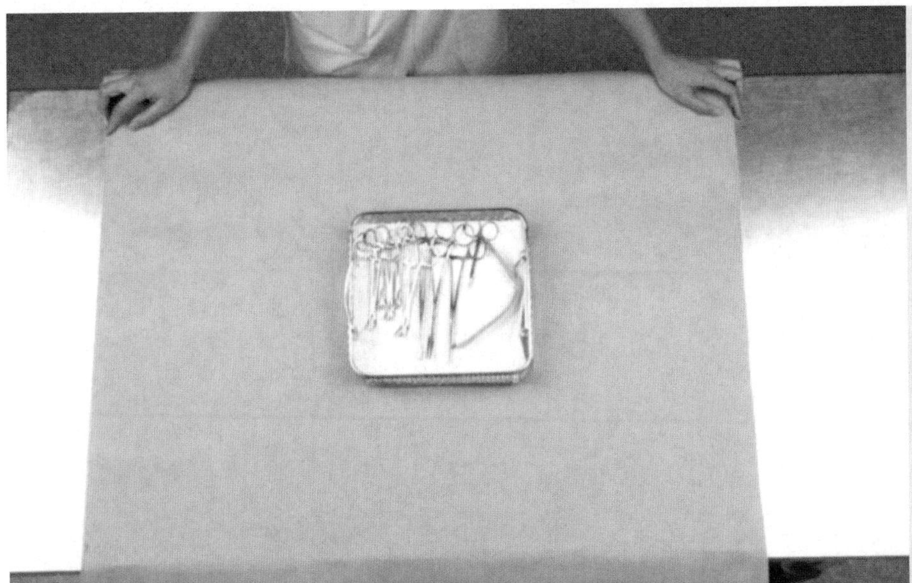

Figure 12.59

Sequential Square: Step 1

The edge of the wrap is placed parallel with the table.

The instrument tray is placed square in the center of the wrap, parallel with the edge of the wrap.

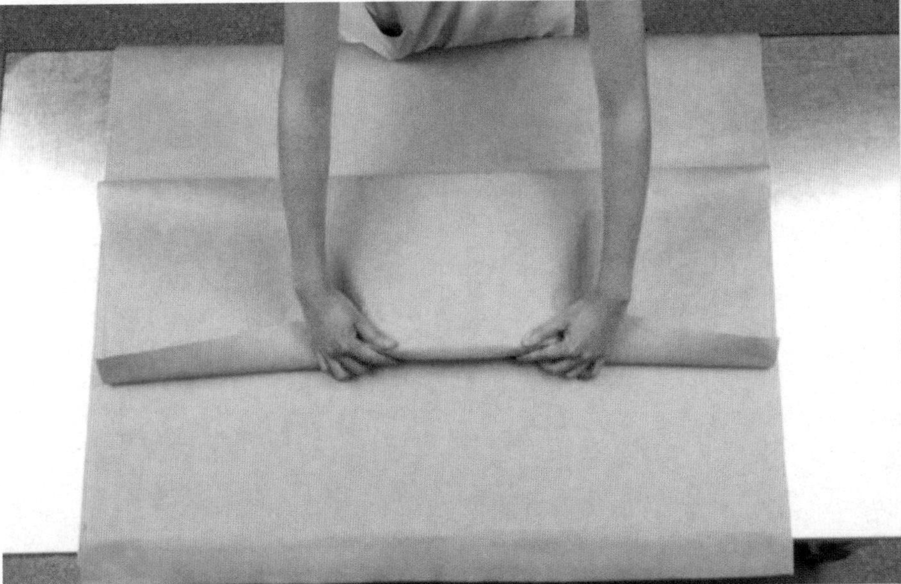

Figure 12.60

Sequential Square: Step 2

The edge of the wrap is folded over the top of the contents. The edge is then folded over itself to form a cuff. This cuff will facilitate aseptic opening of the pack when used. Ensure the entire tray/pack is covered with this fold.

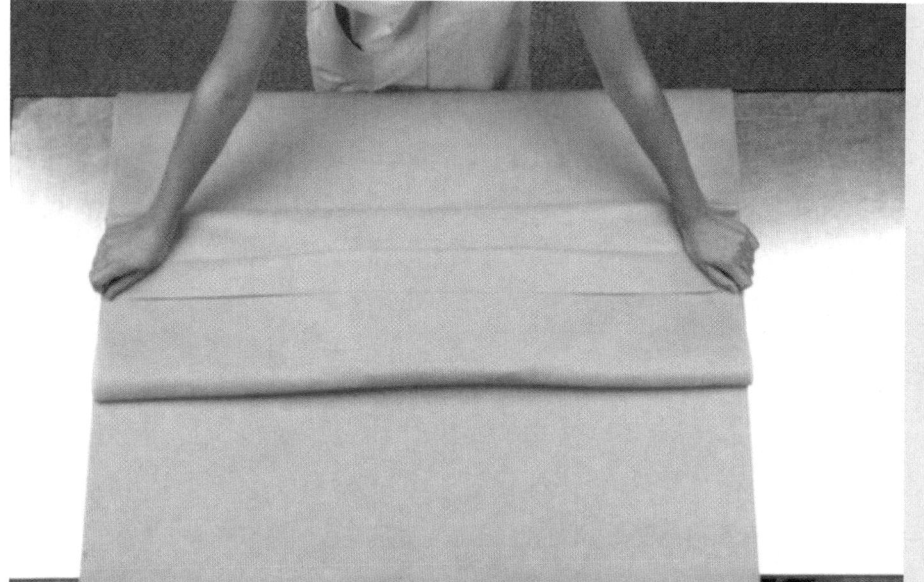

Figure 12.61

Sequential Square: Step 3

The upper edge of the wrap is brought down over the contents and folded back on itself to form another cuff that overlaps the original cuff. Ensure the entire tray/pack is covered with this fold.

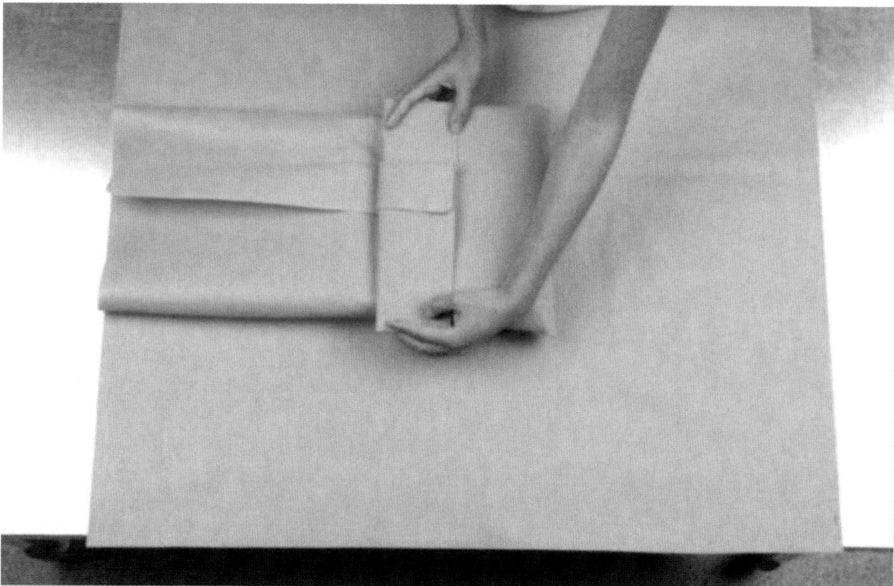

Figure 12.62

Sequential Square: Step 4

The left edge of the wrap is folded over the pack and back onto itself to form a cuff. Ensure the entire tray/pack is covered with this fold.

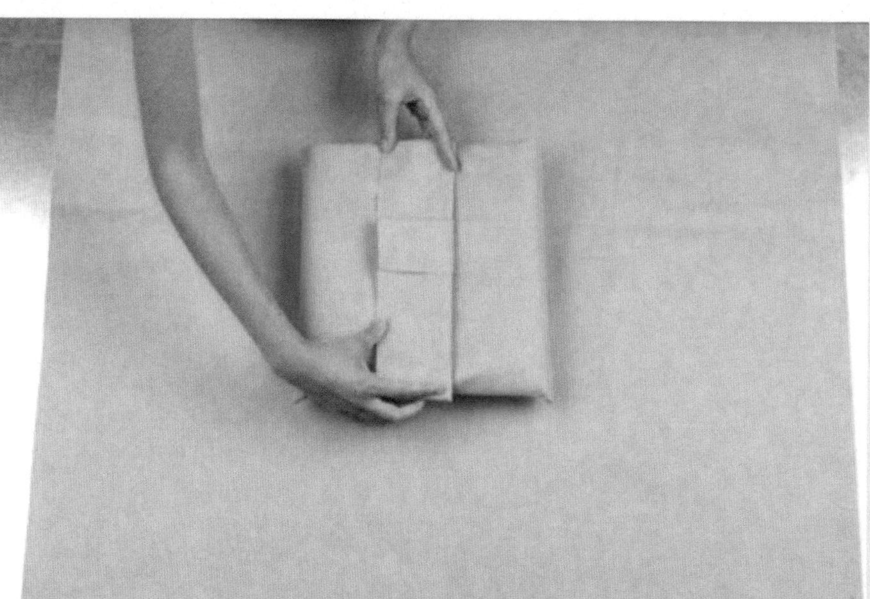

Figure 12.63

Sequential Square: Step 5

The right side of the wrap is folded over the pack, overlapping the previous fold, and folded back to form a cuff. Ensure the entire tray/pack is covered with this fold.

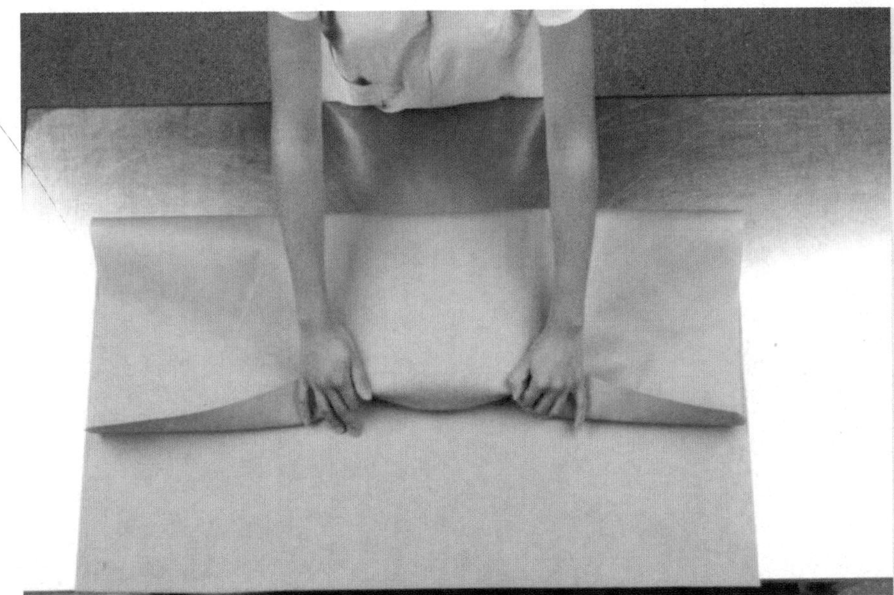

Figure 12.64

Sequential Square: Step 6

The second wrap is applied by placing the single-wrapped item into the center of the wrap and repeating the steps performed for the first wrap to create a package within a package.

The edge of the second wrap is folded over the single-wrapped item. The edge is then folded back over itself to form a cuff. Ensure the entire tray is covered with this fold.

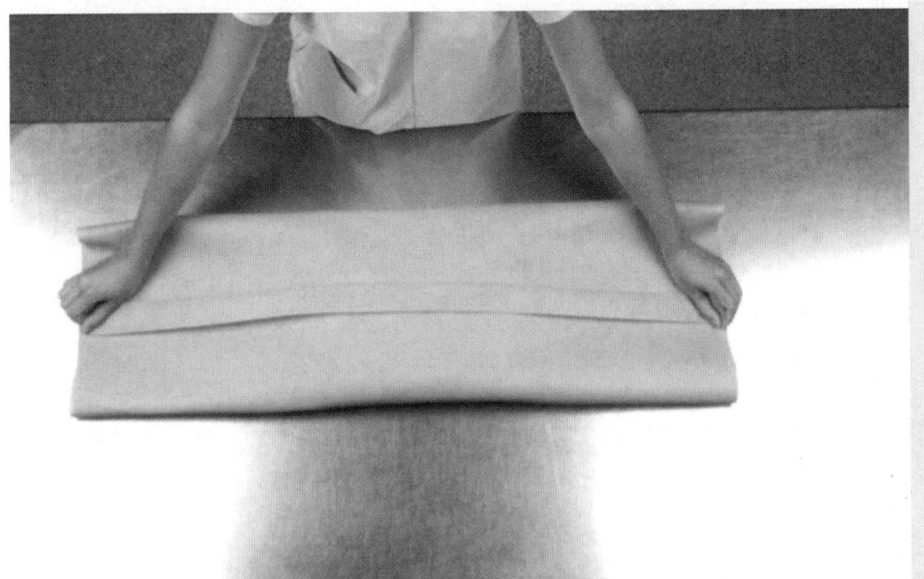

Figure 12.65

Sequential Square: Step 7

The upper edge of the wrap is brought down over the single-wrapped item and folded back onto itself to form another cuff that overlaps the original cuff. Ensure the entire tray/pack is covered with this fold.

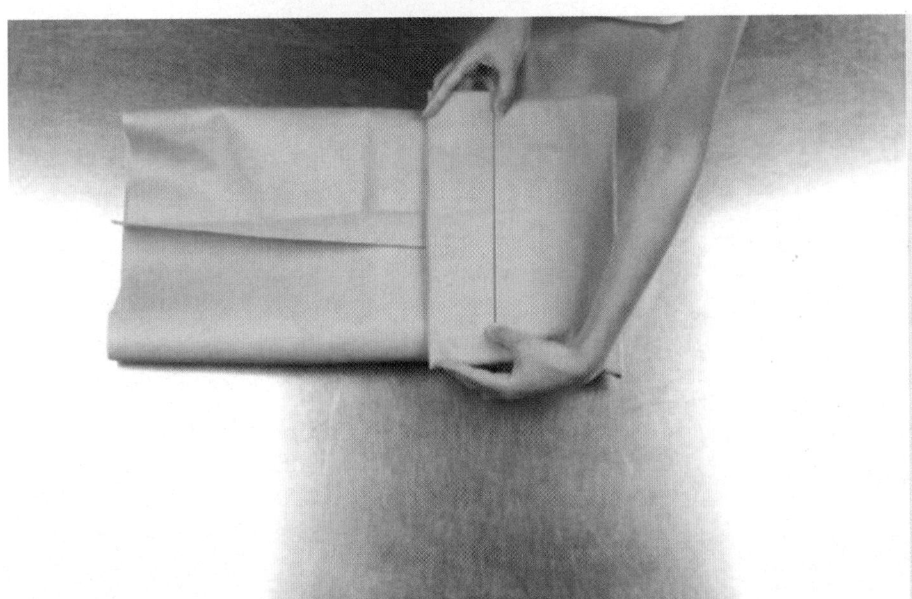

Figure 12.66

Sequential Square: Step 8

The left edge of the wrap is folded over the pack and back onto itself to form a cuff. Ensure the entire tray/pack is covered with this fold.

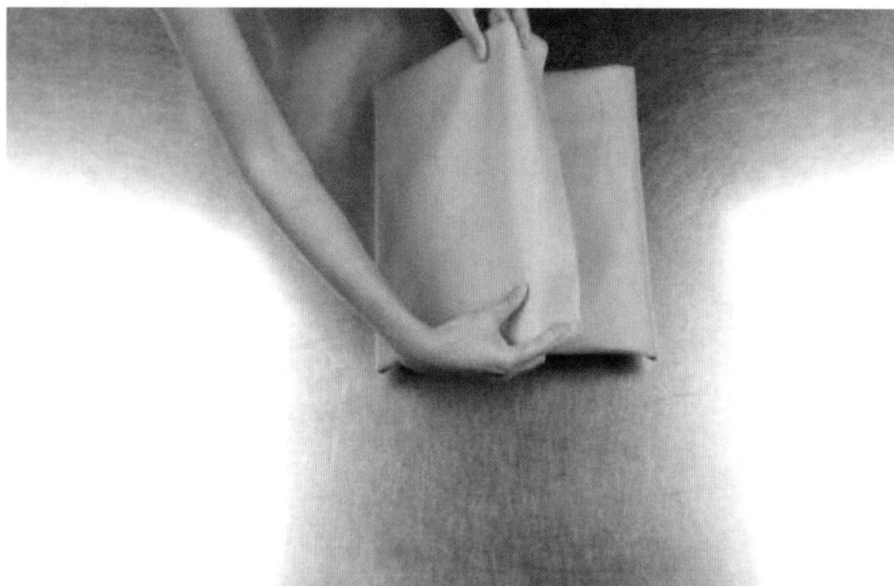

Figure 12.67

Sequential Square: Step 9

The right side of the wrap is folded over the pack, overlapping the previous fold, and folded under. Ensure the entire tray/pack is covered with this fold.

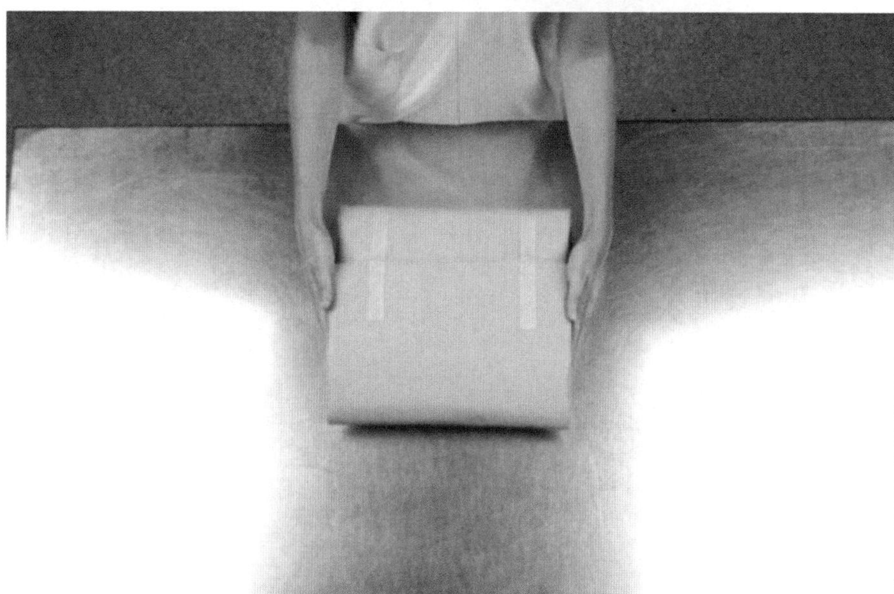

Figure 12.68

Sequential Square: Complete

The package is secured with indicator tape.

Note: ANSI/AAMI ST79 states to secure the wrap with two pieces of tape (one piece for smaller packs). Using excess tape will interfere with the sterilization process and make aseptic presentation of the pack very difficult.

A problem with wrapping instrument trays is that some trays may have sharp edges or corners that cause a hole in the package, thus rendering it unsterile. To prevent holes from sharp corners, tray corner guards may be used following IFU. They are used according to the manufacturers' IFU for the tray corners and the sterile barrier system. The wrapper size should be selected to completely cover the item(s) being packaged. The item is wrapped securely to prevent gapping, billowing, or the formation of air pockets, as these can prevent sterilant contact with the surface of the device or allow contaminates to penetrate the package. Packaging should not be cut to the size of the item; doing so alters a U.S. Food and Drug Administration-approved device.

Simultaneous wrapping uses two layers of synthetic nonwoven material such as SMS bound on two or four edges. Since the material is already double layered, the contents are only wrapped once. Both methods are acceptable, although one may be more appropriate for specific situations.

Figures 12.69 through **12.75** illustrate simultaneous wrapping techniques using the envelope style. In this method, flat wrap is applied together.

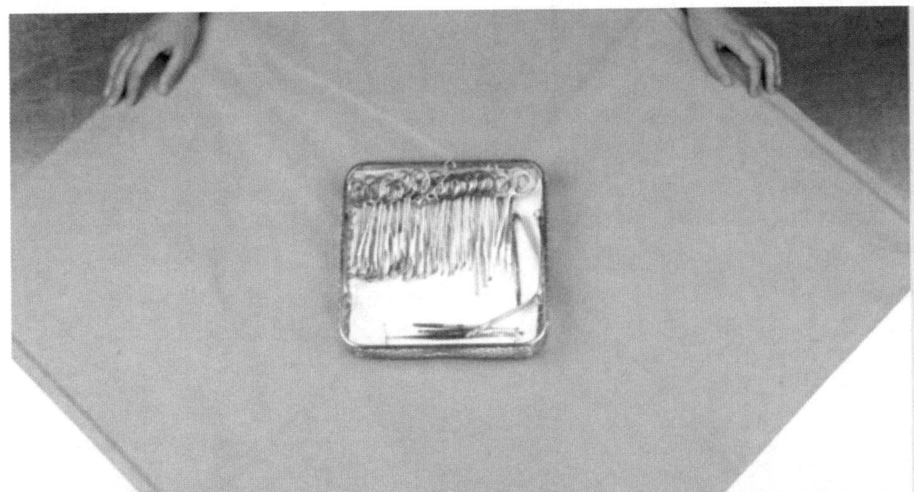

Figure 12.69

Simultaneous Envelope: Step 1

With the simultaneous envelope technique, one application of simultaneous wrap is placed on the table surface in a diagonal or diamond format. Simultaneous wrap is two sheets of wrap bonded together.

Center the instrument tray between the right and left edges of the wrap.

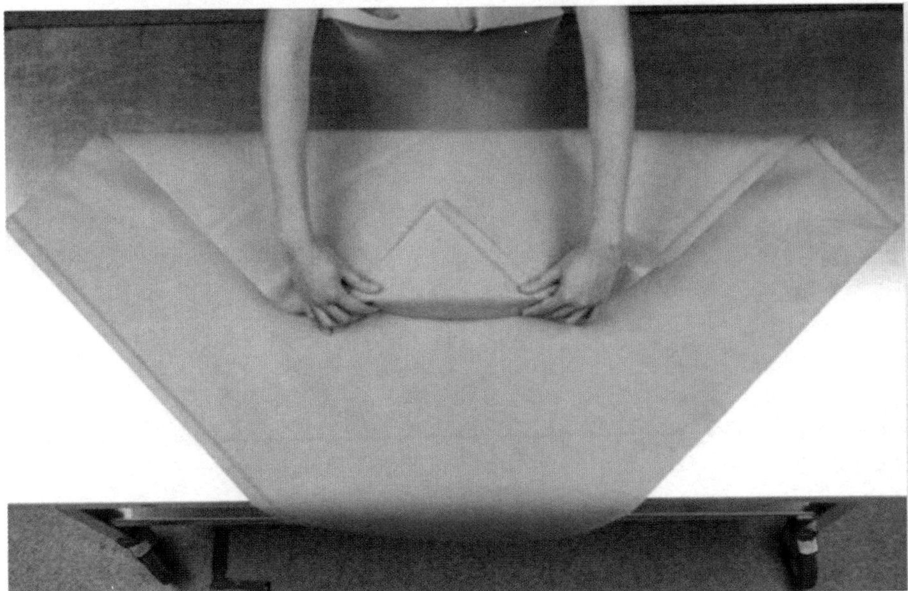

Figure 12.70

Simultaneous Envelope: Step 2

Bring the bottom corner of the wrap up and over to completely cover the instrument tray.

Fold the tip back onto itself to form a flap. This flap is used later to assist in opening the pack aseptically.

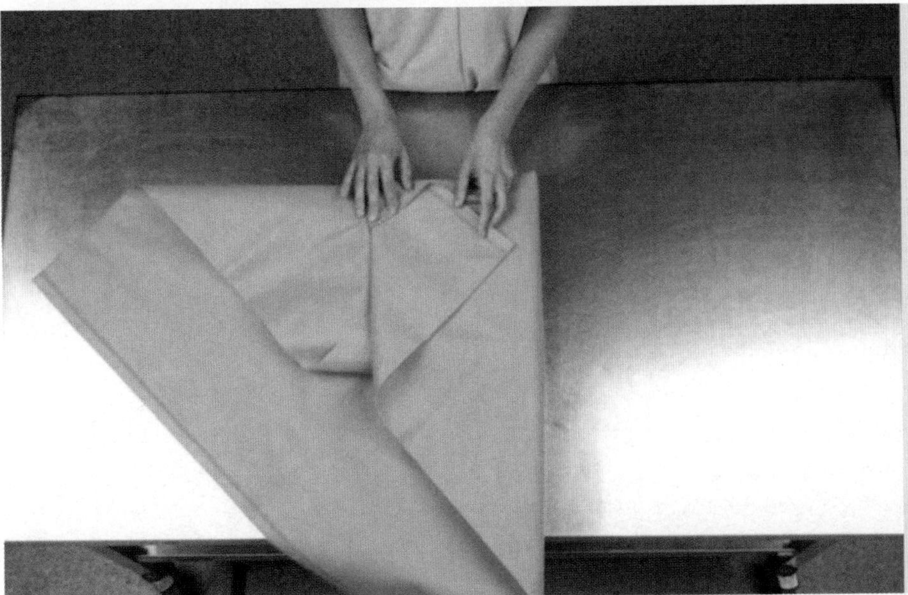

Figure 12.71

Simultaneous Envelope: Step 3

Fold the left corner over the contents and fold the tip back to form a tab. Ensure the entire tray/pack is covered with this fold.

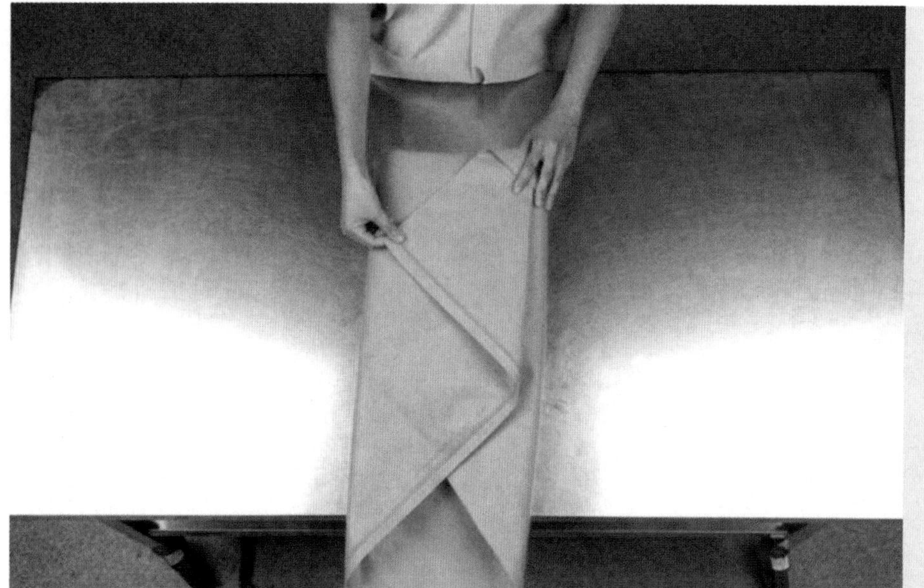

Figure 12.72

Simultaneous Envelope: Step 4

Fold the right corner over the left fold and fold the tip back onto itself to form a tab. Ensure the entire tray/pack is covered with this fold.

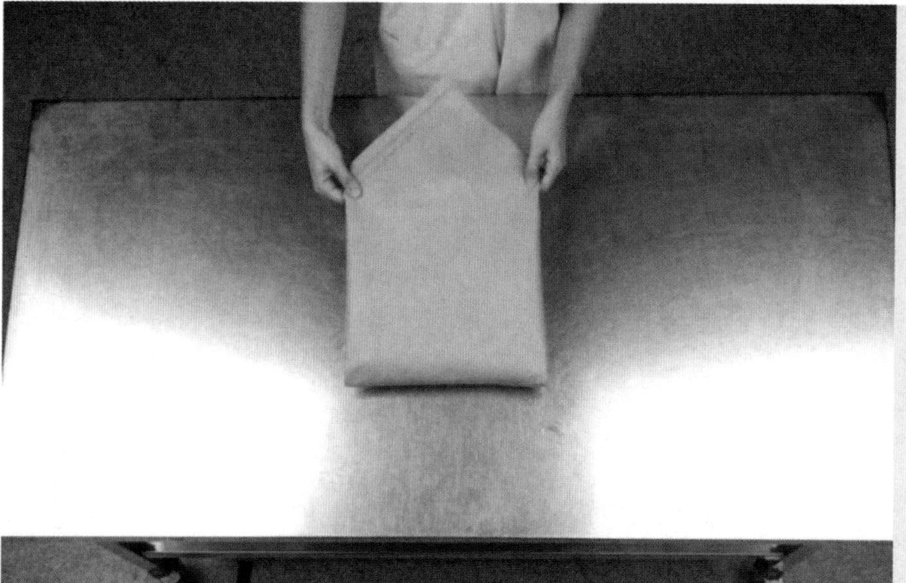

Figure 12.73

Simultaneous Envelope: Step 5

Bring the top corner down over the contents and fold it toward the body. Ensure the entire tray/pack is covered with this fold.

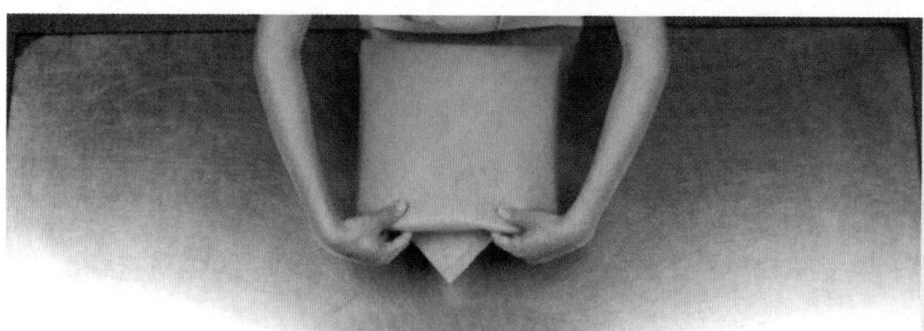

Note: The wrapped package has been turned from the previous slide image to allow for better visualization of the tip

Figure 12.74

Simultaneous Envelope: Step 6

Tuck the corner under the right and left folds. A small tab may be incorporated for easy opening.

Ensure the wrap is not too tight or too loose; either way compromises effective sterilization of the package contents.

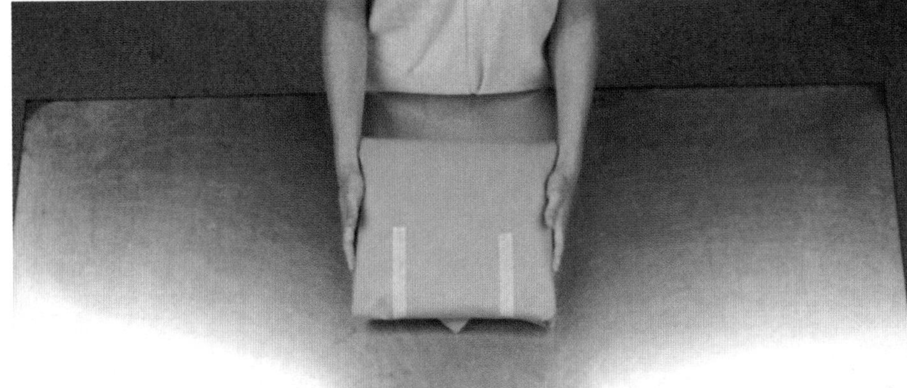

Figure 12.75

Simultaneous Envelope: Complete

The package is then secured with indicator tape to complete the wrap process.

Note: ANSI/AAMI ST79 states to secure the wrap with two pieces of tape (one piece for smaller packs). Using excess tape will interfere with the sterilization process and make aseptic presentation of the pack very difficult.

Figures 12.76 through **12.81** illustrate simultaneous wrapping techniques using the square style. This method is primarily used for large packs.

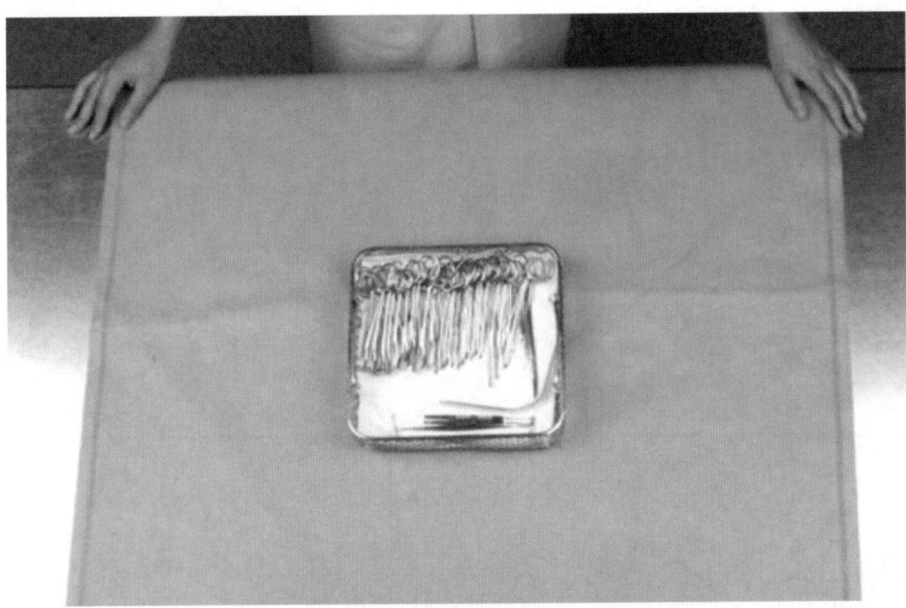

Figure 12.76

Simultaneous Square: Step 1

With the simultaneous square technique, place one application of simultaneous wrap—that is, two sheets of wrap specially bonded together—on the table surface in a rectangular- or square-shaped format.

Center the instrument tray between the left and right edges of the wrap.

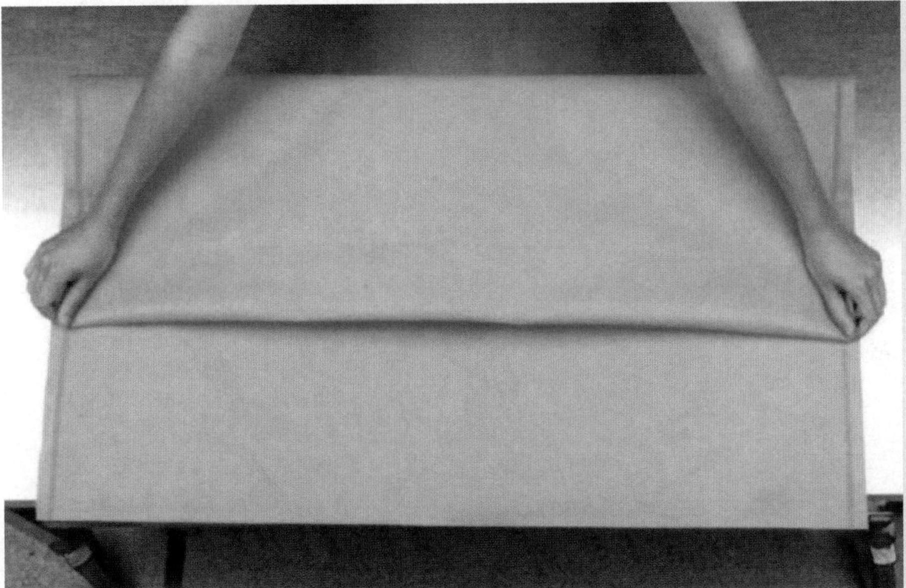

Figure 12.77

Simultaneous Square: Step 2

The edge of the wrap is folded over the top of the contents covering the entire item. The edge is then folded back over itself to form a cuff. This will facilitate aseptic opening of the pack when used.

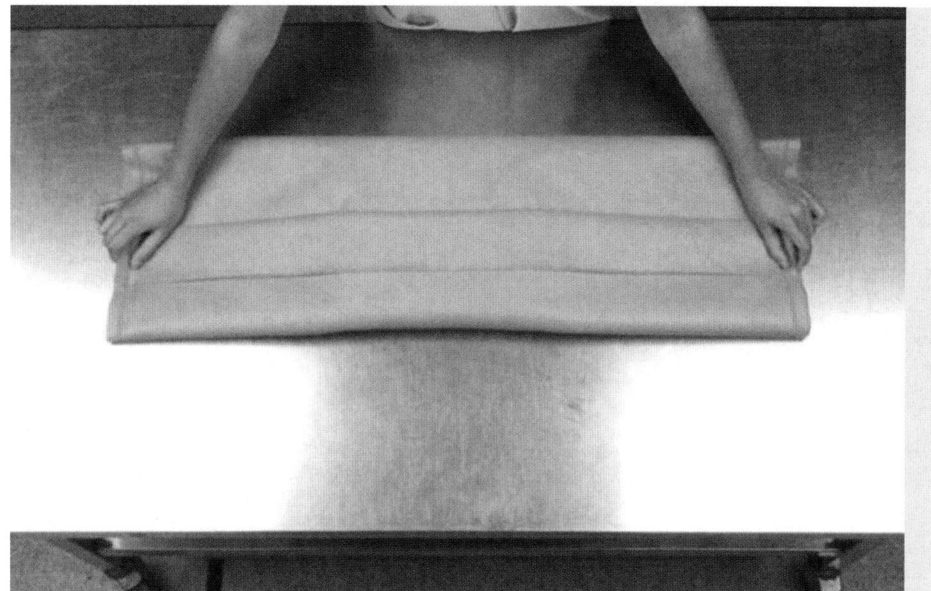

Figure 12.78

Simultaneous Square: Step 3

The upper edge of the wrap is brought down over the contents and folded back onto itself to form another cuff that overlaps the original. Ensure the entire tray/pack is covered with this fold.

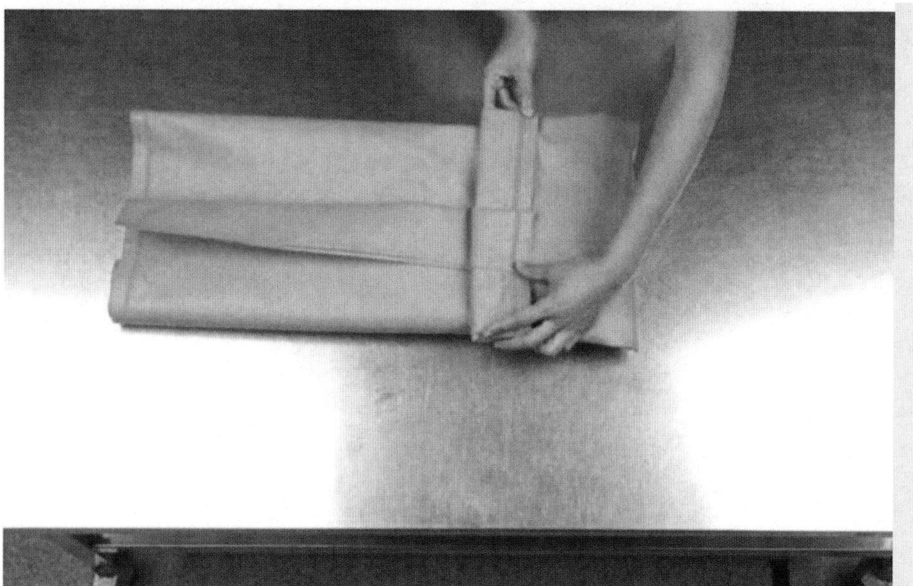

Figure 12.79

Simultaneous Square: Step 4

The left edge of the wrap is folded over the pack and folded over itself to form a cuff. Ensure the entire tray/pack is covered with this fold.

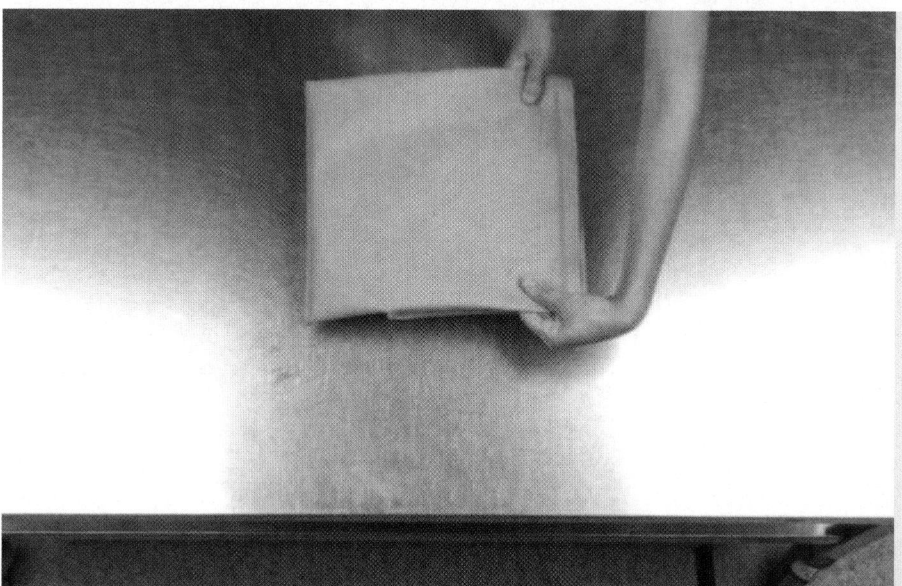

Figure 12.80

Simultaneous Square: Step 5

The right side of the wrap is folded over the pack, overlapping the previous fold. Ensure the entire tray/pack is covered with this fold.

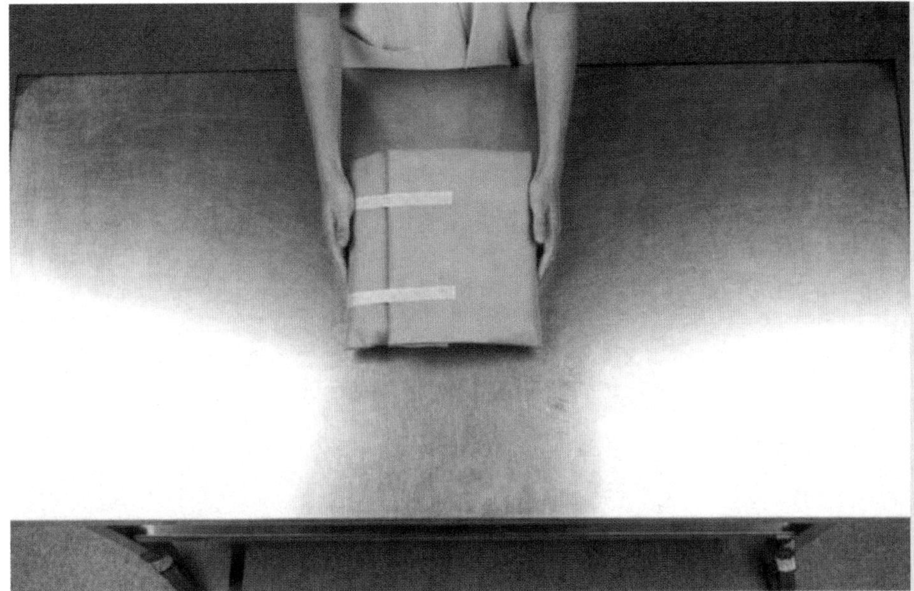

Figure 12.81

Simultaneous Square: Complete

To complete the wrap process, the final fold is tucked under and secured with indicator tape.

Note: ANSI/AAMI ST79 states to secure the wrap with two pieces of tape (one piece for smaller packs). Using excess tape will interfere with the sterilization process and make aseptic presentation of the pack very difficult.

Choose the properly sized wrap for either method. The wrap must be large enough to completely contain the contents without leaving excess material that could inhibit sterilant penetration and release. Wrap must be snug but not so tight as to impede sterilant entry or exit. If the wrap will also be used to create a sterile field, it must be of sufficient size to extend at least six inches below the edge of the surface being covered.

> **Important Note: Be Consistent**
>
> Wrap folding must always be done in the same sequence. This allows the individuals opening sterile packages to establish a pattern, which conserves time and reduces the possibility of error.

METHODS OF PACKAGE CLOSURE

Overview

The purpose of a package closure is to seal the package securely, indicate that the package was processed, maintain the sterile integrity during storage and transport, and prevent resealing if the package is opened or the seal is compromised.

Acceptable Closure Methods

Only approved closure methods should be used to seal a sterile package. There are several types of package closures, and SP technicians must ensure they use the appropriate packaging closure method, including:

- Tape designated as "indicator tape" is considered best practice because it is made specifically to withstand sterilization and change color after being exposed to the sterilization process. It does not, however, provide proof that adequate sterilization of package contents has occurred. Indicator tape or indicator stickers that change color after exposure should be used on every package to avoid mixing processed and unprocessed packages. (See **Figure 12.82**)

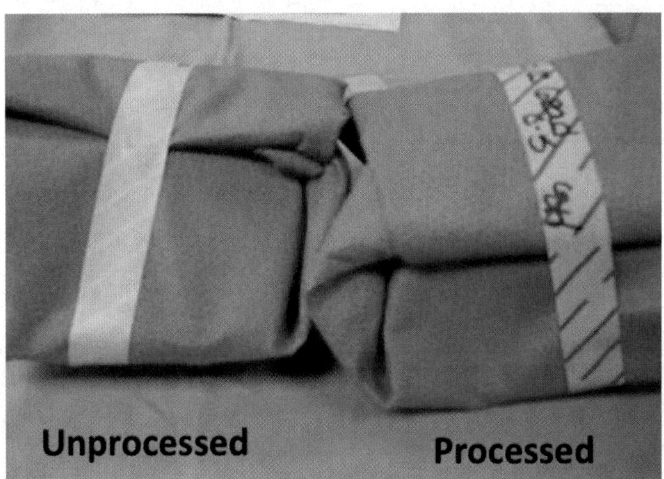

Figure 12.82 External indicator tape

- Specially manufactured elastomer bands or similar closures are only acceptable if the manufacturer of the wrap material explicitly recommends their use. If recommended, care is needed to select the properly sized bands that allow a snug fit, without creating excessive wrinkles or folds in the fabric that may impede sterilant penetration. If bands are used, the label or indicator stickers should be placed in a way that any attempt to remove the band will damage the band and reveal the compromised status of the pack. *Note: Band applications are designed for specific packaging methods and should only be used as recommended by the specific band manufacturer.*

- Rigid container systems have tamper-evident seals, which are secured to the outside of the container and lock the top and bottom of the container together. (See **Figure 12.83**) Ensure the locks are securely in place prior to sterilization. Rigid container seals are designed to break when the seal on the container has been broken. Sterilization containers with broken locks must be reprocessed. The most common types are plastic components that lock in place and must be broken to open the container. Small bands that tighten as they react to heat during sterilization can also be placed on certain types of rigid containers, and these will break when the seal of the container is broken.

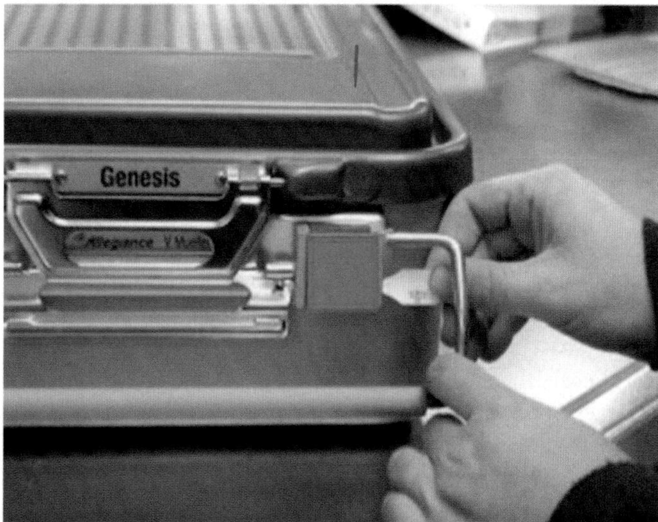

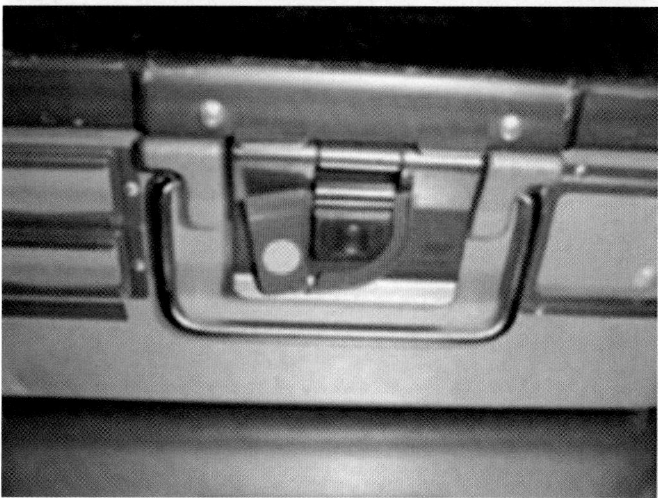

Figure 12.83 Examples of rigid container locks

- Heat sealing is a peel pouch closure method. There are several varieties of heat sealers available. (See **Figure 12.84**) The manufacturer of the sealer and/or pouch material must verify that the two are compatible. If they are not, the seal may not bond, or there may be burn-through; both actions will compromise the seal. Multiple-band or wide-band heat sealers should be used to reduce the possibility of an incomplete seal. The manufacturer's instructions for temperature settings, applied pressure and contact times should be written into procedures and always followed.

- The package is placed inside the jaws of the heat sealer, and the two sides are fused together. Be sure to follow the heat sealer and packaging manufacturers' instructions to ensure appropriate exposure times and temperatures. Inadequate exposure times or temperatures may prevent proper sealing, and those that exceed recommendations may cause package damage. SP technicians should use extra caution when operating heat sealers to avoid burns.

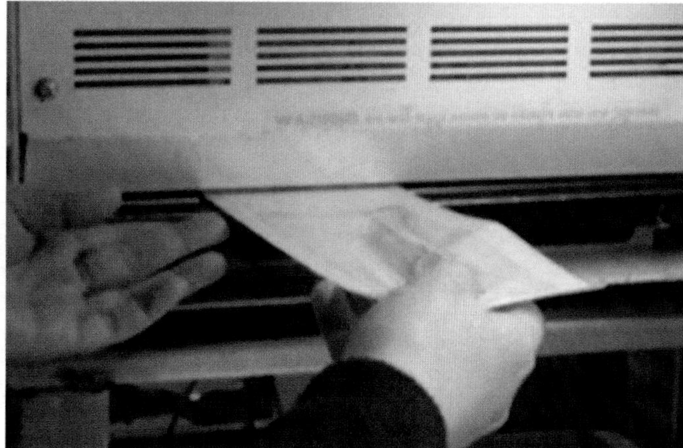

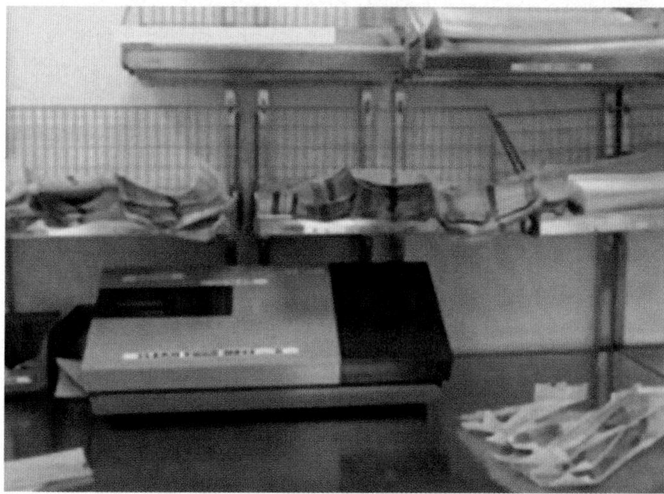

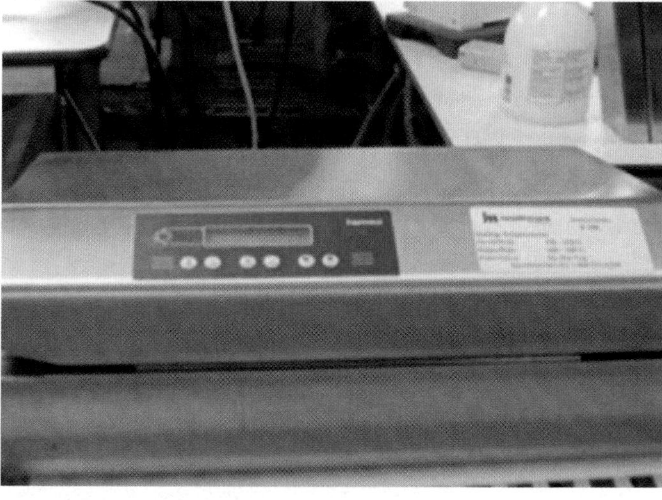

Figure 12.84 Examples of heat sealers

- Heat seals must be observed for bubbles and creases. (See **Figure 12.85**) Seals that are not smooth and complete will allow bacterial contamination after sterilization.

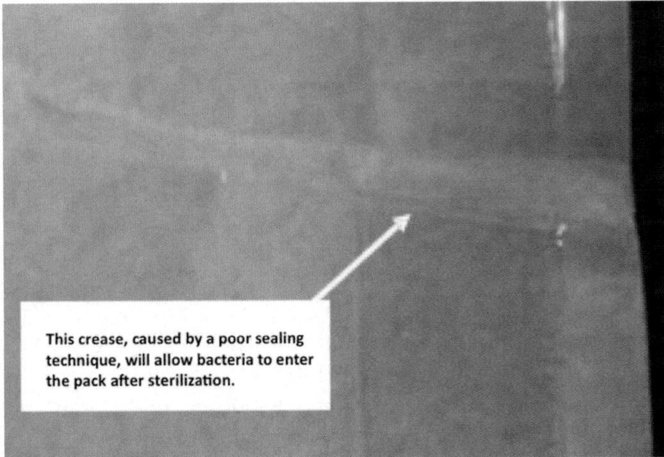

Figure 12.85

- Some paper/plastic and polyolefin-plastic packages contain self-adhesive seals that do not require heat. An adhesive portion is covered with a removable strip at one end of the self-adhesive sterilization pouch. When it is removed, that portion of the seal should be carefully folded over the opening of the package. **Figure 12.86** shows an SP technician sealing a self-adhesive sterilization pouch. Care must be taken to avoid gaps, wrinkles or creases, which compromise the seal integrity for both heat-seal and self-seal closure systems.

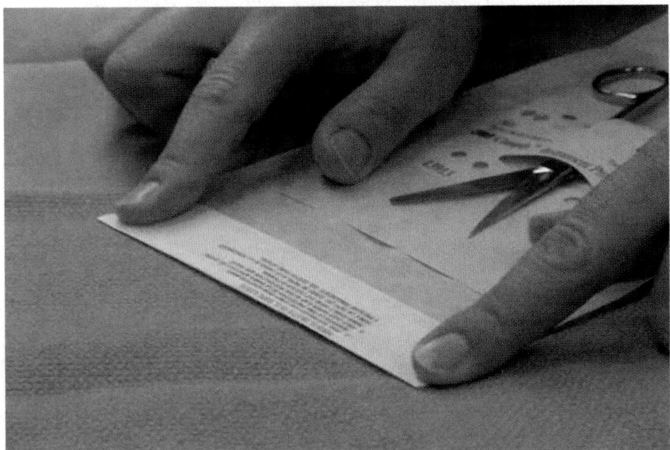

Figure 12.86

- Sealing tape to one end of the pouch is sometimes used to secure pouch openings. Care is needed to ensure that the seal is secure, without compromising gaps. Proper taping technique includes the folding of corners so the side edges of the top corners are parallel to the bottom edge of the pouch. Ensure that the plastic is folded onto the plastic (not paper-to-paper) so sterilant access is not impeded. Then, fold the open bottom edge over the folded corners. Seal with tape overlapping the edge of the pouch by about 1/4". Observe carefully to ensure that there are no gaps, creases or wrinkles, and that the tape has completely covered the pouch's open edge and is securely attached to the plastic. *Note: This method of sealing pouches makes the package difficult to open and presents the contents aseptically.*

> **Do Not Use!**
>
> Several package closure methods are never appropriate for use:
>
> - Do not use safety pins, staples or other sharp objects to seal packages. Punctures create holes that allow contamination. Even the smallest space (hole) is large enough to allow bacteria to pass.
> - Do not use paper clips or binding clips. They can be removed and replaced without evidence of barrier compromise.
> - Do not use tapes that are not designed specifically to withstand the rigors of sterilization.

SP technicians must use closure methods specifically designed for the packaging material selected. They must also check the seals on all packages before dispensing them to user units. Any seals that appear to have been broken or opened should not be issued or used. (See **Figure 12.87**)

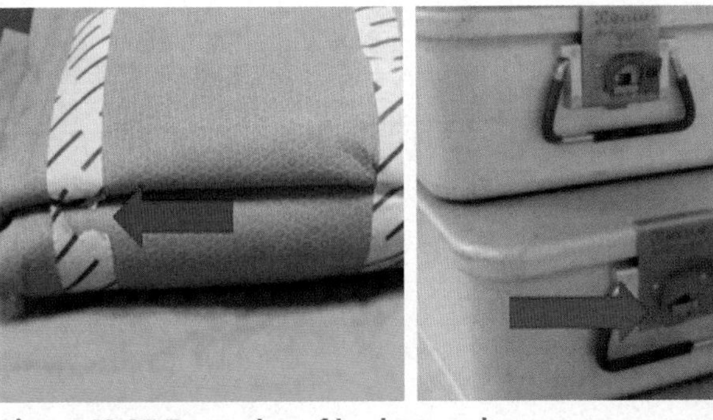

Figure 12.87 Examples of broken seals

PACKAGE LABELING

It is essential that all packages be labeled prior to sterilization. The label must be complete and accurate to ensure that the correct packs are selected and opened.

Label information should include the following:

- Description of package contents
- Identification of the person that performed the packaging (e.g., the initials of package assembler/packager)
- Lot control number

- Identification of sterilizer and cycle to be used
- Date of sterilization (unless contained in the lot control number)
- Assigned storage location
- The requesting department or surgeon's name may also be included on the label for special-request items.

Standardized abbreviations and terms help avoid confusion when labeling packaging. Slang terms and nicknames should not be used. Labeling is necessary for the end user and also for sterilization processing, quality assurance, stock rotation, and inventory control purposes. Correct labeling is also critical in the event of a sterilization load recall.

SP technicians with the responsibility for labeling packages must use clear, legible handwriting and accurate descriptions. Confusion caused by an illegible or inaccurate package label can compromise patient safety because items may be misplaced, or the label may be misread and incorrectly dispensed. Either situation can cause a delay in patient care and treatment.

Labeling should be documented on label-sensitive tape; the indicator tape used to seal the package; commercially available, pre-printed adhesive labels; in-house computer-generated labels (see **Figure 12.88**); or the plastic side of a peel pouch.

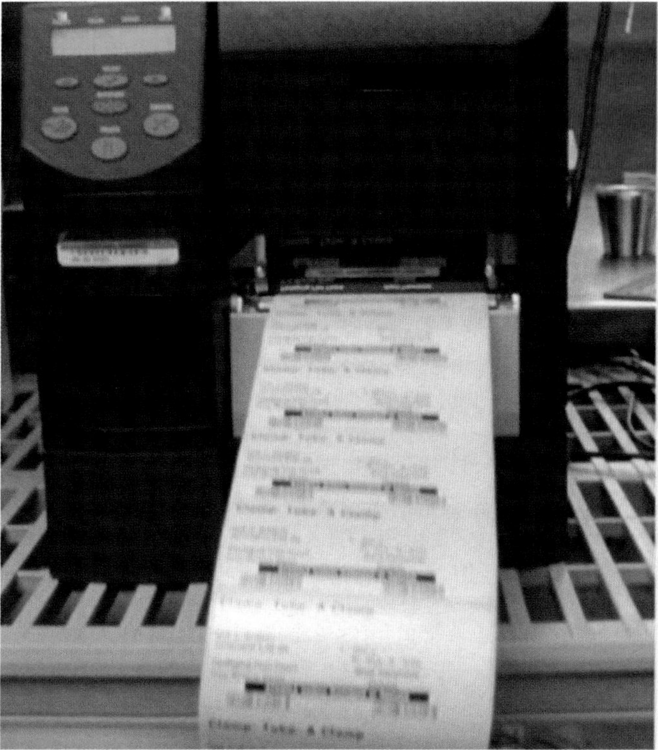

Figure 12.88 Printed pack labels. Computerized instrument systems generate labels that are easy to read and contain barcodes for tracking.

Note: Do not write directly on flat-wrap packaging material.

For pouches, the labels or written information should not be placed on the paper or spunbond polyolefin side, as they may inhibit the microbial barrier properties.

Approved felt-tip pens are generally used for marking packaging material. They should be indelible, non-bleeding, non-fading, non-toxic and able to withstand the sterilization method used.

SPECIAL PACKAGING CONCERNS

Several basic packaging concerns require special mention:

- All packaging materials should be held at a temperature and humidity for a time recommended by the manufacturer. This will permit adequate sterilant penetration and help prevent super heating of the product during sterilization.
- Packaging procedures should be performed only by the department responsible for sterilization. Other departments whose personnel might prepare and package their own instruments and supplies before sending them to SP for sterilization should be discouraged from this practice. Often, SP technicians do not know about all items in the package, and the package could be processed inappropriately. Also, supplying packaging materials to each of these departments is not cost effective. If a facility does allow instrument preparation outside the SPD, personnel must receive training on the proper methods of processing those devices.
- Packages should not be excessively taped because doing so makes opening the package more difficult and may inhibit the sterilization process.
- Paper/plastic pouches should be positioned in the sterilizer standing on edge in loading racks or placed in baskets specifically designed for these packages. They can also be held on edge by an alternate means (e.g., a peel pouch rack or tray pins), and they must be properly spaced. (See **Figure 12.89**) Pouches should be loosely spaced in the basket to ensure the sterilant can reach the breathable paper side of each pouch because the plastic side is not penetrated by air, steam or other sterilants. Arrange the pouches in a paper-to-plastic fashion in a perforated or mesh-bottom tray.
- Paper/plastic pouches should not be placed inside wrapped trays or containers. The plastic portion of the pouch is impervious to sterilants and can prevent a sterilant from contacting and sterilizing instrumentation. The plastic can also hinder circulation and disrupt air removal within the package or tray.
- Pouch packages should not be hung in storage. Placing a hole in the package even outside of the sterilization area can rupture the package.

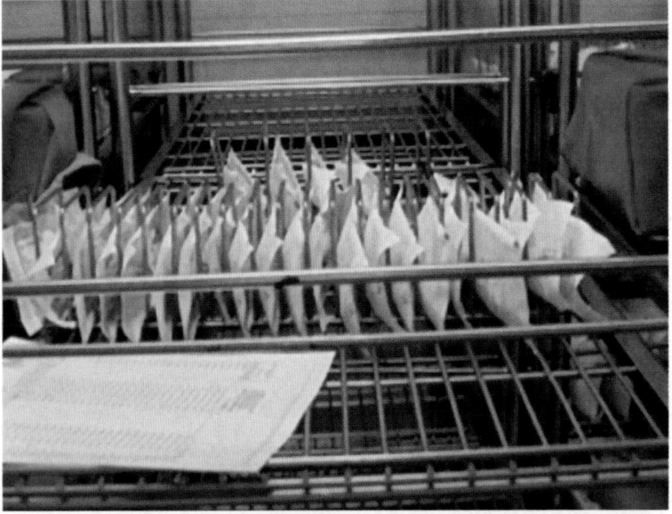

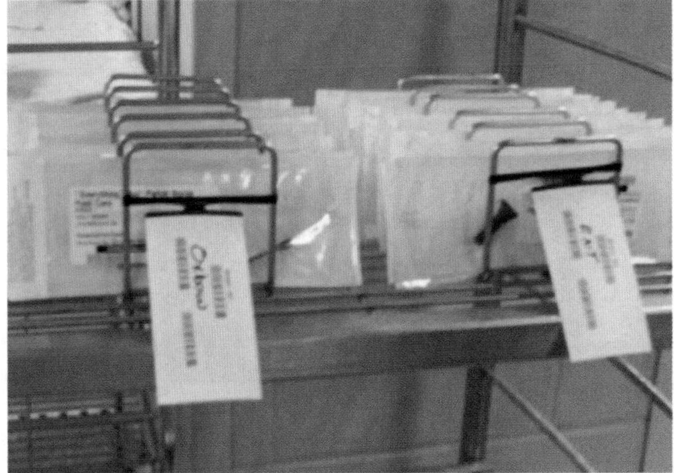

Figure 12.89 Examples of peel pouch loading racks

- All packaging systems must be handled with care. Although they provide protection and a barrier for medical devices, packaging is not impenetrable and can be compromised by rough handling and contact with sharp surfaces. Several devices are on the market to help protect larger trays from damage such as tears in wrap. Facilities may choose to use those devices if they are experiencing issues with wrap integrity. (See **Figure 12.90**)

- Observe pouch contents and outside packaging of flat wrap or containerized instruments for moisture after sterilization and reinspect prior to storage. *Remember: Steam condenses on a metal surface when heat is transferred to the metal. This condensation can allow contamination of the contents.* Prevention of condensation is only possible when sterilizers with heated dry cycle capabilities are used; however, limiting sterilizer contents and following good loading practices can usually prevent the problem.

All sterilized packages, whether sterilized by the facility or purchased as sterile ready-to-use products, should be inspected to ensure the packaging material and/or the seals have not been compromised before placing into sterile storage, prior to dispensing and before opening the package.

Sterility Maintenance

Sterilized packages must maintain their content sterility until opened.

Traditionally, the sterility of a package has been thought of as "**time-related**." That is, the package is considered sterile until a specific expiration date is reached. Then, the package is taken out of inventory and reprocessed. The Joint Commission (TJC) and the Association of periOperative Registered Nurses (AORN) now recognize sterility as "**event-related**."

Sterility (time-related) A package is considered sterile until a specific expiration date is reached.

Sterility (event-related) Items are considered sterile unless the integrity of the packaging is compromised (damaged) or suspected of being compromised, regardless of the sterilization date. This is sometimes abbreviated as ERS.

Tears in wrap

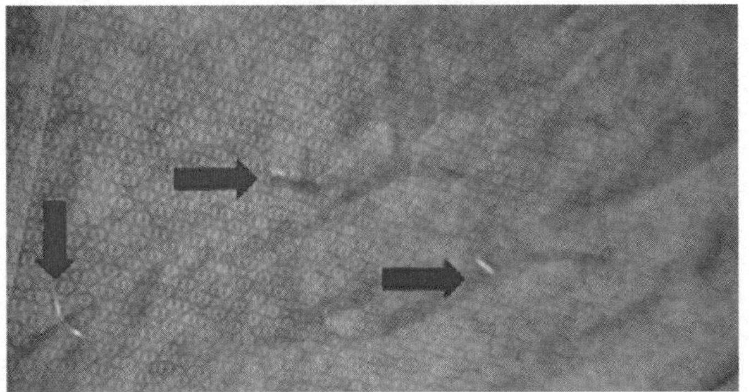

Trays and corner protectors help prevent tears.

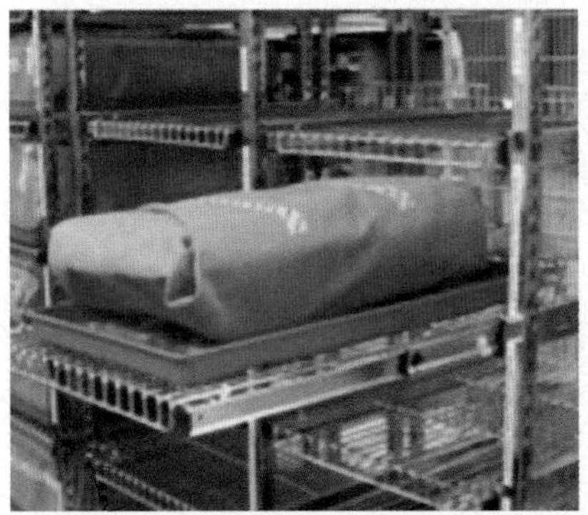

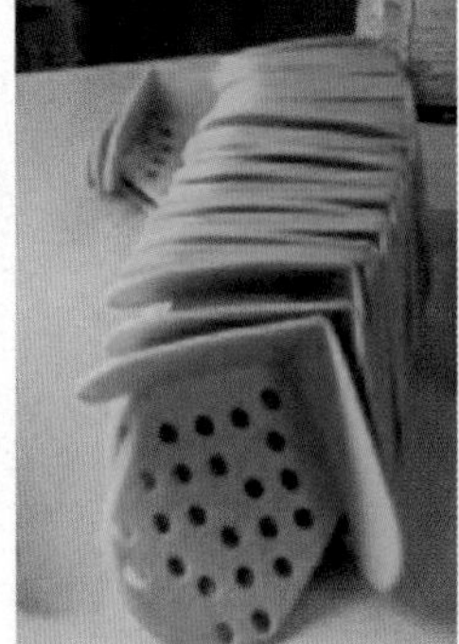

Figure 12.90 Reducing the threat of tears

The concept of event-related sterility acknowledges that microbial contamination of a sterile package is caused by an event, such as improper handling or transport, rather than by time alone. For example, one may purchase a carton of milk at the grocery store with an expiration date that is several days away; however, if he/she forgets to put the carton of milk in the refrigerator, it will become warm and sour. Even though the milk had an expected shelf life, an "event" happened that caused a shorter shelf life.

Event-related sterility (ERS) depends on the quality of the wrapper material, handling procedures, storage and transport conditions, and the number of times the package is handled before use.

By closely controlling the environment and events to which a sterile package is exposed—rather than just the time the package is in storage—the probability of package contamination can be minimized.

Note: Expiration dates on commercial products must be adhered to because they reflect product usability or stability rather than sterility of the contents. Packages that contain dated products must be labeled with the earliest expiration date.

Packaging material may be dated with a "use by date," meaning it must be sterilized prior to that date, which differs from a sterilization expiration date. If the dates are unclear, the manufacturer should be contacted for clarification. In addition, the manufacturer may provide a shelf-life validation study that specifies the length of time the package has been validated to maintain the integrity of the sterilized package after sterilization.

Protective Packaging

Protective packaging plastic overwrap (sometimes called dust covers or sterility maintenance covers) can be applied to packages after sterilization to protect the packages from dust, moisture and other contaminants. (See **Figure 12.91**) The plastic material should be at least 2 to 3 mil thick. Sterilized items must be thoroughly cooled before being placed into the protective package. The seal of the packaging should be secured with either a heat seal or security-tape sealing process. The overwrap should be clearly marked as a "protective packaging" to prevent its use as part of the sterile field. *Note: Protective packaging overwrap is not to be placed in the sterilizer; it should be placed over properly cooled, sterilized items only. Always follow the protective cover's specific IFU for proper application.*

Protective packaging A configuration of materials designed to prevent damage to the sterile barrier system and its contents from the time of their assembly until the point of use.

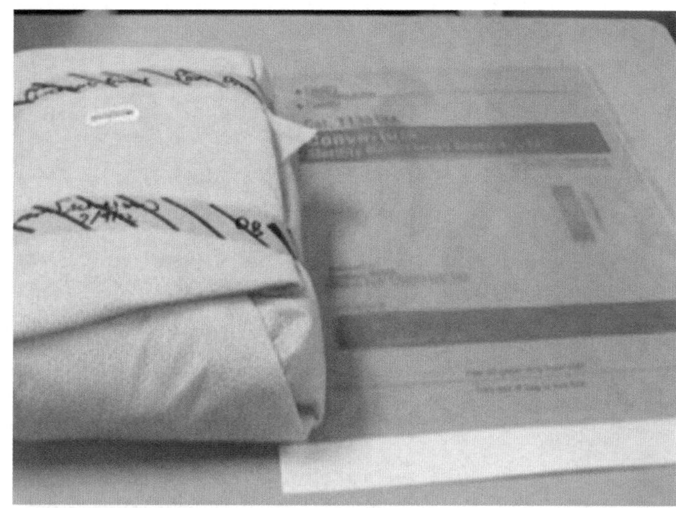

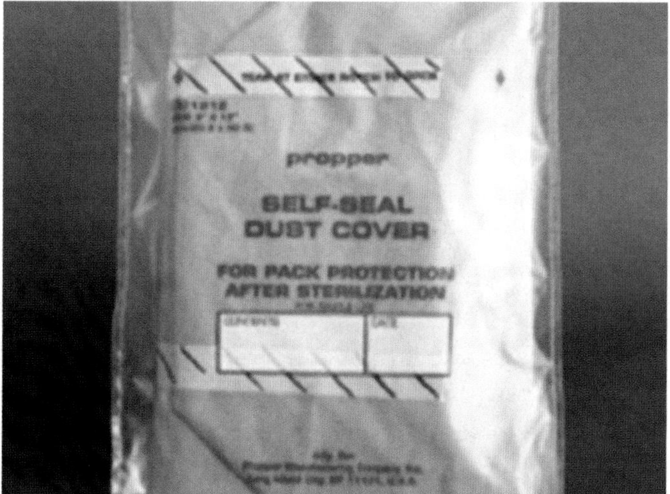

Figure 12.91 Example of protective packaging

Note: The expiration date of any item in a protective packaging cover is not extended by placing the item in the protective cover.

CONCLUSION

Medical devices and supplies used in patient treatment and care are made of various materials and configurations. No single assembly method or packaging system meets all requirements for packaging and sterilization of all devices. SP technicians must understand assembly and packaging concepts and follow best work practices for preparing packages to help ensure that devices dispensed for patients are functional and safe for use.

RESOURCES

Association for the Advancement of Medical Instrumentation. ANSI/AAMI ST79:2017 & 2020 Amendments A1, A2, A3, A4 (Consolidated Text) *Comprehensive guide to steam sterilization and sterility assurance in health care facilities.*

Association of periOperative Registered Nurses. "Recommended Practices for Cleaning and Caring for Surgical Instruments and Powered Equipment." *Standards, Recommended Practices, and Guidelines*. 2022.

Association of periOperative Registered Nurses. "Guidelines for PeriOperative Practice: Packaging Systems." *Guidelines for PeriOperative Practice*. 2022.

Truscott W. "SSI Prevention Pointers from Industry." *Infection Control Today*. 2010.

STERILE PROCESSING TERMS

Preparation and packaging

Super-heated steam

Chemical indicators (CIs)

Process challenge device (PCD)

Tamper-evident seals

Rigid container system

Wet pack

Sterility (time-related)

Sterility (event-related)

Protective package

Chapter 13

Point-of-Use Disinfection and Sterilization

Learning Objectives

As a result of successfully completing this chapter, the reader will be able to:

1. Define immediate use steam sterilization
2. Explain the basic procedures to safely perform immediate use steam sterilization
3. Address point-of-use processing for heat-sensitive medical devices

INTRODUCTION

The majority of instrument processing takes place in the Sterile Processing department (SPD); however, there are times when processing is performed at the point of use. There are two basic types of **point-of-use processing**. The first is **immediate use steam sterilization (IUSS),** which consists of cleaning, steam sterilization and immediate delivery of heat-resistant items to the procedure room. This process is designed for instances when there is not enough time to send the item(s) to the SPD for processing. The second type of point-of-use processing is designed for heat-sensitive items. Regardless of the process used, the goal is to provide an item that is safe for patient use. This chapter examines methods of point-of-use processing.

Point-of-use processing Occurs when a medical device is processed immediately before use.

Immediate use steam sterilization (IUSS) Process designed for the cleaning, steam sterilization and immediate delivery of heat-resistant items for use in the procedure room.

IMMEDIATE USE STEAM STERILIZATION

In patient care, there are always unexpected events that require quick action. Instrument demands become urgent when there is an immediate patient need and the instruments are not ready for use. In previous years, "flash" sterilization was designed for use in the Operating Room (OR) for emergencies and immediate use. The term flash sterilization has since been replaced by IUSS.

Items processed using IUSS are cleaned according to their manufacturers' instructions for use (IFU), placed into containers specifically designated for IUSS, and sterilized according to manufacturer instructions. (See **Figure 13.1**)

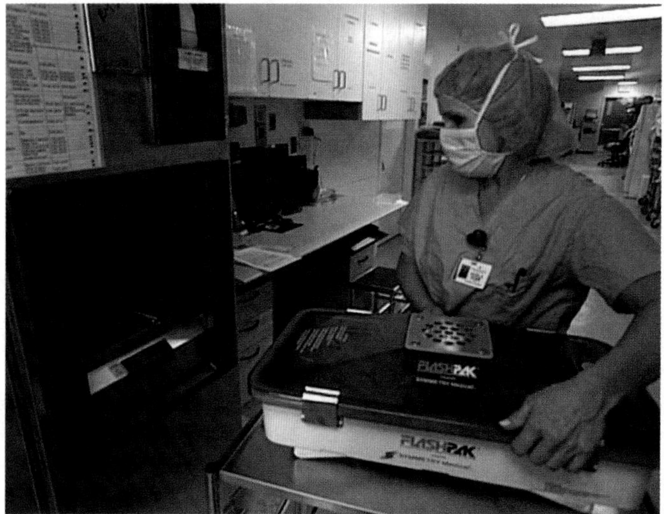

Figure 13.1

Processing devices for immediate use can be safe and effective but only if all steps recommended by the device manufacturer are followed. This includes proper cleaning, decontamination, sterilization using the correct cycle, and aseptic transfer to the point of use. Shortcuts, such as improper cleaning in an effort to save time, can jeopardize patient safety. Following validated manufacturers' IFU and controlling process quality helps protect patients from infections and prolongs the life of instrumentation.

Standards and Recommended Practices

Several associations have developed standards and guidelines to help ensure IUSS procedures are performed properly.

Association for the Advancement of Medical Instrumentation

Standards from the Association for the Advancement of Medical Instrumentation (AAMI) are not law; however, they are the recognized industry standards for sterilization and may be relevant in any legal proceeding. AAMI standards represent a national consensus, and many have been approved by the American National Standards Institute (ANSI).

ANSI/AAMI ST79 *Comprehensive guide to steam sterilization and sterility assurance in health care facilities* is a broad document covering recommended practices for steam sterilization. The document states that IUSS can be performed when deemed appropriate but should not be used for purposes of convenience or as a substitute for insufficient instrumentation. Items processed by IUSS should:

- Only be used in urgent clinical situations
- Be decontaminated according to the manufacturer's IFU, with approved detergents and water to remove soil, blood, body fats and other substances
- Be placed in an approved IUSS rigid sterilization container system
- Be used immediately and not stored for later use
- Be identified as IUSS devices

The Association of periOperative Registered Nurses

The Association of periOperative Registered (AORN) publishes its *Guidelines for Perioperative Practices,* and surveying agencies refer to AORN guidelines. AORN guidelines state that IUSS can be performed only when the following conditions are met:

- The device manufacturer's IFU includes instructions for IUSS.
- Items are placed in a containment device that has been validated for IUSS.

- The IUSS container manufacturer's written IFU are followed.
- Items processed by IUSS are used immediately.
- Staff members are educated on the IUSS process.
- Recordkeeping is maintained to allow tracking of the device after use.

Surveying Agencies

IUSS is designed for urgent situations when there is insufficient time to send an item through the normal **terminal sterilization** process. Surveying agencies closely monitor IUSS to ensure everything is being done by the healthcare facility to decrease IUSS and ensure that wherever and whenever IUSS is practiced, the processes are performed correctly.

> **Terminal sterilization** The process by which surgical instruments and medical devices are sterilized in their final containers, allowing them to be stored until needed.

The Joint Commission

The Joint Commission (TJC) requires that complete documentation be made available for each IUSS cycle so that the device is traceable to the patient if a problem arises. In the past, TJC focused on how many IUSS cycles were run and how to reduce the amount of IUSS sterilization. Now, in addition to focusing on IUSS reduction, TJC surveyors are focusing on the IUSS process to ensure all processes are completed properly. They expect the same safeguards and quality controls to be in place, regardless of whomoperates a sterilizer or where the sterilizer is located. Some areas of focus include:

- Cleaning and decontamination – Before an item can be sterilized, it must be properly cleaned and decontaminated according to the manufacturer's recommendations.
- Sterilization – The manufacturer's instructions must specify the type of IUSS cycle (e.g., gravity displacement and dynamic air removal) and length of time needed for sterilization. Some instruments may require an extended cycle or a specified dry time; some instruments can never undergo IUSS. The manufacturer's IFU must specify that the item can undergo IUSS cycles.
- Transfer to the sterile field – Aseptic transfer from the sterilizer to the sterile field is required to prevent recontamination of the sterilized item.
- Frequency of IUSS use – Lack of instrumentation is not an excuse for using IUSS. A plan should be in place to reduce IUSS cycles.

Centers for Medicare and Medicaid Services

The Centers for Medicare and Medicaid Services (CMS) has established the following requirements for IUSS:

- The same multi-step process used to prepare instruments for terminal sterilization must be completed for IUSS.
- Parameters for all phases of the sterilization cycle must be determined by consulting the IFU for the instrument(s), sterilizer and containment device.
- Each IUSS cycle must use physical monitors and chemical indicators (CIs). At least weekly, the sterilizer must be tested with a biological test for each type of IUSS cycle.
- If IUSS must be used for an implant, a tracking system should be in place to trace the IUSS load to the patient.
- Medical instruments and devices processed using IUSS must be contained in a packaging system labeled for the IUSS cycle(s) used.
- Items sterilized by IUSS must be used immediately.

CMS also indicates that IUSS is *not* acceptable in the following circumstances:

- For implant processing, unless there is a documented emergency situation
- For post-procedure decontamination of instruments used on patients with possible Creutzfeldt-Jakob Disease (CJD) or other prion diseases
- When devices or loads have not been validated for the specific cycle used
- For processing single-use devices

PROCEDURES FOR IUSS

Safe and effective IUSS requires that all steps in the process be performed properly each time to achieve sterilization and maintain sterility of instruments, all the way to the point of use. Improperly sterilized or contaminated instruments used in a surgical procedure can result in serious complications, from surgical site infections (SSIs) to increased costs and legal liability.

Precleaning

Precleaning of instrumentation is a necessary step to help promote effective, thorough decontamination and sterilization. AORN guidelines state that items should be kept free of gross soil during surgery. These guidelines are critical factors when items are to be prepared for IUSS. Soil is easier to remove when items are properly pretreated in the OR.

Decontamination

Thorough decontamination of medical devices is required for safe and effective IUSS. Manufacturers of sterilizers and medical devices assume that the level of contamination has been adequately reduced on the surfaces of instruments before they are placed in the sterilizer. If items are not properly cleaned, they cannot be sterilized.

Standard precautions require that employees who handle contaminated devices wear the appropriate personal protective equipment (PPE). This includes gloves, hair covering, eye protection, masks, fluid-impervious gown or jumpsuit, and shoe covers. PPE should be removed and discarded and not worn outside of the cleaning/decontamination area.

Manufacturer instructions for instrument processing should be available and consulted to ensure proper cleaning and decontamination before IUSS occurs. These may contain special cleaning instructions such as the disassembly process and the recommended use of cleaning solutions and mechanical cleaners. Instruments must be cleaned as thoroughly as they would in the SP decontamination area. Items must be decontaminated in an area designed to clean instruments and never in a scrub or handwashing sink. Surveying agencies will check to ensure that staff members are trained on proper cleaning methods.

Prior to placing instruments in an IUSS-approved sterilization container, instruments must be carefully inspected to ensure they are clean and functional. Instruments must be placed in the sterilization container in a manner that facilitates full steam contact. Sterilization containers should be placed in the sterilizer chamber following the container and the sterilizer's IFU.

IUSS Cycles

Steam sterilizers used for IUSS are usually placed in close proximity to user areas. (See **Figure 13.2**) There are two types of steam cycles commonly used: gravity displacement and dynamic air removal, which includes the prevacuum and steam flush pressure pulse (SFPP) cycles. The type of cycle to be used depends on the manufacturer's IFU.

Consult the manufacturer's IFU for exposure times and cycles when using containment devices or packaging systems.

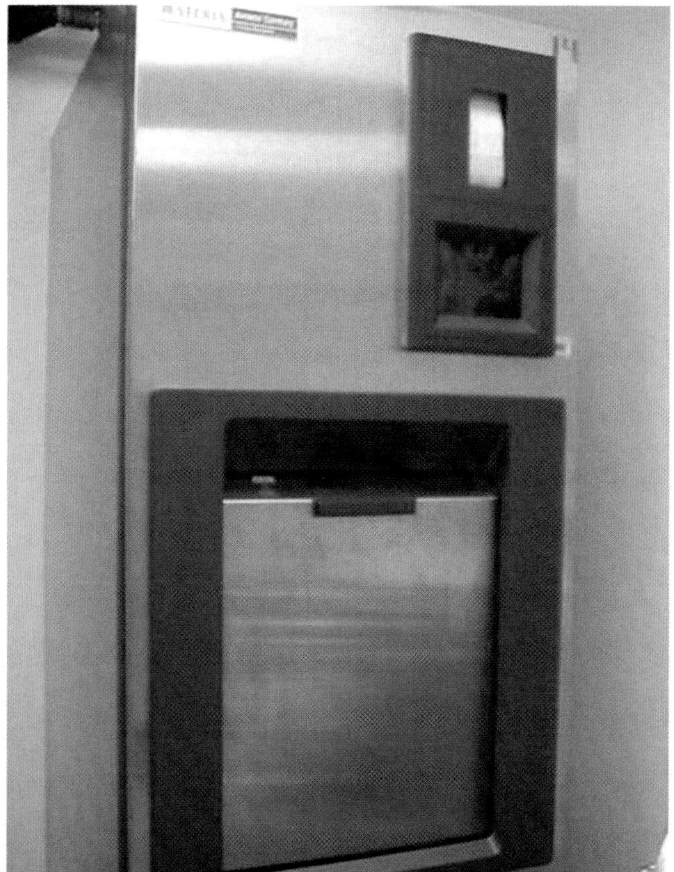

Figure 13.2

Safe Transport After IUSS

Instruments subjected to IUSS should be transported to the point of use in a manner that reduces the potential for contamination. Failure to take appropriate measures to protect IUSS-processed instruments after their removal from the sterilizer and during transport to the point of use will increase the potential for contamination and the patient's risk for acquiring an SSI. *Note: Use of the single-wrapped method helps protect sterile instruments; however, this method cannot be used unless the sterilizer has the "single wrapped" function built into the system.* Utilizing sealed rigid containers approved for IUSS offers the best protection for sterile instruments. Instruments processed in these rigid containers still cannot be stored for later use, unless approved by the U.S. Food and Drug Administration (FDA). The items must be used as soon as possible after the sterilization cycle is complete.

Staff Education

Educating staff members who perform IUSS is important to decrease the possibility of errors that could occur during the process. Staff members should receive initial training, and competency assessment should be performed, followed by continuing education at regular intervals to review and update their knowledge.

QUALITY CONTROL MONITORS FOR IUSS

The efficacy of every sterilization cycle must be monitored. The quality assurance of each process includes physical, chemical and biological monitors. All of these monitors should be carefully watched and reviewed to identify potential issues.

As the name implies, a dynamic air removal test is only performed in dynamic air removal sterilizers. This test should be run each day the sterilizer is used. Biological indicators (BIs) should be run at least weekly and with every implant cycle. A CI should be included in the container with every cycle. All quality monitors should be inspected prior to releasing the contents for use.

Recordkeeping

IUSS records allow for traceability of every sterilized item to the patient. It is important to keep accurate and complete records that include evidence of cycle performance such as sterilization cycle printouts and BI and CI results. Sterilizer cycle records should include:

- Patient identification – There must be a way to identify the patient on whom the items were used in the event of a problem such as sterilization cycle failure or the patient acquiring a healthcare-associated infection (HAI).
- Sterilizer and sterilizer cycle identification
- Instrument(s) sterilized in the cycle
- Cycle parameters
- Reason the IUSS cycle was run (e.g., instrument dropped on floor)
- Operator's signature or other identification

No national standard exists for how long sterilization records should be maintained. Local statute requirements and individual facility policies should be followed.

POINT-OF-USE PROCESSING FOR HEAT-SENSITIVE DEVICES

Low-Temperature Disinfection and Sterilization Processes

Advancing sterilization technologies have changed the way procedures are performed. The medical devices used in many procedures have changed as well. Many of the medical devices used today are heat sensitive. In other words, processing them in a heated process, such as with steam, will lead to damage. Facilities must use low-temperature methods to safely process those heat-sensitive items.

There are several types of low-temperature disinfection or sterilization options for point-of-use processing. Selection is determined by the types of items that will be processed and their compatibility with that low-temperature process. The decision to process heat-sensitive items at the point of use is made based on the medical device IFU and the logistics of the facility.

The level of biocidal process required is based on the intended use of the item. Sterilization is the preferred biocidal method for semi-critical and critical items. If sterilization is not an option for semi-critical items, the items may undergo high-level disinfection (HLD). The most common items are transesophageal echocardiography exam (TEE) probes (See **Figure 13.3**), vaginal probes and flexible endoscopes. Methods used include HLD, liquid chemical sterilization, or a hydrogen peroxide mist unit.

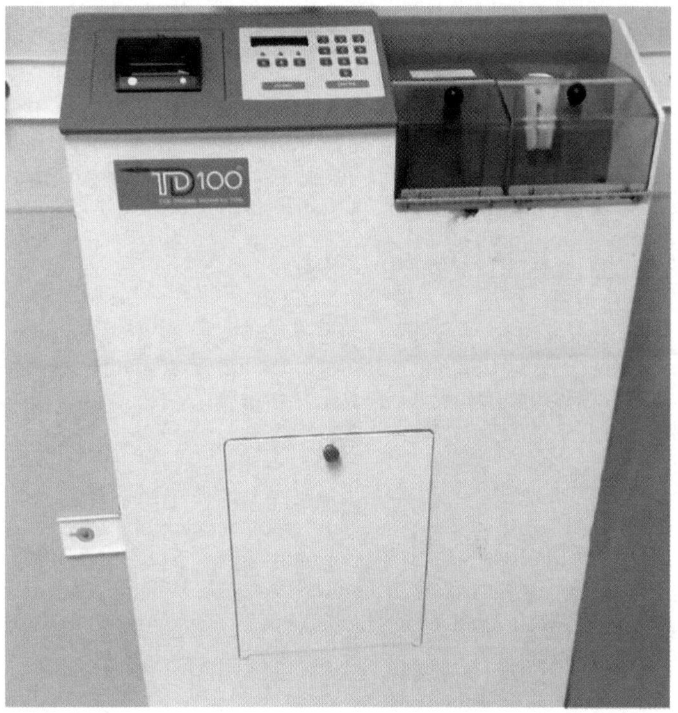

Figure 13.3

All low-temperature processes utilize a chemical process. SP technicians must understand the specific type of process used in their facility and be educated on proper handling and operational procedures, as well as safety protocols for the specific process.

Preparation of Devices for Low-Temperature Processes

As with IUSS processes, proper preparation is critical to the success of the low-temperature point-of-use process. Items must be cleaned thoroughly because any soil remaining on the device will result in a failed process and pose a danger to the patient. Items must be prepared for the low-temperature process according to the manufacturer's IFU.

The device should be protected from environmental contaminants once removed from the processor. After processing, the device should be clearly labeled as "patient ready." As with all HLD and sterilization processes, the medical device manufacturer must have approved the device for the specific biocidal process to be performed.

Quality Control Monitors for Point-of-Use Low-Temperature Processes

Quality control monitors will vary depending on the process used; however, there are some commonalities:

- The process must be monitored
- Items processed must be documented

Monitoring will be unique to each low-temperature process. For manual HLD using a soak process, the solution must be checked for minimum effective concentration (MEC). For mechanical processes, testing should be performed according to the equipment and chemical manufacturer's IFU. That testing may include chemical, biological or diagnostic tests.

All items processed at the point of use must be documented, and those records, along with documentation of quality testing, should be kept on file.

CONCLUSION

Point-of-use processing meets a specific need in procedural areas. Although it is performed away from the SPD, manufacturers' instructions remain the same. When performed properly, point-of-use processing can provide items that are safe for patient use.

RESOURCES

Association of periOperative Registered Nurses. "Guidelines for PeriOperative Practice: Sterilization." *Guidelines for PeriOperative Practice*. 2022.

The Joint Commission. *The Joint Commission Accreditation Manual*. 2013.

Centers for Disease Control and Prevention. *Guidelines for Disinfection and Sterilization in Healthcare Facilities*. 2008.

Multi-Society Statement on Immediate Use Steam Sterilization (AAMI, AAHSP, AORN, APIC, ASCQC, AST, IAHCSMM).

ANSI/AAMI ST79:2017 & 2020 Amendments A1, A2,A3, A4 (Consolidated Text) *Comprehensive guide to steam sterilization and sterility assurance in health care facilities.*

Gillespie S. "Flash Sterilization: Many Users, Many Questions About This Technique." *Biomedical Instrumentation & Technology*. Vol. 44, No. 1. (p 62). 2010.

Nanai P. "Immediate Use Steam Sterilization: It's All About the Process." *AORN Journal*. Vol. 98, No. 1. 2013. pp. 32–38.

Rutala W, Weber D. *Guideline for Disinfection and Sterilization in Healthcare Facilities*. Centers for Disease Control and Prevention. 2008.

Conner R. *Sterile Processing in the Surgical Suite*, 2014 FGI Guidelines Series, Update #4, September 2014.

STERILE PROCESSING TERMS

Point-of-use processing

Immediate use steam sterilization (IUSS)

Terminal sterilization

Chapter 14

High-Temperature Sterilization

Learning Objectives

As a result of successfully completing this chapter, the reader will be able to:

1. Discuss factors that impact the effectiveness of sterilization
2. Discuss the advantages of steam sterilization
3. Provide basic information about the types of steam sterilizers available
4. Discuss basic information about steam sterilizer cycles

6 Describe the conditions necessary for an effective steam sterilization process

7. Explain basic work practices for steam sterilization
8. Review sterilization process indicators and explain the need for quality control

INTRODUCTION

High-temperature sterilization is the process of choice in many healthcare facilities. It is achieved by subjecting items being processed to thermal energy from moist heat (steam). High-temperature sterilization has long been recognized as an effective way to kill microorganisms. Because of its successful record of efficacy, reliability and low cost, steam is the most frequently used sterilant for devices not adversely affected by moisture or heat. In fact, other methods are only used when the object being processed cannot withstand the heat and/or moisture required for steam sterilization.

As with all sterilization methods, devices to be processed must first be thoroughly cleaned, decontaminated and properly prepared. Cleaning involves the removal of all visible soil, and decontamination kills most but not all microorganisms. Sterilization is required to kill any remaining microorganisms, including spores.

Sterilization failure could result in serious, even life-threatening, patient outcomes. A Sterile Processing (SP) technician must learn the components of a steam sterilizer to better understand how it operates and supports quality outcomes and patient safety.

FACTORS THAT IMPACT STERILIZATION

The success of every sterilization process is not guaranteed. Several factors and conditions impact the effectiveness of all sterilization methods, including those using high temperature. These factors include:

- The type of microorganisms present – Some microorganisms are more resistant to the sterilization process than others.
- The design of the medical device – Complex devices present a challenge to the sterilization process.
- The number of microorganisms (**bioburden**) present – When there are more microorganisms on a medical device, the sterilization process becomes more difficult.
- The amount and type of soil present – Soil acts as a shield to protect microorganisms.

Note: The cleaning process is absolutely essential as a first step in sterilization. A device can be cleaned without sterilizing, but sterilization cannot be achieved if a device hasn't been thoroughly cleaned

Bioburden The number of microorganisms on an object; also called "bioload" or "microbial load."

ADVANTAGES OF STEAM STERILIZATION

Steam is the sterilant of choice for several reasons:

- Low cost
- Rapid sterilization cycles
- Relatively simple technology
- Leaves no chemical residues or byproducts

Steam sterilizers date back to the early days of formalized healthcare. Prior to steam sterilization, boiling water was commonly used to kill bacteria. Scientists recognized the need to increase temperatures beyond the boiling point to kill greater numbers of heat-resistant bacteria. **Figure 14.1** is an illustration of an early pressure steam sterilizer (autoclave) developed in 1880 by Charles Chamberlain, a colleague of Louis Pasteur. The autoclave resembled a pressure cooker and was able to use pressurized steam to reach temperatures of 248°F (120°C) and higher. Although it looks primitive by today's standards, it was the first-generation model of the steam sterilizers used today.

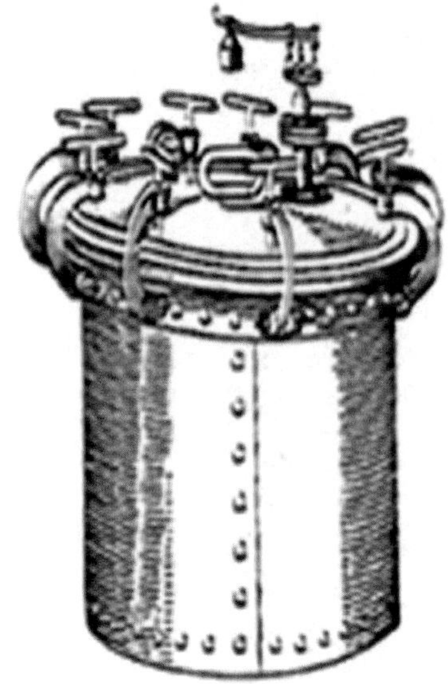

Figure 14.1

ANATOMY OF A STEAM STERILIZER

Steam sterilizers come in many sizes and cycle choices, from small tabletop sterilizers used primarily in clinic and dental settings, to mid-sized and large units designed to sterilize large quantities of items. **Figures 14.2, 14.3** and **14.4** illustrate various sizes of steam sterilizers.

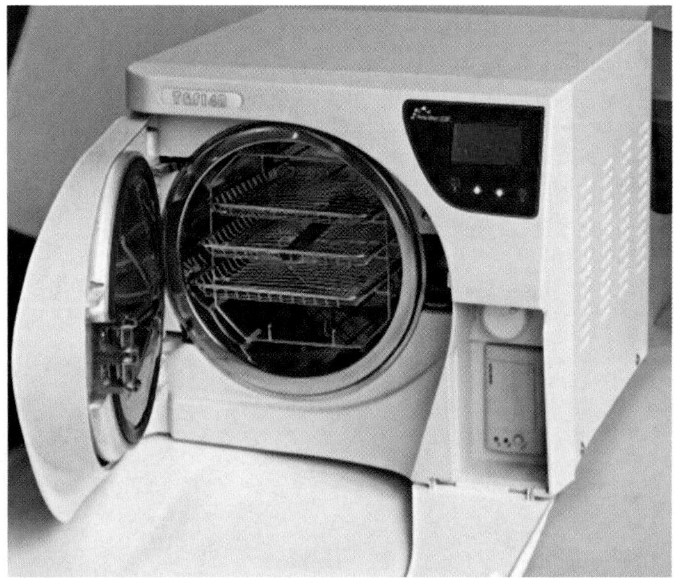

Figure 14.2 Tabletop sterilizer

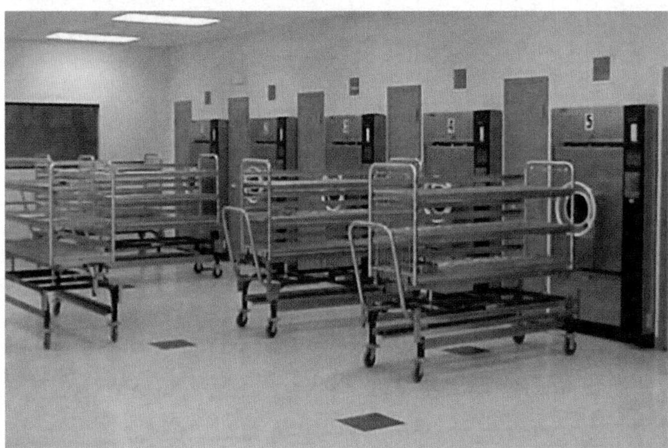

Figure 14.3 Cart and carriage loading sterilizers

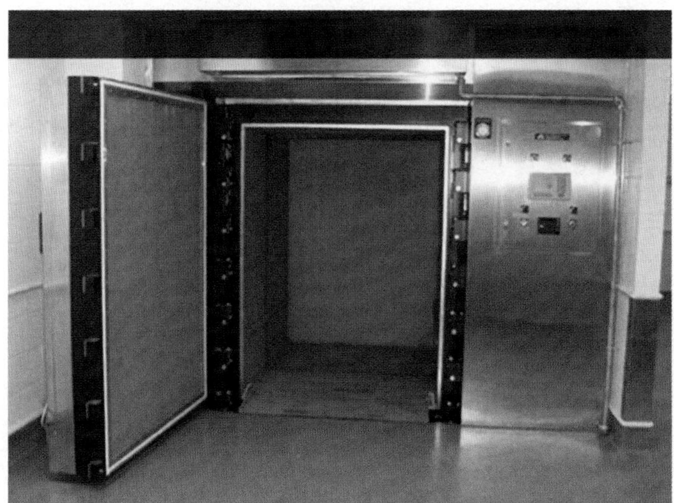

Figure 14.4 Floor-loading sterilizer

COMPONENTS OF STEAM STERILIZERS

An SP technician must know the components of a sterilizer to better understand how it operates.

Jacket

Sterile Processing departments (SPDs) typically use jacketed sterilizers. **Figure 14.5** shows a cutaway diagram of a steam sterilizer and illustrates how steam from an external source enters the jacket. In most hospitals, steam is supplied to the sterilizers from a main steam line; these units themselves do not generate steam. Other sterilizers in clinics, dental practices and some SPDs manufacture their own steam or attain their steam from an independent generator. **Figure 14.6** provides an example of a steam generator.

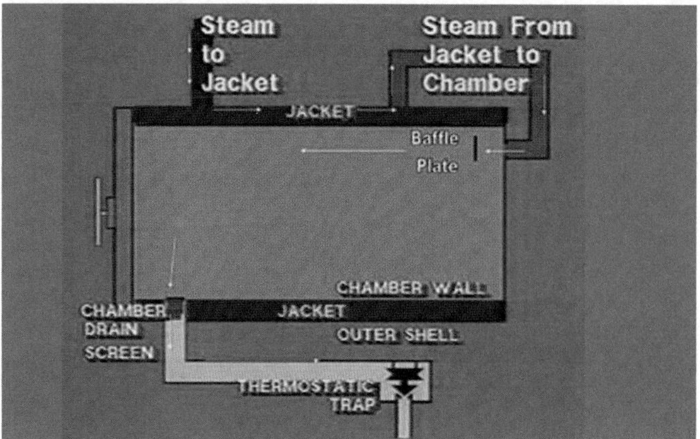

Figure 14.5

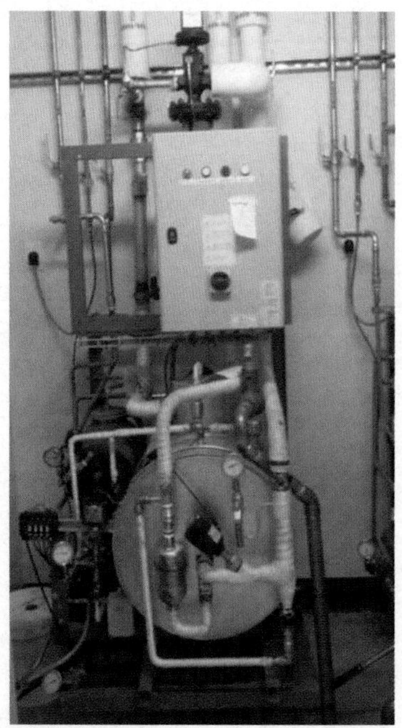

Figure 14.6

The interior chamber walls of the sterilizer are heated by steam in the metal jacket; this helps minimize the amount of condensation (moisture) that forms when hot steam contacts the chamber walls as a cycle begins. **Figure 14.7** shows the condensation that forms during the steam cycle. The jacket surrounds the sides, top and bottom of the vessel, and steam circulates in this space to preheat the interior chamber walls.

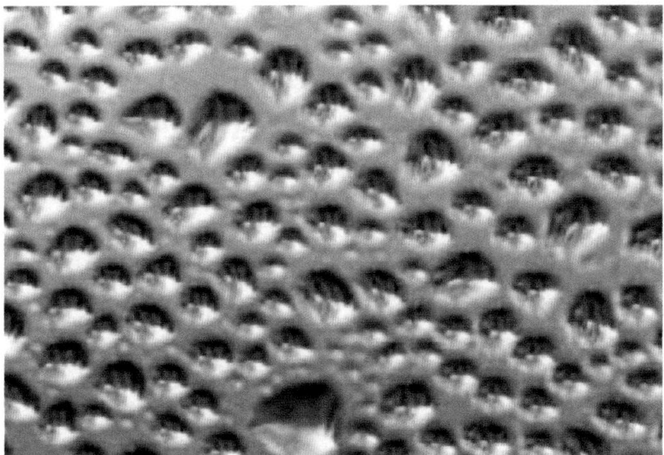

Figure 14.7 Condensation from heat transfer

The outside of the jacket is covered with insulation to help prevent condensation from forming on the jacket's outer and inner walls. This insulation also provides a safety feature because it reduces the likelihood that personnel working behind the sterilizer will be burned. The outer shell is typically located behind a wall and is not readily visible to the sterilizer technician. **Figure 14.8** shows insulation covering the sterilizer outer shell.

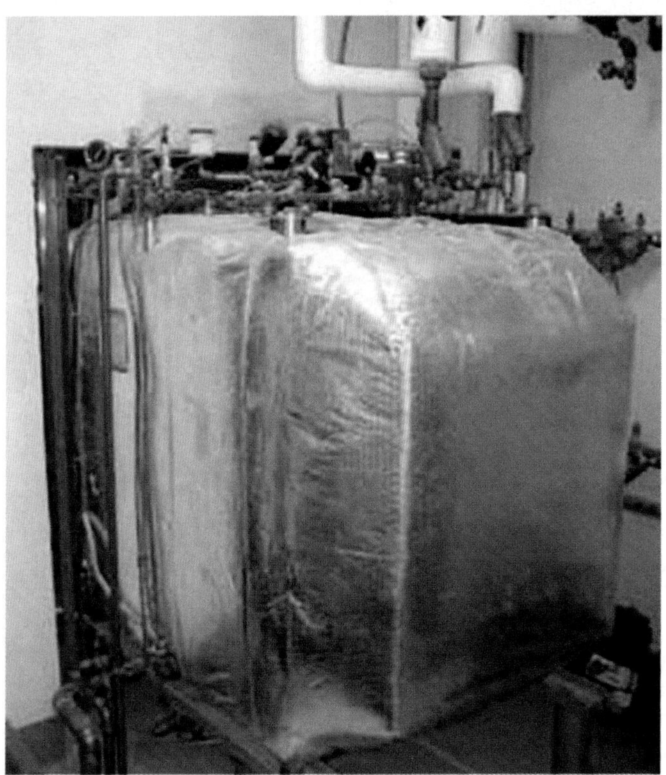

Figure 14.8

Door, Gasket and Chamber Drain

The door is the weakest part of a steam sterilizer. It has a safety locking mechanism that automatically activates when chamber pressure is applied, and it can only be unlocked when pressure is exhausted. Some model sterilizers use radial arm locking doors, which can be tightened but not loosened while the chamber is under pressure. Some sterilizers have active gaskets with pressure behind them to seal the chamber. The door gasket is designed to maintain a tight seal that prevents steam from escaping from the chamber, and air from entering the chamber. (See **Figure 14.9**)

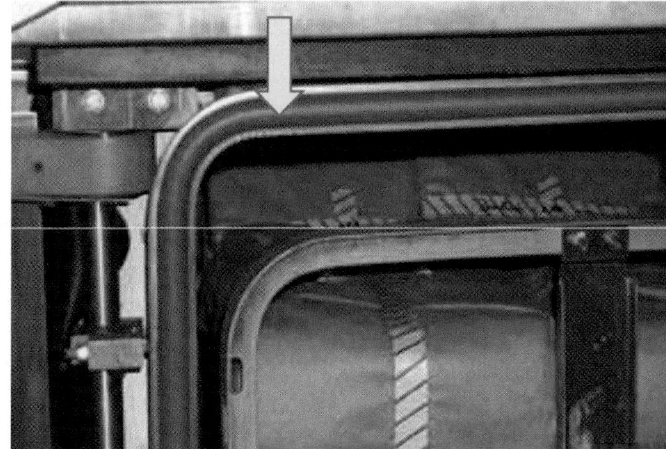

Figure 14.9 Door gasket

On most steam sterilizers, the chamber drain is located at the front or center of the floor. The drain screen must be cleaned at least daily and more often, as needed. Debris in the chamber drain screen can impede cycle performance by blocking the removal of air and steam. (See **Figure 14.10**)

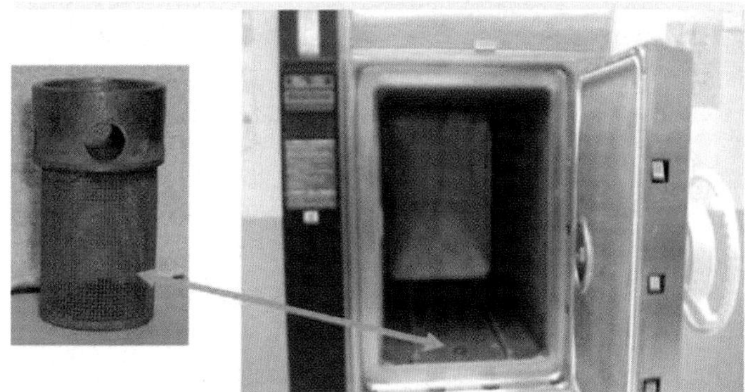

Figure 14.10 Chamber drain and drain screen

Thermostatic Trap

As seen in **Figure 14.11**, the thermostatic trap is located in the drain line. The drain and the area surrounding it are the coolest areas in the sterilizer. A sensor in the chamber drain measures steam temperature and automatically controls the flow of air and condensate from the sterilizer chamber.

Thermostatic trap

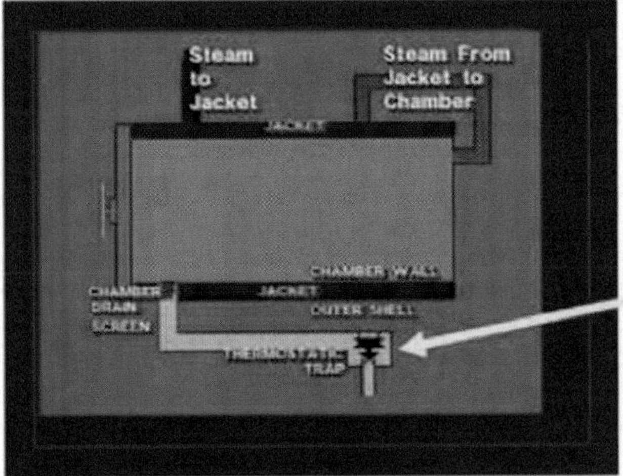

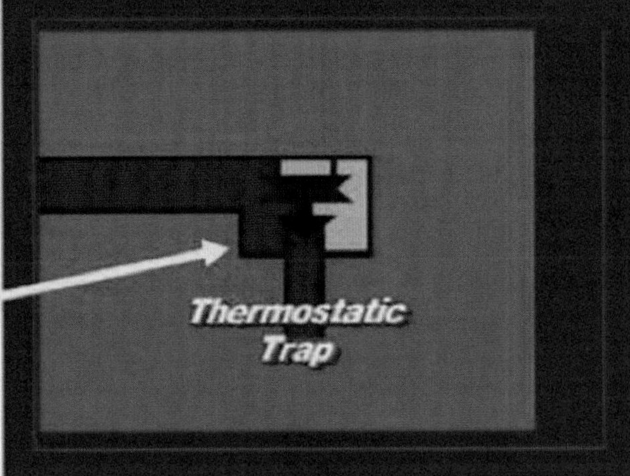

Figure 14.11

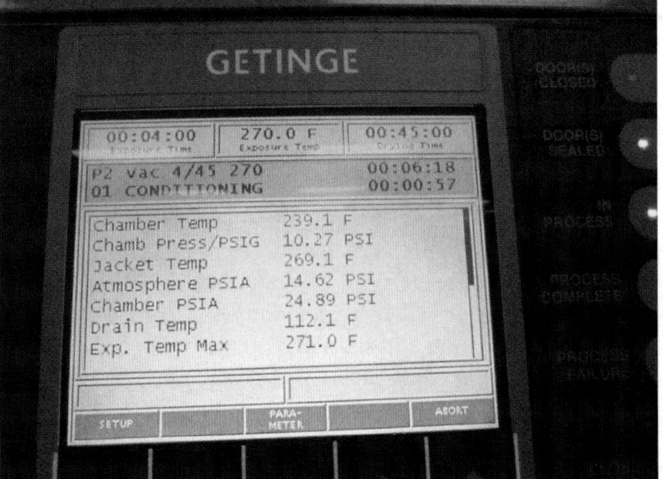

Figure 14.12

Physical Monitors

Physical monitors verify that the parameters of the sterilization cycle have been met. Physical monitors on a sterilizer record the time, temperature and pressure. There are different types of monitors such as digital printouts, electronic recording/data capture, and gauges. These monitors provide a visual and written record of sterilization conditions. SP technicians must check them throughout the sterilization cycle to ensure that necessary parameters are met. A printout from a steam sterilization cycle usually contains the following information:

- Date and time the cycle began
- Selected cycle parameters such as type of cycle, sterilization temperature and dry times
- A written record of actual cycle activities (e.g., temperatures, exposure times and pressure). Some steam sterilizers can also provide the information in a digital format (see **Figure 14.12**) and some can even be integrated into an instrument tracking system. Older steam sterilizers have circular charts that record sterilization activities. Charts are changed daily, and the time listed on the chart is aligned with the recording pen to the correct time of day. The date and sterilizer location are noted on the graph, and the pens are checked daily to ensure they are recording. Charts or printouts are signed by the sterilizer operator, indicating that parameters have been reviewed.

The SP technician is responsible for determining if all sterilization parameters were met and if the load may be released. The physical monitors (recording chart, printer or tape) should be reviewed, signed and dated by the operator to indicate an acceptable cycle. If any steam sterilization parameter was not met, the supervisor should be notified immediately, and the sterilization load should not be released.

TYPES OF STEAM STERILIZERS USED IN STERILE PROCESSING

Several types of steam sterilizers are available today. Healthcare facilities purchase sterilizers that will meet their specific needs, including chamber size, style and available cycle options.

Tabletop Sterilizers

Tabletop sterilizers are frequently used in clinics and dental offices. These units operate by having water poured into the sterilizer, either manually or automatically, through a port or the bottom of the chamber, and are electrically heated until the water turns to steam. Water quality is an important factor and is specified in the sterilizer instructions for use (IFU). In a tabletop sterilizer cycle, steam rises to the chamber's top and as more steam is produced, cooler air is forced out through the drain near the bottom of the chamber. When steam enters the drain, a thermostatic valve closes and causes the steam to build up pressure until the operating temperature is reached. When the proper temperature is reached, the timer is activated. At the end of the cycle, the relief valve opens to allow the steam to escape. The steam passes through the water reservoir where it condenses back to water. After the pressure has dropped to zero, the door can be opened. As with all sterilizers, SP technicians should carefully review the sterilizer manufacturer's IFU for specific operating instructions.

Gravity Air Displacement Sterilizers

Some small- to medium-sized sterilizers have gravity displacement and dynamic air removal cycles. In a gravity displacement cycle, steam enters the chamber and because air is heavier than steam, the steam forces the cooler air to the bottom of the chamber and out the drain. While their operation appears simple, many mistakes can be made, including improper loading or unloading; therefore, thorough knowledge of sterilization theory and practice is essential for those operating these units. Gravity air displacement sterilizers have physical monitoring controls such as temperature-indicating charts and printouts for recordkeeping.

Dynamic Air Removal Sterilizers

Dynamic air removal sterilizers are similar in construction to gravity air displacement sterilizers, except there is a vacuum pump or water ejector that removes air from the chamber more effectively during the preconditioning phase, prior to reaching the exposure temperature. Dynamic air removal sterilizers usually operate at higher temperatures [270°F to 275°F (132°C to 135°C)] than gravity sterilizers. The preconditioning phase increases the speed of operation and reduces the chance of air pockets in the chamber during the cycle. Dynamic air removal sterilizers use different types of preconditioning methods for air removal. These include variations of prevacuum air removal and above-atmospheric-pressure processes, such as the steam flush pressure pulse (SFPP) process. The preconditioning cycle removes air from both the sterilizing chamber and the load before the chamber is pressurized with steam to the exposure temperature. Effective air removal is critical for steam penetration.

Prevacuum Steam Sterilizers

In prevacuum steam sterilizers, the dynamic air removal cycle depends on one or more pressure and vacuum sequences at the beginning of the cycle to remove air during the preconditioning phase. Typical operating temperatures are 270°F to 275°F (132°C to 135°C). To ensure air removal in these sterilizers, the integrity of the sterilizers should be checked daily by processing a Bowie-Dick (or daily air removal) test. Some sterilizers have an automatic cycle (vacuum leak test) to test the vacuum tightness of the chamber.

Steam Flush Pressure Pulse Sterilizers

SFPP sterilizers use a repeated sequence of a steam flush and pressure pulse to remove air from the sterilizing chamber and processed materials. Air removal occurs above atmospheric pressure; no vacuum is required. Like a prevacuum sterilizer, this process rapidly removes air from the sterilizer's chamber and wrapped items.

STEAM STERILIZER CYCLES

Along with understanding the types of steam sterilizers used in the healthcare facility, SP technicians must also understand how these machines function. To begin, SP technicians should be familiar with two basic sterilization cycles: immediate use steam sterilization (IUSS) and terminal sterilization. Items processed using IUSS must undergo the same cleaning and preparation as items that are terminally sterilized. Sterilizers used for IUSS are typically located outside of the SPD. Their intended use is for the emergency sterilization of instruments when there is not enough time for terminal sterilization. These types of sterilization processes have little or no dry time; therefore, at the end of the sterilization process, instrumentation is expected to be hot and wet. **Figure 14.13** is an example of a sterilizer approved for IUSS cycles.

Time is usually shortened due to the reduced dry cycle. Not all items have IUSS instructions from the device manufacturer; consult the medical device manufacturer's IFU to determine if IUSS is possible for the device(s) to be processed and to learn the proper sterilization cycle. Items sterilized using IUSS should be used immediately and cannot be stored for use at a later time, unless such a process has been approved by the U.S. Food and Drug Administration (FDA).

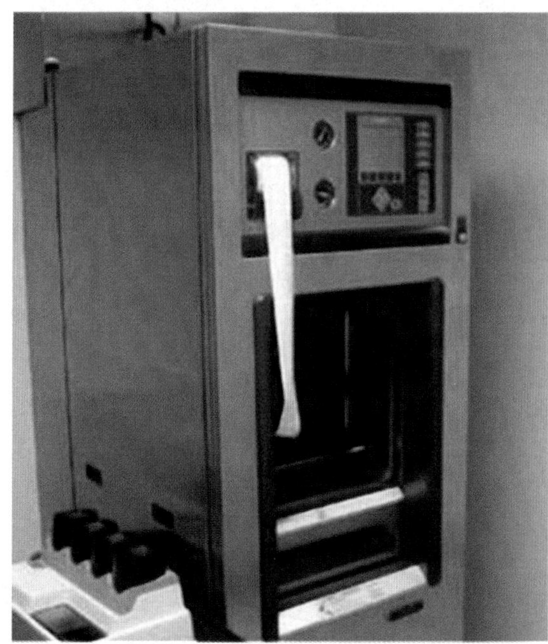

Figure 14.13

By contrast, "terminal sterilization" refers to the sterilization of an item that is expected to be dry upon completion of the sterilization process. Terminal sterilization is most often performed in the SPD.

A saturated steam sterilization cycle has at least three (and possibly four) phases:

- Conditioning
- Exposure
- Exhaust
- Drying (in most instances)

Conditioning

At the beginning of the sterilization cycle, steam enters at the upper back portion of the sterilizer. As steam enters, air is displaced through the drain. As steam continues to enter the sterilizer's chamber, pressure begins to rise, as does the steam temperature.

Exposure

After the desired temperature is reached, the sterilizer's control system begins timing the cycle's exposure phase. *Note: The instrument manufacturer's IFU should be consulted for the specific time and temperature for each instrument/set sterilized to ensure the cycle is appropriate.*

Exhaust

At the end of the exposure phase, the chamber's drain is opened, and the steam is removed through the discharge line. This creates a void in the chamber; filtered air is gradually reintroduced into the chamber and the chamber gradually returns to room pressure.

Steam enters chamber

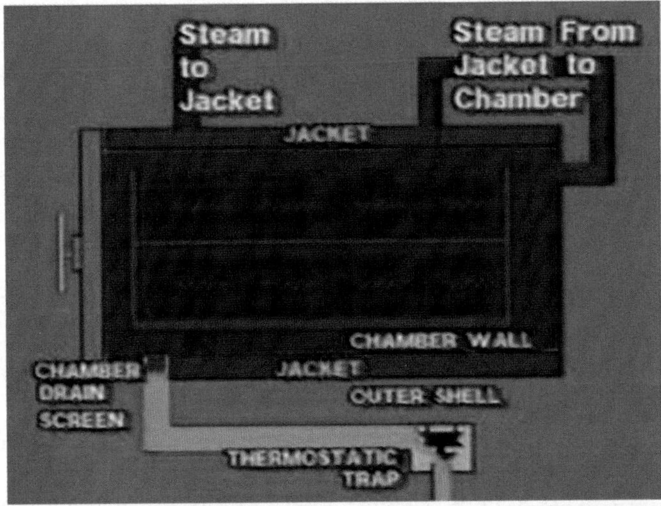

Figure 14.14 shows (in red) steam entering the chamber and air being displaced (in green) down the chamber's drain.

Steam passes through the thermostatic trap

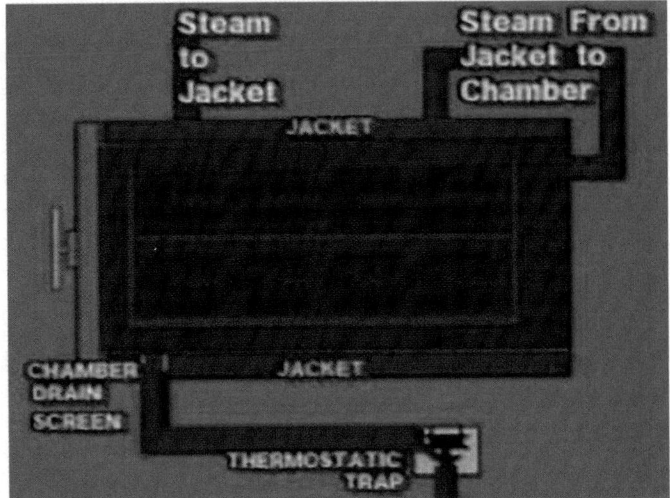

Figure 14.15 shows (in red) steam that has passed the chamber drain screen and the thermostatic trap.

Closed thermostatic trap

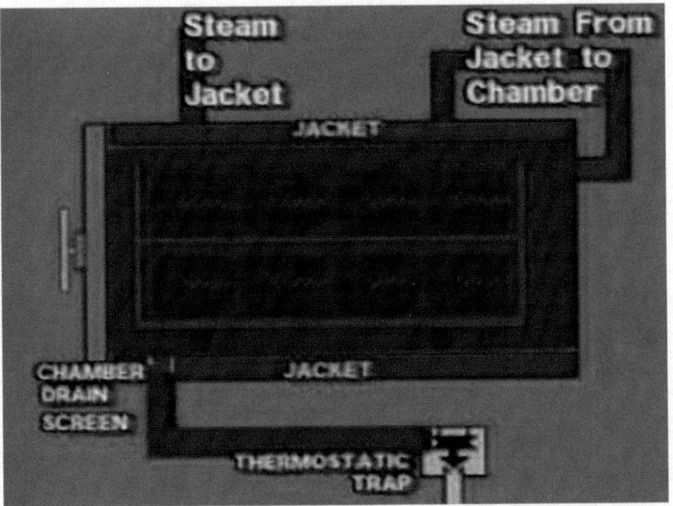

Figure 14.16 shows the thermostatic trap being closed after the desired temperature is reached.

Steam is exhausted from the chamber

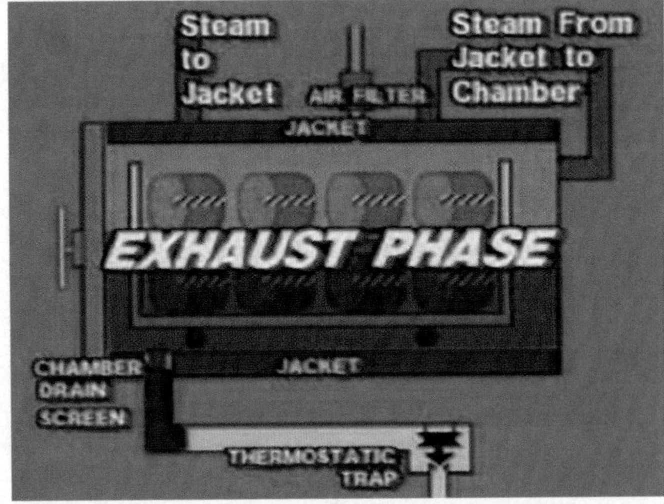

Figure 14.17 shows (in red) steam being exhausted from the sterilizer.

Figures **14.14** through **14.17** provide illustrations of the conditioning, exposure and exhaust phases in the steam sterilization process.

Drying

Drying begins at the conclusion of the exhaust phase. Dry times are based on the device, packaging and sterilizer IFU. At the end of this dry time, the end-of-cycle signal sounds and the door may be opened.

CONDITIONS NECESSARY FOR EFFECTIVE STEAM STERILIZATION

Regardless of the type of steam sterilization method used, the same four conditions—contact, temperature, time and moisture—must be met.

Contact

The most common reason for sterilization failure is the lack of contact between steam and the entire surface of the device being sterilized. This failure may be related to human error or mechanical malfunction. Frequent causes of steam contact failure include:

- Failure to adequately clean the object being sterilized – Any coating of soil, such as protein or oils, can protect the microorganisms from direct steam contact.
- Density – Sets that are too dense, or instruments positioned in a way that does not allow steam contact.
- Packages wrapped too tightly – If packs are wrapped too tightly, air becomes trapped and cannot escape.
- Loads that are too crowded – Packs must be arranged with adequate spacing on the cart. If they are packed too tightly, air may be entrapped, and steam may not be able to penetrate all areas.
- Containers that are positioned incorrectly – Basins and other items that can hold water must be positioned so air can be removed and water (condensed steam) can escape.
- Clogged drain strainer – Most sterilizers have a small drain strainer at the bottom of the chamber to keep lint, tape and other small objects from entering the exhaust line.
- Mechanical malfunctions – Defective steam traps, clogged exhaust lines and similar mechanical malfunctions can occur and cannot be repaired by an SP technician. A qualified service representative should be called to perform the necessary maintenance.
- Utility malfunctions – Boiler or steam delivery system problems can occur, and a qualified service representative is needed to make repairs, as specified in the sterilizer manufacturer's service manual.

Note: While mechanical malfunctions can occur, many sterilization failures are caused by human error and can be prevented by good work practices.

Temperature

To be effective, steam sterilization must occur at specific temperatures. These temperatures are needed to kill heat-resistant bacteria. The two most commonly encountered temperatures for steam sterilization are gravity sterilization 250°F (121°C) and dynamic air removal 270°F to 275°F (132.2°C to 134°C).

Time

The steam sterilization process can only be effective if all items within the load are exposed to the elevated temperatures and steam contact (moisture) for an adequate amount of time. Inadequate sterilization exposure times can lead to failure of the sterilization process.

Steam Quality and Moisture

A specific type of steam quality is required to perform steam sterilization. Steam quality is the steam characteristic reflecting the dryness fraction (weight of dry steam present in a mixture of dry **saturated steam** and entrained water) and the level of **noncondensable gas** (air or other gas that will not condense under the conditions of temperature and pressure used during the sterilization process). Dry, saturated steam is required for effective steam sterilization. Saturated steam acts like fog because it holds many tiny water droplets in suspension. The moisture content of saturated steam should possess a relative humidity (RH) of 97% to 100%. In other words, steam ideally should consist of (by weight) two to three parts of saturated water and 97 to 98 parts of dry, saturated steam.

Saturated steam is similar to air with 100% RH. When saturated steam cools, water condenses as a liquid. The pressure exerted by saturated steam is constant for a given temperature, and the pressure varies in direct proportion to that temperature. In other words, the higher the temperature, the higher the pressure. To increase steam temperature, pressure must be increased; to decrease the steam temperature, pressure must be decreased.

Saturated steam Steam that contains the maximum amount of water vapor.

Noncondensable gases Gases that cannot be liquified by compression under the conditions of temperature and pressure used during the sterilization process.

Temperature		Absolute Pressure	Gauge Pressure (lbs/in)	
F	C	psia	Sea Level	One Mile Altitude
212	100	14.696	0	2.7
220	104	17.186	2.5	5
225	107	18.912	4	7
230	110	20.779	6	9
235	113	22.800	8	11
240	115.5	24.968	10	13
245	118	27.312	13	15
250	121	29.825	15	18
255	125	32.532	18	20.5
260	127	35.427	21	23
265	129	38.537	24	26.5
270	132	41.856	27	30
275	135	45.426	31	33
280	138	49.200	35	37
285	140.5	53.249	39	41

Figure 14.18 Steam table

The atmospheric room pressure at sea level is 14.7 pounds per square inch (PSI) at room temperature. While the pressure gauges on sterilizers at sea level are set at zero, the pressure is really 14.7 PSI. After the sterilizer's door is closed and the sterilization cycle begins, steam is injected into the chamber. Then, the temperature rises, as does the pressure in the compartment. **Figure 14.18** shows the temperature and pressure relationship.

> **Dry or Wet Steam?**
>
> When baking a turkey in an oven with dry heat, it may take hours for the center of the turkey to become cooked compared to one placed in a pressure cooker with saturated steam. Saturated steam is a much better "carrier" of thermal energy than dry steam.

One of the concerns with steam sterilization is super-heated (dry) steam. Superheating can occur if the main steam supply is dry. Super-heated steam reaches higher temperatures than saturated steam, and due to the lack of moisture, it is a poor sterilant. If the steam is not saturated (less than 97% to 100% RH), the following problems can develop (one or all of which will interfere with the effectiveness of sterilization):

- Items in the sterilizer will remain dry, and microorganisms cannot be killed as readily as under wet conditions.
- Textiles and paper become scorched and rubber deteriorates rapidly.

BASIC WORK PRACTICES TO FACILITATE THE STEAM STERILIZATION PROCESS

Medical devices must be properly prepared before sterilization to ensure steam will come in contact with all surfaces. This section provides sterilization preparation guidance for processing some common medical devices.

Preparing Devices and Packs for Steam Sterilization

Effective sterilization requires that the sterilizing agent contact all surfaces of the devices for the prescribed time. Air removal, steam penetration and condensate drainage are enhanced by proper positioning—and by the use of perforated or mesh-bottom trays or baskets. **Figure 14.19** illustrates a mesh-bottom tray. Instrument sets should be prepared in trays large enough to equally distribute the mass, and the configuration of instrument sets should be evaluated to help ensure they remain dry.

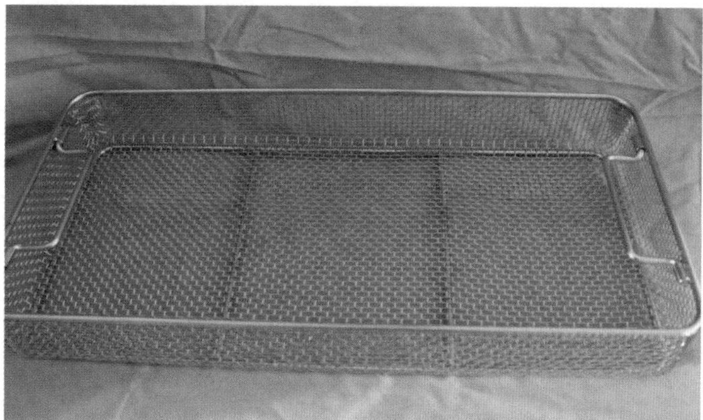

Figure 14.19

Loading a Steam Sterilizer

To ensure full steam contact and removal of air, the sterilizer must be properly loaded to allow adequate air circulation and drainage of the condensate. Care should be taken not to exceed the load requirements for the sterilizer. Prior to loading, refer to the specific sterilizer's IFU for loading requirements.

Basic procedures for loading a sterilizer include:

- Allowing for proper steam penetration and avoiding overloading. Packages must be placed for efficient air removal, steam penetration and evacuation.
- Positioning instrument sets in a way that allows air to exit and steam to enter.
- Ensuring there is a visible space between packs to allow steam circulation and drying.
- When combining loads, placing hard goods, such as rigid containers, on the bottom to prevent condensation from dripping onto lower packs.
- Ensuring that packages do not touch chamber walls.
- Standing basin sets on edge. They should be tilted for drainage so if water is present, it will run out. **Figure 14.20** uses an unwrapped basin to illustrate how basins should be positioned for adequate drainage.
- Positioning textile packs so the layers within them are perpendicular to the shelf. **Figure 14.21** uses two unwrapped towel packs to illustrate how they should be placed on the sterilizer rack to facilitate the sterilization process.
- Standing paper/plastic peel pouches on edge using a basket or rack. Placing them plastic side down may cause moisture to remain inside, and placing them plastic side up may cause water to stand on top of the plastic. Place them so that the sterilization pouches are placed paper-to-plastic for air and steam circulation. (See **Figure 14.22**)
- When possible, sterilizing textiles and hard goods in separate loads. If this is not possible, textiles should be placed on top shelves with hard goods placed below to avoid condensation runoff from the hard goods onto the textiles.

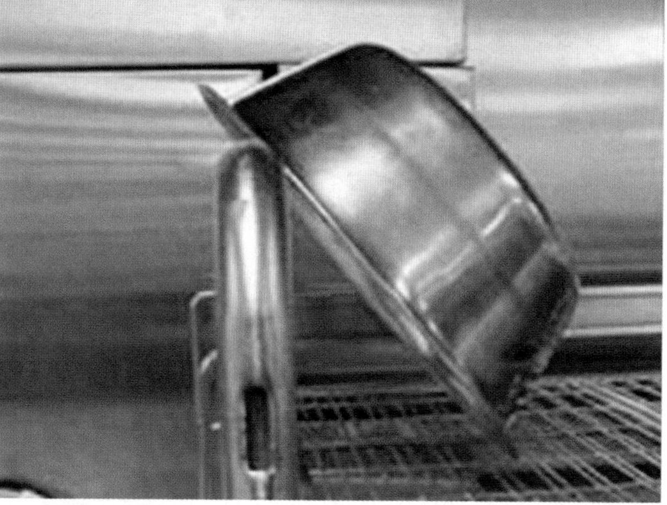

Figure 14.20

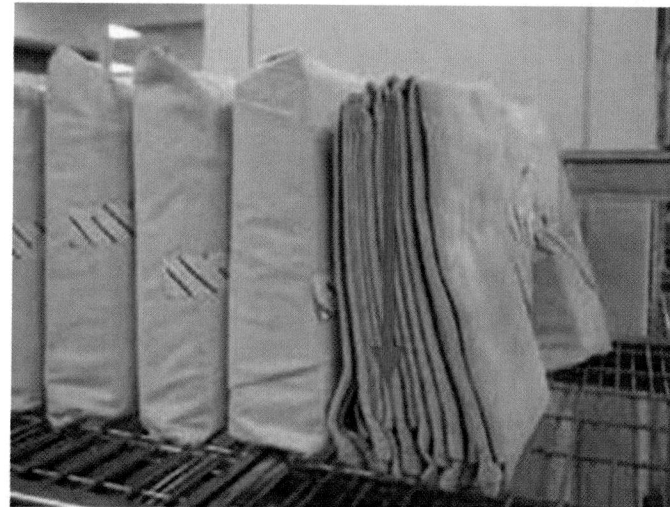

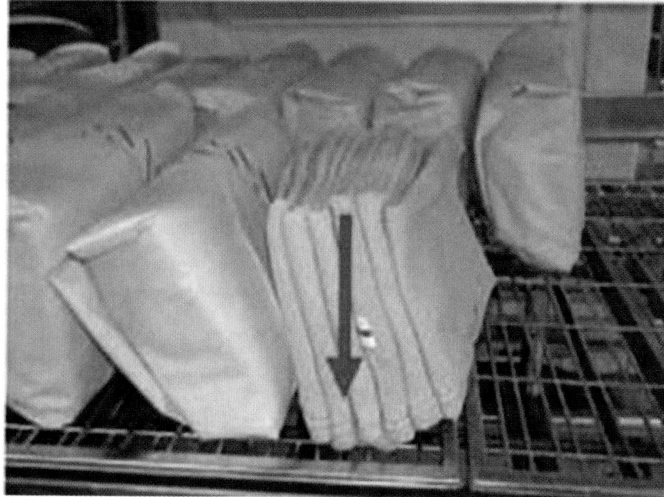

Figure 14.21

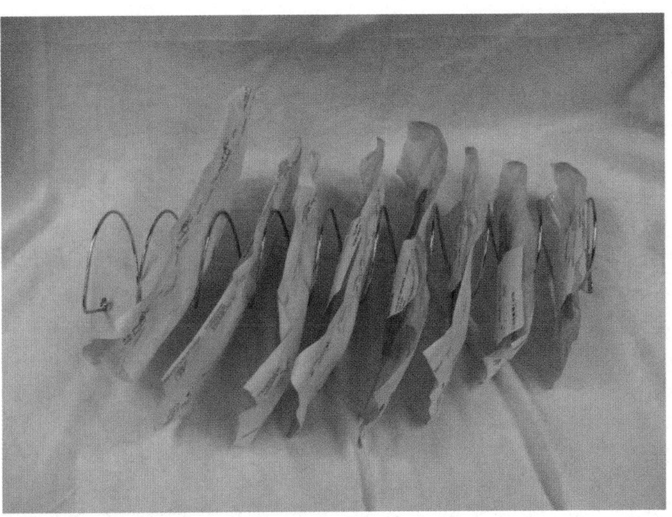

Figure 14.22

- Ensuring that surgical instrument trays with perforated bottoms and most rigid container systems sit flat on the shelf to maintain even instrument distribution and facilitate proper drainage. Standing these instrument sets on their edge permits moisture to collect at the standing edge. **Figure 14.23** uses an unwrapped, perforated instrument tray to illustrate how perforated instrument trays should be placed on the sterilizer rack.

- If a shelf liner is used, it should only be comprised of absorbent material. (See **Figure 14.24**)

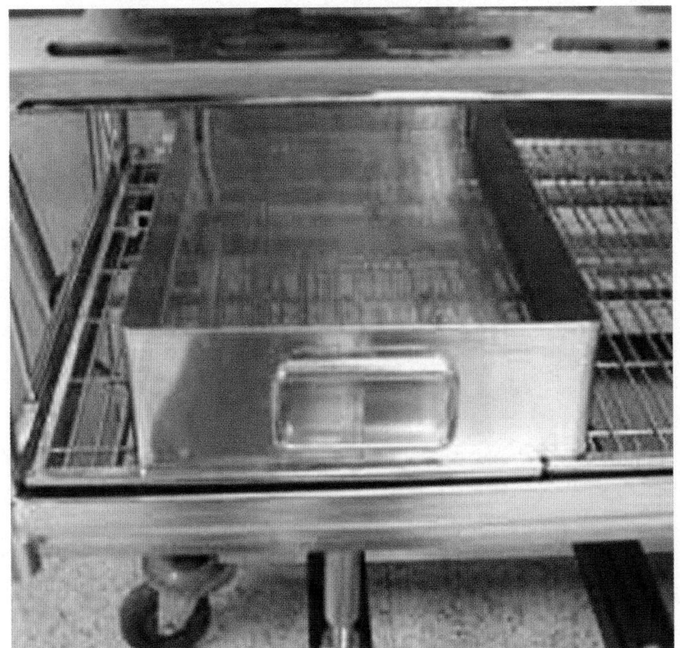

Figure 14.23

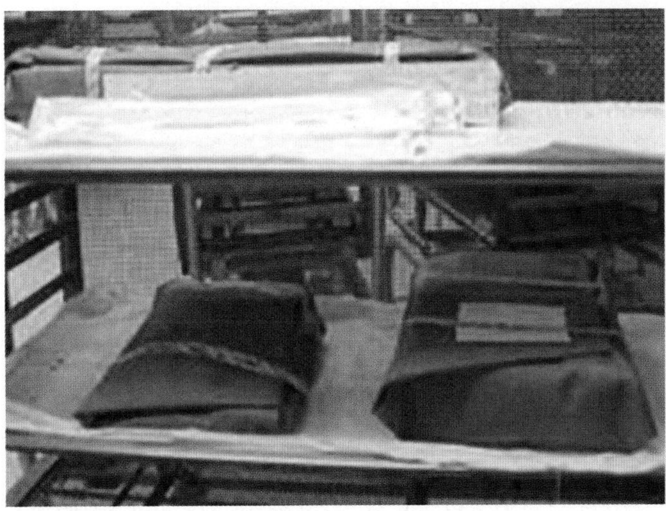

Figure 14.24

Unloading a Steam Sterilizer

When sterilization is complete, follow the sterilizer IFU for opening the sterilizer door. When the cart is removed, it should be placed in a low-traffic area where there are no air conditioning or other cold air vents in close proximity. For sterilizers without carts, items should remain in the sterilizer chamber until properly cooled.

An infrared device or other type of temperature-sensing device may be used to verify that sterilized items have reached room temperature. The cooling time may be only 30 minutes for small sets or peel pouches but can take two hours or longer for larger sets. The cooling time must account for critical factors such as the type of sterilizer used, the design of the device and packaging being sterilized, and the temperature and humidity of the room. The packages may still contain some steam vapor. If packages are touched at this point, the vapor present might carry microorganisms from one's hand through the packaging material, leading to contamination of the item.

The load contents should be visibly free of any liquid. Water droplets on the outside of packages or on the rails of carts signal that every item in the load should be visually inspected. *Caution: Do not touch items during visual inspection.* Wet items should be considered contaminated, even if they have not been touched.

To unload sterile items:

- Do not unload packages before they are cool. Placing hot or warm packages on cold surfaces will cause condensation to develop beneath and/or between them. If warm packages are placed in plastic protective covers, condensate will be trapped until opened, and the moisture may damage items underneath the protective cover.

- Handle the sterile packages as little as possible. Items should not be moved or touched until they have cooled to room temperature.

Controlling Wet Packs

Wet packs may occur when a steam sterilization process is used. Packages are considered wet when moisture in the form of dampness, droplets or puddles of water are found on or within a package after a completed sterilization cycle. Moisture can create a pathway for microorganisms to travel from the outside to the inside of a package. **Figure 14.25** provides an example of condensation (wetness) on the outside of a tray. **Figure 14.26** provides an example of moisture on the inside of a tray. If moisture is present on one pack, the problem may be isolated to that one set. To ensure the problem is isolated to only one pack, other packs in the load may be opened to check for moisture. If there are several wet packs from one load, the entire load should be considered wet. Wet packs cannot be released and should be reported for immediate follow up.

A wet pack is considered contaminated and must be completely reprocessed.

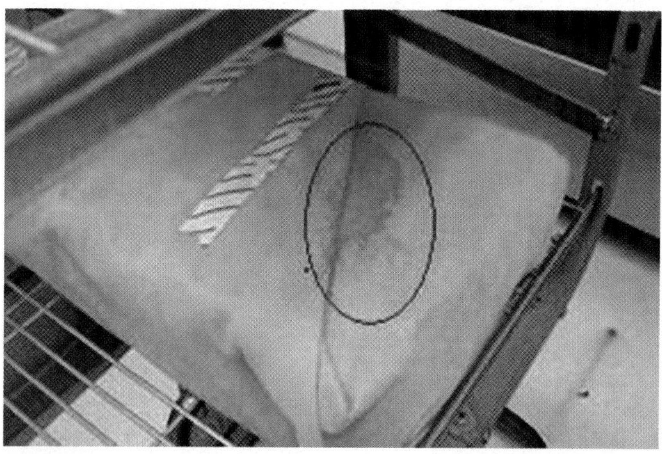
Figure 14.25

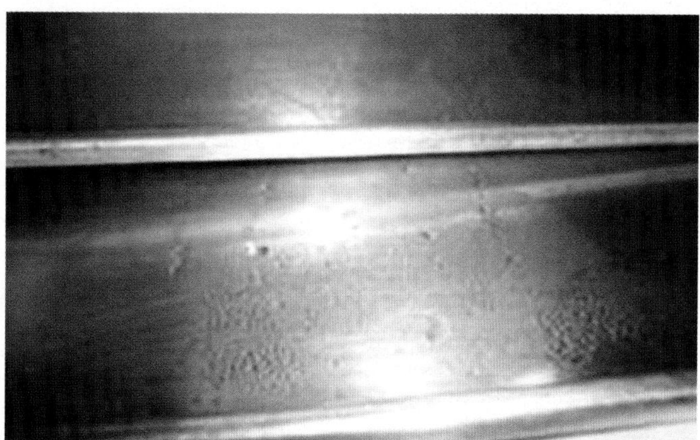
Figure 14.26

Wet Pack Documentation

All wet packs should be documented. Because of the complexity of the issue, finding the cause of and cure for wet packs and/or wet loads can be difficult as there are many factors to take into consideration. Investigation is a multi-step process. Documenting wet pack occurrences may identify a pattern that can pinpoint the root cause. For example, documentation may show that only the plastic instrument sets, specialty devices, packages prepared by another department or processed by a specific SP technician are involved. It may also show a pattern of steam usage within the facility or changes in steam quality during a certain time of year. Identifying the root cause of the wet packs is crucial for preventing additional wet packs. External moisture on packs is usually noticed immediately when the packs are removed from the sterilizer. Internal moisture will not be noticed until the packs are opened for use unless the moisture wicks through the wrap. (See **Figure 14.27**)

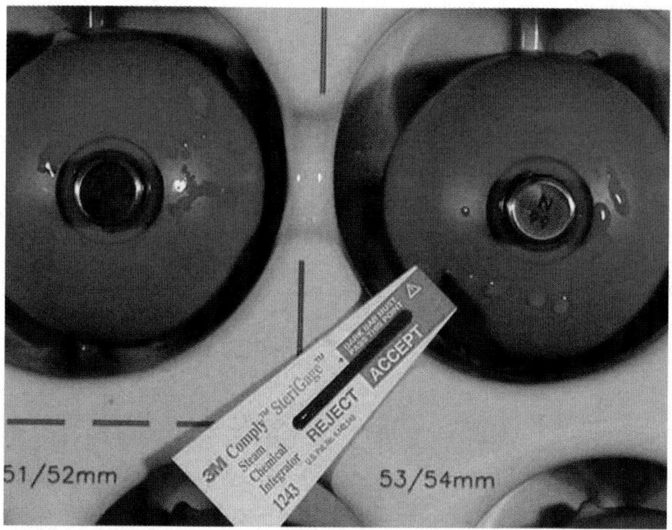

Figure 14.27

Causes of Wet Packs

Primary causes of wet packs arising from SP preparation techniques include:

- Packs that were improperly prepared or loaded incorrectly for sterilization. This is the most frequent cause of wet packs.
- Heavy or dense instrument sets
- Packs wrapped too tightly
- Improperly prepared items such as items wrapped while moist
- Metal items positioned in a way that allows water to pool or trap steam
- Instrument and basin sets that are too dense or overloaded
- Linen packs wrapped too tightly, causing them to retain moisture

- Improper placement of concave items, such as medicine cups, in a position that does not allow for drainage
- Not using correct filters or incorrectly placing the filter on a container

Another reason for wet packs may be the sterilizer itself. Listed below are two of the most common reasons that can be identified by an SP technician:

- Gasket not completely intact. *Note: Door gaskets wear out over time. Regularly scheduled preventive maintenance programs help ensure door gaskets are inspected and replaced prior to deterioration.*
- Clogged chamber drain strainer.

Other causes of wet packs can only be identified and resolved by a qualified sterilizer service technician. Such causes may include:

- Broken valves
- Malfunctioning steam traps or drain check valves
- Faulty sterilizer gauges or controllers
- Clogged drain line
- Faulty drain valves

Wet packs may also be caused for reasons occurring outside the SPD. As previously stated, these reasons can be attributed to the boiler or steam delivery system. Although the SPD does not control these factors, it is important to be aware of some factors from outside the SPD that can contribute to wet packs, including:

- Steam quality that does not meet the requirements of the sterilizer
- Blocked steam lines
- Boiler feed water that contains too many non-condensable gases, including air
- Boiler not properly maintained
- Malfunctioning steam traps or check valves
- Poorly engineered steam piping
- Increased demands for the steam supply

Wet packs can also be caused by environmental factors such as removing a hot load and placing it in an air-conditioned area or an area with humidity exceeding 70%.

Extended Sterilization Cycles

Healthcare facilities typically use standard cycles for a majority of items processed. Occasionally, however, medical instrumentation manufacturers' IFU may include an extended exposure time, which is known as an extended cycle (based on the device's complex design and materials).

SP technicians must obtain, review and consistently follow the manufacturer's written recommendations for all medical devices they process.

Most medical devices require standard cycle times. Damage to some items can occur if items requiring standard sterilizing times are processed with other devices that require an extended cycle. For that reason, extended cycle items should not be sterilized with items that require a different cycle time. Items should never be sterilized in any cycle that deviates from the specific manufacturer's instructions.

Cleaning and Maintaining Sterilizers

The sterilizer manufacturer's written recommendations for sterilizer maintenance must always be followed. The following general cleaning and maintenance guidelines illustrate manufacturer recommendations:

- The chamber drain strainer should be removed at least daily and cleaned thoroughly under running water using a non-abrasive brush and mild detergent. This procedure may be needed more frequently depending on the types of loads processed. If debris is allowed to build up, it may be necessary to soak the strainer before cleaning. **Figure 14.28** shows an improperly maintained strainer that is clogged and will not allow proper air or steam removal.
- The door gasket should be inspected and wiped clean daily with a clean, damp, non-linting cloth. During inspection, look for defects or signs of wear or deterioration, especially if the unit has a vacuum cycle.
- Carriages, carts and loading baskets should be routinely cleaned with a mild solution. Follow the manufacturer's IFU for cleaning and lubrication requirements.
- Carriages, carts and loading baskets should be checked to ensure they are not damaged and can move freely in and out of the sterilizer chamber.
- Follow the manufacturer's instructions about the need and method for cleaning and flushing the chamber's drain. Air and steam will not pass efficiently if the drain line is blocked.

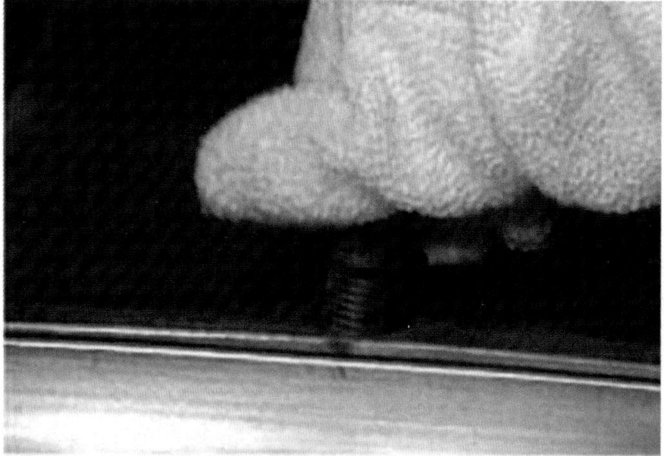

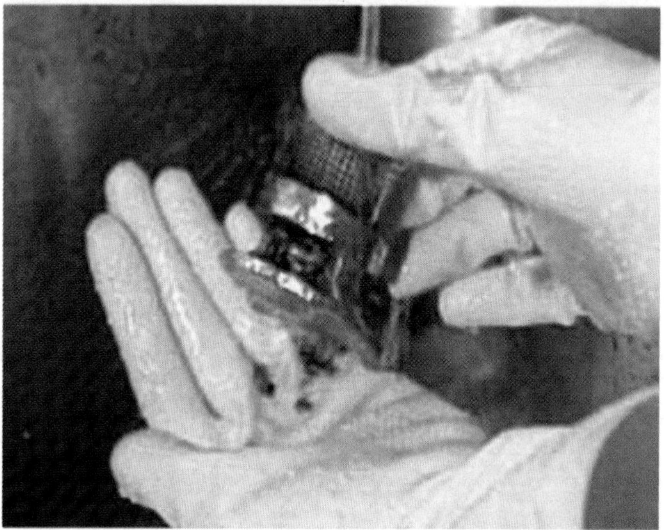

Figure 14.28

- Cool the chamber before performing any cleaning or maintenance procedure.

- The inside of the chamber should be cleaned according to the manufacturer's instructions. Problems with residue buildup on the chamber's interior can affect the cycle's drying ability. Residues in the chamber can leave deposits on instruments and wrappers. **Figure 14.29** illustrates residue buildup in a sterilizer chamber. Clean with non-abrasive and non-linting products. Rinse detergent and residue from the chamber thoroughly to avoid deposits on devices during sterilization.

- Strong abrasives or steel wool should never be used on the sterilizer because they can scratch the surface and encourage corrosion. While sterilizer chambers are made of corrosion-resistant materials, some steam boiler water treatment chemicals can penetrate the chamber if the surface is damaged. Chambers that have not been properly maintained may require professional cleaning.

- Inspect recording devices daily, including paper charts and printer paper.

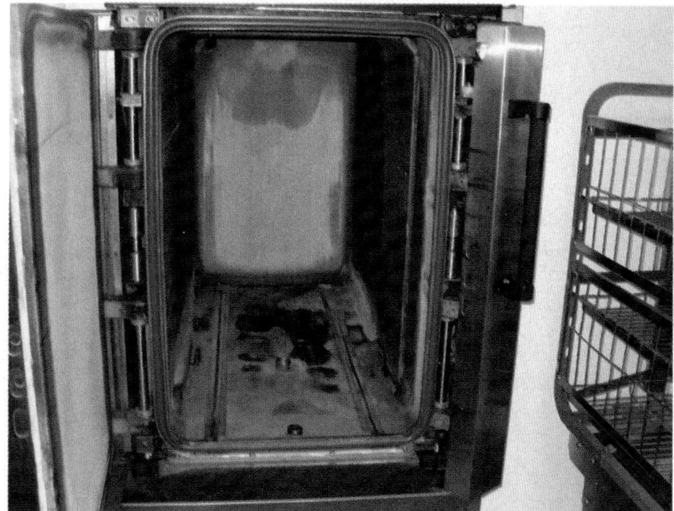

Figure 14.29

CONCLUSION

SP technicians who understand the steam sterilization process reduce the risk of sterilization failure. Knowing when there could be an issue with a steam cycle may allow the load contents to be reviewed and, if necessary, reprocessed before the items are distributed or used on a patient.

RESOURCES

ANSI/AAMI ST79:2017 & 2020 Amendments A1, A2,A3, A4 (Consolidated Text) *Comprehensive guide to steam sterilization and sterility assurance in health care facilities.*

Centers for Disease Control and Prevention. *Guideline for Disinfection and Sterilization in Healthcare Facilities.* 2008.

Huys J. *Sterilization of Medical Supplies by Steam, Volume 1, General Theory.* 2010.

STERILE PROCESSING TERMS

Bioburden

Saturated steam

Noncondensable gases

Chapter 15

Low-Temperature Sterilization

Learning Objectives

As a result of successfully completing this chapter, the reader will be able to:

1. Discuss basic requirements for low-temperature sterilization systems
2. Explain different types of low-temperature sterilization
3. Review parameters of low-temperature sterilization methods

INTRODUCTION

Low-temperature sterilization is important due to the development and growing use of heat- and moisture-sensitive medical devices. Ethylene oxide (EO) and hydrogen peroxide (H_2O_2) are the low-temperature sterilization methods commonly used in healthcare settings. Chemicals used to sterilize instruments have toxic properties, although levels of toxicity and potential for exposure vary widely, based on the sterilization method and sterilant used. As a result, Sterile Processing (SP) technicians must be trained on how to use them safely and effectively. Each low-temperature sterilization method has advantages and limitations, and each type of low-temperature sterilizer has specific process requirements that must be met. This chapter reviews common low-temperature systems and the basic requirements for their use.

BASIC REQUIREMENTS FOR LOW-TEMPERATURE STERILIZATION

Eight basic requirements are important for any type of low-temperature sterilization system:

- Efficacy (effectiveness) – Has the capability of providing the minimum-required **sterility assurance level (SAL)**.

> **Sterility assurance level (SAL)** The probability of a viable microorganism being present on a device after sterilization.

- Safety – There should be no toxic residuals remaining on the packaging or device upon completion of the sterilization cycle.
- Exposure monitoring – Ability to monitor the sterilization process to ensure concentrations of sterilants in the work area remain within any required exposure limits.
- Sterilization performance monitoring – Must be capable of being reliably monitored using physical, chemical indicators (CIs) and biological indicators (BIs).
- Penetration – Must be able to penetrate through packaging materials and into lumens and other the devices other hard-to-reach areas.
- Material compatibility – There should be no changes in the device's functionality.
- Adaptability – Should be compatible with existing healthcare practices.
- Approval – Must be cleared by or registered with the appropriate regulatory agencies.

To be effective in the healthcare environment, a sterilization system must satisfy all requirements; failure to meet even one requirement may pose a significant risk to patients and healthcare workers.

Efficacy

To be legally marketed in the U.S., the U.S. Food and Drug Administration (FDA) requires each sterilant and sterilization technology to be rigorously tested against a broad range of microorganisms. The low-temperature sterilization technologies addressed in this chapter use different sterilization agents and have different processing methods. When used according to the sterilizer's instructions for use (IFU), each sterilization method meets the required minimum SAL, as outlined by the regulations, standards and guidelines.

Safety

Chemicals used as sterilants are designed to destroy a wide range of pathogens; however, the same properties that make them effective sterilants also make them harmful to humans. In sterilization methods, such as EO, significant toxic residues can build up in medical devices and packaging. To ensure a safe work environment, low-temperature sterilization systems should be used according to the manufacturers' instructions, and appropriate work practices, engineering controls, personal protective equipment (PPE), and monitoring should be followed.

Exposure Monitoring

EO has been widely used as a low-temperature sterilant since the 1950s. It has potential health risks that require monitoring, in addition to long aeration times and other precautions. While safer for healthcare workers, newer low-temperature sterilization technologies also can pose health risks. To ensure the safety of healthcare workers, the Occupational Safety and Health Administration (OSHA) has established **permissible exposure limits (PELs)** for all low-temperature sterilants. These exposure limits are expressed as an eight-hour, **time-weighted average (TWA)**: the total allowable worker exposure during an eight-hour period.

> **Permissible exposure limit (PEL)** The maximum amount or concentration of a chemical that a worker may be exposed to under OSHA regulations.
>
> **Time-weighted average (TWA)** The amount of a substance employees can be exposed to over an eight-hour day.

The National Institute for Occupational Safety and Health (NIOSH) also has developed standards for immediately dangerous to life or health (IDLH) concentrations for low-temperature sterilants.

Sterilizer Performance Monitoring

Monitoring sterilizer performance is essential to ensure the successful sterilization of medical instruments and devices. No single monitoring method provides all of the information necessary to ensure effective sterilization; Recommended practices state that available information from physical, chemical and biological monitors should be used to assess the effectiveness of a process before releasing a load. It is essential that SP technicians understand how to handle and use CIs and BIs and also know how to read and interpret their results.

Penetration

Many devices are significantly more complex than their counterparts of just a few years ago. Not only must the sterilant penetrate packaging material (in some cases, multiple layers), it must also reach narrow lumens.

The properties of a chemical sterilant impact its ability to penetrate effectively. For example, EO inactivates microbes by a process called **alkylation**. This allows EO to penetrate packaging and materials to reach remote surfaces where microbes may be located. Hydrogen peroxide destroys microbes through **oxidation**.

Alkylation A chemical reaction where hydrogen is replaced with an alkyl group; this renders the cell unable to normally metabolize or reproduce, or both.

Oxidation Involves the act or process of oxidizing, which is the addition of oxygen to a compound with a loss of electrons.

Materials Compatibility

Medical devices are composed of a variety of materials that may be affected by sterilant ingredients. Sterilizers must be tested to establish compatibility with a wide range of materials. Medical device manufacturers test the compatibility of their devices with one or more of the available sterilization technologies. Compatibility information can be found in the IFU. The manufacturer's IFU should be carefully followed to help ensure successful sterilization and prevent damage that may increase costs and limit instrument availability.

Adaptability

The low-temperature sterilization process should be compatible with existing device processing practices.

Approval

The sterilization system must be cleared and registered with the appropriate regulatory agencies.

ETHYLENE OXIDE

Background

For more than 60 years, EO gas has been an effective sterilization technology for heat- and moisture-sensitive medical devices. **Figure 15.1** shows an EO sterilizer.

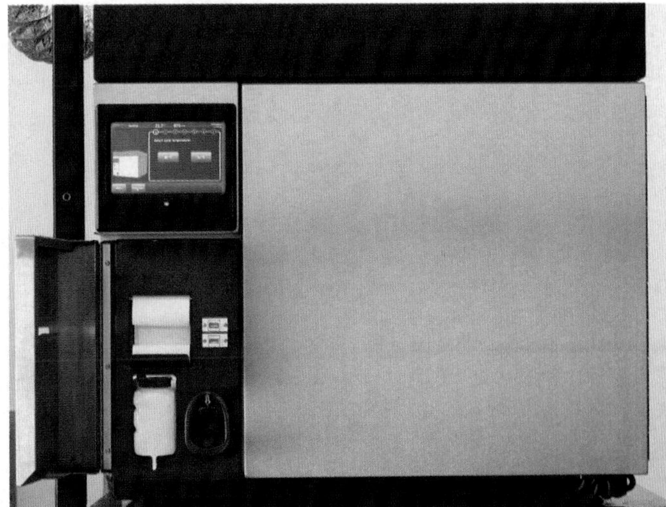

Figure 15.1

Efficacy

EO has excellent microbicidal activity. During the alkylation process, EO destroys the cell's ability to metabolize or reproduce, which leads to the organism's death.

Penetration

EO is a small molecule that vaporizes easily and can permeate throughout a wide range of materials to reach recessed areas. Due to its high vapor pressure and low boiling point, EO is easily maintained in the gas phase.

Sterilization Cycle and Process Parameters

In healthcare EO systems, the gas is provided in individual dose cartridges that are placed inside the chamber. If a leak develops after the cartridge is punctured (see **Figure 15.2**) the ventilation system will pull room air into the chamber rather than allow EO to be released.

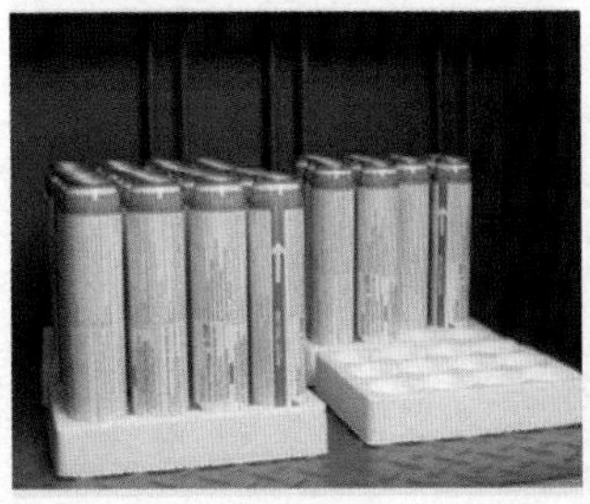

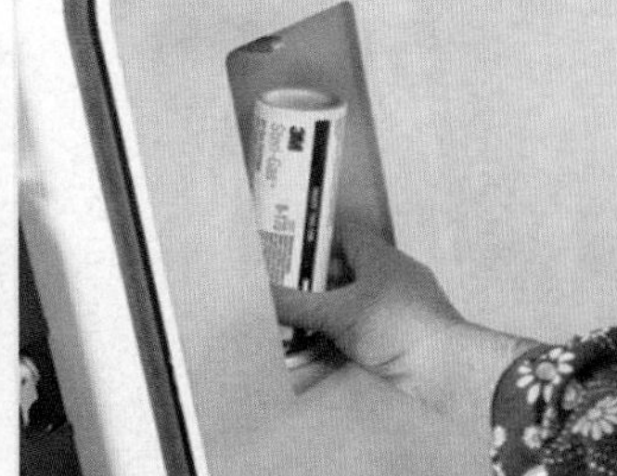

Figure 15.2 100% ethylene oxide cartridges

The basic EO sterilization cycle consists of five stages: preconditioning and humidification, gas introduction, exposure, evacuation and air washes. The cycle takes approximately 2½ to 3½ hours, excluding **aeration** time. Upon completion of the sterilization cycle, the items must go through an aeration process to remove all **residual EO** before the sterilizer can be unlocked and the items can be removed.

Operators should demonstrate competency in all parameters of EO sterilization.

Aeration A process in which sterilized packages are subjected to moving air to facilitate removal of toxic residuals after exposure to a sterilizing agent such as EO.

Residual EO Amount of EO that remains inside materials after they are sterilized.

Safety

EO is a toxic gas classified by OSHA as a carcinogen and reproductive hazard. To protect SP technicians, EO sterilizers should be in a well-ventilated area, with a room air exchange rate of at least 10 changes per hour. The sterilizers are installed in negative-pressure rooms with contained ventilation systems venting to the outside. Ventilation systems, exhaust lines and floor drains should be periodically checked by qualified personnel to ensure they are working properly.

Today's EO sterilizers are designed for safety and have many engineering safeguards to prevent personnel from coming in contact with EO. In addition, environmental engineering controls protect SP technicians. (See **Figure 15.3**)

Cartridges with 100% EO should be stored in a ventilated flammable liquid storage cabinet that is exhausted outside, away from heat, sparks and sunlight.

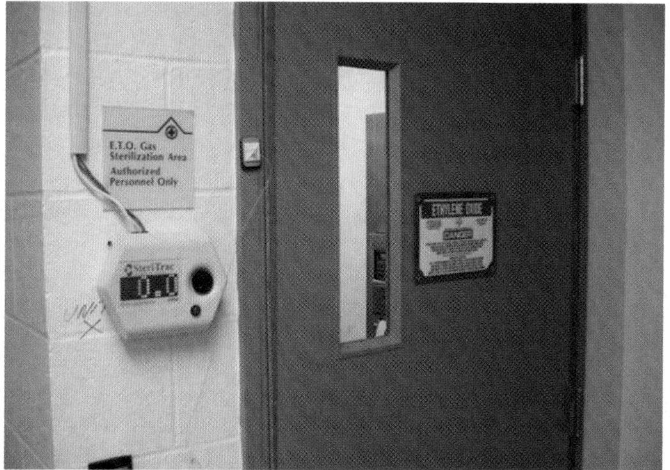

Figure 15.3 Ethylene oxide sterilization room with air monitor

To minimize the safety risks associated with the use of EO, employees should be instructed about:

- EO hazards
- Sterilizer manufacturer and EO supplier IFU
- Processing procedures
- Storage and handling of EO cartridges
- Procedures to reduce employee exposure to EO
- Use of PPE
- Principles of EO monitoring and interpretation of results
- Handling canceled cycles
- Applicable OSHA regulations
- **Safety data sheets (SDS)**
- EO emergency plans

Safety data sheet (SDS) A written statement providing detailed information about a chemical or toxic substance, including potential hazards and appropriate handling methods. An SDS is provided by the product manufacturer to the buyer and must be available in a place that is easily accessible to those who will use the product.

Exposure Monitoring

Personal monitoring involves the use of devices affixed directly to the employee's clothing in the breathing zone (within one foot of the person's nose; See **Figure 15.4**) One limitation of personal monitoring devices is that sampling results are not available until after the actual sampling period has ended. OSHA requires that facilities using EO sterilization have a system or procedure to immediately alert affected employees in case of a leak, spill or equipment failure.

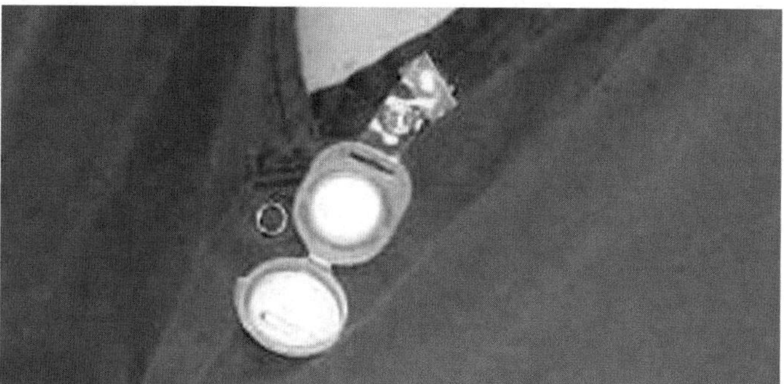

Figure 15.4

Example of an area monitoring system

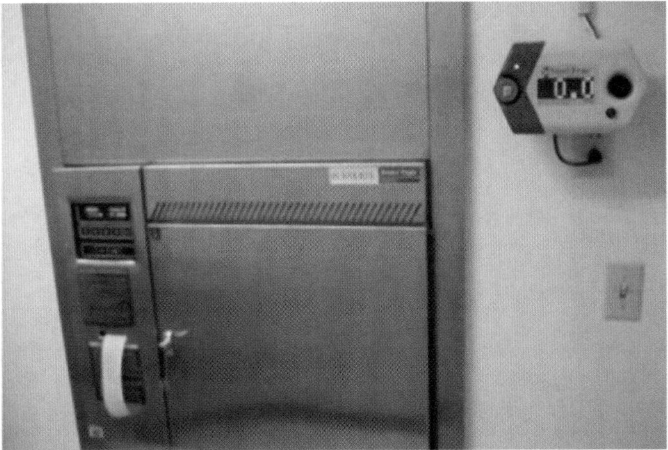

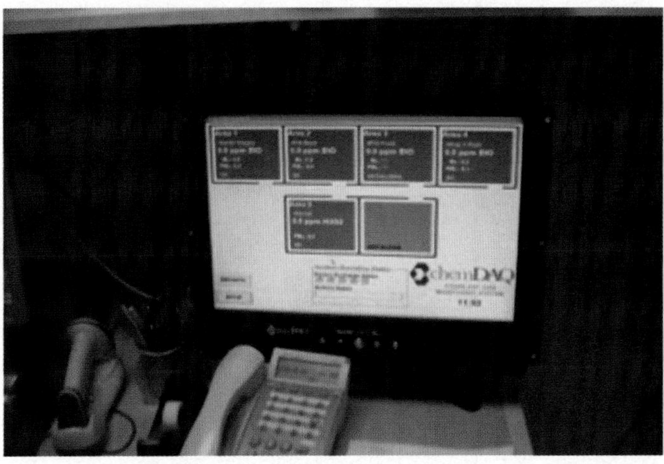

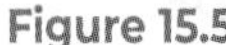
Figure 15.5

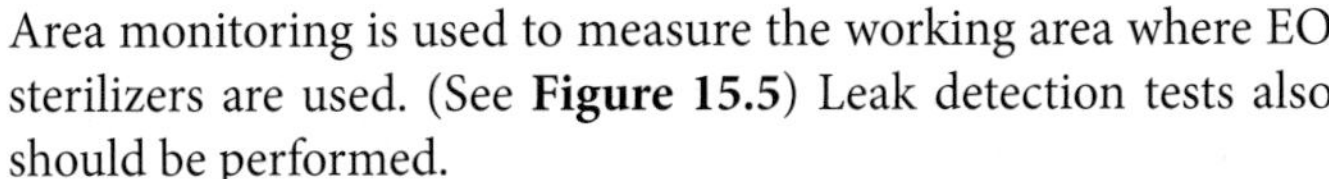

Area monitoring is used to measure the working area where EO sterilizers are used. (See **Figure 15.5**) Leak detection tests also should be performed.

According to OSHA, the employer shall keep an accurate record of all measurements taken to monitor employee exposure to EO. This information includes:

- Date of measurement
- Sampling and analytical methods used and evidence of their accuracy
- Number, duration and results of samples taken
- Type of protective devices worn, if any
- Name of employees whose exposures are represented

The employer shall maintain this record for at least 30 years. OSHA also requires that medical surveillance records for each employee exposed to high levels of EO be kept for the duration of employment, plus 30 years. For specific monitoring requirements, refer to federal, state and local regulations.

Materials Compatibility

EO has excellent compatibility with many reusable medical devices. SP technicians must follow specific device manufacturer recommendations for the appropriate sterilization process.

EO should not be used to sterilize:

- Liquids – EO will combine with liquids and may produce harmful chemical byproducts.
- Devices with energy sources – Energy sources could create a spark in the sterilization chamber during the sterilization cycle.
- Leather items – Chemicals used in the tanning process will combine with EO to form chlorohydrin, which can cause negative health effects.

Packaging

EO sterilization is compatible with a variety of packaging materials, including paper/plastic or Tyvek peel pouches, approved fabric wrappers, medical crepe paper, polypropylene, and most container systems. *Note: Aluminum foil, cellophane, nylon films, polyester, PVC (plastic) films and Styrofoam should not be used.*

Loading and Unloading EO Sterilizers

Proper loading is important since overloading impedes proper air removal, load humidification, sterilant penetration, and aeration. Items should be arranged to avoid contact with chamber walls. Pouches should be placed on edge in wire baskets. Stacking instrument sets should be avoided. *Note: The Environmental Protection Agency requires that EO sterilizers only be operated with full loads of items that share common aeration times. Emergency circumstances may require sterilization of less than full loads. If a less than full load is sterilized due to medical necessity, the operator must record this as well. These records must be kept for five years, and at least the most recent two years must be on site.*

Aeration

Because EO can be absorbed by many materials, aeration is required to remove EO residual gases before instruments and packaging can be safely handled.

Biological testing for ethylene oxide

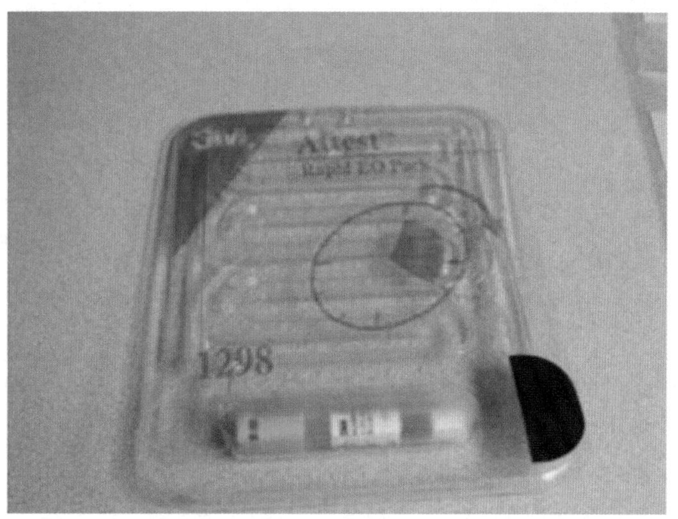

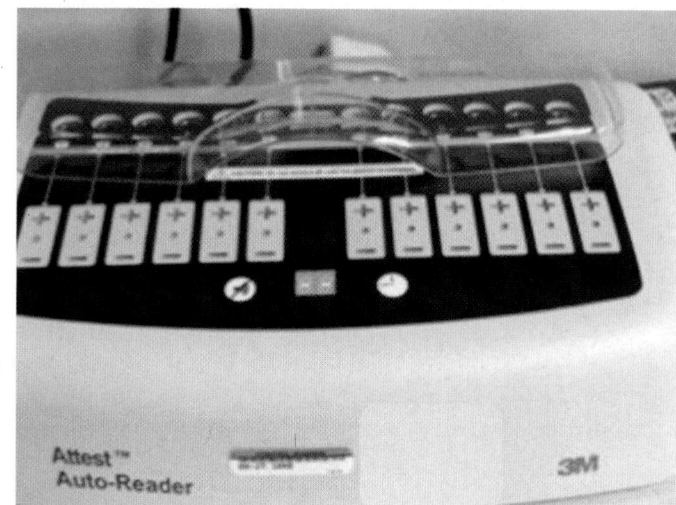

Figure 15.6 Examples of a biological indicator (left) and biological incubator

When the exposure cycle ends, one or more vacuum pulses remove EO from the chamber. The aeration phase then takes place as warm air circulates through the chamber to remove residuals. For aeration recommendations, consult the devices manufacturer's IFU.

Sterilizer Performance Monitors

An EO sterilizer should be monitored with physical monitors and CIs and BIs. While none of these provide conclusive evidence of device sterility on their own, they do provide a high degree of sterility assurance when used in combination.

- Physical monitors – Physical monitors include operating pressure gauges, temperature control/measurement devices, timing recorders, and humidity sensors. Charts, graphs and printouts detailing the measurements made by physical monitors must be carefully examined to ensure the correct parameters were met before devices are removed from the sterilizer.
- Chemical monitoring – External CIs should be used on the outside of every instrument package to demonstrate that each pack has been processed. Internal CIs should be used inside every package to measure whether the sterilant has penetrated the packaging.
- Biological monitoring – Biological monitoring is required for each cycle run in an EO sterilizer. The microorganism of choice for EO is the *Bacillus atrophaeus* spore. Follow the sterilizer manufacturer's IFU for proper BI placement and incubation. (See **Figure 15.6**)

HYDROGEN PEROXIDE SYSTEMS

Several types of low-temperature systems use H_2O_2 as the sterilant. While the systems operate similarly, there are some key differences.

Hydrogen Peroxide Gas Plasma

Background

The more recent low-temperature sterilization technologies includes H_2O_2 gas plasma for the inactivation of microorganisms. This method is popular due to its safety, relative to EO, and its cycle times that allow faster turnaround of medical devices. The byproducts of the cycle (water vapor and oxygen) are nontoxic, eliminating the need for an aeration phase.

H_2O_2 is a highly effective sterilant that sterilizes by oxidation of key cellular components. Plasma is a state of matter distinguishable from a solid, liquid or gas.

Efficacy

H_2O_2 gas plasma—using a hydrogen peroxide solution ranging from 59% to 95% for the sterilization cycle—has been proven effective for killing microorganisms.

Penetration

H_2O_2 gas plasma sterilizers use deep vacuums, multiple pulse additions of the sterilant, and increased concentrations. These systems can sterilize a wide range of devices.

Guidelines have been developed for lumen diameter and length to ensure adequate penetration and efficacy for various cycle parameters. Newer generations of H_2O_2 gas plasma sterilizers utilize a higher concentration of hydrogen peroxide (up to 95%) to shorten exposure time and lessen lumen restrictions. There are still some restrictions involving the size, length and number of lumens, and the type of material and number of devices per cycle. As always, users should closely follow the instrument and sterilizer manufacturers' instructions and recommendations.

Types of H_2O_2 Gas Plasma Systems

There are several types of H_2O_2 gas plasma sterilizers available, ranging from compact systems with 28- to 38-minute processing times to large-capacity systems with 75-minute cycle times. Different models have different cycle times, load capacities and capabilities for processing instruments. (See **Figure 15.7**)

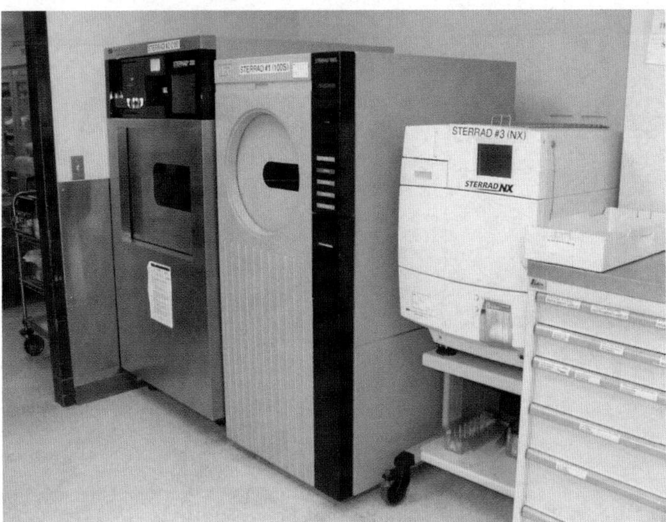

Figure 15.7

Sterilization Cycle and Process Parameters

The phases of H_2O_2 gas plasma include:

- Vacuum – The load is heated while the vacuum system removes air from the chamber and packages until the pressure is reduced to below atmospheric pressure.
- Injection – Once the correct pressure has been reached, a pre-measured amount of concentrated H_2O_2 is pumped into the chamber.
- Diffusion – This phase drives hydrogen peroxide vapor into the small crevices and lumens of devices.
- Plasma – A vacuum decreases the pressure, and radio frequency (RF) energy is radiated within the chamber from an electrode screen. The RF energy creates H_2O_2 gas plasma. The injection and plasma phases are repeated a second time.
- Vent – At the end of the second plasma sequence, air is vented into the chamber through bacterial high-efficiency particulate air (HEPA) filters, returning the chamber to atmospheric pressure. The process byproducts are water vapor and oxygen. Aeration is not required, and instruments can be used immediately after cooling.

Operators should demonstrate competency in all parameters of hydrogen peroxide (H_2O_2) gas plasma sterilization.

Safety

Concentrated H_2O_2 liquid can irritate skin and is damaging to eyes if direct contact occurs. A number of safeguards built into H_2O_2 sterilizers are designed to minimize the likelihood of personnel contacting H_2O_2.

The H_2O_2 is packaged in sealed containers (See **Figure 15.8**), with a chemical leak indicator on the outside of the package. These indicators change color when exposed to liquid or vapor H_2O_2.

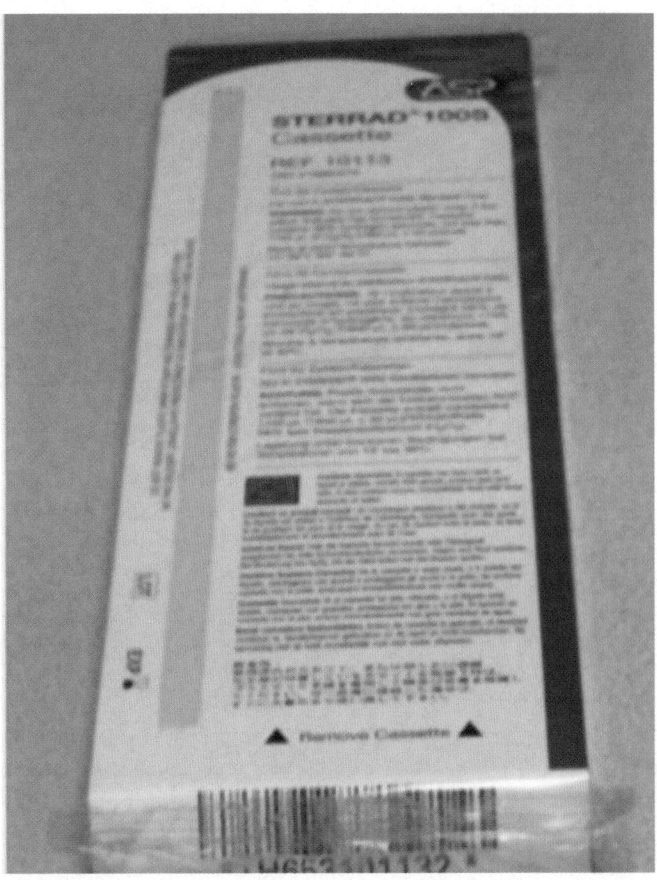

Figure 15.8 Example of a cassette for H_2O_2 gas plasma sterilization

To minimize the likelihood of exposure to H_2O_2 when removing items from a canceled cycle, SP technicians should always wear the recommended PPE. As with any chemical used for sterilization, healthcare workers should consult the SDS and follow all manufacturer recommendations and departmental procedures.

To minimize H_2O_2 risks, employees should be instructed about:

- Hazards of H_2O_2
- Storage, handling and disposal of H_2O_2
- Handling canceled cycles
- Applicable OSHA regulations
- Use of PPE
- SDS

Exposure Monitoring

Monitoring the area around the system during operation should be conducted according to the manufacturer's IFU and established guidelines.

Materials Compatibility

H_2O_2 gas plasma sterilization is compatible with a wide variety of materials found in medical devices; H_2O_2 gas plasma is not compatible with:

- Liquids and powders
- Any material that absorbs liquids
- Items that contain cellulose, such as cotton, paper or cardboard, textiles or any item containing wood pulp

Packaging

Packaging materials can affect the penetration of H_2O_2. Packaging materials used in the sterilizers should be designed to optimize diffusion of the H_2O_2 and not interfere with the RF energy or absorb H_2O_2.

Approved trays and container systems, polypropylene wrap and Tyvek pouches are compatible with H_2O_2 sterilization.

Cellulose-containing packaging materials, such as paper/plastic pouches, cellulose-based disposable wrappers, and muslin wraps, should not be used with H_2O_2 gas plasma sterilizers because they absorb the peroxide and inhibit effective penetration.

Excess moisture remaining on devices can cause the cycle to abort. Consult the manufacturer's IFU for suggested drying methods.

Loading H_2O_2 Gas Plasma Sterilizers

As with other low-temperature sterilization technologies, H_2O_2 gas plasma sterilizers must be properly loaded for effective sterilization. If the available amount of H_2O_2 is reduced because it reacts or is absorbed before reaching all surfaces, a sterilization failure could occur; therefore, the chamber should not be overloaded. (See **Figure 15.9**)

NEED A DUPLICATE
PRINTOUT?
PUSH THE CANCEL
BUTTON.
NEVER THROW ANY
PRINTOUT AWAY.
STERRAD

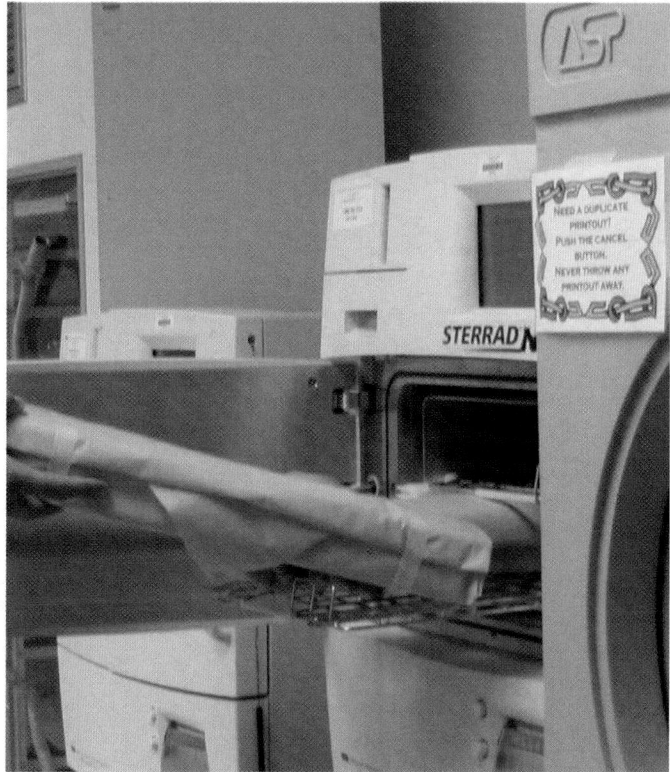

Figure 15.9

Sterilizer Performance Monitors

H_2O_2 gas plasma sterilizers should be monitored with physical indicators, CIs and BIs. Sterilizer performance monitors include:

- Physical monitoring – H_2O_2 gas plasma sterilizers operate on a fixed automatic cycle controlled by a microprocessor. All critical parameters are monitored during the operation of the cycle, and a printed record documenting the process parameters is provided at the end of each cycle. All physical monitors must be carefully examined to ensure the correct parameters were met before devices are removed from the sterilizer.
- Chemical monitoring – External CIs should be used on the outside of every package to demonstrate exposure to H_2O_2 gas plasma. Internal CIs should also be used to demonstrate exposure to H_2O_2. Internal CIs should be placed at challenging locations inside each pack.
- Biological monitoring – The microorganism of choice for H_2O_2 gas plasma BIs is the *Geobacillus stearothermophilus* spore. Biological monitoring should be performed at least daily, but preferably with each load. (See **Figure 15.10**) Follow the sterilizer manufacturer's IFU for proper BI use.

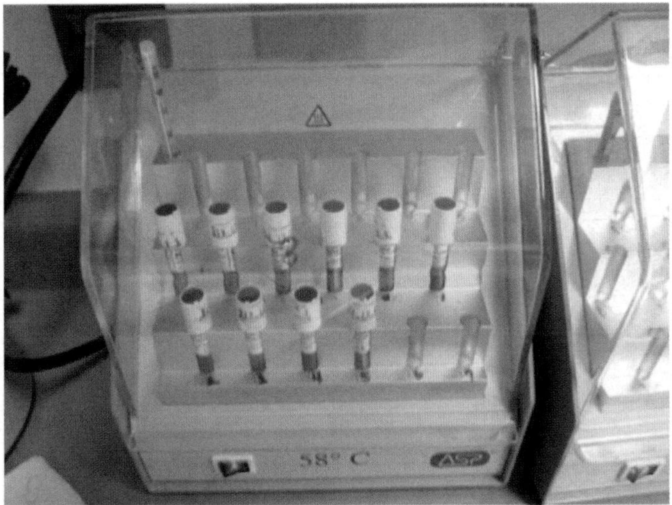

Figure 15.10 Example of hydrogen peroxide gas plasma biologicals and an incubator

Vaporized Hydrogen Peroxide

Background

Low-temperature sterilization technology utilizing vaporized hydrogen peroxide (VHP) has been available to hospitals in the U.S. since 2007. As with H_2O_2 gas plasma, VHP systems utilize an oxidative process and provide a cycle time that improves the throughput of medical devices. (See **Figure 15.11**)

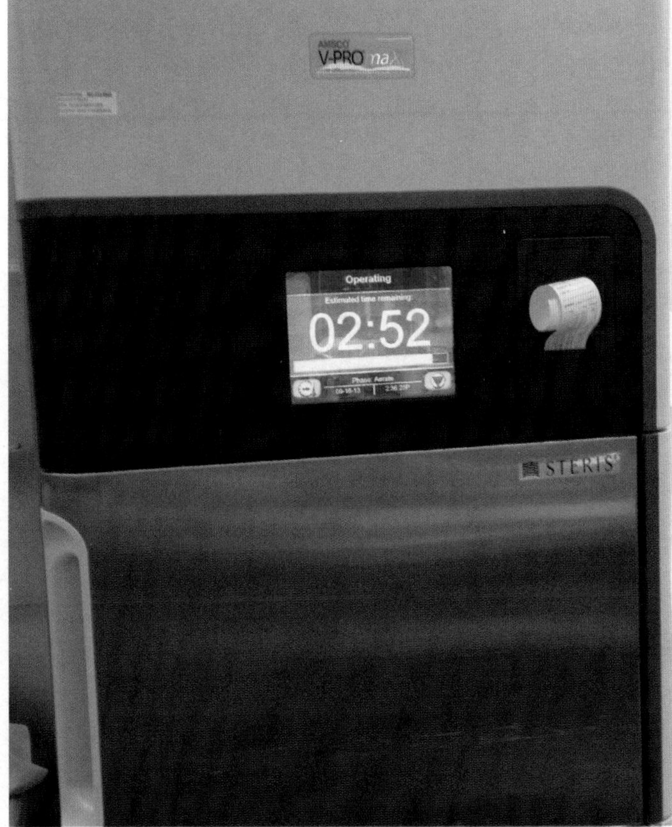

Figure 15.11

Efficacy

VHP sterilization uses a 59% H_2O_2 solution that is shown to be effective against a broad spectrum of microorganisms.

Penetration

VHP is injected four times during each sterilization cycle. Upon completion of the fourth injection hold period, the load is automatically aerated in the sterilizer. The VHP is exhausted from the chamber through a catalytic converter that converts the VHP to water and oxygen.

Types of VHP Systems

There are different types of VHP sterilizers. One system has a single, pre-programmed, 55-minute sterilization cycle for use with both lumened and non-lumened instruments and devices. Another system offers two pre-programmed cycles: a 28-minute cycle for non-lumened instruments and a 55-minute cycle used to sterilize instruments with lumens and non-stainless steel mated surfaces.

These sterilizers use different technologies, and the cycles have different sterilant injection numbers, sterilant exposure times, H_2O_2 concentration levels, and cycle pressure profiles. VHP sterilization processes are based on a fixed amount of sterilant for each cycle type and for every load placed in the chamber. This fixed amount of sterilant is delivered in different manners such as an ampule contained in a cassette, or cup, depending upon the type of sterilizer used. It is important to note that by having a specific fixed amount of sterilant there is little room for error since no additional sterilant is added during the sterilant exposure phase; therefore, a small load (or a very large load) is exposed to the same amount of sterilant during the sterilization exposure phase.

Always follow the manufacturer's IFU for sterilizer operation.

Sterilization Cycle and Process Parameters

The sterilization cycle of many types of VHP systems operate at low pressure and temperature and is suitable for processing heat- and moisture-sensitive medical devices. VHP is generated by injecting a fixed amount of aqueous H_2O_2 into a vaporization chamber (see **Figure 15.12**) where the solution is heated and converted to a vapor and then introduced into the sterilizer chamber under negative pressure. The phases of VHP systems include:

- Conditioning – To remove air and excess moisture from the chamber and packaging, the chamber is evacuated and then recharged with dry, filtered air.

- Leak test – Vacuum is held to ensure a leak-tight chamber.

Vaporized hydrogen peroxide sterilant

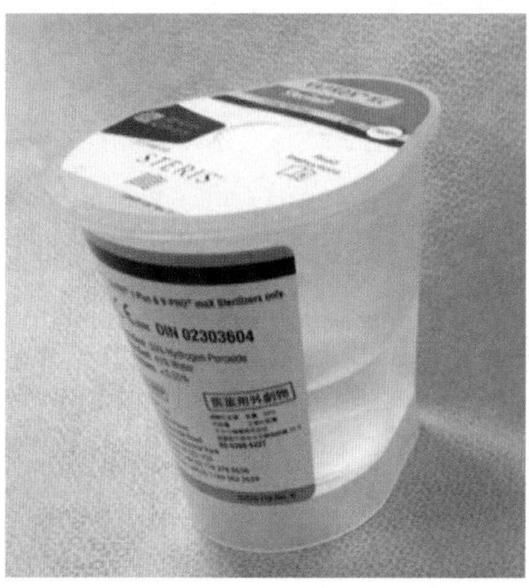

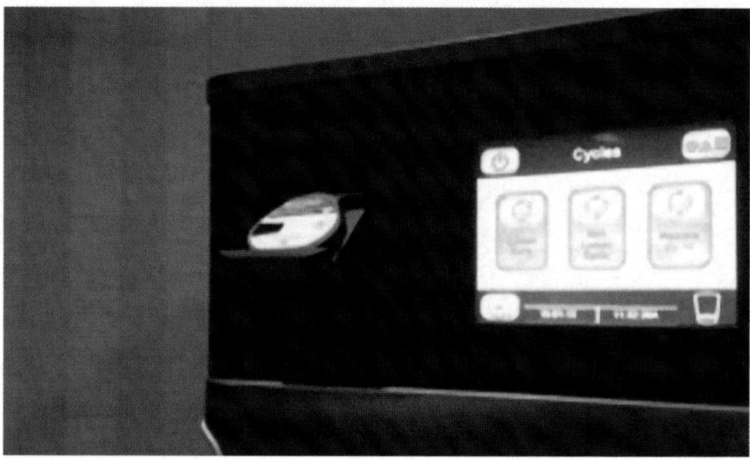

Figure 15.12

- Sterilization – Enhances penetration by injecting VHP into the chamber with a series of pulses, each followed by a hold period.
- Aeration – Upon completion of the last VHP injection hold period, the load is automatically aerated in the sterilizer. The chamber VHP is exhausted through a catalytic converter that changes the VHP to water and oxygen. No special venting is required.

As with all methods of sterilization, operators must demonstrate competency in all parameters of VHP sterilization.

Safety

Concentrated H_2O_2 is corrosive to skin, eyes, nose, throat, lungs and the gastrointestinal tract. Under normal conditions of use, the VHP sterilizer operator is not exposed to the contents of the sterilant container. The sterilizer automatically dispenses and injects liquid hydrogen peroxide (LHP) into the chamber. After each sterilization pulse, VHP is removed from the chamber and converted to water and oxygen. An aeration phase facilitates the removal of H_2O_2 residuals from devices and packaging. To avoid exposure to H_2O_2 when removing items from a canceled cycle, SP technicians should always wear the appropriate PPE.

To minimize risks, employees should be instructed about:

- H_2O_2 hazards
- Applicable SDS
- Handling canceled loads
- Applicable OSHA regulations
- PPE use
- Storage, handling and disposal of H_2O_2 cartridges

Exposure Monitoring

No personal or area monitors are required. Testing to check for H_2O_2 vapors in the environment around the sterilizer has shown acceptable VHP levels during typical sterilization cycle conditions.

Materials Compatibility

VHP sterilization is compatible with a wide range of medical devices being processed. The VHP system is not intended to process liquids, linens, powders or any cellulose materials.

Packaging

Packaging materials can affect the penetrating capability of VHP. Packaging materials approved for use with VHP sterilization include polypropylene. Tyvek and some sterilization containers are also validated for H_2O_2 sterilization.

Loading VHP Sterilizers

VHP sterilizers must be loaded properly for effective sterilization. Sterilizers are cleared by the FDA, with a maximum weight limit for individual loads for each cycle type. Always refer to the sterilizer's IFU for specific restrictions on devices for each cycle type. During the loading process of a low-temperature H_2O_2 sterilizer, the following details should be taken into consideration:

- Ensure the devices are approved for a specific VHP sterilizer model and cycle type.
- Ensure the total load weight is below the stated weight limit.
- Select the packaging type acceptable for use in the VHP sterilizer.

Always follow the sterilizer IFU for lumen size, length and quantity. **Figure 15.13** shows a properly loaded sterilization chamber.

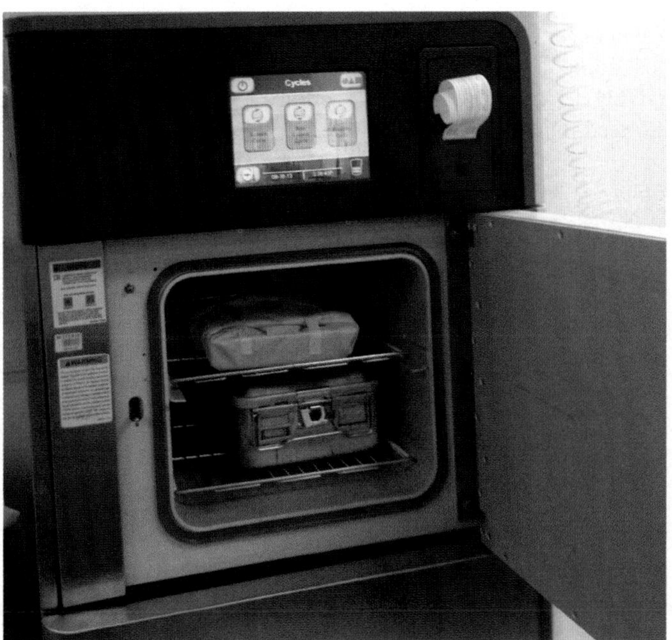

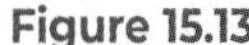

Figure 15.13

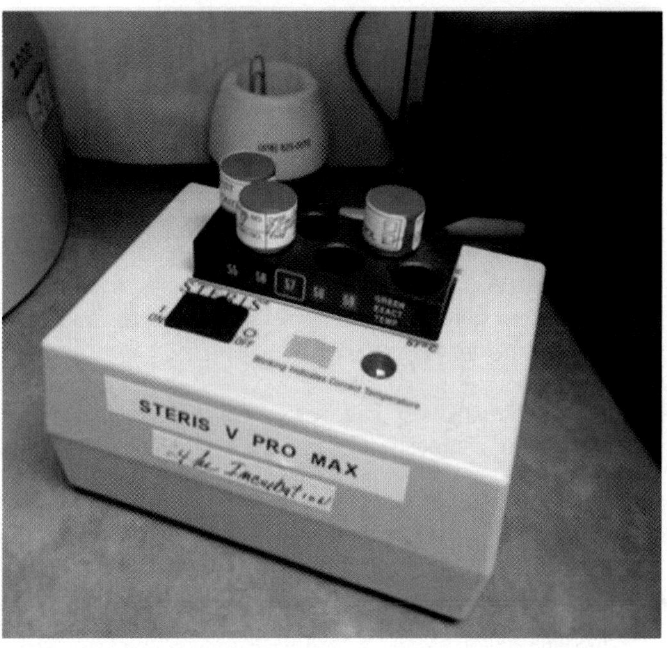

Figure 15.14 Example of vaporized hydrogen peroxide biologicals and an incubator

Advantages and Disadvantages of Low-Temperature Sterilization Technologies		
Sterilization Method	**Advantages**	**Limitations**
100% ethylene oxide (EO)	· Penetrates medical packaging, many plastics and device lumens · Compatible with most medical materials · Simple to operate and monitor · Single-dose cartridge and negative-pressure chamber minimizes the potential for EO exposure	· EO is toxic, flammable, a carcinogen and a mutagen · Requires lengthy aeration time to remove EO residue · Requires personal and area monitoring · EO emission regulated by states · EO cartridges should be stored in a flammable liquid storage cabinet
Hydrogen peroxide (H_2O_2) gas plasma	· Safe for the environment · Leaves negligible toxic residuals – no aeration required · Compatible with most medical devices · Cycle times vary with model type · Used for heat- and moisture-sensitive items · Sterilant contained in a multi-use cassette to prevent user contact with H_2O_2	· H_2O_2 may be toxic at levels greater than 1 ppm time-weighted average (TWA) · PPE should be worn when removing items from a canceled load · Cellulose (paper), textiles, liquids and powders cannot be processed
Vaporized hydrogen peroxide (VHP)	· Safe for environment · Leaves negligible toxic residuals · Compatible with most medical devices · Used for heat- and moisture-sensitive items · Cycle times vary with model type · Sterilant contained to prevent user contact with hydrogen peroxide · Simple to operate and monitor	· H_2O_2 may be harmful at levels greater than 1 ppm TWA · PPE should be worn when removing items from a canceled load · Cellulose (paper), textiles, liquids and powders cannot be processed

Figure 15.15

Sterilizer Performance Monitors

VHP sterilizers should be monitored with physical monitors, CIs and BIs.

Sterilizer performance monitors include:

- Monitoring all critical parameters during the operation of the cycle and the printing of a record at the end of each cycle to document the process parameters. All physical monitors must be carefully examined to ensure the correct parameters were met before devices are removed from the sterilizer.
- CIs – External CIs should be used on the outside of every package to demonstrate exposure to H_2O_2. Internal CIs should also be used to demonstrate exposure to H_2O_2. Internal CIs should be placed at challenging locations inside each pack.
- BIs – The microorganism of choice for VHP is the *Geobacillus stearothermophilus* spore. Biological monitoring is required each day the sterilizer is used but recommended for every cycle. Follow sterilizer manufacturer's IFU for proper BI placement. (See **Figure 15.14**)

REVIEW OF LOW-TEMPERATURE STERILIZATION PROCESSES

Figure 15.15 compares the three low-temperature processes discussed in this chapter.

CONCLUSION

Today's instrumentation is far more sophisticated and complex than devices of even the more recent past, and many of the materials cannot withstand the high temperatures or moisture required for steam sterilization. For these types of medical devices, low-temperature sterilization can be used. Low-temperature sterilization uses chemicals in the process, and a significant amount of detail goes into sterilizing each load. The SP technician must be knowledgeable of all factors involved in this process. When procedures are carefully followed, these methods are safe for patients, medical devices, and personnel.

RESOURCES

Center for Devices and Radiological Health, U.S. Food and Drug Administration. "Updated 510(k) Sterility Review Guidance K90-1; Guidance for Industry and FDA." 2011.

Rutala W, Weber D. *Guideline for Disinfection and Sterilization in Healthcare Facilities*. 2008.

Occupational Safety and Health Administration. "OSHA Fact Sheet: Ethylene Oxide." 2002.

Centers for Disease Control and Prevention. "Documentation for Immediately Dangerous to Life or Health Concentrations (IDLH): NIOSH Chemical Listing and Documentation of Revised IDLH Values." 1994.

OSHA. "Understanding OSHA's Exposure Monitoring Requirements." 2007.

OSHA. *Guideline for Hydrogen Peroxide.*

Chaunet M, Dufresne S, Robitaille S. "The Sterilization Technology for the 21st Century." TSO3. 2007.

Carter P, Wright M. "The lowdown on low-temperature sterilization for packaged devices." *Healthcare Purchasing News.* July 2008.

Reichert M, Schultz J. "Is new ozone sterilizer right for your OR?" *OR Manager*. 2003.

Scheider MS. "New Technologies for Disinfection and Sterilization. Principles, Practices, Challenges, and New Research." Association for Professionals in Infection Control and Epidemiology. 2003.

HSPA. "Vaporized Hydrogen Peroxide Sterilization." *PROCESS,* Lesson No. CRCST 164. 2019.

Conway RA, et al. "Environmental Fate and Effects of Ethylene Oxide." *Environmental Science & Technology*. 1983.

Environmental Protection Agency. 40 CFR Part 63 [EPA–HQ–OAR–2005–0171; FRL–8512–1] RIN 2060–AM14. "National Emission Standards for Hospital Ethylene Oxide Sterilizers." *Federal Register*. Vol. 72, No. 248. Friday, December 28, 2007.

Kobayashi H, Yoshida R. "Hydrogen Peroxide Vapour in the Proximity of Hydrogen Peroxide Sterilisers." *Japanese Journal of Environmental Infection*, Vol. 26, No. 4. 2011.

Kobayashi H, Yoshida R. "Hydrogen Peroxide Vapourised from Surface of Fiberscope after Low-Temperature Hydrogen Peroxide Sterilisation." *The Japanese Journal of Medical Instrumentation.* Vol. 83, No. 3. 2012.

Robinson NA, Eveland RW. "Using HPG sterilization for heat-sensitive devices." *Healthcare Purchasing News.* STERIS Self-Study Series. January 2015.

Association of periOperative Registered Nurses. *Guidelines for Perioperative Practice.* See "Sterilization" section (pp. 1061–1087). 2022.

STERILE PROCESSING TERMS

Sterility assurance level (SAL)

Permissible exposure level (PEL)

Time-weighted average (TWA)

Alkylation

Oxidation

Aeration

Residual ethylene oxide (EO)

Safety data sheet (SDS)

Chapter 16

Sterile Storage and Transport

Learning Objectives

As a result of successfully completing this chapter, the reader will be able to:

1. Review basic sterile storage requirements
2. Explain the concept of event-related sterility
3. Discuss protocols for sterile storage and transport

INTRODUCTION

A great deal of work goes into ensuring items are sterile and ready for patient use. Once items are sterile, they can easily become contaminated. Extreme caution must be used to keep each sterile item safe until it is used. While **barrier packaging** protects sterile items from contamination, it is not an impenetrable barrier. Sterile packages must be protected from events that can cause them to become unsterile. This is accomplished by keeping the items in a safe environment and consistently practicing good protocols when handling a sterile package. This chapter examines strategies to help keep items sterile until use.

Barrier packaging Packaging that provides a barrier from microorganisms and allows aseptic presentation of the product at the point of use.

STERILE STORAGE CONSIDERATIONS

After sterilization, or after purchased sterile items are received from an outside vendor, the items are stored until needed. The activities of personnel in the storage area and the environment itself affect the maintenance of item sterility.

Just like at home, if items are not properly protected or something unexpected happens, stored items may become unusable. If the kitchen floods, for example, food items like flour or sugar in their original packaging could become ruined by the water. If water is present in sterile storage, some or all of the packaged items may become ruined. Healthcare sterile storage areas need to be well planned and continually maintained to keep items sterile until use.

The sterile storage process starts as soon as the sterilizer door is opened at the end of a cycle or when purchased sterile supplies are received into the facility. (See **Figure 16.1**)

Protecting sterile items from contamination begins with considering the environment where the items will be stored. Providing the proper environment is critical for maintaining sterility. The following are all considerations that must be addressed when determining an appropriate sterile storage area.

Location

The sterile storage area should be located next to or near the sterilization cooling area. This area should ideally be an enclosed room easily accessible from the sterilization, **break out** and case cart staging areas, while being out of the facility's main traffic areas. The storage location should be removed from general traffic flow patterns to minimize airborne contaminants and keep items away from untrained personnel. (See **Figure 16.2**)

Break out The process of removing commercially sterilized items from their outer shipping containers in an area adjacent to the storage area to prevent contamination that is present on the containers from being introduced into the storage area.

STOP
STERILE AREA
PROPER ATTIRE MUST BE DONNED BEFORE ENTERING.
THIS INCLUDES SCRUBBS, JUMPSUIT, AND SHOE COVERS.

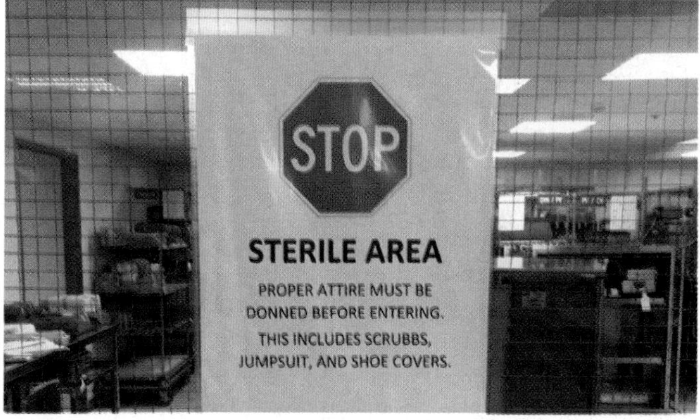

Figure 16.2

Sterile storage begins as soon as in-house items are sterilized and commercially sterilized items are received.

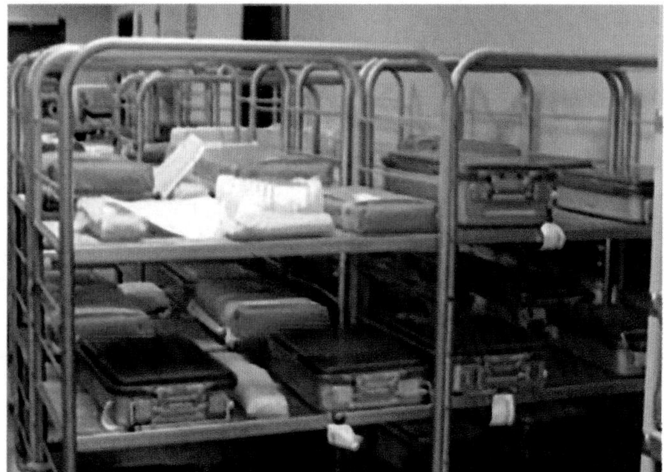

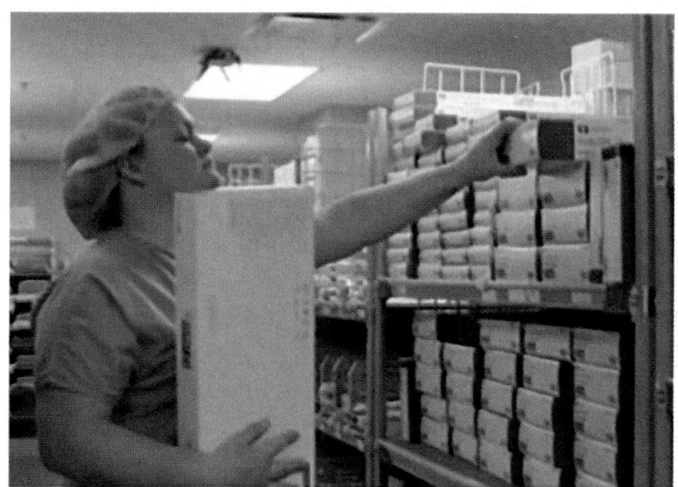

Figure 16.1

Appropriate storage space is important.

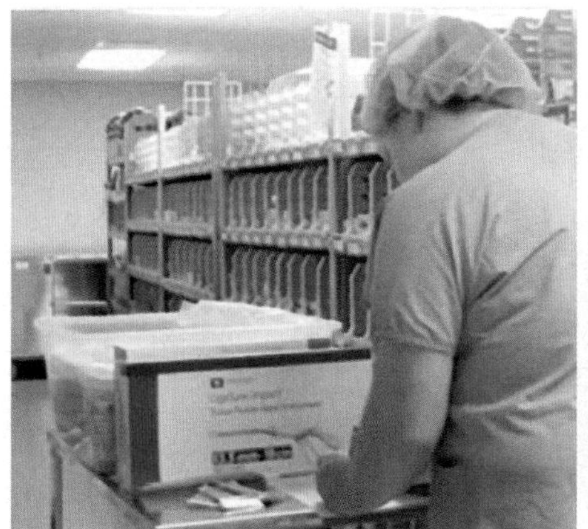
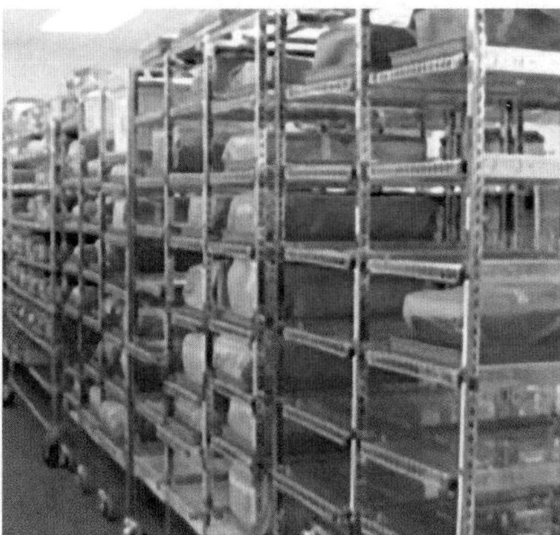
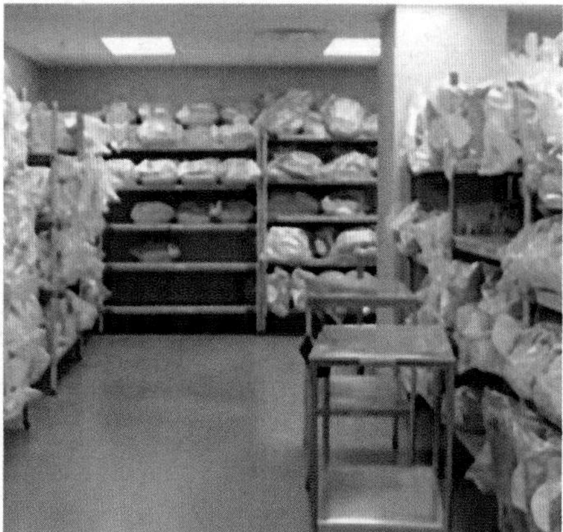

Figure 16.3

The area should be designed and designated for storage of sterile items only. (See **Figure 16.3**) While it may be impossible to create a separate sterile storage area, every effort should be made to place items in a location that meets criteria for sterility maintenance. It must be noted that sterile items may be stored in other areas of the healthcare facility such as nursing units, clinics, special procedure departments, etc.

Storage Conditions

Sterile storage areas should have no exposed water, sewer or air conditioning lines that could leak and contaminate the items. Work surfaces should be made of easy-to-clean, smooth and durable material. There should be no exposed light fixtures, pipes or ducts that can collect and shed dust. The location should be physically separated from other areas of the department. If this is not possible, extra care is required so that air and traffic always flow from sterile to clean to dirty. No pass-through traffic should be permitted.

Air supply to the storage areas should be as clean and free from dust as possible, and this usually requires filtration. Because this area stores sterile items, air pressure should be positive in relation to surrounding areas so air flows out of the area when a door is opened, reducing the chance of airborne contamination. Doors and dispensing windows should remain closed when not in use. The room should also have at least four complete air exchanges per hour.

ANSI/ASHREA/ASHE 170 *Ventilation of Health Care Facilities* recommends that temperature in the sterile storage area may be as high as 75°F (24°C), with less than 70% relative humidity (RH). This recommendation depends on when the healthcare facility last installed or upgraded the heating, ventilation and air conditioning (HVAC) system. Very dry air can affect seals and cause plastic materials to become brittle. Excessive humidity can cause tape and labels to lose their adhesion, loosen seals or affect package content identification. It is important to keep packs at least two inches away from exterior walls, windows and window seals where condensation can form on interior surfaces of exterior walls. Temperature and humidity levels should be checked and recorded at least daily. (See **Figure 16.4**)

Temperature, humidity and air pressure should be monitored in the sterile storage area.

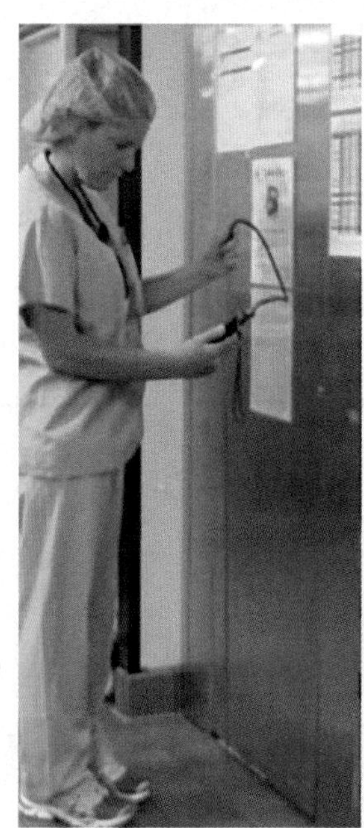
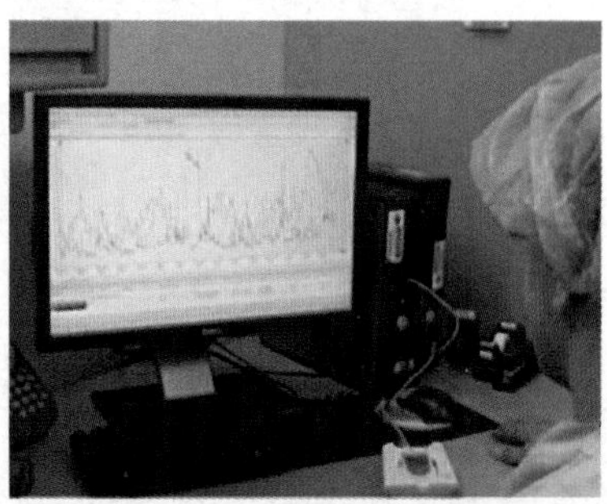
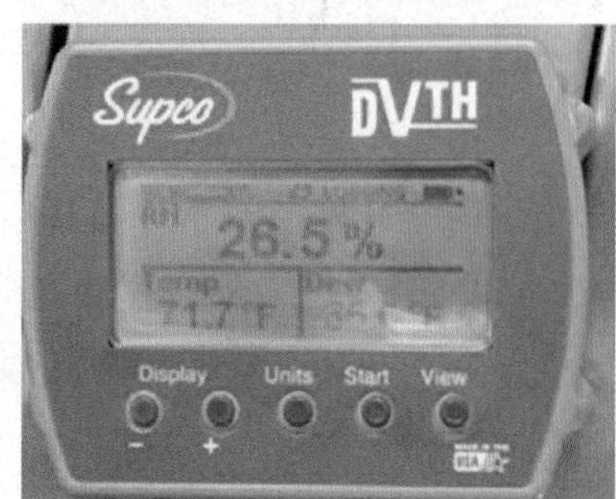

Figure 16.4

This area should have proper lighting so package labels can be easily read. There should be no dark corners or blind spots, which could lead to improper product identification and misplaced or forgotten inventory. Adequate lighting is also critical for personnel safety. Hand hygiene stations should be located in this area.

Storage Shelving

Many companies manufacture shelving that is appropriate for storing sterile supplies. Some facilities have custom-made

Proper shelving can prevent contamination and staff injury.

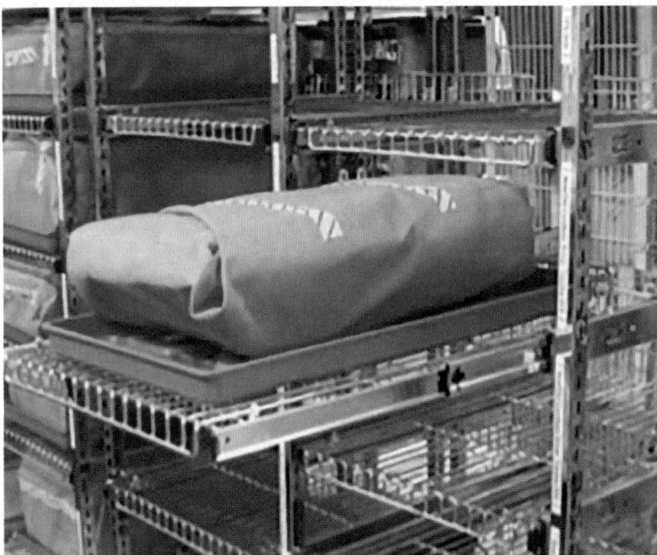

Figure 16.5

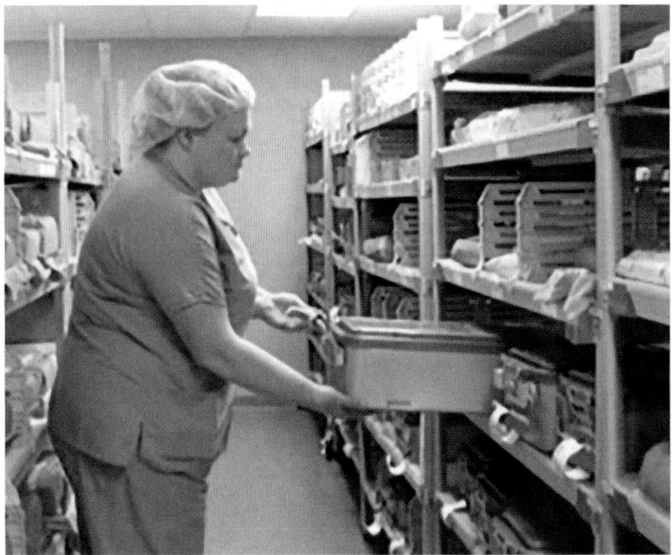

shelving units to fit their allotted space properly. Regardless of the shelving type (see **Figure 16.5**), there are several factors to consider when choosing or replacing shelving:

- Storage shelving should be designed to protect the sterile product.
- Shelving should be sized to properly fit the stored items, without product overhang. Trays that do not properly fit on the shelf pose a safety hazard to all who work in the area. Trays that overhang shelving may also become contaminated by people walking by and brushing against them.
- Shelving must be designed to easily hold the total weight of the trays to be stored.
- Shelving should also be ergonomically friendly to prevent injuries.
- Shelving should be clearly labeled.
- Adequate space should be allocated to prevent package damage.
- Shelving must be easily cleaned. Metal or plastic shelving is recommended for this reason. Porous materials, such as wood, should not be used because it cannot be properly cleaned and can harbor microorganisms.

Closed Shelving

Closed shelving is the preferred type of shelving because it protects the sterile packaging from dust, traffic and air flow as well as other environmental and physical challenges within the storage area. Shelves are usually constructed as solid units, allowing for secure storage and easy cleaning. Closed shelving is expensive, so many facilities do not use this system (or it is used only for the most delicate and expensive items.)

Doors should always be kept closed unless items are being accessed. When opening the doors, they should be opened slowly to avoid causing swift air currents that could potentially contaminate the sterile product.

Semi-Closed Shelving

Semi-closed shelving is shelving with at least three solid sides (top and two sides) that forms a closed unit when the shelves are moved together; these units are usually on tracks or have independent wheels. (See **Figure 16.6**) This type of shelving is also expensive; however, it is very versatile, user friendly and offers good protection for shelved items. Shelves may be solid or open wire. The bottom shelf must be solid to protect the stored items from contamination. The units should be pushed to the closed position when not accessing sterile products.

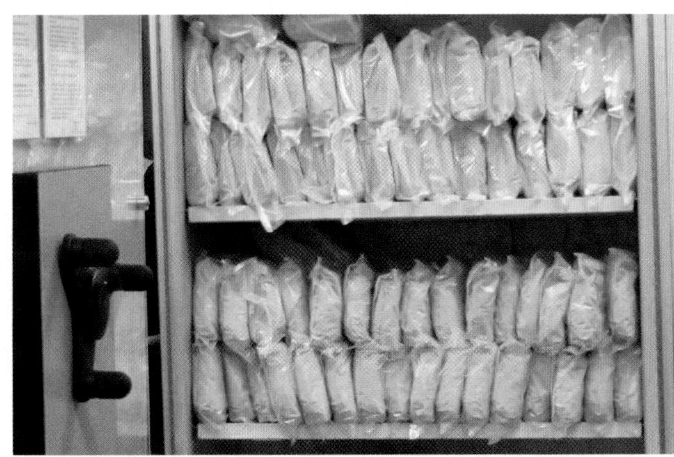

Figure 16.6

Open Shelving

In open shelf storage systems, items are placed on shelves that are not enclosed. Shelves usually have open-wire racks to prevent dust accumulation; however, the bottom shelf must be solid to protect the stored items from contamination. Open shelving is convenient and less expensive than closed shelving; however, packages are more vulnerable to physical hazards (usually accidental) and environmental challenges from cleaning solutions and microorganisms.

Regardless of the system in use, a few standards must be followed:

- The bottom shelf of each unit must be between eight and 10 inches from the floor. This protects stored items from contamination due to floor cleaning and dust.
- The bottom shelf must be solid to protect items from environmental cleaning. If the shelf itself is not solid, commercially purchased shelf liners may be used to line the bottom shelf. (See **Figure 16.7**)
- Although not required, having solid top shelves will help protect sterile items from dust.
- All shelves must be cleaned regularly.

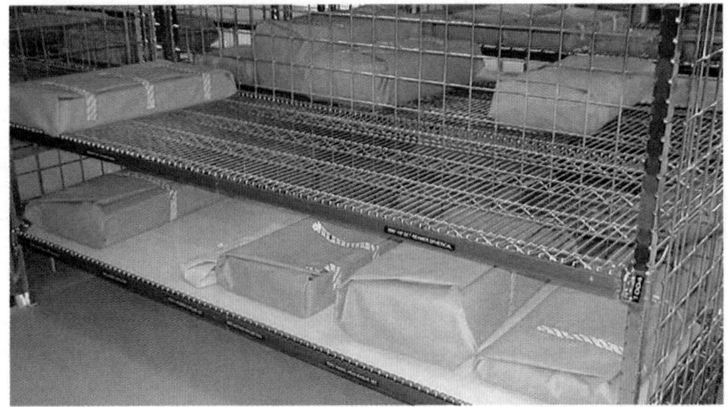

Figure 16.7

RECEIPT OF STERILE ITEMS INTO STORAGE

As previously stated, the sterile storage process starts when the sterilizer door is opened after a cycle or upon receipt of purchased presterilized items.

In-House Sterilized Items

Once items are removed from the sterilizer, they should be moved to a designated cooling area. (See **Figure 16.8**) This area should be close to the sterilizers because moving the warm cart causes air currents to flow over the warm items. Since the room air is cooler than the sterilized items, this movement can cause condensation, making the items unsterile. Air currents can also help microbes penetrate the warm packaging material, again contaminating the sterilized packages.

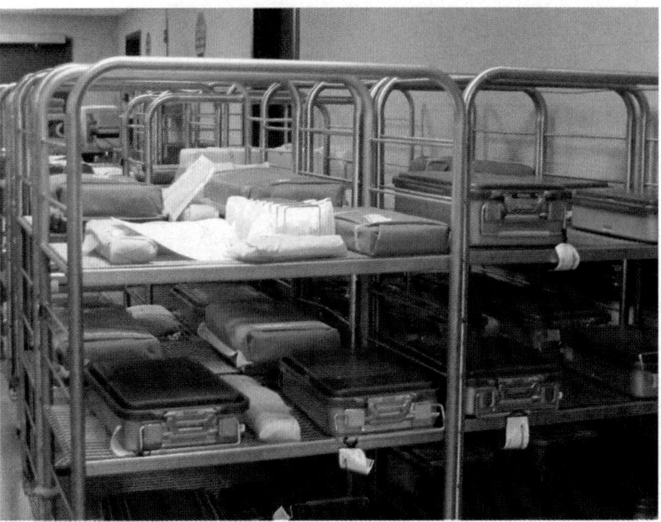

Figure 16.8

Packages should not be touched until they reach ambient (room) temperature. Touching warm packages can cause the packages to become contaminated from microbes on the skin transferring through the warm packaging material.

A temperature meter, such as an infrared device, can be used to determine the temperature of a package without touching the package. (See **Figure 16.9**)

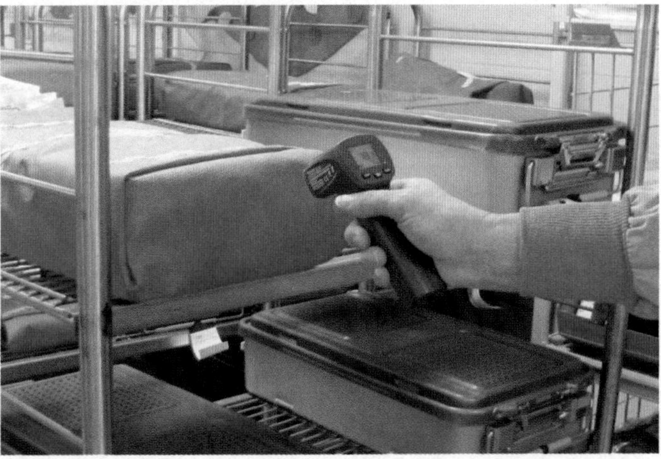

Figure 16.9

Once items are properly cooled, they may be placed on the storage shelf. Carefully check each item prior to placing it on the shelf. Ensure the indicator tape, peel package seal or container locks are intact. Visible chemical indicators (CIs) should show appropriate color change. There should be no holes, visual moisture or tearing of the package material.

Lift (do not drag) wrapped trays; dragging will cause holes or tears in the packaging material. Wrapped trays should not be stacked on top of each other because stacking causes the lower trays to compress. (See **Figures 16.10** and **16.11**) When the upper trays are removed, air will be pulled into the lower packages, causing contamination. Stacking wrapped trays may also cause holes in the wrapper of the lower trays.

Rigid container systems may be stacked, if approved in the instructions for use (IFU).

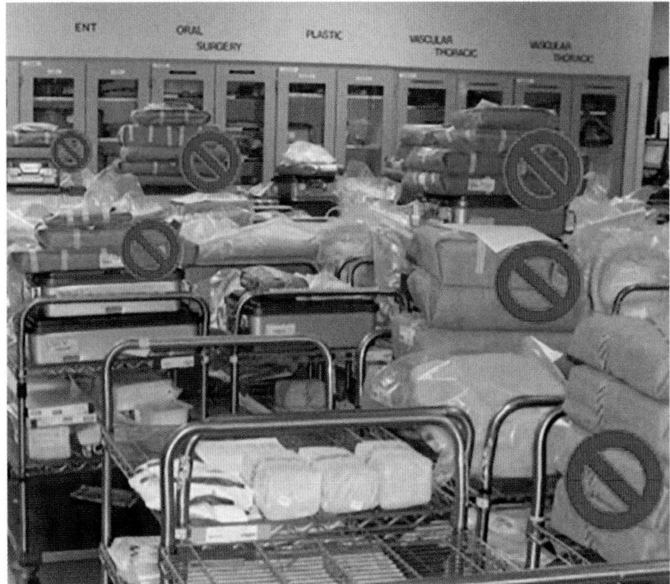

Figure 16.10 Do not stack wrapped trays

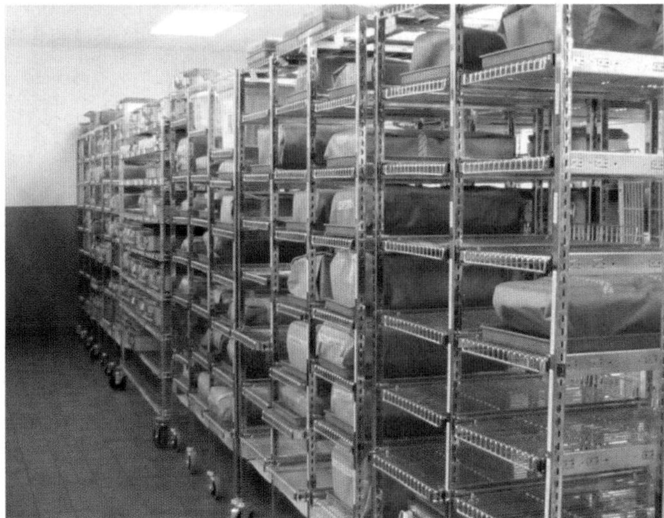

Figure 16.11

Storage of High-Level Disinfected and Liquid Chemically Sterilized Items

Storage of items that have undergone high-level disinfection (HLD) or liquid chemical sterilization (LCS) is an important aspect of processing to ensure the devices are safe for the patient. Identification of patient-ready devices is important because it distinguishes LCS- or HLD-processed devices from non-processed devices.

Endoscopes must be completely dry and stored in a cabinet that is clean, dry, well-ventilated, and dust free to prevent exposure to potentially hazardous microbial contamination. They should be stored in a way that protects them from damage or contamination and in accordance with the item and storage cabinet manufacturers' written IFU.

Other LCS- or HLD-processed devices, like laryngoscope blades, must be stored in a manner that protects them from unintentional handling.

Items that have undergone LCS and are intended to be used as critical devices should be used immediately after processing. If they are stored, they must be reprocessed immediately before use.

The acceptable storage time for LCS or HLD items differs according to each facility and item. Each facility should have a policy that specifies acceptable storage times.

Purchased Pre-Sterilized Items

Sterile storage areas are also used to store pre-sterilized products from outside vendors. These products are typically received in shipping containers. These outer shipping containers should be removed in a controlled break out area because the outside box has been exposed to environmental challenges, including weather, insects and microorganisms. (See **Figure 16.12**) Sterile items should not be removed from their outside box on the receiving dock unless there is an area protected from the outside environment that has been designed for this purpose.

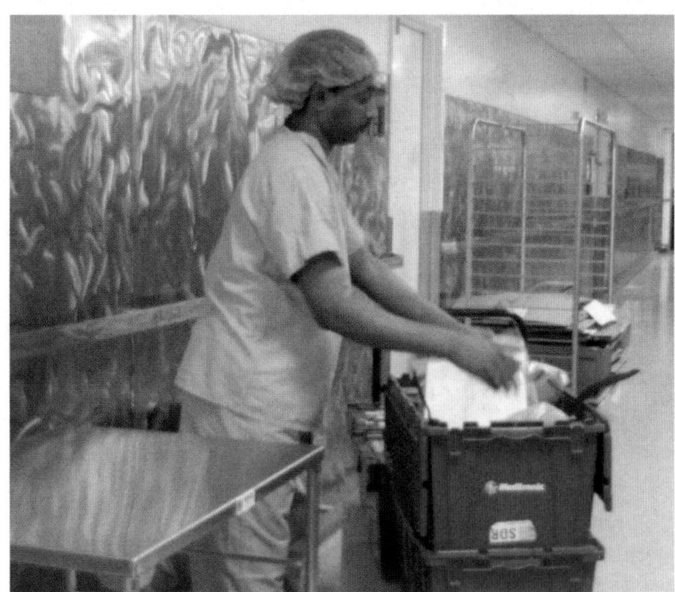

Figure 16.12

Some items are shipped in shelf cartons. Shelf cartons are commonly contained within an outer shipping box and are designed to store sterile items in a sterile or clean storage environment.

Shelf cartons can be removed from the outer shipping cartons in the break out area and placed onto a sterile storage shelf. Using shelf cartons to store sterile items on shelves reduces the handling of the sterile items and provides protection.

Received items should be delivered to an area close to the sterile storage area, where the items can be removed from the outside box. Sterile items should be placed inside a clean, enclosed transport cart, tote bin, or container so the items can be delivered to the storage area. Outside shipping cartons should never be allowed in the storage area because they are a major source of contamination. Transfer bins and carts must be cleaned regularly to help keep the sterility of the items intact.

Items should be handled gently when transferring them from the box to the transport cart or container. Place items loosely; packing items tightly may compromise the items' sterility.

Transport items directly to the sterile storage area. Never leave sterile items unattended where others may have access to the items. Curious staff or visitors may handle items and unintentionally damage the packaging, causing the items to become unsterile.

Carefully place items on the shelves. (See **Figure 16.13**) Do not pack items tightly, as doing so will compromise the package sterility and may damage items inside the package. Always follow proper stock rotation procedures.

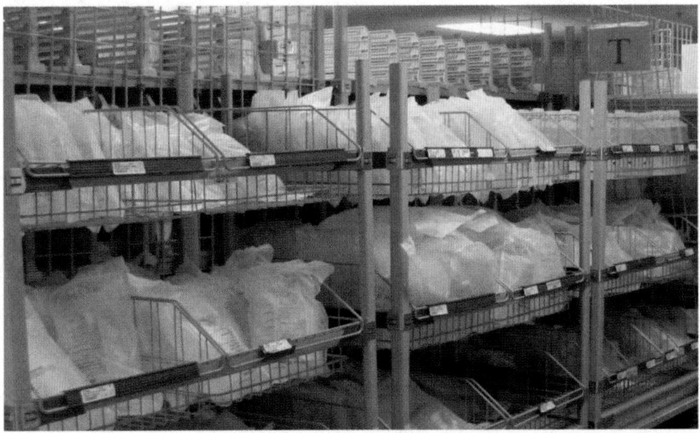

Figure 16.13

EVENT-RELATED STERILITY

Shelf life is related to events that may compromise the pack sterility. Event-related sterility is the concept that sterile products remain sterile until an event occurs to make them unsterile. This section describes events that may render a package unsterile. This is not inclusive, as there are many events that can compromise sterility.

Type of Packaging Material Utilized

Many packaging materials have a defined useful life. SP technicians must be sure to follow the manufacturer's recommendations for shelf life before and after sterilization because the product's ability to perform properly diminishes after the stated expiration date. One of the events that could occur after the expiration date is loss of microbial barrier protection of the packaging. When this occurs, items will not remain sterile.

Condition of Package

Package integrity is very important. Rough handling, poor storage practices, moisture, dust, and poor transportation procedures are some of the events that can occur and damage a package. Once a package is damaged, the items inside must be considered unsterile. (See **Figure 16.14**)

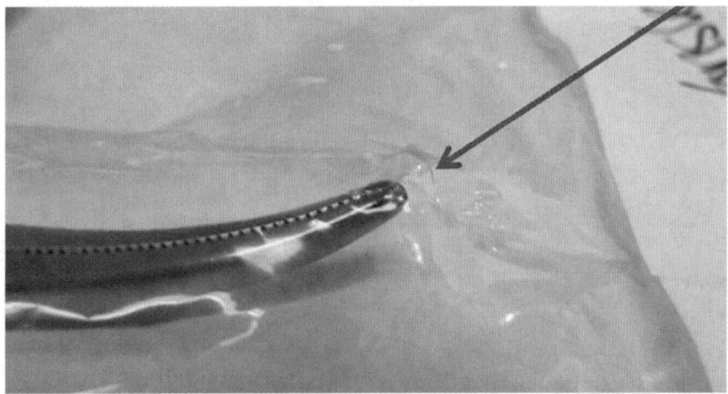

Figure 16.14 Package condition can compromise sterilit.y

Storage and Transportation Conditions

Clean, dry shelving in the storage area or in the transportation carts is required to keep items sterile. Whether the shelving or carts are open or closed can affect item sterility. Open shelving allows for a greater chance of contamination from the environment or personnel working in the area. Temperature and humidity must be monitored, and ensuring the absence of dust and insects helps maintain package integrity.

Handling

The following are all considered events: handling items while they are still warm, handling items excessively, and personnel engaging in poor hygiene when handling sterile items. Below are techniques to reduce the opportunity for contamination:

- Practice good hand hygiene when handling sterile packages. Hands must be clean and completely dry before handling packages.
- Handle sterile packages gently.
- Containerize items when possible.
- Keep items in shelf cartons to reduce extra handling of the sterile packaging.
- Maintain an appropriate inventory, and practice **first in, first out (FIFO).**

All sterile items should be monitored for events that may render them unsterile. If any event occurs to jeopardize an item, the item in question must be removed and processed or disposed of according to the facility's policy. Whenever there is doubt regarding the sterility of a package, the item should be considered unsterile.

> **First in, first out (FIFO)** A stock rotation system whereby the oldest product (that which has been in storage the longest) is used first.

BASIC STORAGE GUIDELINES

Once items are delivered to the sterile storage area, they need to be carefully placed in their designated storage space. Regardless of whether the items are processed in-house or purchased outside the facility; the guidelines for storage of sterile items remain the same.

The primary conditions that can adversely affect a sterile package's ability to maintain its sterility until it is opened by the user at the point of use include:

- Moisture and liquid/fluid contamination
- Dirt and dust
- Physical damage to the package, including abrasions, cuts, tears, punctures, broken seals and the breakdown of packaging material (e.g., some plastics become brittle). Holes should not be put into packages for hanging because it can affect the package seals.

Storage environments should be clean, dry and easily accessible by authorized personnel.

Stored items should be arranged so packages are not crushed, bent or compressed. If the air inside a package is forced out, it can potentially rupture closures and seams. As previously stated, by forcing the air out of the pack, a void is created. When the source of compression is released (i.e., the weight on its top is removed), a slight suction can be created by the void. This can potentially establish conditions for the packs to "suck in" contaminated air.

Per fire codes, stored items should be placed at least 18 inches below the ceiling or the level of the sprinkler heads to allow for proper air circulation and for water to flow unimpeded during a smoke or fire emergency. Spacing must also be planned and maintained to prevent packages from being touched, bumped or leaned upon when the room is cleaned or when personnel are storing or retrieving packs.

Sterile packages should not be stored near or under sinks, exposed water pipes, sewage lines or air conditioning drains.

Always place sterile items on clean surfaces. Do not trust the package barrier to protect contents from soil.

When placing items on shelves or when removing them from the shelf, always check package integrity, including the filter area of rigid containers, and ensure all external CIs have turned to the proper color. If sterilized in house, be sure the load (lot) control label is still intact and all seals are securely in place. (See **Figure 16.15**) If the item has an expiration date, ensure the item has not expired. Do not place anything on the shelf until the items have been checked and verified to be intact.

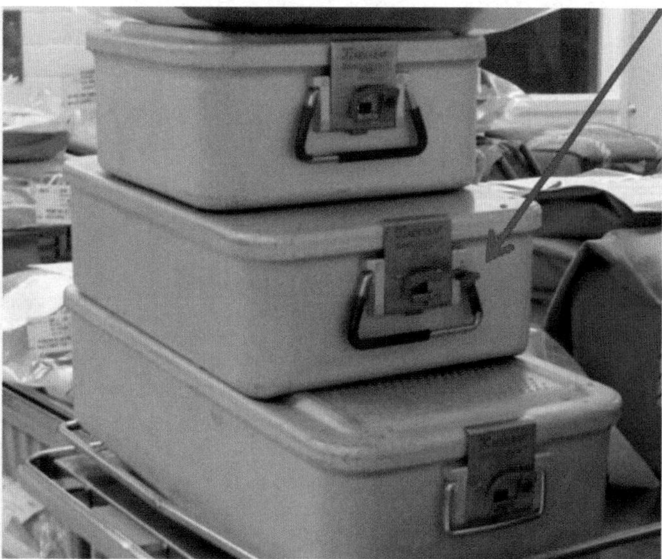

Figure 16.15 Be certain seals and locks are intact.

Sterile items should fit on the shelf; they should never overhang the edge of the shelf. The shelf edge may cause damage to the item, and the overhang can create a safety hazard.

Place heavy items on middle shelves to allow for safe lifting. Lightweight packages should be placed on the higher shelves.

Always lift items across the shelf; dragging them will damage the packaging.

Handle all items gently. Rough handling of sterile packages can damage the packaging, causing the items to become unsterile.

Arrangement of Instruments and Supplies

Storage areas for instruments and supplies must be carefully planned. The goal is to help ensure that items are easy to locate and are protected from events that may cause them to become unsterile. Proper use of stock rotation principles is also important to ensure that older items are used first and that supplies with time-sensitive expiration dates are used before they must be discarded.

The logical arrangement of stock improves efficiency, decreases staff injuries and facilitates appropriate stock rotation.

SP technicians should review the manufacturer's IFU to determine if there are any special storage requirements.

Locator systems help SP technicians manage large numbers of supplies and instruments.

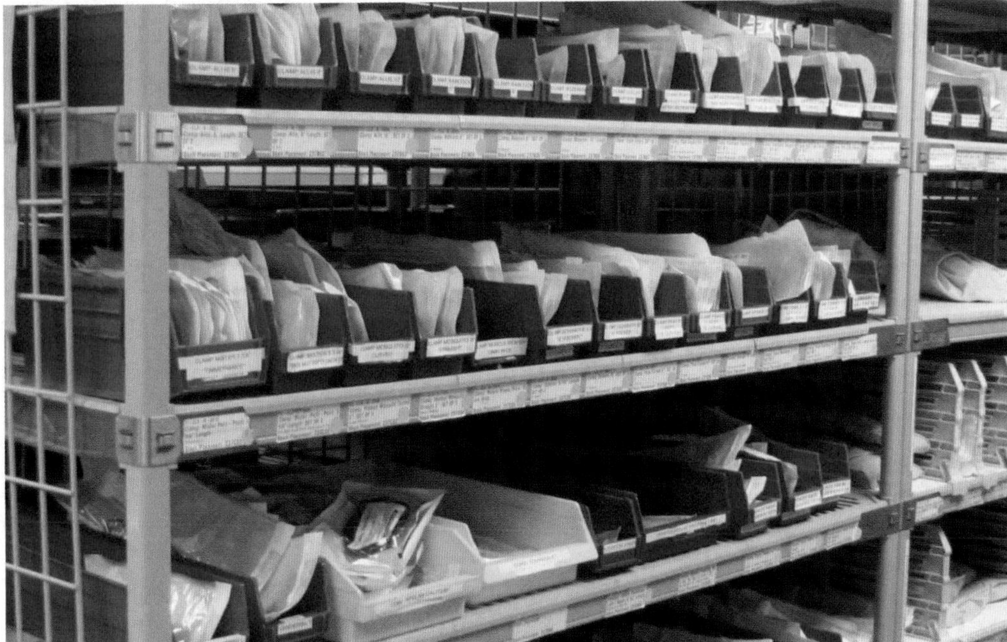

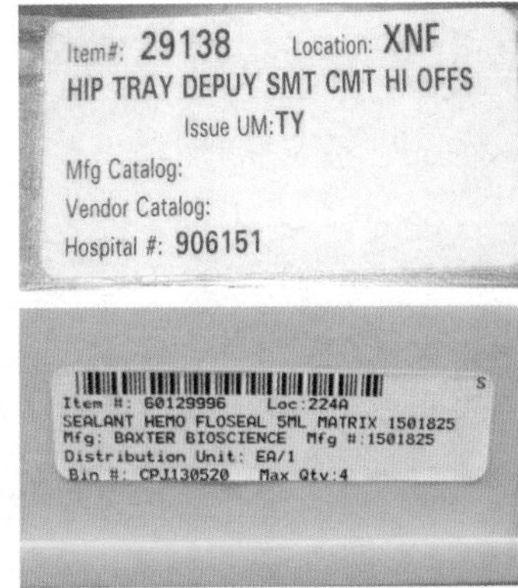

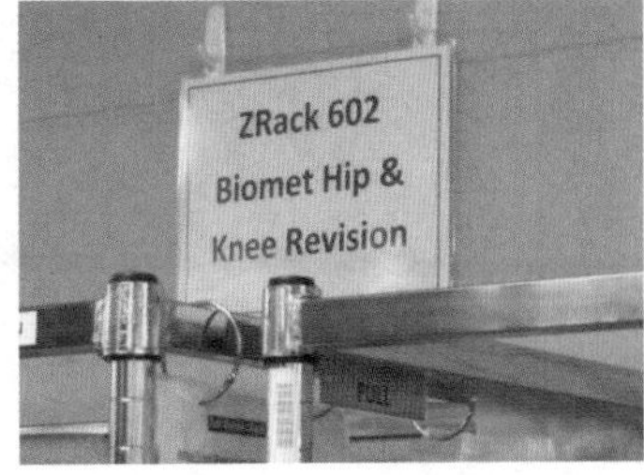

Figure 16.16

Sterile items should be arranged so they are easy to locate. This may be best accomplished by organizing them alphabetically by name, functionality or specialty (related items shelved together), or numerically, based on stock codes. Shelves should be clearly labeled, designating where items should be stored, and include pertinent ordering and dispensing information. (See **Figure 16.16**)

Stock Rotation

Sterile packages should be arranged and maintained to allow stock rotation with a FIFO system. This ensures that the oldest items are used first. The longer a sterilized item remains in storage, the greater the chance the item can become contaminated due to handling and environmental issues such as dust. Even if the item does not become contaminated, it may not be able to be opened aseptically. Practicing a FIFO inventory control system prevents a "neglected packs syndrome" where hard-to-reach packs remain in storage much longer than others and are more likely to become damaged or contaminated. *Note: Items with expiration dates should be used in the order of their expiration dates, with newer items that will expire being used first.*

The goal of a stock arrangement system is to provide minimal pack handling, while allowing FIFO rotation. Many facilities use a left-to-right system: the newest item is placed on the left and the older items move to the right. The pack on the far right is the first to be picked up for use. Other facilities place the new packs in from the back of the shelf and pick up the oldest from the front of the shelf.

Satellite Sterile Storage

Many facilities store sterile items in user departments. Storage areas for sterile supplies located outside the SP department (SPD), such as in the Operating Room (OR), must follow the same guidelines as stated previously and be included in quality assurance and infection prevention audits conducted for the sterile storage area in the department. Regardless of where a sterile item is stored, it must be protected from events that can render it unsterile. If satellite storage sites are used, personnel responsible for the areas should be trained about requirements for sterility maintenance.

CLEANING

To maintain product sterility, it is important to keep the sterile storage area clean and free from dust and debris. Standards for environmental cleaning should be the same as those for an OR or Labor & Delivery suite.

The floors should be damp mopped, and trash should be emptied at least daily. Walls and vents should also be on a routine schedule for cleaning.

Shelving, racks and other storage devices should also be routinely cleaned. The frequency depends on several factors. Closed shelving usually does not need to be cleaned as frequently as open shelving. The air filtration system in the storage area is also a factor in determining cleaning schedules. The better the filtration system functions, the less frequently the area must be cleaned.

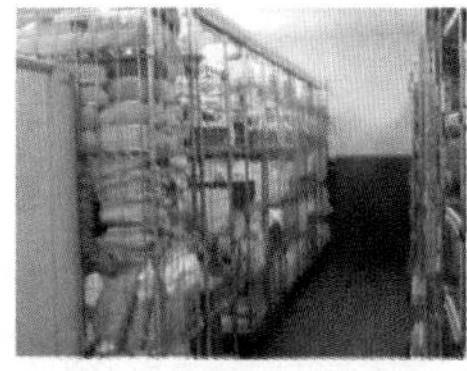

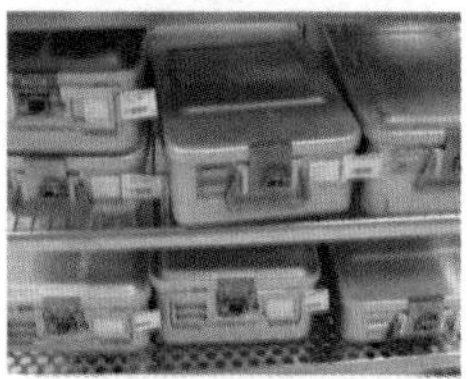

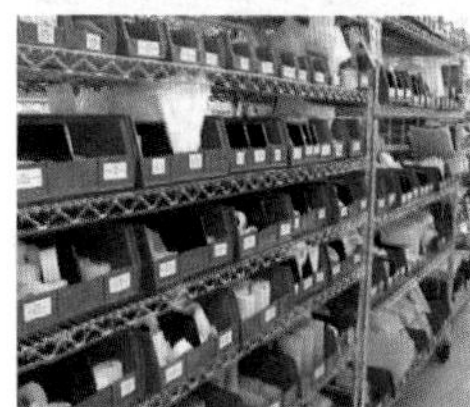

Shelf Cleaning

1	Remove all items from the shelves and storage bins.
2	Wipe entire shelf, including sides and top, using a facility-approved solution.
3	Clean all bins and shelf organizers using a facility-approved solution.
4	After cleaning surfaces touched by sterile packages, clean the shelf base, under the bottom shelf, and wheels.
5	Allow to dry thoroughly. *Note: Alcohol may be used as a drying agent, if approved by facility protocols.*
6	Wait until shelves, bins and organizers are completely dry.
7	Place items back in their assigned location. Check items for package integrity, external indicator change, expiration dates and lot control numbers for in-house sterilized items.
8	Document cleaning per the facility's quality assurance requirements.

Figure 16.17

When cleaning shelves, all items should be carefully removed from the shelf. Using a facility-approved solution, wipe the entire shelf, including the sides and top. Alcohol may be used as a drying agent, if approved by the facility's protocols. After the shelves, base and shelf bottom have been cleaned, the wheels should also be cleaned. Be sure the shelves are completely dry before placing items back onto the shelf. Also, clean and completely dry all storage bins before placing them back on the clean shelf. Carefully check each item for package integrity and ensure seals are intact. Look for proper external indicator color change and check expiration dates. Ensure the load control number is still on the in-house processed items. As with most processes, sterile storage cleaning should be documented, and the documentation maintained for use in the department's quality assurance program. The process for sterile storage shelf cleaning is outlined in **Figure 16.17**.

STERILE STORAGE HYGIENE

All SP technicians should maintain a high level of personal hygiene, including clean hair, body, nails (no artificial nails) and clothing at all times. SP technicians should frequently perform hand hygiene.

Fingernails should be short to reduce the microbial load under the nails, and to minimize the potential for rupturing packages and pouches.

Jewelry of any kind (including wedding bands and wristwatches) should not be worn. If badge lanyards are worn, they should be cleaned on a regular basis.

Personnel working in the sterile storage area must be trained properly in all aspects of the storage process.

Authorized individuals entering a storage area must follow hand hygiene policies, wear proper attire, be in good health and maintain good personal hygiene.

TRANSPORTING STERILE ITEMS

Transportation of sterile packages should be done in a manner that protects the sterility of the items. It is important to follow the department's established procedures to ensure the items are delivered intact and ready to use. There are several ways to transport sterile items. Regardless of the method used, it is important to protect the items from crushing, bending, falling or other damage. (See **Figure 16.18**)

Hand Carry

It is often faster and easier to carry small, lightweight items to the point-of-use area by hand. Items being delivered should be protected from the environment and air currents from hallway traffic. Carefully place the items to be delivered in a protective cover, or a clean closed bin. Keep items away from the body to avoid contaminating them. The sterile items should be held with both hands, while keeping the items flat so instruments and products do not shift and become damaged.

Cart Transport

Transporting items by cart is easier and safer than hand carrying items. As with shelving, transport carts can be opened or closed. The bottom shelf should be solid to protect the items from dirt and dust contamination. When transporting with open carts, including wheeled tables, items should be covered and protected against the hallway traffic. Items should be placed flat on the cart to protect contents. Trays and packs should not overhang the edges of the cart.

Sterile item transport

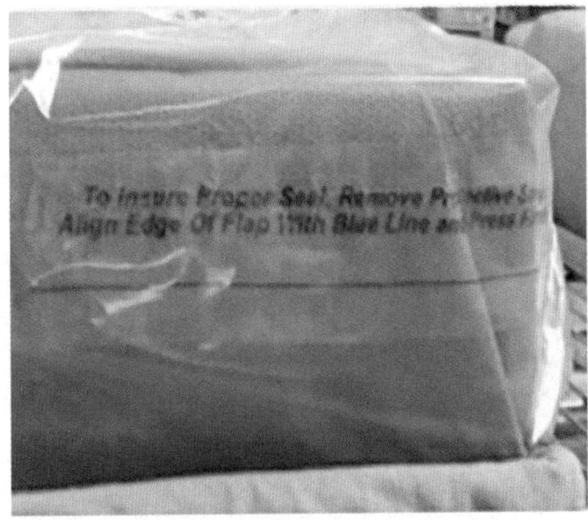

Protective covers

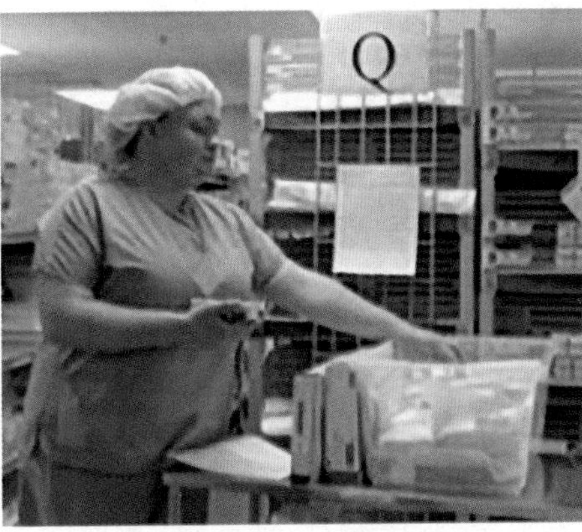

Open cart with bins

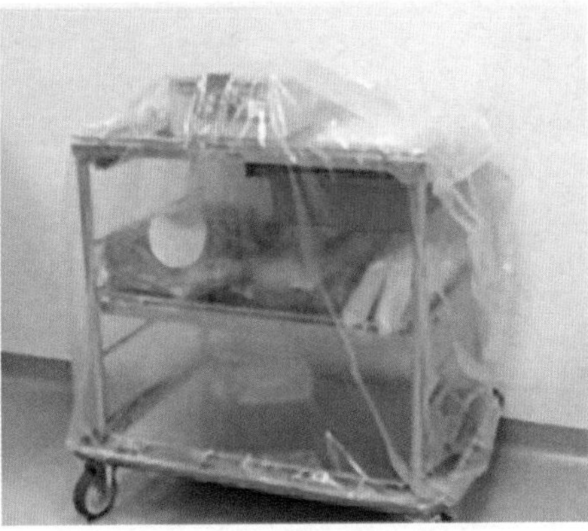

Open cart with covers

Figure 16.18

Closed carts are the transportation method of choice because they provide the best protection for sterile items. (See **Figure 16.19**) Carefully place items inside the cart. Do not overcrowd the cart. The cart doors should close and latch without touching the sterile item.

All carts should be kept in good working order, and cart doors should be free from damage. Wheels should be properly maintained so the cart will move easily and quietly.

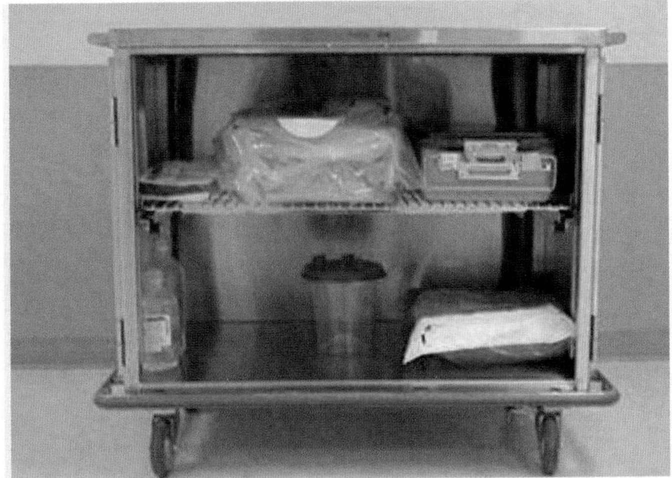

Figure 16.19 Enclosed cart transport

Elevators and Lifts

Many facilities have dedicated clean elevators for sterile product transportation. These elevators should be used for clean and sterile transportation only. Soiled items should be returned using an elevator designated for soiled items. When using a dedicated lift, items must still be contained because air currents from outside the lift can contaminate the sterile items.

Vehicles

Healthcare facilities today may transport sterile items between sister facilities and to offsite clinics and physician offices. Items should not be transported in the trunk of a car because temperature and humidity levels cannot be controlled properly. There must be clear separation of clean and soiled items within the transport vehicle. The vehicle must be completely enclosed and in good repair, with no holes in the walls that will allow outside contaminates to enter. Sterile items should be placed inside clean, protective bins or carts. Protect the items from movement within the device, as packaging and instruments can be damaged from movement during transport. The cart or bin must be properly secured inside the vehicle to keep it from shifting. Temperature and humidity levels should be monitored. When the vehicle is not running, items should not be left inside the vehicle for extended periods of time, as condensation may form inside the sterile packages, rendering them unsterile. The transport vehicle should be cleaned on a regular basis.

CONCLUSION

Maintaining product sterility during storage and transport is one of the most important tasks for SP technicians. If unsterile instruments or supplies are used, patients could be put at risk. Carefully following written storage and transport procedures and keeping the area clean and maintained will help keep patients safe.

RESOURCES

ANSI/AAMI ST79:2017 & 2020 Amendments A1, A2,A3, A4 (Consolidated Text) *Comprehensive guide to steam sterilization and sterility assurance in health care facilities.*

ANSI/AAMI ST91:2021 *Flexible and semi-rigid endoscope processing in health care facilities.*

Association for PeriOperative Registered Nurses. *Guidelines for PeriOperative Practice: Guideline for Sterilization Packaging Systems*. 2022.

STERILE PROCESSING TERMS

Barrier packaging

Break out

First in, first out (FIFO)

Chapter 17

Monitoring and Recordkeeping for Sterile Processing

Learning Objectives

As a result of successfully completing this chapter, the reader will be able to:

1. Discuss the importance of monitoring work areas and processes within the Sterile Processing department
2. Discuss the importance of recordkeeping
3. Explain the types of monitoring required in each area of the Sterile Processing department
4. Explain the need for monitoring and review of the sterilization process indicators that help assure quality control
5. Discuss the importance of employee training and continuing education records

INTRODUCTION

Much planning and effort goes into every aspect of the Sterile Processing department (SPD). From the decontamination area to the storage area, rigid requirements must be met to help ensure the safety of patients and healthcare workers.

Documentation is required to provide a record that those requirements were met; if requirements were not adequately met, documentation provides a record to assist with performance improvement.

Sterile Processing (SP) technicians are involved in the recordkeeping process across many different functions of their jobs. Records provide evidence that processes were routinely checked, and the information collected provides a quality framework that will be examined by surveying agencies, such as The Joint Commission (TJC), the Centers for Medicare and Medicaid Services (CMS), and state agencies. If the healthcare facility is involved in a legal claim regarding any products that were dispensed from (or processed through) the SPD, records can help demonstrate that a specific standard of practice was followed.

This chapter provides information about SP recordkeeping requirements and addresses methods used to **monitor** and document conditions and processes to meet established requirements. Special emphasis is placed on the methods used to monitor sterilization processes and the recordkeeping required for those processes.

Monitor To watch, observe, listen or check (something) for a specific purpose over a period of time.

THE IMPORTANCE OF ACCURATE RECORDS

Records are kept to document many processes and conditions in the SPD, including sterilization cycles, preventative maintenance, and routine equipment testing and cleaning. It is important to note, however, that records are only as good as the information they contain. Having incomplete records is as detrimental as having no records at all. The following are some facts about SPD records:

- Recordkeeping is mandatory – SPD recordkeeping is not optional. It is as much a part of the job as assembling instruments or operating sterilizers.

- Records must be accurate – Information must be documented as it is, even if the information indicates a process has failed to meet the expected standard.

- Records must be legible and understandable – Handwritten records should be legible to anyone who needs to review them. Slang, unapproved abbreviations and nicknames should not be used, as that terminology may confuse the reader.

- Records must be complete – All information should be documented according to the department's specific requirements.

- Records should be audited routinely – Routine audits ensure that documents contain all necessary information.

Accurate and complete records provide documentation that the SPD is following standards, regulations and its own procedures to help ensure ongoing adherence to best practices.

GENERAL MONITORING

SP technicians should continually monitor their environment to help ensure that the integrity of each work area and the processes performed in those areas are maintained. Some monitoring is informal such as watching to ensure that everyone who enters the area is dressed appropriately, practices good hand hygiene and follows established traffic control guidelines. This type of informal monitoring is not recorded, but each employee is expected to identify and correct breaches in established protocols. Visual monitoring is especially important when monitoring dress codes in the decontamination area. Visitors, such as loaned instrument vendor personnel or facility employees from other departments [e.g., Facilities Maintenance, Biomedical Engineering, Environmental Services (EVS) and etc.], may not be familiar with or understand the importance of personal protective equipment (PPE) and may endanger themselves if they enter the area without proper attire.

Formal monitoring of the physical environment is also required. For example, room temperature and humidity must be monitored at least daily to ensure they meet the established standard.

Note: Standards for temperature and humidity can be found in the ANSI/ASHRAE/ASHE Standard 170, Ventilation of Health Care Facilities. *Temperatures and humidity for sterile processing are determined by the initial installation of the heating, ventilation and air conditioning system (HVAC) or last system upgrade.*

That data must be recorded, along with actions taken when temperature and humidity deviate from established parameters. Some departments use electronic devices to collect the data and transfer the data to an electronic record, while others collect the data manually. In either case, SP technicians must have that data recorded and accessible. **Figures 17.1** and **17.2** illustrate examples of manual and computerized data collection methods used to monitor temperature and humidity. *Note: Temperature and humidity in some facilities are monitored, documented and maintained by Facilities Maintenance.*

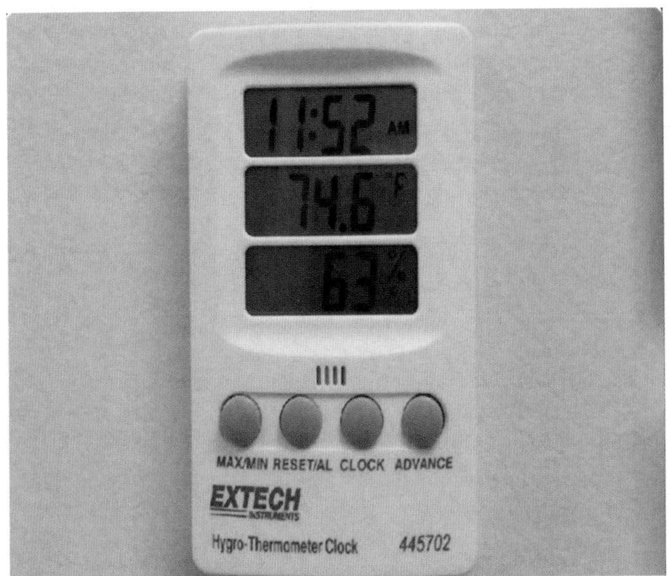

Figure 17.1

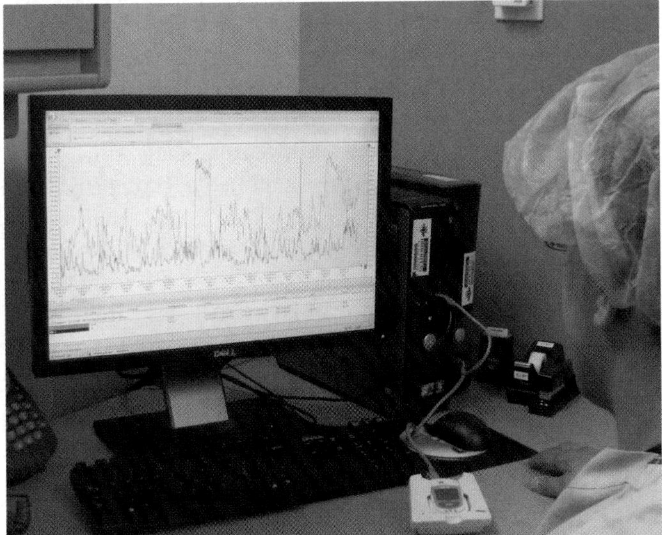

Figure 17.2

SP technicians also monitor their work areas for safety hazards. They learn to keep a watchful eye for unsafe conditions, broken or unsafe equipment, and other issues that may put themselves and others at risk. Once identified, they remedy the situation, if possible (e.g., wiping up a spill), or report it to the appropriate person to initiate a repair or replacement process.

Departmental cleanliness is also monitored by SP technicians.

Routine cleaning usually is performed by the EVS department. Cleaning should be scheduled, documented and available in either the SPD or by request from the EVS department. There are several areas in the SPD that staff are required to maintain (i.e., SP technicians are responsible for keeping their work area clean). This not only means cleaning their work areas at designated times (i.e., at the end of their shift), but also involves cleaning the area whenever it becomes contaminated or soiled.

SP technicians are often assigned specific cleaning duties within the SPD. For example, they are often responsible for cleaning cabinets, racks and carts in the sterile storage area. SP staff are assigned to clean those areas because of their understanding of sterile package handling and their ability to handle sterile items, clean storage shelves, and return those items to their proper location without compromising the integrity of the sterile packs. The cleaning process in this very important area must be documented to provide a record of routine cleaning. This may be done by using a cleaning checklist to demonstrate compliance with the cleaning schedule. Monitoring and documenting cleaning outcomes provides feedback to improve the thoroughness of the cleaning process.

SP technicians are also responsible for cleaning transport equipment in their area. Every effort must be made to limit the presence of dust, lint and microbial contamination in the work area. Microbial contamination must be kept to a minimum in all work areas. Excess dust can easily be transported to items being prepared for sterilization or onto sterile packages. In either case, that dust may then become airborne and be introduced into an open wound during a procedure.

Figure 17.3 provides an example of a sterilizer loading cart that has not been cleaned recently. The dust and lint pose a significant threat to patient safety.

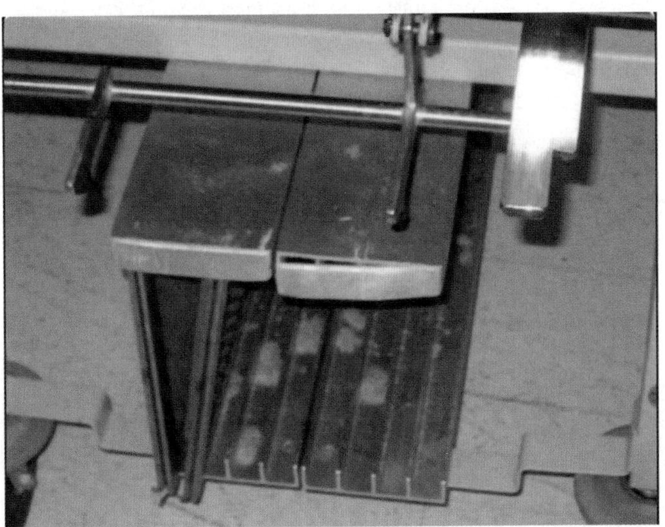

Figure 17.3

SP staff also monitor equipment within their work areas. Some monitoring is informal, such as checking the sterilizer carts for dust; other monitoring is formal; for example, small electrical equipment has a current preventive maintenance (PM) sticker. Items falling outside of their PM date should be rechecked by qualified personnel, such as biomedical engineers, according to facility policy.

In addition to general guidelines for all work areas, there are unique requirements for each area. The following sections review those requirements.

DECONTAMINATION AREA MONITORING

Monitoring of the decontamination area is important to ensure all cleaning equipment is working properly. If the equipment is not working properly, instruments will not be clean and safe to handle.

Automatic Dose Units

If an automated chemical delivery system or dose unit is used, it should be routinely verified or calibrated to verify it is dosing the correct amount.

Water Quality

Poor water quality will impact every process in the decontamination area. Cleaning chemicals must be used with the recommended water pH and will not function as designed if the water's pH is incompatible with the chemical. Hard water will cause scale to form on equipment, reducing the equipment's cleaning effectiveness. Water quality should be monitored to ensure that the appropriate chemical dilution is utilized.

Commercially prepared water testing products may be purchased to test water on a weekly or daily basis.

Mechanical Cleaning Equipment

Specific tests are available for each type of equipment. SP technicians must follow the equipment manufacturer's instructions for use (IFU) for inspection and testing. If the machine does not meet the inspection requirements outlined by the manufacturer, or if the test fails, the SP manager should be notified immediately. All test results should be documented.

Ultrasonic Cleaners

Ultrasonic cleaners use a process called cavitation to remove soil from instruments. Commercially prepared tests are available to test the efficacy of the ultrasonic. Tests can help identify issues with internal transducers that are not producing sufficient energy to create cavitation and remove soil as intended.

Irrigating Ultrasonic Cleaners

Irrigating ultrasonic cleaners are used to help clean lumened instruments. These units also use a cavitation process but employ irrigating tubes that flush solution through each lumen. In addition to the cavitation test, the irrigating tubes should be checked to ensure water is flowing freely through them. Test results should be documented.

Washer-Disinfectors

Washer-disinfectors should be visually checked at least daily to ensure screens are clean and that rotating arms are properly attached, rotating and unclogged.

Washer-disinfectors can use several solutions during a processing cycle. Enzymatic solutions, detergents, and instrument lubricators can be dispensed during a single cycle. Steps must be taken to ensure chemicals are placed in the correct dosing dispenser and the dispenser's dosing rate is correct. Visual checks and dosing results should be documented per facility policy.

Washer-disinfectors should be tested for proper cleaning ability. Commercially prepared products are available to assist with the testing process.

At the end of each cycle, physical monitors should be checked. On a washer, the physical monitor is the cycle printout or data log. The printout should be verified by the operator to ensure that the thermal disinfection temperature set by the manufacturer was attained and all other cycle parameters were met.

Cart Washers

Cart washers must be monitored to ensure they are working properly. Floor screens should be checked at least daily to ensure they are free of debris. Check rotating arms or cables to make certain they are operating as intended by the manufacturer.

Cart washers must also be tested to ensure they are cleaning effectively. This can be done using a commercially prepared test.

Some cart washers have an instrument cycle which is validated to wash and disinfect surgical instruments. If used, this cycle should be tested at least weekly, preferably daily, on the instrument cycle program.

HIGH-LEVEL DISINFECTION MONITORING

Many items processed today, such as flexible endoscopes, some respiratory therapy equipment, and other heat-sensitive, Class II semi-critical items, are high-level disinfected. The high-level disinfection (HLD) process contains many variables that can render it ineffective; therefore, it is important to carefully monitor the process. Surveying agencies review disinfection records as carefully as they review sterilization records.

Chemical Disinfection Monitoring

Test strips are used to ensure the minimum effective concentration (MEC) of the disinfectant solution. When a new bottle of test strips is opened:

- Test the efficacy of the strips, according to the manufacturer's IFU.
- Document the date the test strips are opened and the final date the strips may be used, per the manufacturer's IFU.
- Document the test results, per facility policy.

Endoscope Processing Equipment

Cleaning medical devices intended for HLD is a complicated process that may require different equipment. Equipment must be monitored for functionality prior to use, and the test results should be documented. The following are some examples of equipment that must be checked daily or prior to use:

- Leak testers
  - › Manual
  - › Automated
- Automated irrigation flushing devices
- Cleaning device **verification**

> **Verification** Procedures used by healthcare facilities to confirm that the validation undertaken by the equipment manufacturer is applicable to the specific setting.

Manual Disinfection

Documentation of the manual disinfection process should include the following:

- Date
- Time in HLD solution
- Time out of HLD solution
- Test strip results (MEC)
- Expiration date of test strips and disinfecting solution
- Items disinfected

Note: Some products also require solution temperature to be recorded.

If the disinfected item is a flexible or rigid endoscope, the following must also be documented:

- Name of the technician who cleaned the endoscope
- Patient identifier for whom the endoscope was used

Automated Endoscope Reprocessor Monitoring

As the name implies, an automated endoscope reprocessor (AER) is used to disinfect endoscopes using an automated process. While this process is less labor intensive than the manual method, monitoring is still just as important.

As with manual disinfection, the disinfecting solution in the AER must be tested for each cycle. The AER manufacturer's IFU must be followed to ensure proper testing of the disinfecting solution.

Most types of AERs have a physical printout of the cycle available after the cycle is complete. This printout should be reviewed to ensure all parameters were properly met. Technicians should then sign the printout to show the cycle has been reviewed.

Some AERs have a computerized control panel that allows the input of items sterilized in each cycle. If this feature is not available, the items must be manually documented. With the exception of the printout, documentation for AER disinfection is the same as with the manual system.

Most AER processors use a water filtration system with micron filters that require changing periodically. Filter changes may occur monthly, quarterly or annually. Responsibility for changing filters may lie solely with the SPD or with Biomedical Engineering, or it may be a shared responsibility. Regardless of ownership, documentation of filter changes should be recorded and easily retrievable.

STERILIZATION AREA

The sterilization process requires a monitoring system to help ensure parameters needed for sterilization are met. Sterilization of medical devices is difficult to prove without culturing the sterile items, which would contaminate the device during the process. Because it is difficult to prove an item's sterility, SP technicians must rely on sterility assurance factors needed to achieve sterilization [e.g., physical parameters, chemical and biological indicators (CIs/BIs)]. By carefully monitoring the parameters needed for sterilization, SP technicians can determine which items have been sterilized and are safe for patient use.

These sterilization monitoring protocols are an important part of the SPD's monitoring and quality assurance systems. Several control measures must be used to ensure the conditions within the sterilizers are adequate to achieve sterilization.

Chemical Indicators

Sterilization CIs help to confirm that packages have been properly exposed to the sterilization process. ANSI/AAMI ST79 states, "Chemical indicators are designed to respond with a chemical or physical change to one or more of the physical conditions within the sterilizing chamber."

There are two basic types of CIs: internal CIs that are placed inside a package to be sterilized, and external CIs that are placed on the outside of packages.

CIs provide a visual indication to help identify possible sterilization failures. They can detect problems with incorrect packaging, loading or other procedures, and can also detect certain equipment malfunctions such as air leaks, wet steam and inadequate temperature. CIs are an integral part of the sterilization monitoring program and are used in conjunction with physical monitors and BIs to demonstrate the efficacy of the sterilization process.

After sterilization, process indicators are examined by the SP technician to ensure complete exposure. If processes, such as packaging and loading, have been performed correctly, the CI will have changed color. By contrast, an incomplete color change indicates a failure in the sterilization process and may provide the first sign that part or all of a load has not been properly sterilized. While CIs do not verify sterility, they are an important part of the larger sterilization monitoring system. When a CI fails, SP technicians must follow established policies and procedures, which should include an investigation and documentation of the failure and any action taken.

External CIs

External CIs are often the first performance test the user sees upon removing a package from the sterilizer. They provide instant results and visual evidence that the package was exposed to a sterilant. Every item sterilized in a healthcare facility should have an external CI. Items processed that do not have an external CI must be processed again with the appropriate indicator. *Note: External CIs do not indicate that the item is sterile.*

External process indicators, including tape, load cards or labels on the outside of the packages, are also examined before the items are dispensed or opened to ensure that proper processing has occurred. (See **Figure 17.4**)

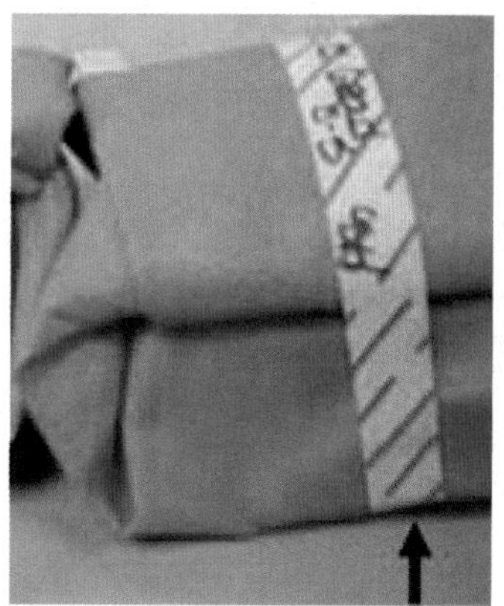

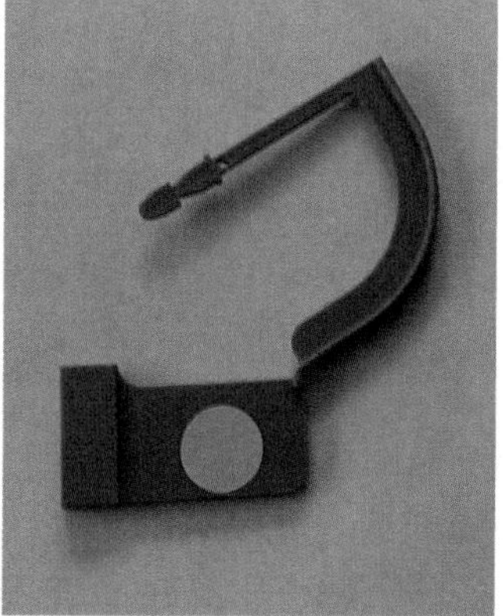

Figure 17.4

Internal CIs

Internal CIs are placed inside a package and provide evidence that the sterilant penetrated the package. *Note: Internal CIs do not prove sterility.* **Figure 17.5** provides examples of some CIs.

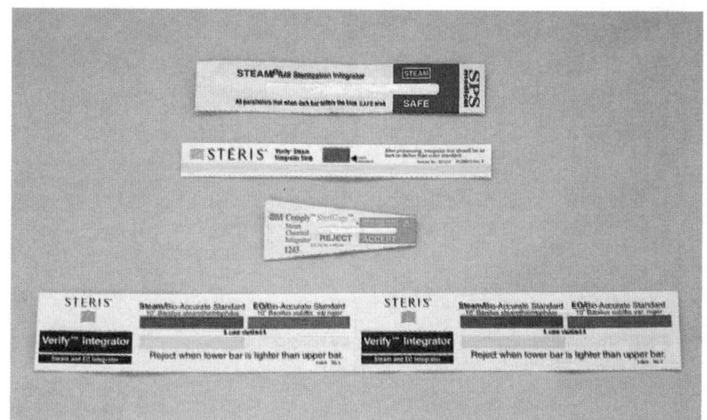

Figure 17.5

CIs should be placed in the area of the package, tray or container considered to be least accessible to sterilant penetration. *Note: This location is not necessarily at the center of the package, tray or container.*

If the interpretation of the CI in a package, tray or container suggests inadequate sterilant penetration, the contents cannot be used and should be returned to the SPD for investigation. If there is no CI found in the tray or container, the item must not be used and it should be sent to the SPD for processing. *Note: It is possible to have one unacceptable indicators in a load because of improper packaging or loading, with the remainder of the load being acceptable.*

CIs showing a "fail" result require further investigation to determine the cause. The following could cause a CI test failure:

- Utility or sterilizer malfunction.
- Inappropriate sterilizer loading techniques.
- Not using the correct CI monitor.
- Wrong cycle selected.
- Poor storage of the CI indicator.
- Improper packaging techniques.

Some facilities use CIs that consist of heat-sensitive dye applied to a cardboard strip, or a dye that moves along a window. When exposed to a sterilant, these devices gradually change color, thereby integrating a time component to the measurement. These types of CIs are called integrators.

Physical Monitoring

Physical monitors include time, temperature and pressure recorders, displays, digital printouts, and gauges. (See **Figure 17.6**) During and at the end of the cycle, and before items are removed from the sterilizer, the operator should review the monitor to ensure all cycle parameters were met.

Examples of physical monitors

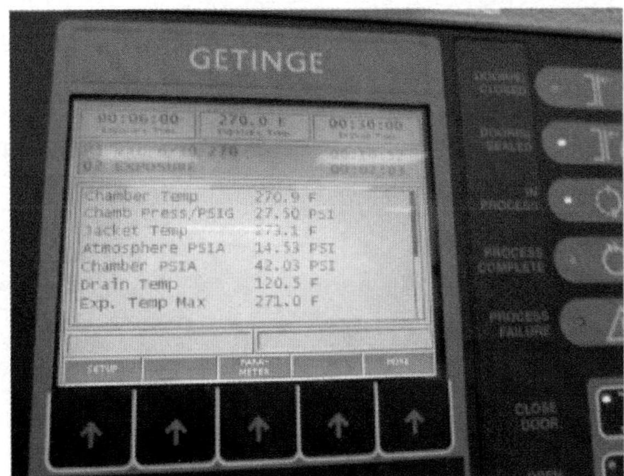

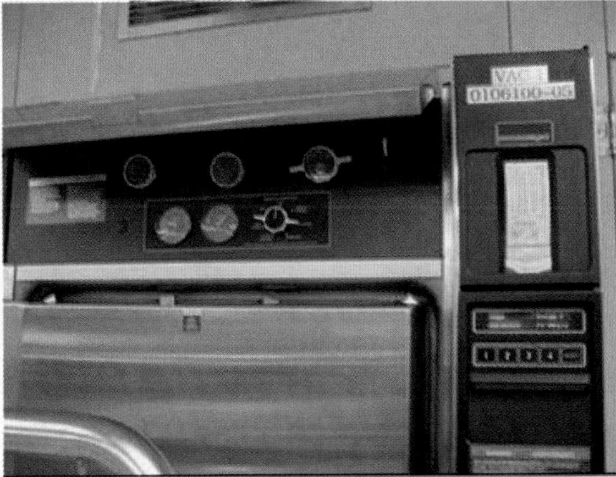

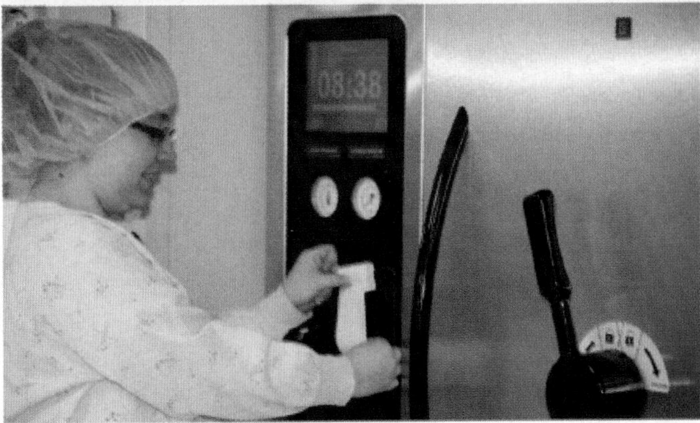

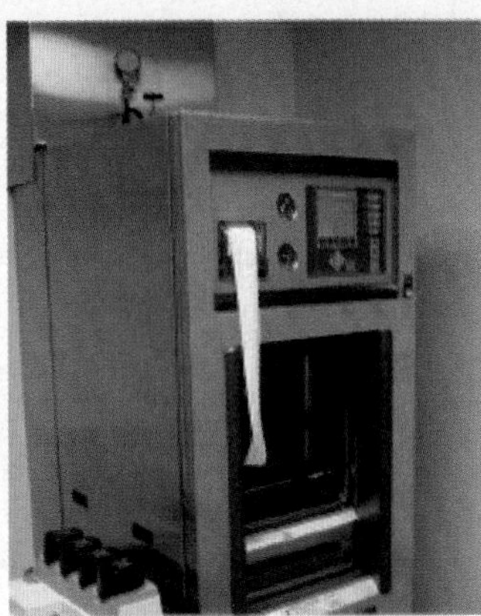

Figure 17.6

Upon completion of the cycle, the operator must sign the chart as proof that it was monitored and that all sterilization parameters were met. Physical monitors are needed to detect equipment malfunctions as soon as possible so appropriate corrective actions can be taken. (See **Figure 17.7**)

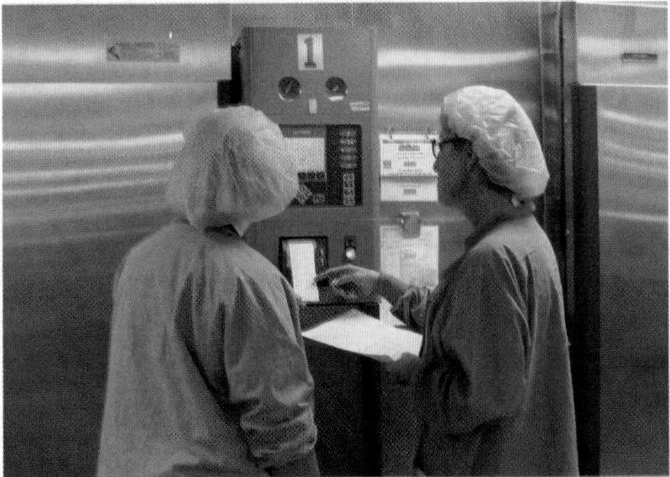

Figure 17.7

If there is any indication of malfunction, the department manager or designee must be notified immediately. The load should be considered unsterile, and the sterilizer should be removed from service. It should not be reused until the problem is corrected. SP technicians should document the failure and recall actions taken and verify that all items in the load were retrieved.

Biological Indicators

BIs are one of the most important sterilizer monitors available to the SP technician. BIs are usually ampules that contain a paper strip impregnated with a predetermined amount of live bacterial spores and a solution of growth media. The growth media provides a source for any remaining live bacteria to feed on after sterilization, thus allowing bacteria to grow and be detected. The type of bacteria varies with the method of sterilization. Spore-producing bacteria that are most resistant to the specific method of sterilization are used. This test directly determines whether the conditions have been met to kill these resistant organisms. If the most resistant organisms are killed, then less-resistant organisms should also be killed. If the proper conditions are not met to kill the spores, the test organism will grow when incubated after the sterilization cycle.

Biological tests should be run weekly, preferable every day that the sterilizer is in use, and with every implantable device. Some facilities may choose to run a BI with every load; this can be beneficial when recalling failed loads and identifying sterilization failures sooner.

At the completion of the sterilization cycle, the BI should be incubated according to the manufacturer's IFU. The load-identifying information must be identified on the BI in a manner consistent with the IFU. If the bacterial spores have been killed, there will be no color change or indication of life during incubation. This is known as a negative test result (no growth). If there is a color change in the ampule or there is indication of life through the incubator reading, it is known as a positive test (live bacteria), and items within the load should be recalled and reprocessed. **Figure 17.8** provides an example of a BI (left lower front) and an incubator.

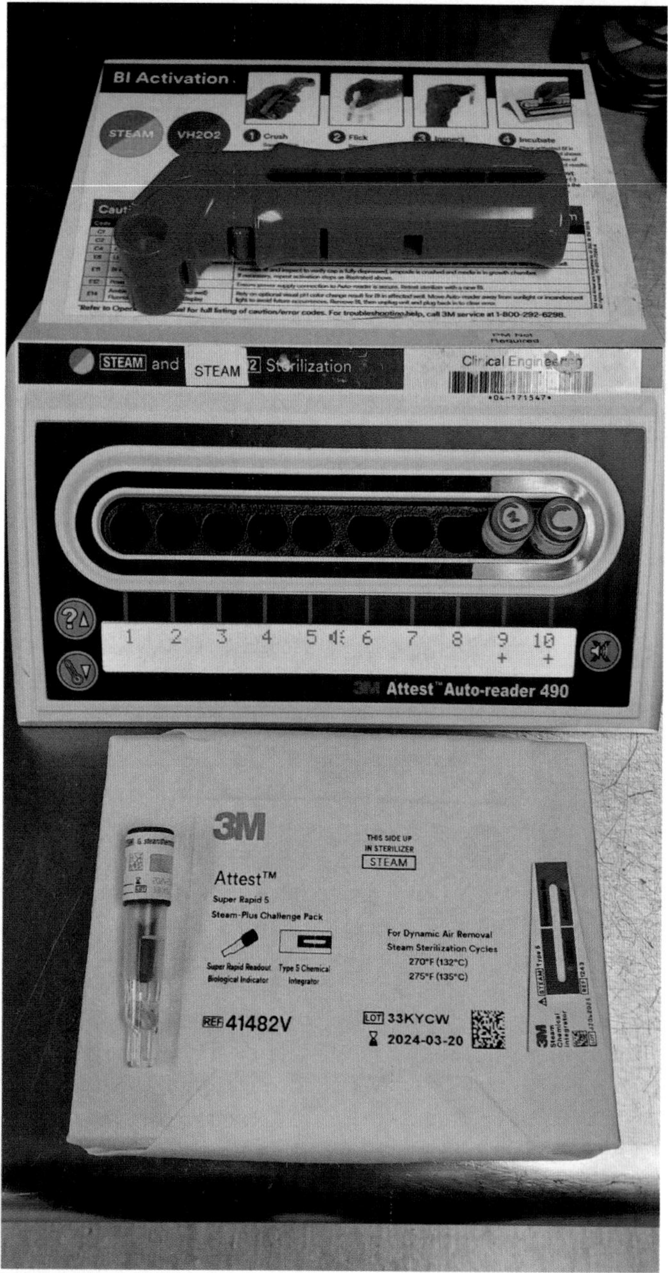

Figure 17.8

When incubating BIs, users must follow the manufacturer's IFU for interpretation of results. Some BIs may have shorter incubation times and others may require longer incubation times. Incubation times for BI tests may differ from the incubation times for the corresponding BI control.

A test ampule, called a control, should be run at least daily when a BI is run. The control and BI must come from the same lot and have the same lot number. When documenting, the records must reflect both lot numbers. A control test is the same as the BI, except it has not been put through a sterilization cycle; therefore, the impregnated bacteria will grow when incubated (positive test results). This demonstrates that the ampules in that specific lot are still viable (alive). If the control ampule does not show bacterial growth when incubated (negative test), that means the impregnated bacteria were likely dead before sterilization; therefore, the BI test run with the items being sterilized is inaccurate and will give a false negative reading.

A negative BI result does not prove that all items in the load are sterile or were all exposed to proper sterilization conditions. Instead, it shows that all conditions required for sterilization were met. SP technicians must follow proper preparation, packaging and loading procedures to help ensure proper sterilization parameters will result.

Reasons for Positive Biological Monitors

Positive BI results can be due to an operator error or a sterilizer or utility malfunction. Whenever a positive BI result occurs, it must be investigated to determine its cause.

An operator error can be caused by:

- Using the wrong BI – BIs must be validated for the mode of sterilization being used.
- Incorrect placement of the BI in the sterilizer load – BIs placed in the wrong section of the sterilizer, under trays or on their sides may give inaccurate results.
- Not following the BI manufacturer's IFU.
- Incorrect storage of the BI – BIs stored in temperatures that are too cold or too warm can be damaged and lead to incorrect results. Storing BIs where there is inadequate humidity can also impact results.
- Incorrect cycle selection.
- Not loading the sterilizer cart to allow for air removal and sterilant penetration around and through the load. Placing items too closely together (overloading) or placing items on top of the BI can cause an inaccurate test result.

If the cause of the positive BI is not determined, the facility, department or outside agency responsible for sterilizer maintenance should be contacted for further investigation. The sterilizer should not be used until the issue is corrected.

Process Challenge Devices

A process challenge device (PCD) is designed to challenge a sterilization cycle. Commercially prepared PCDs are available. PCD packs may contain only a CI, but more frequently, they contain a BI and a CI/integrator. For those cycles where a PCD has been developed, the PCD should be used to challenge the sterilization cycle. (See **Figure 17.9**)

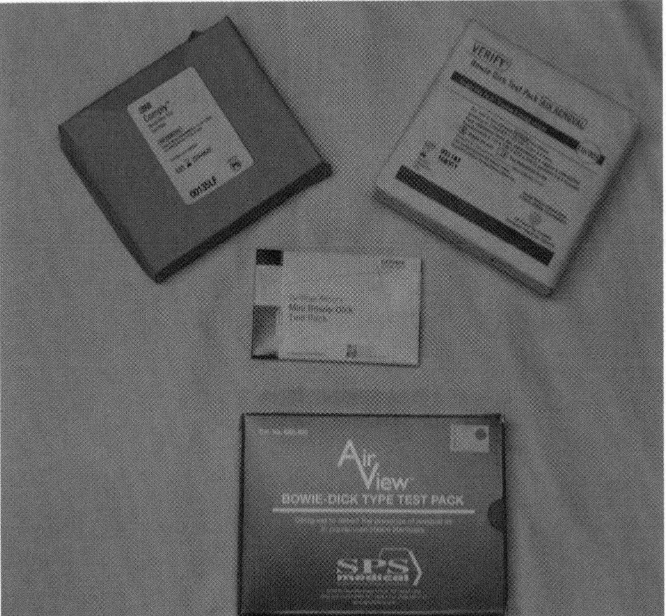

Figure 17.9

Protocols for using PCDs include:

- The PCD should be labeled with sterilizer load information before being placed into the sterilizer.
- The PCD should be positioned in the chamber according to the sterilizer manufacturer's written recommendations.
- The sterilization cycle should be run. Check the sterilizer and PCD's IFU for specific instructions.

Implants

Every load containing implantable devices should be monitored with a PCD that contains a BI and a Class 5 integrating CI. An implantable device should not be released before the BI results are known. As with all cycles, the sterilizer operator should review the sterilizer printout and the results of other indicators used to monitor the sterilization process.

Implants should be quarantined until the results of the BI testing are available. In the case of a documented emergency, an implant may be released before the result of the BI is known; however, the BI must continue to be processed to obtain and document a final result. If, due to an emergency, the implantable items must be released before the BI has been read, SP leadership, Operating Room (OR) leadership, the infection preventionist (IP) and physicians involved should be notified of the release, the facility policies and procedures should be followed, and the reason for the release must be documented.

Sterilizer Printouts

Sterilizer printouts should be reviewed and signed by the SP technician responsible for cycle monitoring. If all sterilization parameters were met, the load may be released. It is important for the SP technician to know and understand the parameters that must be met by each type of sterilizer in order to properly monitor the cycles.

Sterilization Load Control Numbers

All items to be sterilized should be labeled with a **load control (lot) number** that identifies:

- Sterilizer identification number
- Sterilization cycle number
- Date sterilized
- Some facilities use a **Julian date** on their packages. The Julian date is the number of days that have lapsed since January 1. For example, January 1 is day #001 and December 31 is day #365.

Load control (lot) number Label information on sterilization packages, trays or containers that identifies the sterilizer, cycle run and date of sterilization.

Julian date Number of days that have elapsed since January 1; also known as Julian day number (JDN).

Load control information is applied to each package with a labeling applicator gun to place an identification sticker containing the load information. (See **Figure 17.10**) Lot control numbers can also be placed manually on each package.

All packages sterilized by the SPD should contain load (lot) information. Load information helps to retrieve items during recalls and trace problems such as a positive CI test result.

The following information should be recorded on a load log sheet and maintained for each sterilization cycle:

- Load control number date and time (cycle number) of the sterilizer load
- Specific items sterilized, including quantity, department and item description (e.g., minor pan 1 OR, towel pack 10 SPD, or sternal saw 1 CVOR)
- Exposure time and temperature

Load information

Load stamp labeler

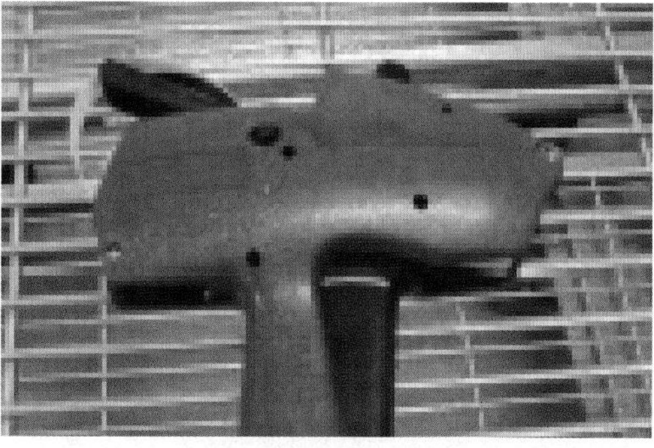

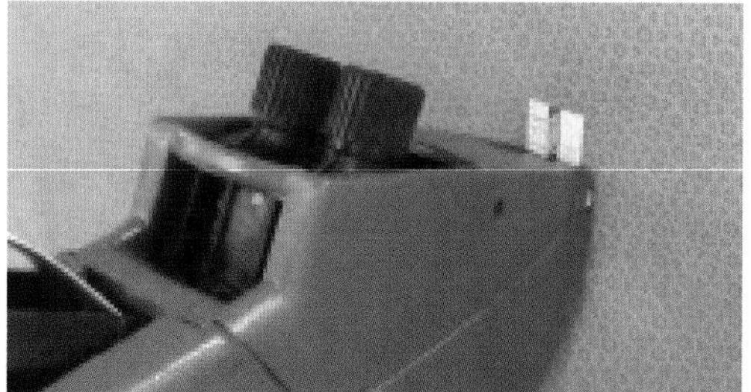

Scanner

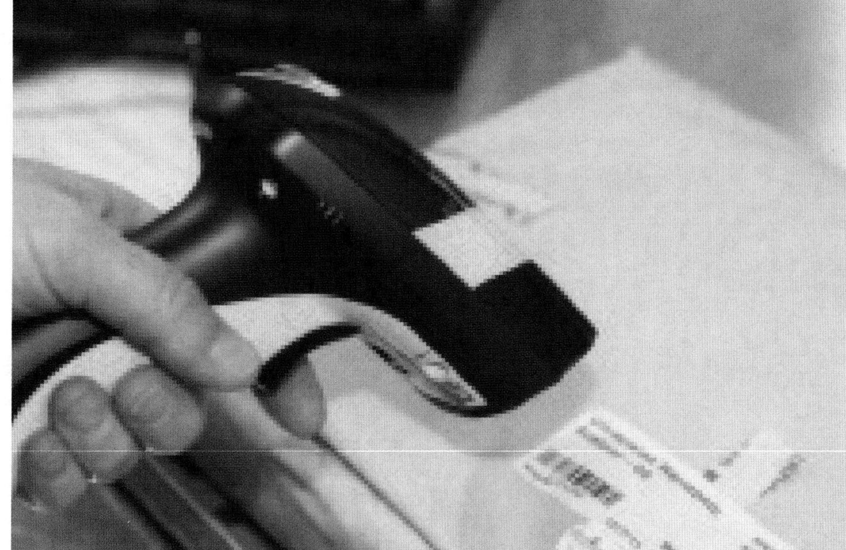

Figure 17.10

- Sterilizer operator identification
- Results of biological testing (if applicable)

This documentation ensures that cycle parameters were monitored and met and helps personnel determine whether a recall is necessary. *Note: A recall is initiated for a positive BI or nonresponsive CI, wet packs, or other sterility problems. Knowing the contents of the load enables personnel to know where to go to reclaim the packages. This documentation can be compiled manually in a sterilization logbook, or there are computer software programs available to compile and maintain these records.*

Validation and Verification

No discussion of sterilization monitoring can be complete without mention of **validation** and verification processes. There is a significant difference between "validation" and "verification." Validation is done by the device manufacturer using a documented procedure to obtain, record and interpret the testing results required to determine a process consistently produces a sterile product. Validation requires extensive laboratory testing and retesting of the processes that will be recommended, and the results must be appropriate and reproducible. Testing must also show that the validated sterilization process will not jeopardize the integrity of the product.

Validation Procedures used by device manufacturers to obtain, record and interpret test results required to determine that a process consistently produces a sterile product.

By contrast, verification is performed by the healthcare facility to confirm that the validation undertaken by the manufacturer is applicable to the specific equipment and settings in their facility.

SP technicians perform verification by documenting the procedures to obtain, record and interpret the healthcare facility's test results.

Important Note

While product verification can be accomplished in a healthcare facility, the parameters validated by the manufacturer cannot be changed and properly verified. For example, if a manufacturer has validated a device to be steam-sterilized in a 10-minute 270°F cycle, a facility cannot test this item in a five-minute 270°F cycle. Healthcare facilities do not have the proper products or equipment to correctly test and ensure the item is sterile in the shorter cycle. Also, the U.S. Food and Drug Administration (FDA) has approved the manufacturer's cycle, not the healthcare facility's cycle.

Sterilizer Qualification (Verification) Testing

Qualification testing is performed to verify that the sterilizer is in good working condition in the location in which it is being used. This testing also ensures that the sterilizer performs to manufacturer's specifications.

Qualification testing is performed after sterilizer installation, relocation, malfunctions, major repairs, or any time there is a significant change to the utilities connected to the sterilizer. A major repair is considered outside the scope of normal repairs. The replacement of a door gasket is considered a normal repair; however, weld repairs, chamber door replacement, vacuum pump repairs, major piping assembly repairs or rebuilds or control upgrades are considered major repairs. Qualification testing consists of three consecutive passing BI tests. For dynamic air removal sterilizers, the BI tests are followed by three consecutive passing dynamic air removal tests commonly referred to as Bowie-Dick tests.

STERILIZER-SPECIFIC MONITORING

In addition to the previously discussed monitoring parameters, each sterilization method may have specific parameters that must be monitored to help ensure it is performing correctly.

Dynamic Air Removal Sterilizers

Dynamic Air Removal Test

This test is a Class II CI, also known as a Bowie-Dick test and specialty indicator. Class II indicators are designed for specific procedures such as monitoring the effectiveness of the steam sterilizer to remove air from the chamber. **Figure 17.11** provides an example of a failed Bowie-Dick test. The indicator paper has not turned a uniform color and the light area indicates a failure.

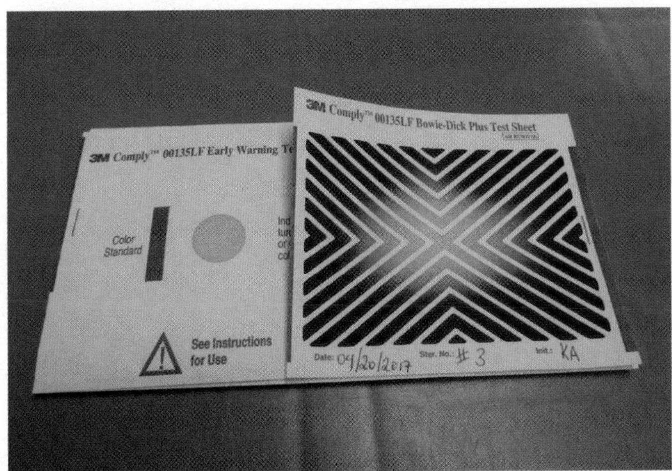

Figure 17.11

This test should be performed each day the sterilizer is used, at the same time of day and after major repairs. The only items that should be in the chamber during this test are the sterilizer loading carriage (to hold the test), and the test itself. The dynamic air removal test should be placed over the chamber drain and run per the manufacturer's IFU.

Some sterilizers have a designated air removal test cycle; check to ensure this cycle matches the air removal test manufacturer's instructions. When the cycle is complete, remove the test pack. If the chemically impregnated sheet has a complete uniform color change, the test is considered negative, and the sterilizer is ready to use. If the color change is not uniform and there are blotchy areas of unchanged color, the test is considered positive, and the sterilizer should be removed from service until the issue can be determined and corrected.

Leak Testing

Leak testing of dynamic air removal sterilizers is performed to ensure there are no air leaks within the chamber. This test checks the sterilizer's ability to hold a vacuum by testing all of the sealed areas and piping to ensure air is not allowed into the chamber during a cycle's vacuum phase. Leak tests should be performed at least weekly in an empty sterilizer chamber. Leak testing is more sensitive than a dynamic air removal test, so it will detect problems before the air removal test might detect the leak. *Note: Refer to the manufacturer's operating manual to determine the acceptable leak test.*

BIs/PCDs

The spore-producing microorganism used in steam sterilizer testing is *Geobacillus stearothermophilus*. This bacterium is used because it is heat-loving and, therefore, resistant to the temperatures used for steam sterilization.

It is recommended that commercially prepared PCDs be used; the materials utilized in the packages remain consistent because they are manufactured for single use, so there is no wear or erosion of the product.

Gravity Sterilizers

BIs/PCDs

The spore-producing microorganism used in gravity steam sterilizer testing is *Geobacillus stearothermophilus*.

It is recommended that commercially prepared PCDs be used; the materials utilized in the packages remain consistent because they are manufactured for single use, so there is no wear or erosion of the product. Ensure that the PCD to be used is designed for gravity sterilizers.

Immediate Use Steam Sterilizers

BIs/PCDs

The spore-producing microorganism used in steam sterilizer testing is *Geobacillus stearothermophilus*.

BIs are processed in immediate use steam sterilizers (IUSS), without a PCD. This is because items are processed unwrapped or in special containers designed for IUSS. BI ampules should be run in IUSS per the manufacturer's IFU. BIs should be run at least weekly, preferably each day the sterilizer is used, and with every load containing an implantable item. Similar to the processing of BIs in SP, BI tests in an IUSS cycle should be performed with a control of the same lot.

IUSS monitoring includes detailed recordkeeping so patients can be monitored if necessary. When an IUSS cycle is run, the following information should be documented:

- Date and time of sterilization cycle
- Sterilizer identification (ID)
- Cycle temperature and sterilization time
- Item(s) being sterilized
- Patient ID
- Reason for sterilizing the item using IUSS
- CI results
- BI results, if appropriate

Multiple Cycle Testing

Some dynamic air removal and immediate use steam sterilizers have the ability to operate in either a dynamic air removal mode or gravity mode. If a sterilizer is used in both sterilization methods, then BI/PCD testing must be done at least weekly (preferably daily) in both modes.

Tabletop Steam Sterilizers

BIs/PCDs

The spore-producing microorganism used in tabletop steam sterilizer testing is *Geobacillus stearothermophilus.*

Commercially prepared PCDs are currently not available for tabletop sterilizers. Types of items sterilized vary greatly from facility to facility, so creating a standard PCD would be extremely difficult. To create a PCD for the tabletop sterilizer:

- Select a tray of instruments or package that represents the most difficult item routinely sterilized in the tabletop sterilizer.
- Once the tray or pack has been identified, it should be used for each test performed.
- Place at least one BI and at least one CI in the most challenging area of the tray or pack to sterilize.

After a major repair to a tabletop steam sterilizer, three consecutive test cycles with a PCD should be run, and the results should be read before the sterilizer is put back into use.

Ethylene Oxide Sterilizers

BI/PCDs

BIs are the most acceptable means of providing quality assurance monitoring for ethylene oxide (EO) sterilization. Like BIs used in steam sterilization, an EO BI has a carrier that has been inoculated with a known population of a microorganism that is highly resistant to the sterilant. The microorganism of choice for EO is the *Bacillus atrophaeus* spore. It is assumed that killing all spores on a standardized BI indicates a successful sterilization cycle; this is because the BI's population and resistance exceeds that of the bioburden on items being sterilized. *Note: This assumption only applies to properly cleaned, prepared, packaged and loaded supplies. It is required that a PCD be run in every EO load.*

Remember the four Rs

Process monitoring consists of the four Rs: run, read, record and retain. No single monitoring product provides all information necessary to ensure effective sterilization; therefore, recommended practices state that available information from physical, chemical and biological indictors should be used to assess the process before releasing a load.

Hydrogen Peroxide Sterilizers

There are several different types of hydrogen peroxide (H_2O_2) sterilizers available in today's healthcare market; however, the basic monitoring requirements remain the same for all types of H_2O_2 sterilizers.

BIs/PCD

BIs are the most accepted means for providing quality assurance for hydrogen peroxide (H_2O_2) sterilizers. The microorganism of choice for H_2O_2 is the *Geobacillus stearothermophilus* spore because this bacterium is the most difficult to kill using H_2O_2 methods. A BI PCD should be run at least each day the sterilizer is used, but preferably in every load.

Commercially prepared PCDs are available; however, they are sold to monitor specific sterilizer models. Ensure the correct PCD is being used for the sterilizer.

PERSONNEL MONITORING

Personnel monitoring can involve several different types of devices. One type of monitoring system uses a badge-type monitor that affixes directly to the employee's clothing in the breathing zone (within one foot of the person's nose). Area monitors are also commonly used. These measure the quality of air in a specific area and alarm if air quality levels are breached.

STAFF EDUCATION

Tasks performed by SP technicians require specific knowledge and skills. The safety of both staff and patients depends on proper execution of specific skills. New instruments, equipment, standards and regulations make ongoing education necessary for even the most experienced SP technicians.

SPDs must provide evidence of the training and education provided for staff. That evidence is usually contained in training documents, competencies and continuing education records.

Training Documents

When a new employee enters the SPD or when an existing employee moves to a new position within the department, the formal process of orienting and training the staff member to their new responsibilities begins. That process should follow a carefully designed training plan that will prepare the employee to correctly perform the required duties. Training and/or orientation documents must be kept on file for each employee as evidence that formal training occurred.

Competencies

Employee competency records are an important monitoring tool for the SPD. Competencies provide evidence that the employee understands specific tasks and is qualified to perform them. Competency records are important for the growth of the department and serve as a basis for a quality improvement program.

Detailed, step-by-step lists should be developed and utilized for each task performed within the SPD. Competencies should be done during initial orientation, whenever a new device is received, when updated instructions are received, and on a routine basis for daily SP tasks. Some competencies will need to be done annually (i.e., tasks pertaining to sterilizer operation and documentation and when processing endoscopes), while other job duties, such as wrapping techniques, may only need to be done when issues arise or on a rotating basis.

Competency records can be reviewed to determine areas where each employee excels or where more training is needed. They can also be used to show process improvement.

Continuing Education Records

The SP discipline is constantly evolving, and SP technicians must evolve with it. Continuing education provides a means of staying abreast of changes in regulations, standards, technology, scientific knowledge, and equipment. Continuing education records provide evidence that the employee has kept current and is aware of new best practices. **Figure 17.12** provides an example of an employee inservice, a common method used to help educate SP staff.

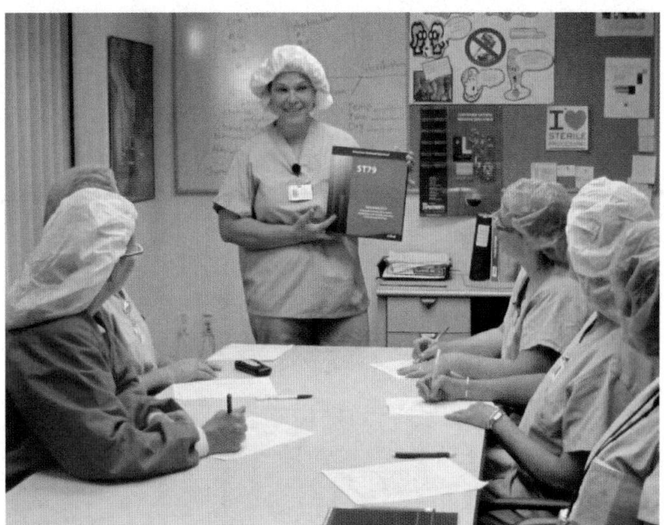

Figure 17.12

Education records should be kept on file for all SP employees and should be monitored to help ensure they are current.

CONCLUSION

Properly and consistently monitoring the SPD and processing equipment helps ensure patient and staff safety. It also helps ensure the consistent production of high-quality products.

Every member of the SPD must monitor the environment, work practices, mechanical processes, and training and education to ensure that standards, regulations and best practices are properly and consistently followed.

RESOURCES

Occupational Safety and Health Administration. OSHA Standard 29 CFR 1910.151(c).

OSHA Standard 29 CFR 1910.1047. Ethylene Oxide.

Centers for Disease Control and Prevention. *Guideline for Disinfection and Sterilization in Healthcare Facilities.* 2008.

ANSI/AAMI ST58 *Chemical sterilization and high-level disinfection in health care facilities.* 2013

ANSI/AAMI ST79:2017 & 2020 Amendments A1, A2, A3 and A4 *Comprehensive guide to steam sterilization and sterility assurance in health care facilities,* Section 13.

AAMI TIR34:2014/(R)2021 *Water for the reprocessing of medical devices.*

STERILE PROCESSING TERMS

Monitor

Verification

Load control number

Julian date

Validation

Chapter 18

Quality Production and Monitoring

Learning Objectives

As a result of successfully completing this chapter, the reader will be able to:

1. Define quality and process monitoring in the context of Sterile Processing operations
2. Explain common quality programs
3. Discuss how to manage quality

INTRODUCTION

Healthcare consumers demand **quality** in the products and services they receive. They expect nothing less than the best for themselves and their loved ones while using healthcare services. Sterile Processing (SP) technicians must establish and monitor appropriate quality levels for the products and services they produce and ensure that these levels are consistently maintained.

SP technicians directly serve **internal customers** (physicians, nurses and other professionals working in the facility). The success of SP depends upon satisfying the needs of these internal customers so caretakers can best serve the patients. Quality (or lack of quality) can have dramatic consequences on the health and safety of both patients and facility personnel. Providing quality products and services directly impacts patient outcomes and significantly impacts the success of the department and healthcare facility.

> **Quality** The consistent delivery of products and services according to established standards. Quality "integrates" the concerns for the customers (including patients and user department personnel) with those of the department and facility.
>
> **Customer (internal)** The physicians, nurses and other professional personnel served by Sterile Processing personnel.

SP technicians are an integral part of quality service throughout the healthcare facility. SP technicians are now processing medical devices for surgery centers, physician's offices, off-site clinics, nursing rehabilitation facilities, dental offices, and third-party reprocessors. With antibiotic-resistant bacteria, deadly viruses, ever-increasing complexity of surgical instrumentation and increasing news coverage of poor quality services and outcomes, it has never been more challenging and rewarding for SP personnel to consistently provide quality products and services.

This chapter addresses several established quality SP indicators and how to increase and maintain quality processes within SP departments (SPDs). The ultimate goal is high-quality patient care. This can best be achieved through comprehensive training programs and ongoing quality monitoring.

QUALITY IN SP OPERATIONS

Quality requires SP technicians to look at what they do from their customers' perspectives. In many respects, SP production is only as good as the last device processed or the most recent service provided. A complex surgical instrument set can be processed 100 times, with 99 sets being perfect but the final set missing an instrument that was not noted. Not only is the 100th set below the department quality standard, but the customer now remembers the defective tray and may assume the entire department is negligent. While this may seem unreasonable, it is important to understand that just one error can cause significant harm to patients and employees.

What Is Quality?

The concept of quality relates to the degree or grade of excellence of a product or service. For example, a procedure cart that was not properly stocked may be sent to the Emergency Department (ED). Even if the ED staff had everything they needed, they may still notice that items were missing from the carts. In short, quality is measured through the eyes of the customers, and their concerns relate to both products and service. Quality monitoring requires the department maintain and/or improve their quality process constantly.

The patient must be at the center of every quality concern. SP technicians must provide properly processed products when they are needed. Just being "good" is not good enough. A surgical tray delivered to the Operating Room (OR) on time but with incomplete or incorrect instruments does not represent quality service and can cause a patient to have a less-than-desirable outcome due to instrumentation problems. SP technicians accept this responsibility and the challenge to consistently meet requirements.

Looking at functions from customer' perspective allows the SP team to critically review its processes to determine where improvements can be made. Remember that:

- Increased education should help staff provide a higher quality of service.
- Quality takes time, effort and participation from everyone in the healthcare facility.
- When measuring quality, best practices provide a good starting point.
- SP staff can use their knowledge to increase efficiencies.

How Is Quality Identified?

Products and services might be considered "excellent" if they meet one's needs (they do what they are supposed to do). If a new washer-disinfector is used properly, but instruments are still dirty after a complete cycle, the equipment will be judged inferior; however, if the equipment meets expectations (produces clean and decontaminated instruments), it is easier to assume that, "This is a great manufacturer, and I would purchase from this company again."

Such assumptions provide a subjective view of quality that provides no basis for measurement. What's more, they do not consider the customers' service levels. Branding is another subjective form of quality identification. If one has a great experience with specific equipment, a future purchase from that manufacturer is more likely than if negative experiences occur.

What Is Quality Monitoring?

Products processed by SP technicians should always be complete and properly assembled, with no errors. Quality monitoring is the process of maintaining or improving the department's quality outputs. An internal department system should be implemented to identify inferior products before they leave the area. External department information can be obtained from customers by using the count sheets for trays, pick tickets for case carts and requested items, and/or by formal surveys designed to learn about quality dimensions from customers' perspective. Statistics from both internal and external sources should be analyzed, errors should be studied, and corrective actions should be implemented to best ensure quality improvement.

COMPONENTS OF QUALITY

Quality is not a quick fix for healthcare facilities. Achieving world-class (best in the industry) quality requires a multi-year plan to move a facility from its current quality level to the ideal (highest achievable) quality.

Top-level administrators must emphasize quality because their support is critical for success. Most problems affecting employees' ability to accomplish work are caused by systems and procedures that have, in some way, been required or implemented by leadership.

Departmental quality should be multidisciplinary as well as intradepartmental. A true quality program utilizes all SP technicians and a cross section of its customers. (See **Figure 18.1**)

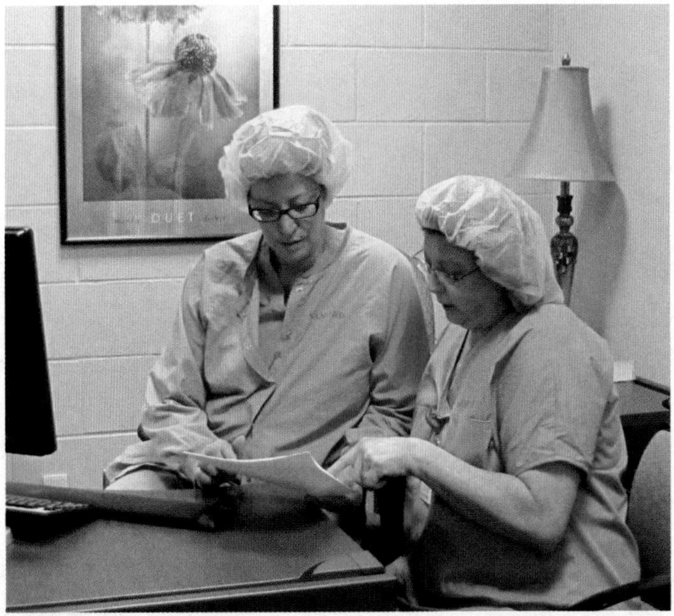

Figure 18.1

Many technicians believe quality initiatives are leadership's responsibility when, in fact, the SP staff should be an integral part of the team selected to develop the program (and the technicians should follow the program they developed as a team). There are many components, like planning and environmental conditions, that are leadership's responsibility; however, these quality components, as well as many others, are a critical part of the quality input all technicians should add to the program on a daily basis. **Figure 18.2** shows many of the quality input items that technicians should incorporate into their daily work.

Empowerment

Empowerment is another component of a quality program. It drives the process of decision making and implementation down the facility's chain of command. In other words, some decisions that have traditionally been made by managers or higher-level departmental staff or administrators are now made by supervisors or frontline staff members. Empowerment is typically limited to well-defined areas such as **process improvement** changes within the employee's defined areas of responsibility.

Empowerment The act of granting authority (power) to employees so they may make decisions within their areas of responsibility.

Process improvement Activity to identify and resolve task-related problems that yield poor quality; the strategy of finding solutions to eliminate the root causes of process performance problems.

Employees assigned to specific work areas must know how to perform all tasks properly before they can be empowered. Managers must provide training about the concept of empowerment, and encourage the sharing of ideas and suggestions that can lead to improvements.

It is important to remember that with empowerment comes responsibility. Decisions should be based on the standards and best practices, not on changing something that is a completely correct process for one that is incorrect but convenient.

Leadership

Quality requires committed leaders to help manage the data, plan opportunities, establish priorities and empower people to implement process improvements. Effective leaders define standards to be attained in quality products and services. Those standards will drive the development of strategies that address customer satisfaction and the attainment of the facility's goals.

Departmental leaders, including shift supervisors and lead technicians, should be the first line "guardians" of the quality program to ensure that all department personnel consistently

Quality Input	Knowledge Needed
Administrative	· Planning · Knowledge of critical items · Prioritization · Shift organization · Safety policies · Standards, guidelines, best practices · Communication (verbal and written) · Teamwork
Environmental	· Air/humidity policy · Dress code for each area · Needed equipment available and functional · Preventative maintenance compliant · Emergency policies
Education	· Continues to grow · Maintains competencies · Formal education classes · Informal education classes · Mentors others · Accepts mentors for self

Risk Management	· Assists with assessments
	· Instrument traceability
	    o Instruments/sets
	    o Implants
	    o Loaned instruments
	· Departmental mitigation practices
	· Knows and always follows regulations, standards, best practices
	· Assesses and uses IFU in every area

Decontamination/Assembly	· Cleanliness inspection of all devices · Function testing · Verification testing · Quality assurance procedures
Sterilization	· Load weights for each sterilizer and type of cycle · Cycle monitoring · Verifications · Expiration dating/lot control
Storage/Transport	· Storage policies · Rotation/expiration · Inventory policies · Sterility maintenance
Quality Assurance	· QA process · QA processes for sets, single instruments, equipment
Documentation	· Required documentation for each area · Attended education · Incidents

Figure 18.2 Quality inputs

adhere to the standards and priorities set by senior managers. Technicians should help their teammates follow established guidelines. Technicians can accomplish this by following policies and procedures, applying the education received in the department and interacting with new or less-qualified staff members, assisting in ongoing training and participating in daily quality control checks.

Data Collection

Each department must select the data that will be used to monitor its quality processes. **Figure 18.3** provides an example of data that has been collected and compiled for analysis. Data for data sake is not useful; data points should be carefully selected and reported in a standardized format so it shows a realistic picture of the existing department status and where the department is headed.

Measurement	Goal	Actual	Color
Avg. Trays Backlogged 7am	< 15	42	
Avg. Trays Backlogged 11pm	< 25	76	
# Errors Reported	< 3	2	
% Case Carts Complete Supplies	99%	97%	
% Case Carts Complete Instruments	95%	91%	
% Complete Instrument Trays	98%	94%	
Total Hours per Tray Processed	1.80	2.03	
Staff Productivity	90%	92%	

Figure 18.3

Sterile Processing Department Dashboard												
	Goal	Apr-22	May-22	Jun-22	Jul-22	Aug-22	Sep-22	Oct-22	Nov-22	Dec-22	Trend	Desired Trend
Immediate Use Sterilization Rate (IUSS): Month	< 0.5%	1.1%	0.8%	0.9%	0.5%	0.3%	0%	0.14%			↓	↓
Immediate Use Sterilization Rate (IUSS): YTD	< 0.5%	1%	1%	1%	0.5%	0.3%	0.4	0.28			↓	↓
QA Set Monitoring Accuracy Program	> 95%	98%	100%	98%	99%	98%	98%	97%			–	↓
SPD Set Accuracy Rate	> 90%	No data	No data	No data	93%	95%	96%	94%			↑	↑
Tray Audit into Decontamination	> 90%	No data	No data	No data	93%	96%	94%	96%			↑	↑
SPD/Surgical Tech Tray Audit: % Compliance with IFU	100%	No data	No data	No data	100%	100%	100%	100%			↑	↑

Figure 18.4 Quality dashboard

Quality Planning

Quality planning can reduce existing problems and prevent potential problems. It involves studying other facilities, thinking about how to improve, and remembering that the process (not people) is the cause of most problems. Steps of quality planning include identifying the customer's needs, comparing how the department functions to today and how it should be functioning, and system improvement. Error measurement is important to determine the current state of the department and where the department should go from there.

While tracking and improving quality are important components to an overall quality department, todays' focus is on managing the quality improvement process.

Several principles of quality management form the foundation of a quality process:

- Patient focus – Assuring that patients' needs are the driving force in decision making, problem solving and other activities.
- Process management – Placing the emphasis on managing the process rather than upon managing the employees.
- Continuous quality improvement – Believing that things can always be done better and then undertaking improvement efforts.
- Fact-based decisions – Basing decisions on facts rather than assumptions.

Staff Members

To have a successful quality program, all departmental staff members must be fully engaged with the program. While management may set the standards and goals, technicians, for the most part, carry out the processes to achieve success. Providing all staff members with a solid education foundation will help ensure they use critical-thinking skills on the job.

Employees must be empowered to address solutions to immediate problems within their realm of expertise. For example, technicians should be allowed to stop what they are doing to help another employee, or they should be able to enlist the assistance of other workers in problem-solving tasks, when necessary. Technicians who desire additional responsibilities should be allowed to work on longer-term problem-solving projects. This may be done with the use of **cross-functional teams** that select a process problem, analyze it, develop alternatives, offer solutions and make implementation suggestions. It is important for senior leaders to recognize superior staff.

Cross-functional team Group of employees from different departments within the healthcare facility that works together to resolve operating problems.

Process Management

Studying processes is critical because process problems cause errors. If errors are identified and resolved, patients and customers will experience fewer problems. (See **Figure 18.4**) Also, SP technicians will have greater success in consistently delivering products and services that meet quality standards. Some processes commonly studied for improvement are:

- Instrument set turnaround times
- Instrument set accuracy
- Surgical case cart accuracy
- Inventory fill rates

The highest levels of quality are difficult to attain and maintain. When quality is not emphasized, inconsistent products, service delays, negative patient outcomes, and employee conflicts can arise. These problems contribute to higher costs for the facility and the patient, and lower revenues for the healthcare facility.

QUALITY CONTROL INDICATORS

Purpose of Quality Control Indicators

SP quality control indicators are often used to determine how well the department is meeting its objectives. Several quality indicators should be monitored periodically. (See **Figure 18.5**) Some examples of SP quality indicators are:

- Customer departments receive STAT (urgent) medical supplies within five minutes of the request.
- Only sterile supplies with current dates are available on unit supply carts.
- Sterilization processes are acceptable, based upon results of physical indicators and chemical and biological indicators (CIs/BIs).
- Instrument sets contain clean, functional and correct contents.
- Patient care equipment and supplies are available and in proper working condition.
- Instruments are available for scheduled procedures to avoid the use of IUSS.
- BIs accompany every load that requires biological monitoring.
- Case carts contain correct contents.

Failure Mode and Effects Analysis

Failure mode and effects analysis (FMEA) has its origins in the military and industrial fields and is a method of identifying and preventing problems with products and processes before they occur. For new processes, it identifies potential bottlenecks or unintended consequences prior to implementation. It is also helpful for evaluating an existing system or process to understand how proposed changes will impact the system. The FMEA process seeks to accomplish several things. First, it aims to define the topic that must be addressed (e.g., replacing a hospital boiler) and then a group of multidisciplinary staff is assembled to identify possible hazards and causes (e.g., poor steam quality, pipe ruptures, and service disruption). Finally, the team identifies actions and outcomes for each potential problem. For example, before replacing the boiler, it may be important to rent a temporary steam generator to use if problems arise so the food service department, OR and SP may remain.

Root Cause Analysis

Root cause analysis (RCA) is a reactive process that looks at an adverse outcome (error) to help prevent its recurrence. Assume, for example, that a washer-disinfector's pump malfunctioned and caused instruments to be cleaned improperly. Each event after the pump failure would be examined to determine what could have occurred and what can be done to prevent this issue in the future.

Another example is the tip of a carbide insert on a needle holder breaking during surgery. All members involved with the set will meet to determine what happened and how to prevent a recurrence. Members of this group should include:

- Surgeon (How was the instrument used?)
- Scrub technician and circulating nurse (What happened? Was the instrument checked before giving it to the surgeon?)
- SP manager and the technician who assembled the tray (What are the set policies and procedures for instrument assembly/testing? Was the instrument checked properly?)
- Risk manager (usually serves as meeting facilitator)

Step	Explanation
Select a process to analyze	Choose a process that is known to be problematic in your facility or one that is known to be problematic in many facilities.
Select team facilitator and team members	Leadership should select a project facilitator to launch the team. Team members are people who are directly involved in the process to be analyzed.
Describe the process	Clearly define the process steps, so everyone on the team knows what is being analyzed.
Identify what could go wrong during each step of the process	Here is where the people directly involved in the process describe the problems that can or do occur.
Pick which problems to work on eliminating	The focus of improvements will be on those problems that happen quite often and/or have a significant impact on safety when they do occasionally occur.
Design and implement changes to reduce or prevent problems	The team determines how best to change the process to reduce the risk of harm.
Measure the success of process changes	Like all improvement projects, the success of improvement actions is evaluated.

Figure 18.5

- Any other interested parties (instrument repair technician, Infection Prevention personnel)

RCA is widely utilized in the medical field to examine contributing factors to adverse events. *Note: The Joint Commission (TJC) standard LD 04.04.05 requires facilities to conduct an RCA on any recurring* ***sentinel event***.

Failure mode and effect analysis (FMEA) A process designed to predict the adverse outcomes of various human and machine failures to prevent future adverse outcomes.

Root cause analysis (RCA) A method of problem solving that "looks backward" to identify the root cause of a problem to help prevent its future occurrence.

Sentinal event An unexpected occurrence involving death, serious physical or psychological injury, or the risk thereof.

QUALITY PROGRAMS

Quality assurance programs should be comprehensive and pertinent to the individual SPD. The type of data collected should reflect the areas where SP needs improvement, or the high-risk processes performed by the department's technicians.

Because of the wide variety of tasks that are performed in SPDs, many facilities develop their own quality program utilizing a combination of several of the different types of programs. As long as the program works for the facility and emphasizes the main focus of quality patient care, it doesn't matter which program or combinations of programs are used. **Figure 18.6** provides examples of some of the most popular quality programs used in healthcare today.

Quality assurance A comprehensive and measured effort to provide total quality. Also, a technical, statistical sampling method that measures production quality.

Total quality improvement (TQI) The concept of measuring the current output of a process or procedure and then modifying it to increase the output, increase efficiency, and/or increase effectiveness.

Processes (work) A series of work activities that produces a product or service.

Continuous quality improvement (CQI) A scientific approach that applies statistical methods to improve work processes.

Total quality management (TQM) A quality management approach based on participation of all members aimed at long-term success through customer satisfaction and benefits to all members of the organization and society.

Six Sigma A quality process that focuses on developing and delivering near-perfect products and services.

Lean A quality process that focuses on eliminating waste in the production of products.

Quality Assurance Program	Program Focus
Total Quality Improvement	· Measures current output · Modifies the program to increase output · Improvement can occur with one person or a group
Continuous Quality Improvement	· Statistical method to improve **work processes** · Uses input from staff and a multidisciplinary team · Identifies where more training is needed
Total Quality Management	· Success through customer satisfaction · Ensures work tasks are performed correctly · Eliminates operational wastes and defects
Six Sigma	· High performance · Reliability to end customer · Near-perfect products · Process improvement · Variation reduction
Lean	· Production focus · Fast implementation · Error reduction · Financial improvement · Increased customer satisfaction and staff morale

Figure 18.6

SPD Missing Instruments

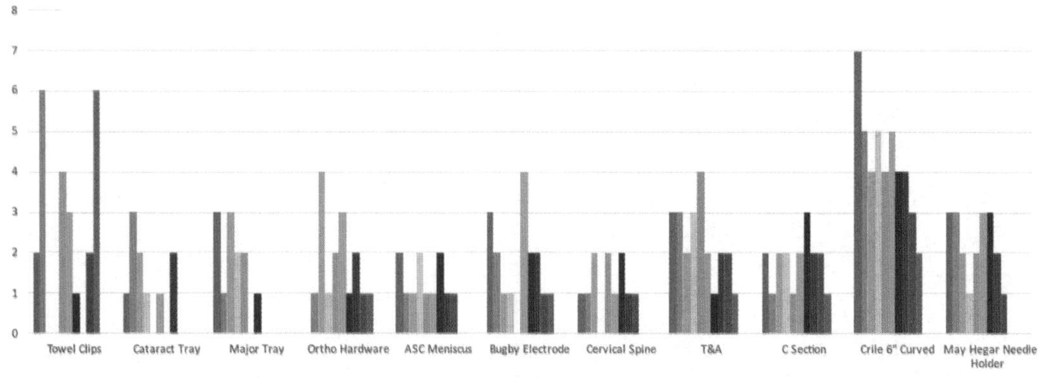

Figure 18.7

SPD Missing Instruments

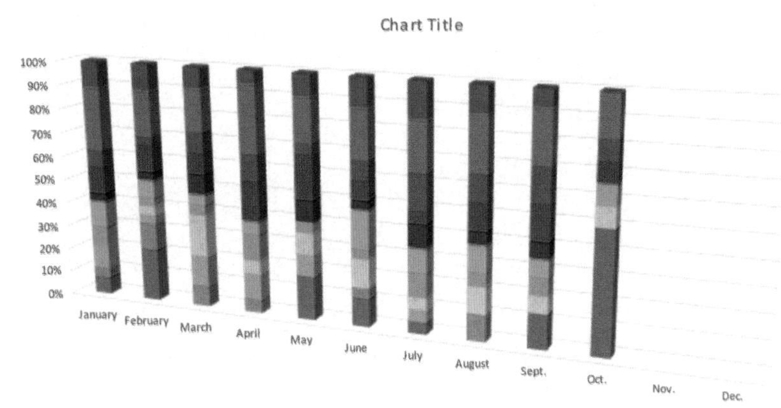

Figure 18.8

SPD IUSS Cycles

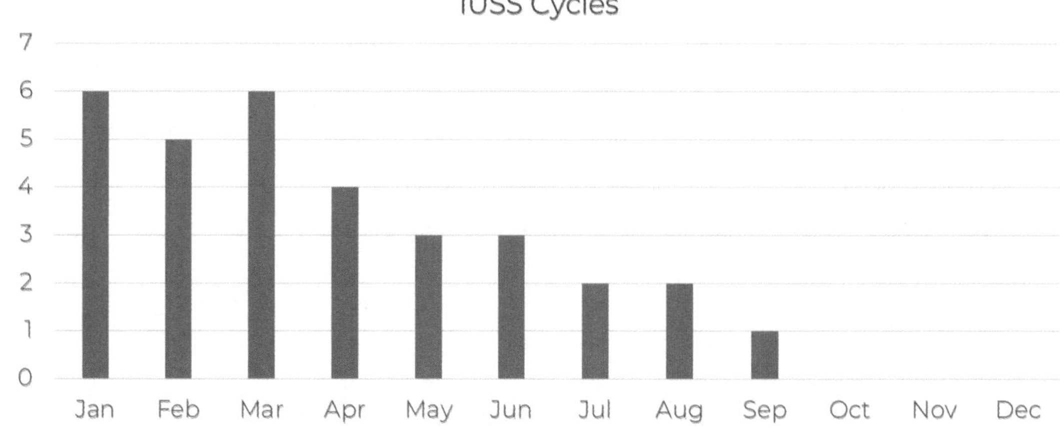

Figure 18.9

Problem Analysis Charts for Missing/Incorrect Instrument Trays

Trays sent from OR to SP

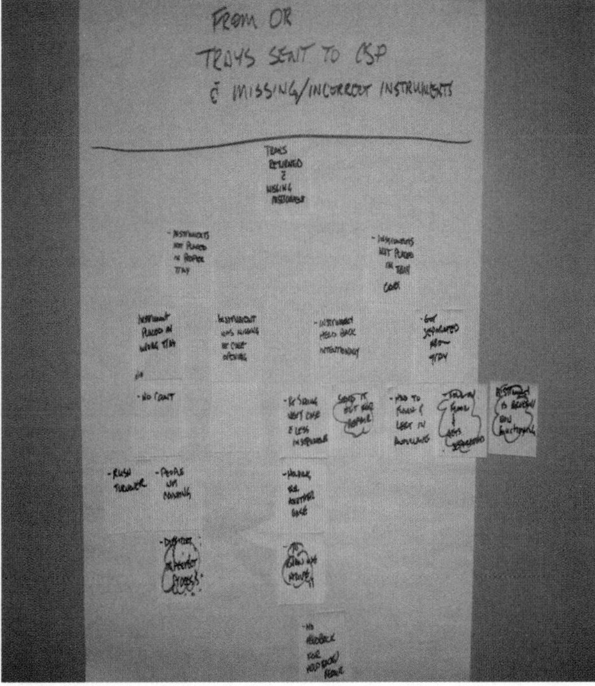

Trays sent from SP to OR

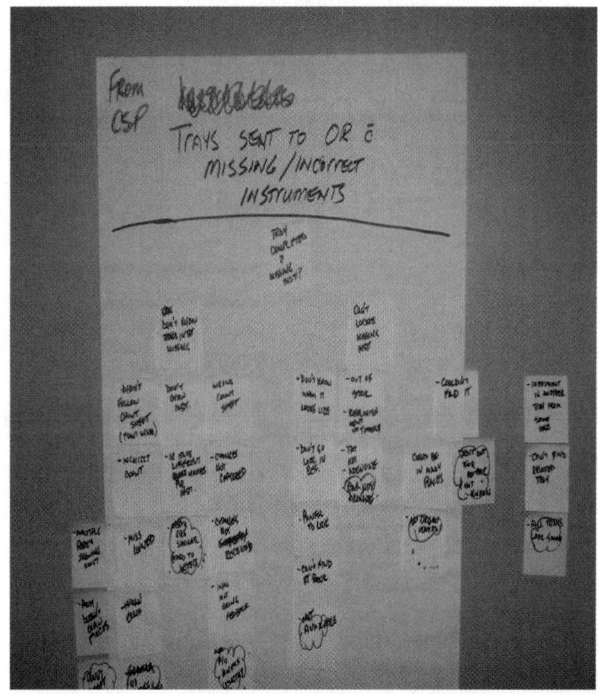

Figure 18.10

Figures 18.7 and **18.8** provide examples of a quality report that identifies the types of instrument errors made in one department. **Figure 18.9** provides an example of a report indicating progress in an effort to reduce IUSS.

Quality at Work

Being an active participant in any quality process helps ensure the solutions generated are workable for everyone involved. Whether the activity involves the SP workgroup or a broader, cross-functional team, taking the time to examine processes and identify opportunities for improvement is worthwhile.

This section provides examples of some common methods to identify quality issues and improve them. **Figure 18.10** illustrates a simple process where representatives from two workgroups, OR and SP, identified issues with trays sent to the OR and SPD. Using a simple problem analysis chart fostered better communication, captured issues and gave the group information to make changes to improve their processes.

Figure 18.11 shows the result of a workgroup's efforts to identify waste in their processes. This information was then used to simplify processes, reduce waste, and educate staff.

Figures 18.12 and **18.13** address labor trends and processing volumes for the SPD. Each provides a tool to address quality issues.

WASTES
74
LARGER lock ON PAN
PLACEMENT OF LABEL ON OUTER Container
BARCODE NOT ON BOTH END OF TRAY
HEAVY TRAY ON DELICATE LIDS
LIDS NOT ON TRAYS

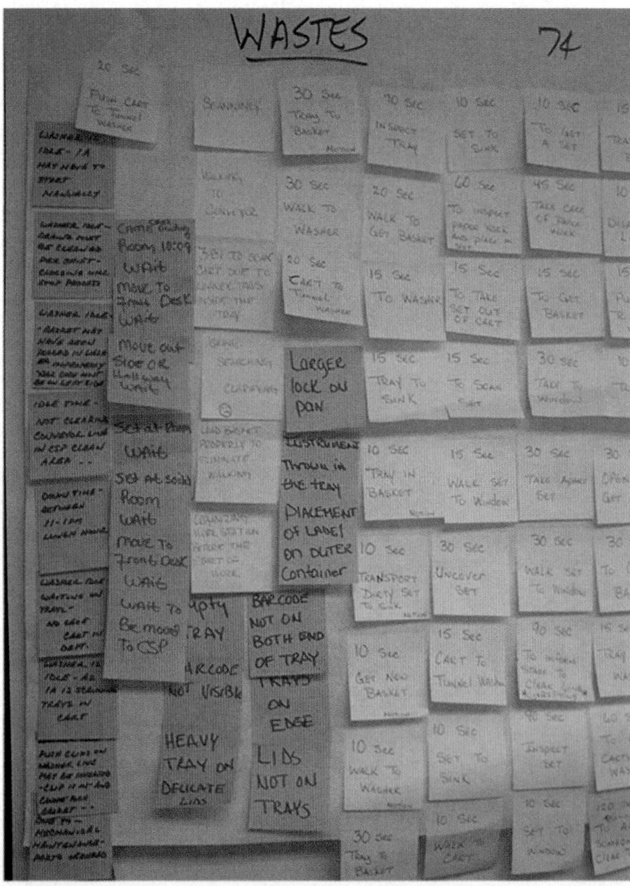

Figure 18.11

		SPD Labor Hour Needs				Cycle Starts	
		Decontam	Assembly	Sterilize	Total	Washer Loads	Sterilizer Loads
1st Shift	7:00	0.3	0.8	0.1	1.2	0.4	0.2
	8:00	0.2	1.0	0.0	1.2	0.3	0.1
	9:00	0.2	0.7	0.0	0.9	0.3	0.2
	10:00	1.8	0.7	0.0	2.5	3.0	0.1
	11:00	3.0	7.4	0.0	10.4	4.9	0.1
	12:00	4.4	12.0	0.3	16.8	7.3	1.2
	13:00	4.2	17.8	0.5	22.4	6.9	2.0
	14:00	4.1	16.7	0.7	21.5	6.7	2.9

Figure 18.12

Quality-Centered Organizations and Standards

Quality efforts of healthcare facilities are also impacted by external agencies whose requirements must be addressed. SP technicians should be familiar with the following:

The Joint Commission

The Joint Commission (TJC) is an accreditation organization that ensures quality standards are set, monitored and maintained by member healthcare facilities. It has established many health and safety program requirements for patients and staff using recommended practices and guidelines from agencies and associations, including the Occupational Safety and Health Administration (OSHA) and the Association for the Advancement of Medical Instrumentation (AAMI). Routine and unannounced inspections are used to monitor standards, and each member facility is graded on its performance. TJC requires that any sentinel event be reported and thoroughly investigated to correct the causes. *Note: There are several approved accreditation agencies like the Healthcare Quality Association on Accreditation (HQAA) and American Association for Accreditation of Ambulatory Surgery Facilities (AAAASF).*

Centers for Medicare & Medicaid Services

The Centers for Medicare & Medicaid Services (CMS) is a government agency that focuses on quality in healthcare as well as patient safety and security. Like TJC, CMS performs announced and unannounced surveys of healthcare facilities to ensure industry standards and regulations are being followed and maintained, and that high quality patient care is the outcome.

National Committee for Quality Assurance

The National Committee for Quality Assurance (NCQA) is a nonprofit organization dedicated to improving healthcare quality. The organization is known for assisting healthcare facilities in identifying how to prioritize quality goals, measure them and promote ongoing quality improvement.

Hospital Consumer Assessment of Healthcare Providers and Systems Survey and Value-Based Initiatives

The Hospital Consumer Assessment of Healthcare Providers and Systems (HCAHPS) (pronounced "H-caps") is a standardized survey tool. Hospitals utilize survey results to measure the patient's perception of their experience during hospitalization. Three broad goals shape HCAHPS:

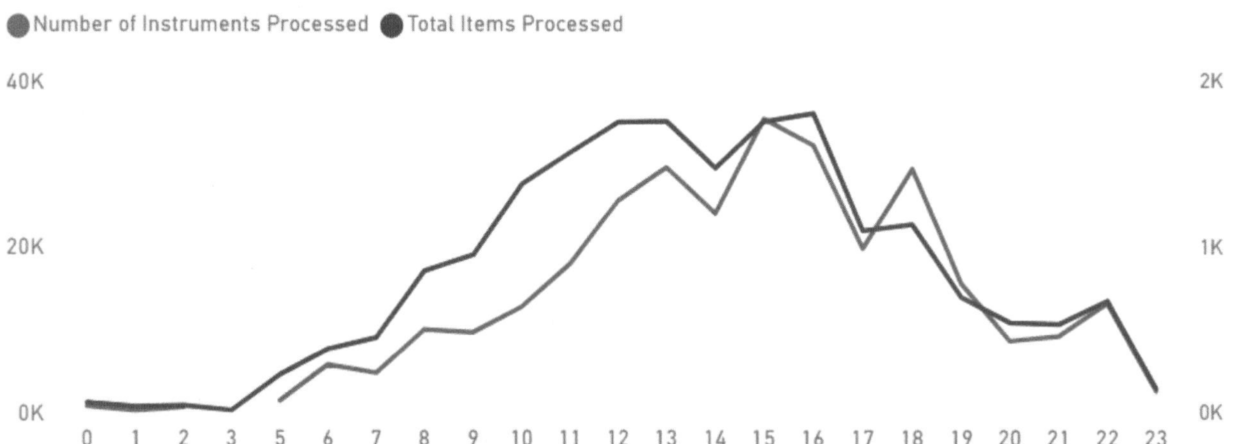

Figure 18.13

1. The standardized survey allows meaningful comparisons of hospitals from the patient's perspective.

2. Public reporting of HCAHPS results creates new incentives for hospitals to improve their quality of care.

3. Public reporting serves to enhance accountability in healthcare.

The value-based purchasing (VBP) initiatives compare a hospital's HCAHPS scores in a baseline period to those in a later performance period. Healthcare facilities that do not reach HCAHPS goals are penalized through reduced government reimbursement.

International Organization for Standardization

The International Organization for Standardization (ISO, commonly referred to as the International Standards Organization) provides ISO 9000 and 9001, international standards that companies use to ensure their quality system is effective. This process is believed to guarantee that a company consistently delivers quality services and products. ISO 9000 is the definition of quality management system; ISO 9001 are the requirements needed to meet ISO 9000. While many healthcare organizations have subscribed to ISO standards, few SPDs have applied or qualified for ISO status.

QUALITY IN SP WORK AREAS

There are many quality processes that all SP technicians must consistently practice in their daily routine. This section reviews some of these processes on an area-by-area basis within the department.

Decontamination Area

- Always wear personal protective equipment (PPE) when working in this area to protect oneself, other staff, and patients when leaving the area.
- Document the temperature humidity of the area, if not done electronically, and verify negative pressure flow.
- Disassemble all items, where applicable, to ensure all instrument parts are accessible for cleaning.
- Measure chemicals properly. Improperly measured chemicals are not effective cleaners or disinfectants.
- Load and operate equipment properly. Improperly loaded or operated equipment cannot effectively clean instruments.
- Follow all written procedures for cleaning and disinfection. Ensure that items are cleaned and disinfected according to the manufacturer's instructions for use (IFU).
- Check processing equipment before use to ensure it is in proper working order. Improperly working equipment can harm staff and patients.
- Check quality monitoring devices, such as leak testers, for functionality.
- Check all equipment monitors, like printouts, to help ensure all required parameters were met; do not release any instrument from a failed load.
- Check each manually cleaned item for cleanliness prior to sending it to the preparation and packaging area.
- Perform cleaning verification:
    - › Ensure all cleaning equipment has been properly tested and verified as ready for use. Different pieces of equipment may have different tests that need to be performed each day of use to verify that the equipment is in proper working order. Run each test per facility policy and both the equipment and the verification tests' IFU.
    - › Although cleanliness verification of most devices is performed in the preparation and packaging area, there are devices that should be tested in the decontamination area before moving the device to the next step in the process. Always use the correct verification test and follow the test's IFU. Do not avoid or rush this process because an unclean device can harm co-workers and patients.
    - › Legibly and accurately document all test results per the facility's policy.

Preparation and Packaging Areas

- Perform cleaning verification testing following facility protocol for instrument type and frequency. There are different types of cleaning verification tests available [protein, hemoglobin and adenosine triphosphate (ATP)], so always ensure the proper test is used correctly and document all results.
- Check instruments for functionality, cleanliness, alignment, proper assembly, and sharpness. Failure to do so could result in patient harm.
- Always follow count sheets. Even if a technician has extensive experience performing the assigned task, changes may have occurred to a case cart or instrument set. Remember, patient care personnel require the correct supplies and devices as requested for the procedure.
- Only use U.S. Food and Drug Administration (FDA)-cleared items, like tip protectors, in any set.

- Place the appropriate internal indicator(s) per facility procedure.
- Use only FDA-approved wrappers and containers cleared for the specific method of sterilization utilized.
- Check for holes in all wrappers and disposable filters to ensure they are intact before sterilization. Even normal handling can sometimes cause a small percentage of wrappers and filters to become damaged prior to use. Be sure containers are undamaged and the correct size for the amount of instruments in the set.
- Never use towels unless stated in the container's IFU.
- Always launder towels between uses to avoid superheating.
- Never reuse disposable foam. Clean reusable foam between uses per the IFU.
- Never use a wrapper, filter or instrument that has fallen on the floor. If this occurs, instruments should be recleaned, and disposable wrappers and filters should be discarded.
- Use the proper external indicator on each package.
- Document the temperature and humidity of the area and verify positive pressure flow.

Sterilization Area

- Perform any sterilizer diagnostic testing or dynamic air removal tests, such as the Bowie-Dick test, prior to use.
- Always load sterilizer carts as trained. Improperly loaded carts can result in wet or nonsterile loads.
- Ensure each package contains the expiration date, if appropriate, and lot number.
- Ensure the sterilizer parameters are set properly for the load contents. This should include proper temperature, exposure and dry time.
- Always verify physical indicators and CIs after a sterilization cycle to ensure the process was completed properly.
- Run and incubate BIs per facility policy and the manufacturer's IFU.
- Do not touch sterilized items until cool.
- Properly complete all documentation, including load, biological and implant logs.

Storage and Distribution Areas

- Check product packaging for compromised integrity, expiration dates and appropriate color changes of all indicators prior to placing items on shelves or removing items for distribution.
- Ensure all shelves are clean and in good repair before placing items on them.
- Always follow established pick sheets to ensure that all items are collected and delivered.
- Ensure transport and case carts are clean and dry before placing items on or inside them.
- Document all issues, returns and damaged or expired items.
- Document the temperature and humidity for the area and verify positive pressure flow (if not captured electronically).

All Sterile Processing/Distribution Areas

- Pay attention to the job at hand. Excessive visiting or other distractions, like a loud radio, can lead to errors.
- SP technicians should not do anything they have not been trained to do. They must always inform someone when they are asked to perform a process or function in which they lack training.
- An SP technician who is unsure about a completed project should ask someone to check their work. This is much better than to have an incomplete or incorrect item leave the department.
- If distracted, check the entire project to ensure it was done correctly.
- If SP technicians cannot perform at 100%, they should not do the project. Also, they should not start a project if they know someone else will need to finish it.
- Recheck all work. The short time required to do so can eliminate an incident in a patient care area.
- Remember that neatness counts.
- Always help other staff members.
- If something appears wrong, speak up.
- Report inoperative or damaged equipment.
- Attend as many educational inservices, seminars, infection prevention- or service technician-provided training. The more education SP technicians can attain, the better they will become on the job.

Quality Improvement Results				
Measure	**Before**	**After**	**% Improvement**	**Lean Tools**
Daily capacity and demand	378 trays per day	437 trays per day	14% increase	Visual management layout
Rewashes	96 rewashes per day	34 rewashes per day	64% reduction	Standardized work, visual management
Reduction in walking	30 secs per tray	15 secs per tray	100% reduction	Layout
Receiving errors	14 trays per day	9 trays per day	35% reduction	Standardized work, visual management

Figure 18.14

- Always follow the established departmental policies, procedures and protocols. They are in place for a reason, which typically is to protect staff and patients.

Remember that quality is the responsibility of every employee, and every employee must be involved, motivated and knowledgeable if the SPD is to consistently produce and deliver quality products and services. (See **Figure 18.14**)

QUALITY MANAGEMENT

Attaining and maintaining high quality SP standards is everyone's responsibility. Every technician should play an active role in the department's quality program. It is also each technician's responsibility to help or report others who are struggling with a process. Keeping the patient as the focus means helping ensure everyone is properly trained and performing at optimum levels while working in the department. Allowing a known defective product out of the department is inexcusable and can be very dangerous for patients. There are several tools that can be used by technicians to help ensure quality is always addressed:

- Performing departmental audits of each area of the department on a regular basis helps to keep the department and its functions at optimal levels – Audits can be performed by outside departments, such as Safety or Infection Prevention and Control, or they can be done by the SP staff or a combination of these. Technicians are a valuable asset to these audits because they know the environment and processes better than anyone else. SP technicians should always take the initiative to report sub-quality work or departmental areas that do not meet existing quality standards.

- Following the departmental policies, procedures and processing protocols – These documents were developed to help ensure the safety of all SP members and ensure that all products produced are of the highest quality. Not following policies, procedures and protocols will result in a lower-quality product (i.e., missing, incorrect or soiled instruments), which may harm a patient.

- Keeping current with new technology and appropriately sharing what has been learned with co-workers and supervisors – As technology advances, the ability to check work becomes more effective. New products are continually being developed to help check for residual blood and protein. Better products are on the market to check for lumen cleanliness, as well as products that help ensure processing equipment is working properly. As instrumentation becomes more complex, it becomes more important to utilize technology to make certain quality products are being delivered. If there is any doubt about the functionality of processing equipment or any medical device, remove the item from service until it is properly repaired.

- SP technicians should take an active role in all process improvement projects – Technicians are very familiar with all department activities and can be a vital asset in helping determine problems and how best to resolve them.

- Assuming responsibility for survey readiness – As part of the SP team, each person is responsible for keeping the department ready for all facility surveys. Cleanliness, following set practices and knowing the required information about safety, disaster and department processes is a year-round practice.

- Adopting a team mentality – Help co-workers and accept help from them. No one is an expert on all processes within the department. Seek help where skills are not as strong and help those who need assistance.

- Attaining SP certification – Certified technicians demonstrate a baseline knowledge in SP processes and know why they perform procedures a specific way. This knowledge of the science behind the practices helps ensure practices will be followed correctly, thus helping ensure a quality product.

SP technicians are expected to consistently attain desired quality standards as they undertake their normal responsibilities. While this is a difficult goal to attain, it is a necessary one. SP technicians play a significant role in implementing quality within their facilities. They can, for example, consistently follow all instrument procedures discussed throughout this manual. They do not, however, work by themselves. Technicians are an integral part of the entire healthcare team. To ensure the highest quality of patient care, all staff members must work together. The sum of all contributions by all personnel in all departments represents the facility's accomplishments.

One of the most important tasks of quality management is to keep the department's quality numbers in the forefront of everyone's mind. If the numbers are sliding in the wrong direction, each technician should bring the issue forward, offer assistance as to why the problem is occurring and suggestions on correcting the issue.

When the quality numbers seem to stall or hold in one position with no improvement, study the numbers and help identify why the quality is not getting better. Technicians are in the active work area all shift and can see potential issues. Share concerns and ideas for helping improve the quality output.

If quality levels are dropping, be open about any issues that may be causing the decrease in quality. Keep in mind, excuses don't help; however, actively working to find the reason does. Engage fellow workers to work together to find the issue.

Study departmental errors to help find the cause and a resolution. Suggestions from the technicians working in the affected area will help develop a working solution.

It is also important to keep a close eye on the department's statistics. It is easier to fix a problem before it becomes a habit. Work together with co-workers to help develop corrective actions.

Last but not least, be sure to celebrate the department's successes. When a goal is met, patting each other on the back for a job well done increases morale and helps the statistics remain in the forefront.

CONCLUSION

Improving quality may seem easier than it is. Maintaining and improving quality takes work and pride and commitment in one's job. Quality is everyone's responsibility in the healthcare environment and must remain at the core of SP operations. Paying careful attention to all policies, procedures and protocols, actively participating in all quality projects, and helping co-workers are critical cornerstones of SP quality.

A team-based approach to quality can provide measurable results that improve patient care and on-the-job satisfaction. Technician ownership of departmental quality is the key to maintaining and improving quality and being part of a well-functioning, efficient department in which everyone can be proud to work. Remember, quality improvement begins and ends with each departmental team member.

RESOURCES

ISIXSIGMA. What is Six Sigma? http://isixsigma.com.

Centers for Medicare and Medicaid Services. *Guidance for performing root cause analysis.* https://www.cms.gov/medicare/provider-enrollment-and-certification/qapi/downloads/guidanceforrca.pdf

STERILE PROCESSING TERMS

Quality

Customer (internal)

Empowerment

Process improvement

Cross-functional teams

Failure mode and effects analysis (FMEA)

Root cause analysis (RCA)

Sentinel event

Quality assurance

Total quality improvement (TQI)

Processes (work)

Continuous quality improvement (CQI)

Total quality management (TQM)

Six Sigma

Lean

Chapter 19

Supply Chain Management Within the Sterile Processing Department

Learning Objectives

As a result of successfully completing this chapter, the reader will be able to:

1. Explain the importance of supply chain management in the healthcare facility
2. Define the role of Sterile Processing technicians as it relates to supply chain management
3. Explain basic inventory terms used in healthcare facilities
4. Explain the cycle of consumable items
5. Discuss the partnership between Sterile Processing and Supply Chain Management
6. Describe guidelines for handling commercially sterilized packages
7. Describe common inventory replenishment systems
8. Discuss the role of healthcare facilities in sustainability efforts and waste reduction

INTRODUCTION

A patient enters the healthcare facility for a surgical procedure. Throughout the admission process, the patient wonders, *"Will the procedure go as planned? Will there be much postoperative pain? How long until I can return home? How long before I can go back to my normal activities?"* The patient does not typically wonder if the healthcare facility has all the supplies needed for the surgery and postoperative care. The patient assumes that these supplies will be available and safe for use in their procedure(s).

Providing procedural support requires a vast amount of instrumentation, supplies and equipment. Every surgery requires both reusable items, such as surgical instruments, as well as disposable (consumable) items such as suture, bandages, syringes, needles, etc. Failure to provide items needed for patient care and treatment directly affects patient safety; therefore, supply chain management in the healthcare facility is critically important.

It takes a tremendous amount of communication, coordination and planning to ensure that every patient has all items needed for their procedure. In most facilities, supply purchasing, receiving and distribution is the responsibility of the Supply Chain Management (SCM) department. To ensure that needs are always met, the overall inventory management and distribution process requires input from users and from dispensing areas like Sterile Processing (SP). SP technicians play an essential role in inventory management due to the many inventory items that pass through the SP department (SPD).

Inventory items that arrive in the SPD can be classified under two basic categories: **operational supplies** and **patient care supplies**. Operational supplies are defined as items needed for the SPD to operate effectively. Examples include detergents, sterilization wrap and sterilization testing products. Patient care supplies are those that will be dispensed for patient treatment and care. Examples include catheters, implants and bandages. **Figure 19.1** provides examples of products in basic SP inventory categories.

Operational supplies Supplies needed for SPD operations. Examples include detergents, sterilization wrap, sterilization testing products, etc.

Patient care supplies Supplies dispensed for patient treatment and care. Examples include catheters, implants, bandages, etc.

Both supply categories are especially important to patient care. It is easy to see how a shortage of patient care supplies would impact patient care; however, it is also important to realize that the same would be true of a shortage of operational supplies. Imagine trying to provide clean and sterile instruments without detergents or sterilization wrap. An SPD's scope of service (responsibilities) varies. Some departments provide supplies for the entire facility; other SPDs may only provide supplies for surgery. Regardless of the department's scope of service, all SP technicians are involved in the inventory management process in some way.

Case cart technicians work with consumable and reusable inventory supplies dispensed for each procedure. Decontamination technicians must ensure they have an adequate stock of personal protective equipment (PPE) and a

SP Inventory

Patient care supplies

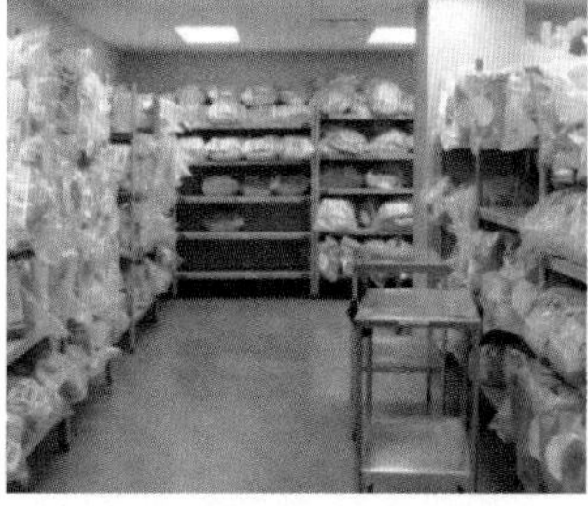

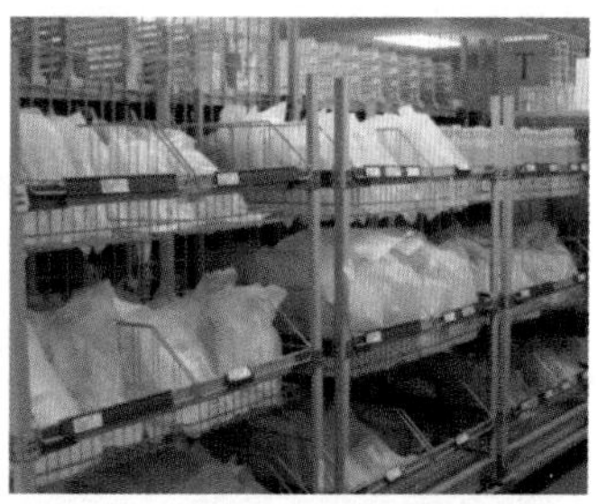

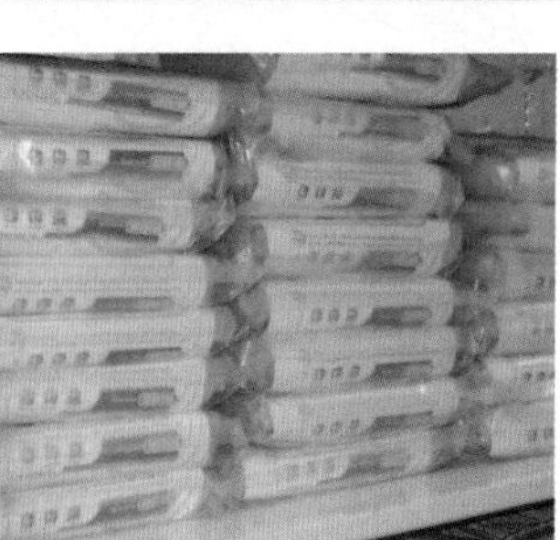

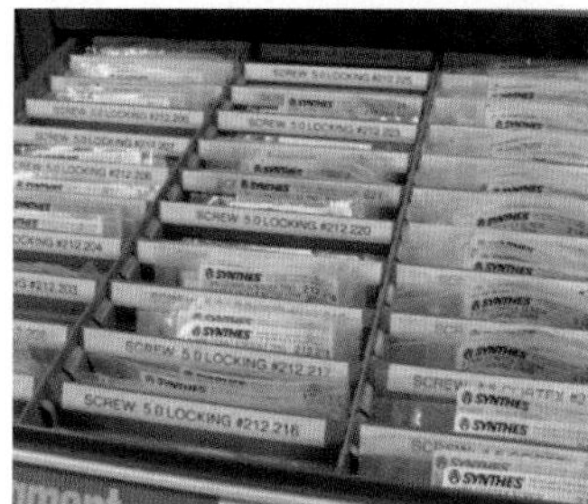

Operational supplies

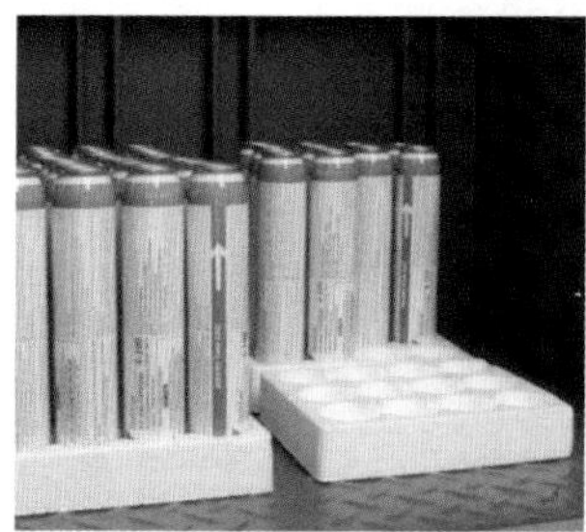

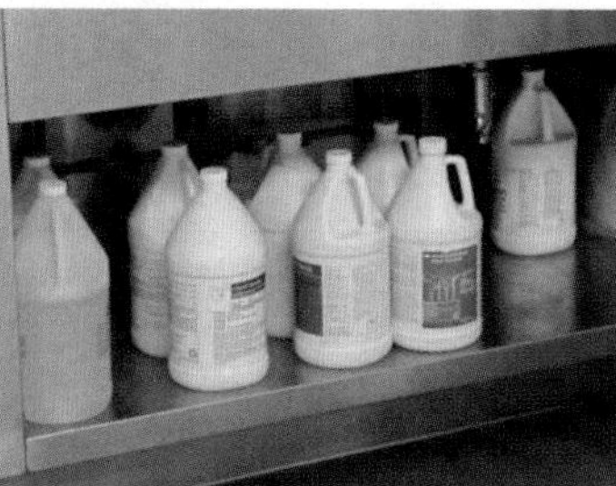

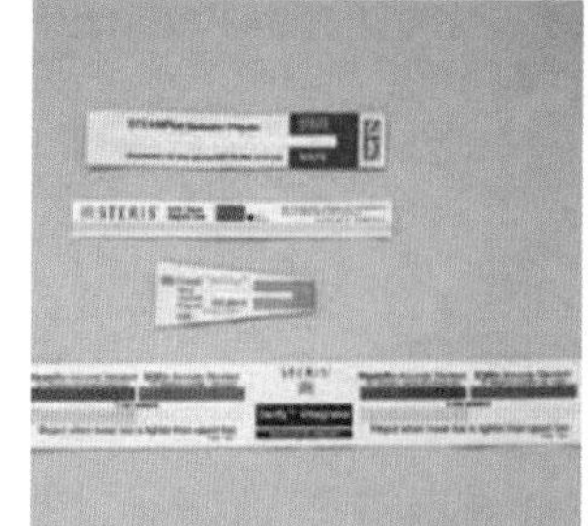

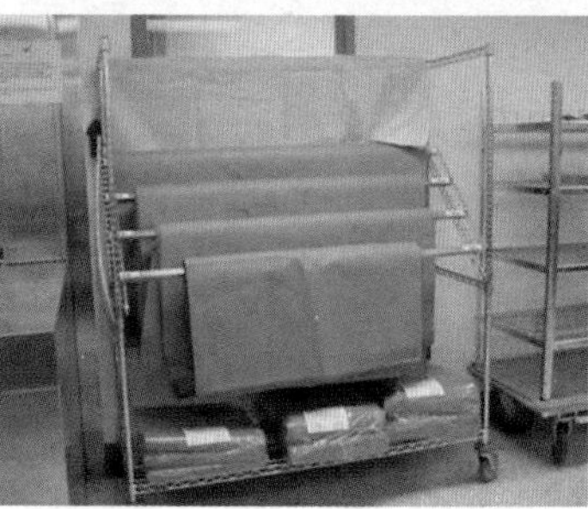

Figure 19.1 To provide proper support, the SPD must ensure the availability of hundreds of inventory items.

sufficient supply of detergents, disinfectants, brushes and other decontamination supplies. Instrument assembly technicians must ensure they have an adequate supply of packaging materials, chemical indicators (CIs), package closure supplies and other assembly supplies. In some cases, SP professionals may need to ensure they have replacement components, such as screws, plates and pins, for implant trays. Sterilizer operators must make certain they have sterility assurance tests, such as biological indicators (BIs) and Bowie-Dick tests. For some types of sterilizers, they must maintain an adequate supply of the sterilant.

WHAT IS INVENTORY?

The term **inventory** has a broad meaning in healthcare facilities. It refers to both **reusable** and **consumable** items. Before beginning a discussion about inventory, it is important to become familiar with some key terms and concepts.

> **Inventory** Reusable equipment and consumable items used to provide healthcare services for patients.
>
> **Reusable (inventory)** Assets, such as medical devices and sterilization containers, that can be reused as healthcare services are provided to patients.
>
> **Consumable (inventory)** Assets, such as wrapping supplies, processing chemicals, and other items that are consumed as healthcare services are provided to patients.

There are two specific inventories in the SPD:

- Reusable inventory items that include items such as transport carts, rigid sterilization containers, and many instruments. Reusable inventory also includes items such as mechanical washers and sterilizers. In the healthcare facility, high-cost, reusable inventory items are called capital equipment.

- Consumable inventory items that include supplies such as detergents, disposable wraps and sterility assurance products. Consumable inventory also has a specific life cycle. It is purchased, stored until use, used and replaced. (See **Figure 19.2**)

Consumable and reusable items are considered assets. They represent a significant financial investment by the healthcare facility and must be managed in a way that enables the facility to benefit from them at the lowest cost possible. This chapter focuses on the management of consumable assets as they relate to the SPD.

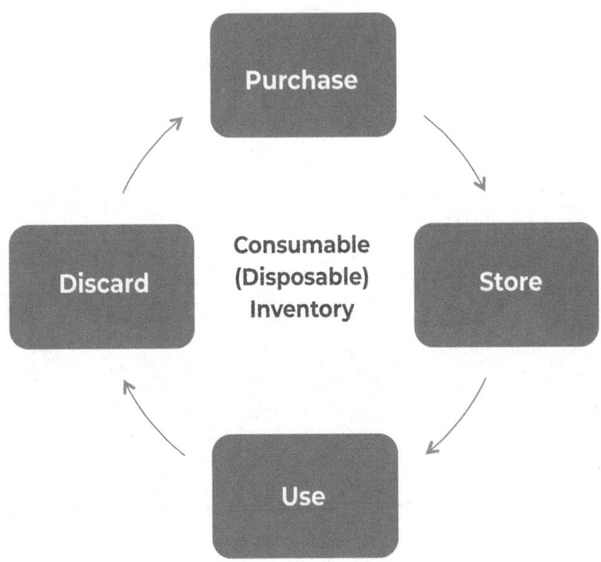

Figure 19.2

WHERE DOES INVENTORY COME FROM?

Every healthcare facility has hundreds and often thousands of items in inventory. Each item serves a specific purpose. Some inventory items are used regularly, such as detergents for the decontamination area. Others, like certain specialty catheters, are used less often but must always be available when patient safety may become jeopardized by delaying treatment or care. All of these items represent a financial investment and must be managed properly to keep costs down. Managing inventory is one of the primary responsibilities of the SCM department.

The SCM department is responsible for the purchase, receipt, and delivery of items to user departments. It oversees the flow of supplies and equipment coming into the healthcare facility. Buyers in the SCM department search for and procure (purchase) items using a variety of tools and strategies to ensure they are able to meet the facility's needs at the lowest possible cost.

Most health systems belong to purchasing groups that enable them to purchase items at pre-negotiated discount pricing. These group purchasing organizations (GPOs) represent many healthcare facilities; they are able to negotiate contracts for products and services that enable facilities (members of the GPO) to receive special, reduced pricing.

SCM plays an important role in the supply chain by helping ensure that everything necessary to support patient care is available when needed.

Once items are received at the healthcare facility, they are checked in to verify that what was ordered was received. From there, items are placed into storage. In most facilities, a large portion of inventory items is stored in the SCM department. Then, items are delivered to various areas, as needed. **Figure 19.3** reviews the four steps in the flow of materials through the healthcare facility.

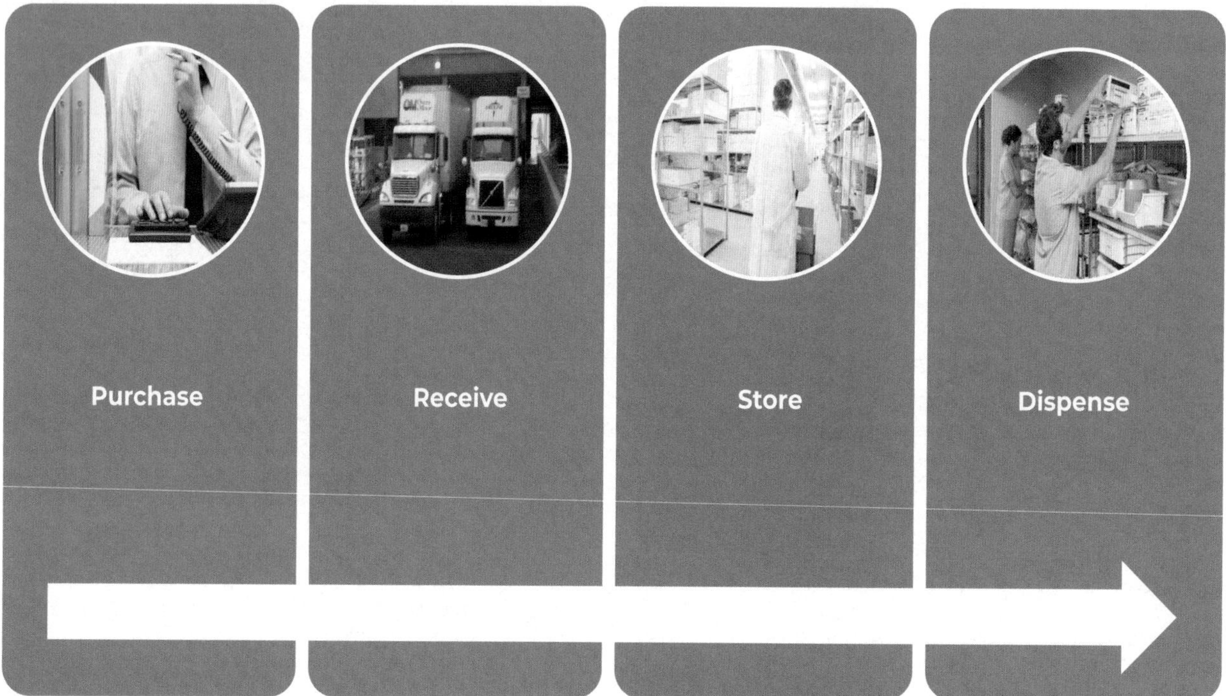

Figure 19.3

Consignment Inventory

In addition to purchasing inventory items, SCM may use an inventory system called consignment. Consignment is an inventory system where items are provided to the healthcare facility by the vendor but not charged to the facility until the items are used. For example, a total hip procedure will usually require several sizes of hip implants to be available for each case. Even though there are several sizes available, only one will be used once the final measurements are made during the procedure. The facility will pay for the implant used, while the remaining implants will remain on the shelf (still owned by the vendor).

Managing consignment inventory is important to SP technicians because any implant not accounted for when the vendor inventories their product will be charged to the facility.

HANDLING COMMERCIALLY STERILIZED ITEMS

When commercially sterilized items are brought into a healthcare facility, care must be taken to ensure that those items are not compromised during shipping, storage, handling and distribution. That means that those items must be stored in a manner that will protect each package from events that may render it unsterile.

Although the types of packaging may differ in appearance and feel, commercially sterilized packages are vulnerable to the same potential contaminants as in-house sterilized items. Items should be stored in a clean area—away from moisture, dust and other contaminates that can compromise packaging. Dust on the outside of a package can be easily transferred to the Operating Room (OR) and introduced into that clean environment, contaminating it.

As with every sterile package, care must be taken to ensure that the integrity of the package is maintained until use. Sterile packages should be handled gently and as little as possible. Technicians must understand storage and handling requrequirements and the basic information provided on each commercially sterilized package.

Commercially Sterilized Package Information

Unlike in-house sterilized items, commercially sterilized packages come with printed instructions that contain pertinent information for SP technicians. Most product packaging contains information regarding product manufacturer, sterility, storage and safe use. **Figure 19.4** reviews the types of information commonly found on commercially sterilized packages and labels and explains why that information is important to SP.

Manufacturers employ several symbols to convey information on package labels. Those symbols are designed to provide information that is easily understandable in the small space of a product label. **Figures 19.5** and **19.6** provide common commercially sterilized symbols and their meanings.

Important Information Provided on Package Labels

Category	Type of information	Why it is important
Manufacturer information	1. Manufacturer's name 2. Product name and specifics (size, etc.) 3. Product reference number 4. Date of manufacture 5. Batch (or lot) number 6. Product serial number 7. Expiration information	**#1–#3** Important for: · Reordering purposes · Verifying that the correct product is being dispensed **#4–#7** Important for: · Tracking product to patient · Product recalls · Stock rotation
Sterility information	1. Sterility statement 2. Expiration date	**#1** Important for determining if a product was supplied sterile **#2** Important for determining the shelf life of the product
Storage information	1. Storage temperature limits 2. Moisture or humidity limits 3. Fragility	**#1–#3** Important for ensuring that items are stored as required by the manufacturer
Safe use instructions	1. Identification of single-use items 2. Notification of latex contents 3. References to product instructions for use	**#1** Important for ensuring single-use items are not processed **#2–#3** Important for providing patient safety information

Figure 19.4

Symbol	Meaning	Symbol	Meaning
REF	Reference number (catalog number)	LOT	Lot number (batch code)
SN	Product serial number	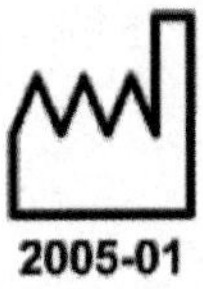 2005-01	Date of manufacture
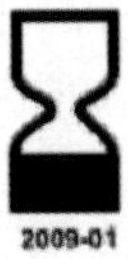 2009-01	Use by date	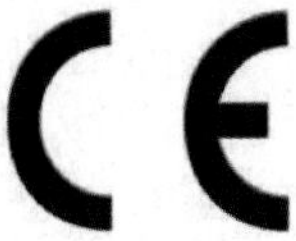 CE	The CE mark is an identification mark that indicates that a product has complied with the health and safety requirements, as published by European directives.
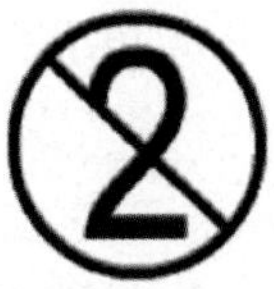 2	Do not reuse	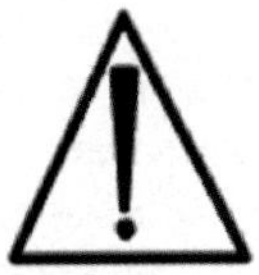 !	Attention; see instructions

Figure 19.5

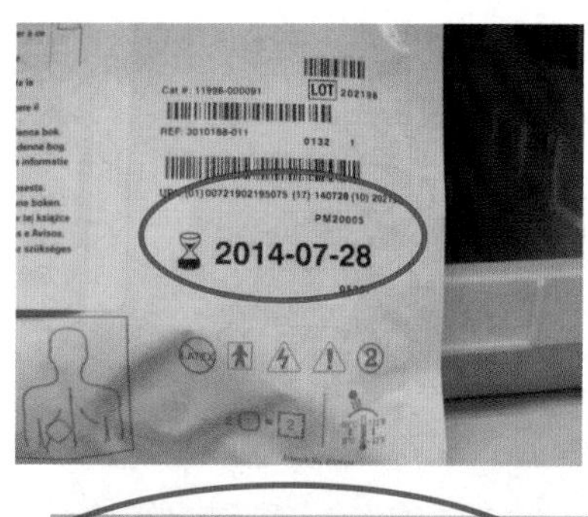

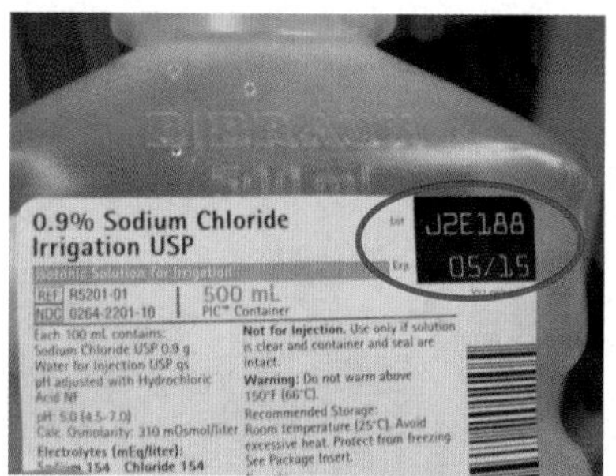

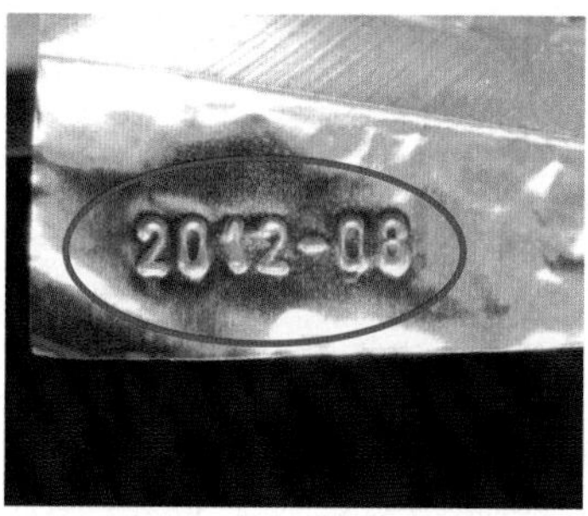

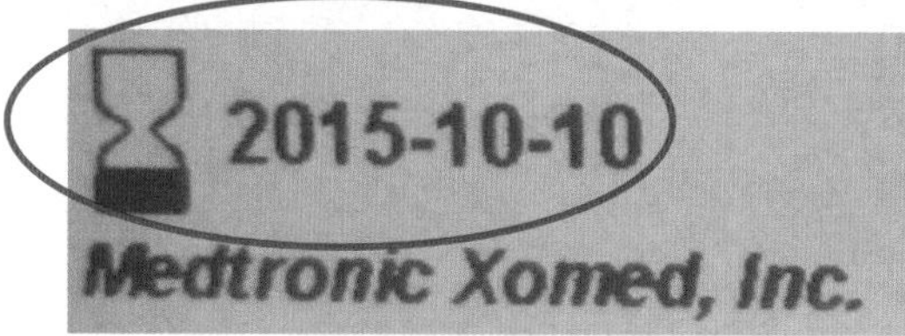

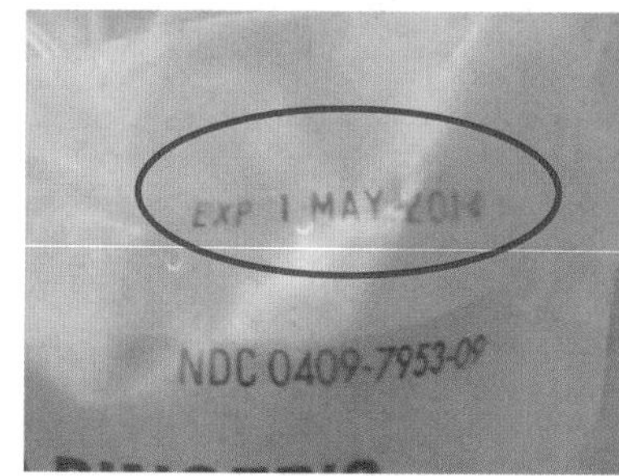

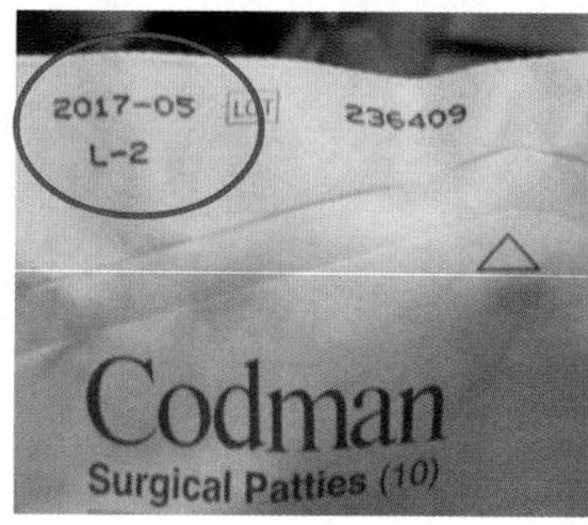

Figure 19.6 Expiration date format and placement are not the same on all packages.

Expiration Dates

Many medical products on the market today have expiration dates, sometimes referred to as outdates, and these are very important for SP technicians. It is important to recognize that even if a healthcare facility uses an event-related shelf-life policy, expiration dates on medical products must be checked, and items that have reached the end of their stated shelf life must not be used. *Note: When practicing event-related shelf life, expiration dates are considered an event.*

Identifying expiration dates can be difficult because there is no standard requirement for where they are placed on a package. For that reason, SP technicians must be diligent when checking packages for expiration dates. When new products that have expiration dates are received, all staff who handle the packages should be educated on the existence and location of the expiration information. **Figure 19.6** provides examples of locations of expiration date information on commercially sterilized packages.

Sometimes, a single package will contain several items within the package but will only have a single expiration date identified on the original outer package (e.g., a box of sterilization wraps or a pouch of indicators). The pouch of indicators may contain hundreds of indicators. If those indicators are poured into a bin at a workstation and the outer pouch is thrown away, the expiration date could be lost. SP technicians must be aware of those items and have a plan or process that identifies the items' expiration dates and ensures that no expired item is unintentionally used.

Not all packages have an expiration date. Such items do not have materials that will degrade or decompose in an established, normal-use timeframe. The packages will have a statement indicating that the package is sterile, unless opened or damaged. In a storage area filled with commercially sterilized items, there will most likely be a combination of items with expiration dates and items with event-related sterility statements. It is important to know which items have expiration dates, and to check those dates each time a package is dispensed. Regularly scheduled checks for outdates, ideally monthly, can also help SP staff identify and remove expired items from inventory.

Inspection

Regardless of whether an item uses event-related or date-related shelf life, it must be inspected before being dispensed. That inspection is part of a multi-check safeguard. While it is true that the package will be inspected at the point of use, SP can reduce delays by identifying package integrity issues before they reach the point of use.

Inspections should include a visual check to ensure that the packaging has no holes, tears, signs of moisture, dust, or other visible damage. Packages that show excessive handling (wear) should also be identified. Expiration dates (if present) should be checked. **Figure 19.7** shows an SP technician checking a package before dispensing it.

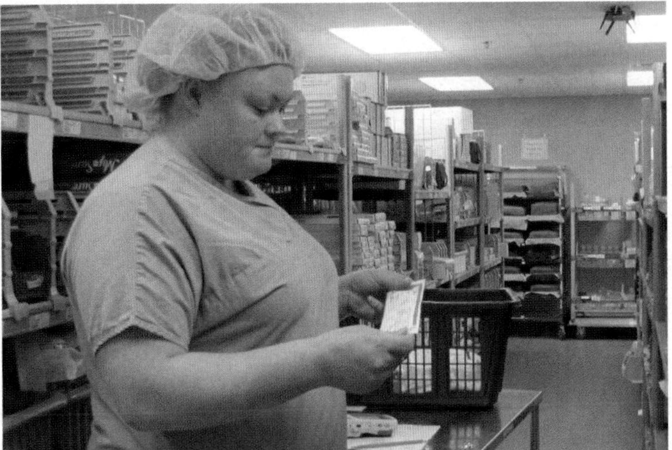

Figure 19.7

ITEM LOCATOR SYSTEMS

Every healthcare facility has hundreds and perhaps thousands of medical supplies. Each one can impact patient safety if it cannot be located when needed. Poorly organized storage can also lead to loss or damage, which can impact a facility's budget.

Every medical supply storage area must have a system in place that enables all employees who handle supplies to locate a specific product quickly.

Unique Device Identifier

The unique device identifier (UDI) system was first introduced in the U.S. in 2013 by the U.S. Food and Drug Administration (FDA). This multi-year planning/implementation system, when fully implemented, will be a worldwide method for identifying medical devices. As the name indicates, each medical device will have its own identification number that also identifies the manufacturer and other important product information. This system will allow:

- Tracking of medical devices
- Easy identification of an item being recalled
- More accurate reporting and analysis of adverse events caused by a medical device
- Identification of counterfeit medical devices

Currently, UDI labeling of medical devices is required for manufacturers. The FDA has stated that healthcare facilities will eventually be included in this program.

LOSS OF STERILE ITEMS

Ideally, disposable items are purchased, used and replaced; however, there are times when a disposable item may fall out of that sequence. When that happens, the item is lost, which may delay patient care and treatment and cost the facility money for replacement. **Figure 19.8** lists some common causes for the loss of sterile items.

Common Causes of Waste (Loss)	
Expiration	The item was not used before the end of its designated shelf life.
Contamination	The item suffered an event that rendered it unusable.
Obsolescence	The item was replaced by a newer, different item.
Loss	The item was lost and cannot be located.
Theft	The item was taken by an unauthorized individual.

Figure 19.8

Each of the examples in **Figure 19.8** represents a financial loss to the healthcare facility. Helping control losses for the facility is everyone's responsibility. Some of the ways technicians can assist in lowering losses are:

- Always placing items back on the shelf in their proper location
- Always following the facility's policies for stock rotation to help ensure items are used before they expire
- Ensuring hands are clean before touching medical devices
- Not handling items unless they need to be handled; the fewer times items are touched, the greater the chance they will remain clean/sterile.
- Using the facility's tracking system when receiving/issuing items. Document all issues.
- Keeping storage areas closed to non-departmental staff
- Not giving items to unauthorized people
- Never taking items for personal use

It is easy to get in the mindset that the facility can afford to lose a few of these "low-cost" items; however, each loss adds up over time and can create a significant financial loss for the facility.

TRANSPORT OF COMMERCIALLY STERILIZED PACKAGES

Transporting commercially sterilized packages follows the same process as transporting in-house processed items. Care should be taken to protect packages from contamination during transport. Items should not be exposed to conditions that may compromise the sterility of the package, such as excessive temperatures, humidity or moisture.

Items should be protected from the environment during transport. The best method of transport is using closed case carts; however, covered case carts, approved transport bins and bags may also be used.

Equipment, such as carts and totes used to transport devices and supplies, must be frequently cleaned and inspected for damage. Items that are to be transported outside the facility must be contained in appropriate containment devices.

DISTRIBUTION OF SUPPLIES

Distribution involves moving supplies throughout the facility, usually from their storage location to the point of use. In most facilities, this activity includes distributing consumable supplies from the storeroom or SPD to clinical units, including the OR.

Distribution The movement of supplies.

The goal of distribution is to move the correct items in appropriate quantities to the right places at the right times and in the most cost-effective manner possible. The method of supply distribution used will vary depending on frequency or volume of use, peak activity times, the amount of storage space available in the areas to which the supplies are distributed, and other factors. For that reason, it is important to note that no single distribution method is the best choice for all facilities. Each healthcare facility will need to assess its particular needs and develop a system that will best suit those needs. In most cases, different methods of distribution will be used to meet the needs of different departments.

Carts and totes used to transport sterile items must be kept clean.

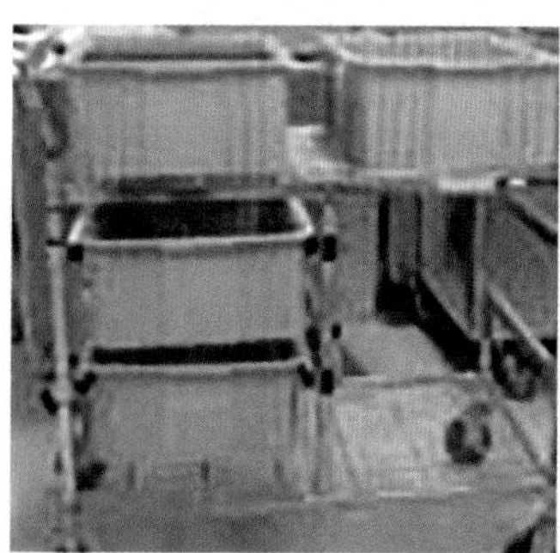

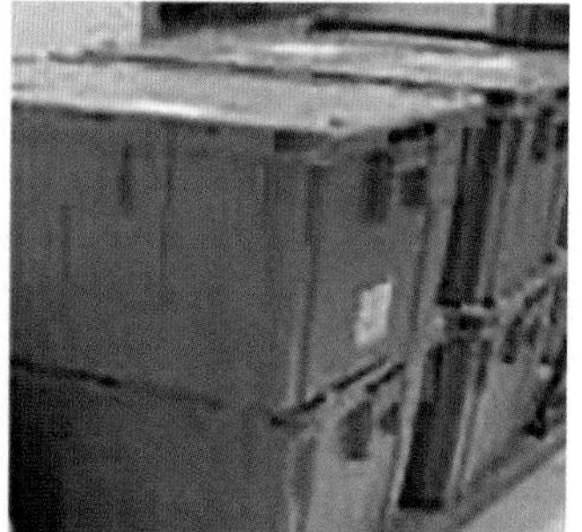

Figure 19.9

Inventory Replenishment and Distribution Systems

The methods used to replenish needed consumable supplies throughout the healthcare facility must be carefully considered and planned to best manage costs, have items available when needed and minimize the supply efforts of responsible staff members. Effective systems are, to the extent possible, automatic.

The following are examples of inventory replenishment and distribution systems commonly used in healthcare facilities:

Periodic Automatic Replenishment Level Systems

Periodic automatic replenishment (PAR) systems establish a standard level (PAR) for each supply item stored in a specific department. This level is usually jointly determined by the user department and SCM staff. After these levels are set, there is typically no need for items to be ordered by clinicians. Instead, SP/SCM personnel inventory (count) each area where supplies are housed. They check the current on-hand supply and note the quantity of each item still available. The amount needed to bring the quantity of supplies to the agreed-upon standard (PAR level) is determined and automatically transmitted to the SCM department (or vendor) who will send the required supplies. **Figure 19.10** shows the checking and restocking of PAR levels on a shelf.

Periodic automatic replenishment (often called PAR level or PAR system) An inventory replenishment system in which the desired amount of products that should be available is established, and inventory replenishment returns the quantity of products to this level.

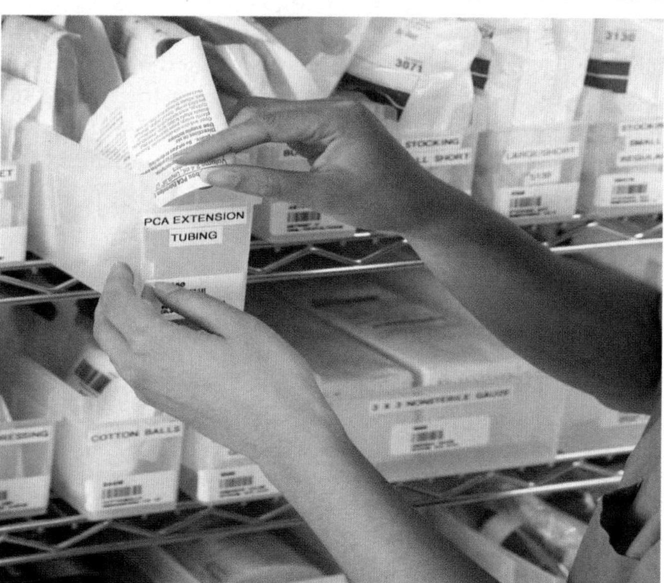

Figure 19.10

Automatic Supply Replenishment Systems

Automated supply replenishment systems use a computerized system to gather and track the issuing of patient items. (See **Figure 19.11.**) PAR and reorder levels for each item are established. Clinical staff scan or push a button to account for each item removed from the inventory location. An order is generated at a scheduled time for all items that are at or below their reorder point, and the order for the entire location is placed. The supply pick list is printed and used to gather replacement products to refill the unit.

> **Automated supply replenishment system**
> Replenishment system in which items removed from inventory are automatically identified and tracked. When a reorder point is reached, item information is generated on a supply pick list in the central storeroom, or with a contracted vendor. Items are then issued and transferred to the appropriate user area.

Usually, automated systems are interfaced with the healthcare facility's SCM system for managing inventory. The use of these interfaces reduces the number of staff required to perform these functions.

Examples of Automated Replenishment Systems

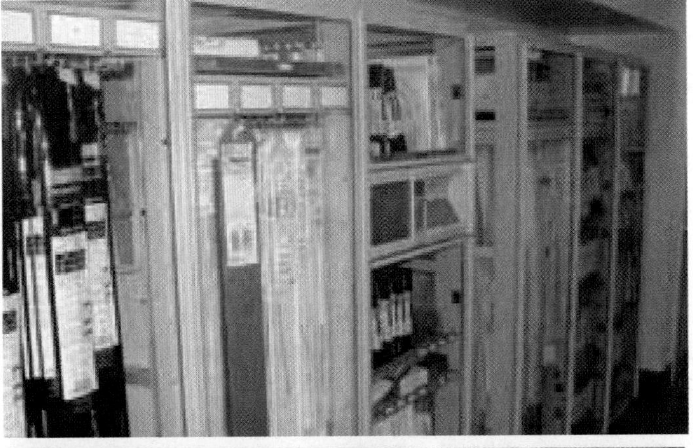

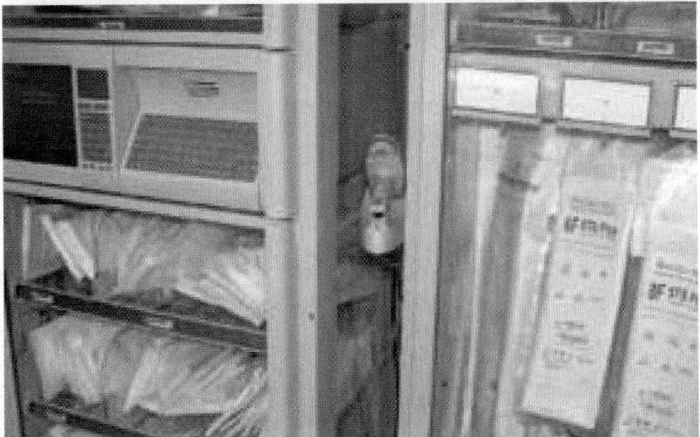

Figure 19.11

Exchange Cart Systems

An **exchange cart system** is an inventory replenishment method that involves the exchange of a freshly filled supply cart on a user unit. Supply items and quantities on the exchange cart, as well as its location, are determined by user unit staff and SP/SCM personnel. At a pre-determined time, a full cart is brought to the unit. The partially depleted cart is returned to the replenishment area, and remaining items are inventoried to determine the supplies and quantities used. The cart is then replenished with the supplies needed to return the cart back to full inventory. As supplies are removed from inventory and added to the cart, they are charged to the budget of the unit that "owns" the cart. At the scheduled time, this full cart is delivered to the unit, the depleted cart is retrieved for restocking, and the cycle repeats. **Figure 19.12** provides an example of exchange carts designed to stock anesthesia supplies.

> **Exchange cart system** An inventory system where desired inventory items are placed on a cart assigned to a specific location. A second duplicate cart is maintained in another location and exchanged on a scheduled basis to ensure sufficient supplies are available at all times.

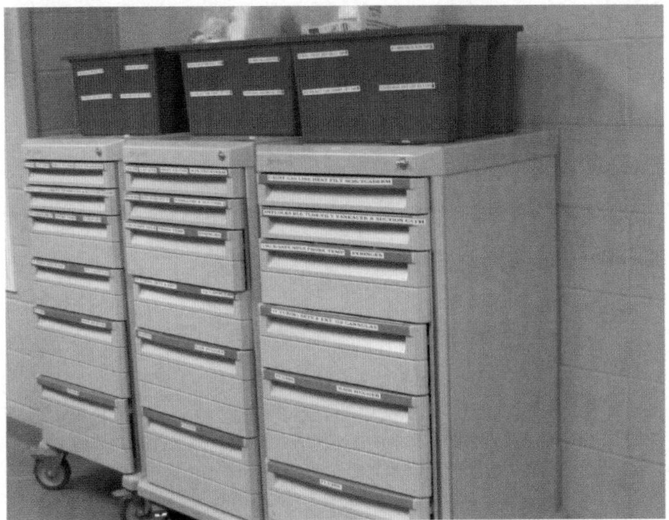

Figure 19.12

An advantage of an exchange cart system is that it is "automatic" unless there is a need to change the cart's items or quantities. Clinical staff do not need to order these items, and SCM staff do not have to determine which supplies are needed.

Disadvantages associated with exchange carts include the need for duplicate inventory and carts. The system is labor intensive and requires adequate space to stage the carts. In addition, unless the system is well managed, numerous unused supplies will be transported back and forth each cycle. This system does work well for emergency medical supply carts (code carts), which are exchanged for a newly restocked cart each time they are used. (See **Figure 19.13**)

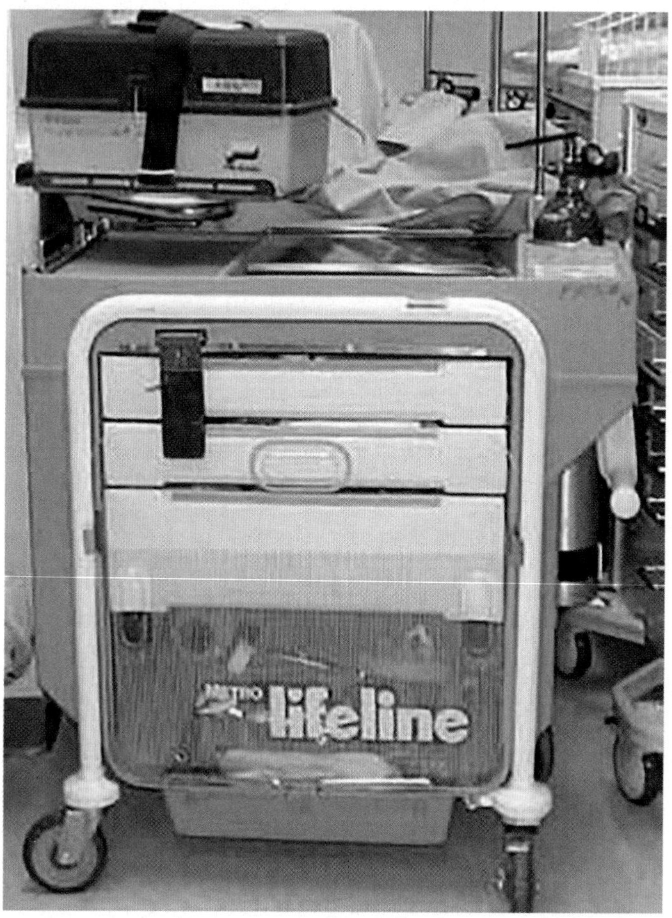

Figure 19.13

Procedure Carts

Procedure carts are specialty carts designed to supply a specific type of procedure. Examples of procedure carts include crash carts, urology carts and case carts. Procedure carts may be stored on the using unit and exchanged when a procedure is complete, or the cart may be stored in the SPD and delivered to the user area when needed. Each cart must be carefully cleaned, inventoried and restocked after each use.

Requisition Systems

Even when PAR level or exchange cart systems exist, it will still be necessary to order additional supplies. That usually happens because of insufficient quantities on hand or because a specific item is not included among those routinely provided. **Requisition systems** exist in every facility.

Requisition system A method of inventory distribution where items needed are requested (requisitioned) by user department personnel and removed from a central storage location for transport to the user department.

Requisition systems require users to request (order) needed supplies by completing a requisition. Requisitions may be manually created or computer generated. Manual systems do not offer the productivity advantages of computerized systems. Requisition systems that electronically requisition supplies typically eliminate the need for SCM personnel to re-enter ordering information from a paper order form. Accuracy and productivity improvements associated with automated data entry are lost when manual requisition systems are used. **Figure 19.14** provides an example of a technician completing a requisition for special-order catheters.

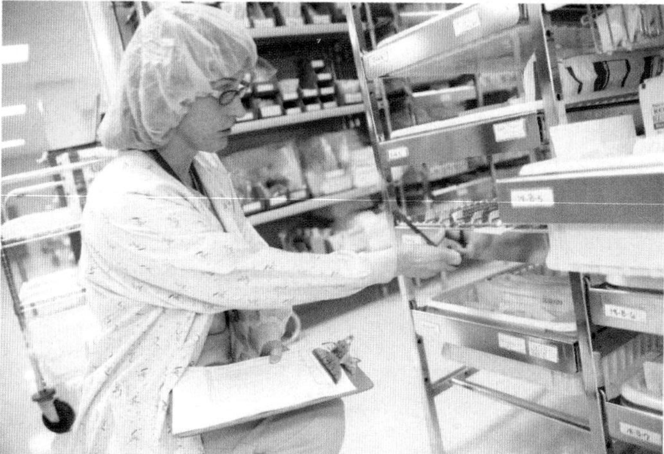

Figure 19.14

Specialty Items

Every facility has a need for patient-specific and infrequently ordered specialty items that are not maintained in the routine replenishment system. SP technicians must understand the requisition, ordering, tracking and replenishment processes used by their facility for these items. If a patient is scheduled for surgery and a specialty item is needed, it may need to be ordered several days before surgery to ensure that it is available. If an item is not available when needed, patient safety may be compromised.

Case Cart Systems

In case cart systems, items needed for each specific procedure are assembled in individual carts and delivered to the department where the procedure will be performed. There are several benefits to case cart systems, including:

- Reducing the amount of space needed for supply storage in the user department
- Promoting more standardized infection prevention practices

- Reducing operational costs associated with supply and instrument management
- Allowing more efficient equipment and supply tracking

In a case cart system, specific needs for each procedure are identified by users. These needs are compiled on a requisition form, called a preference card (or pick list). The preference card usually contains two components: the first is a list of instruments, supplies and implants needed for the specific procedure; the second component contains notes that are helpful to the procedure room staff.

When a procedure is scheduled, a copy of the list of needed items is sent to the SPD, and the case cart is assembled. (See **Figure 19.15**) That case cart is delivered to the OR (or other user unit) before the procedure. Additional unanticipated needs are communicated to SP professionals, as necessary, and the SPD responds to those additional requests.

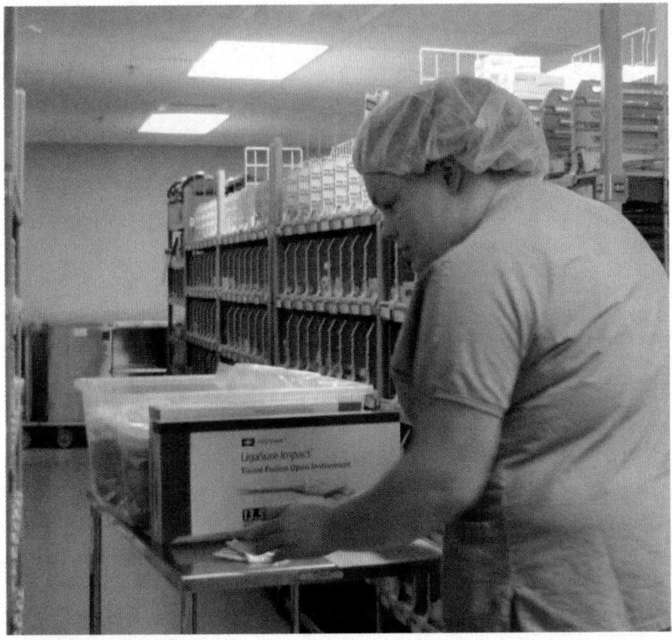

Figure 19.15

Case cart systems can also provide effective control of supplies and instruments. Because a separate case cart is assembled for each individual procedure, it is easier to track what is actually used and identify supplies and instruments that are often requested but seldom used. Quantities of supplies can then be reduced, which can reduce the amount of inventory that must be on hand as well as reducing unnecessary repetitive handling. Close monitoring of instrument usage allows the facility to shift instruments that are not being used to other areas where they are needed. Monitoring can also identify instrument shortages, which may be addressed with scheduling changes or the purchase of additional instrumentation.

Case cart systems rely on user input to be effective. Physicians and other healthcare personnel utilizing the case cart must identify their specific needs in advance. These needs are then transferred to pick lists that SP staff use to assemble each cart. Care should be taken when developing requisitions to ensure that products are standardized whenever possible. Routine follow up is needed to adjust requisition quantities to actual usage. Properly stocked case carts should be delivered to the user unit. Personnel assigned to the case cart area must maintain direct contact with user staff so additional items can be supplied as needed.

While case cart systems typically use carts assembled as needed for specific procedures, most systems also utilize some form of preassembled carts that remain assembled and "on standby" for emergency situations. These carts are used for STAT situations (e.g., emergency cesarean sections) when there is no time for cart assembly.

An effective case cart system requires effective communication between OR and SP personnel. As cases are performed, SP and OR staff must be in constant communication to ensure that items are correct and arrive on time. Personnel in each department must be familiar with one another's routine duties and workflow patterns. Frustration can be eliminated if, for example, OR personnel understand the steps involved in processing instruments for another case. Instead of questioning instrument turnaround times, they will understand that this time is required for safe, effective cleaning, inspection, assembly and sterilization/cooling.

SP technicians working with case cart systems should have good medical terminology skills and a thorough understanding of surgical instruments so they can easily communicate with their OR counterparts. They must also remain up to date about new products because they serve as the link between the inventory system and the user department. Along with effective oral communication skills, case cart systems rely heavily on written procedures and communications. Personnel from all user departments must establish procedures for product handling, outage notification, and scheduling. Even the best-planned case cart system will be substandard without effective communication.

Case cart systems also require upkeep. As instruments and supplies are added to or removed from the system, physician's preference cards must be updated to reflect changes in the system. (See **Figure 19.16**) Failure to update preference cards to reflect current needs can result in unavailability of supplies and instruments, which can then lead to compromised patient safety and user frustration.

Case cart systems require significant input from SP professionals, and to be efficient, they require a full array of processing skills and inventory management methods.

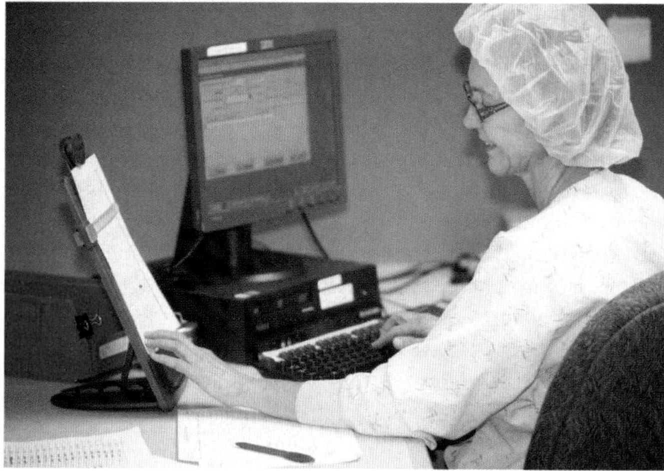

Figure 19.16

STAT Orders

Emergency supply orders requiring immediate action (STAT orders) are a reality in every facility. STAT orders can also occur for a procedure scheduled for the next day if the item is unavailable. These orders are time consuming and costly to fill, and they usually disrupt routine inventory management activities. Consider, for example, times when additional external resources, such as overnight air shipments or borrowing from another facility, may be required. All reasonable efforts to minimize the need for STAT requests should be made; these efforts include reviewing why they occur and how they can be prevented.

Many STAT requests result from deficiencies in a poorly managed daily supply and distribution system. STAT requests can become a patient safety issue if the root cause is not addressed, and routine reviews may determine if PAR level adjustments will help ensure appropriate inventory levels. When STAT requests result from improper planning by clinical staff, SCM and SP managers should assist in the planning and education efforts to resolve the issue. While OR staff cannot predict that an emergency patient will require a specific **non-stock item**, they may be able to plan for such a need and ensure that the item is available.

Non-stock items Items not carried in the central storeroom or in the Sterile Processing storage area but that are purchased from an outside vendor, as needed, and then delivered to the requesting department.

SUSTAINABILITY

The SCM department is often involved in **sustainability** efforts. Increasingly, healthcare facilities are taking sustainability into consideration when selecting supplies. Items that can be recycled or otherwise help reduce waste can benefit patients, healthcare facilities and the environment.

Sustainability Processes designed to reduce harm to the environment or deplete natural resources, thereby supporting long-term ecological balance.

Many facilities are moving toward systems that allow them to reduce the amount of waste being generated. SPDs may be involved in those efforts. (See **Figure 19.17**)

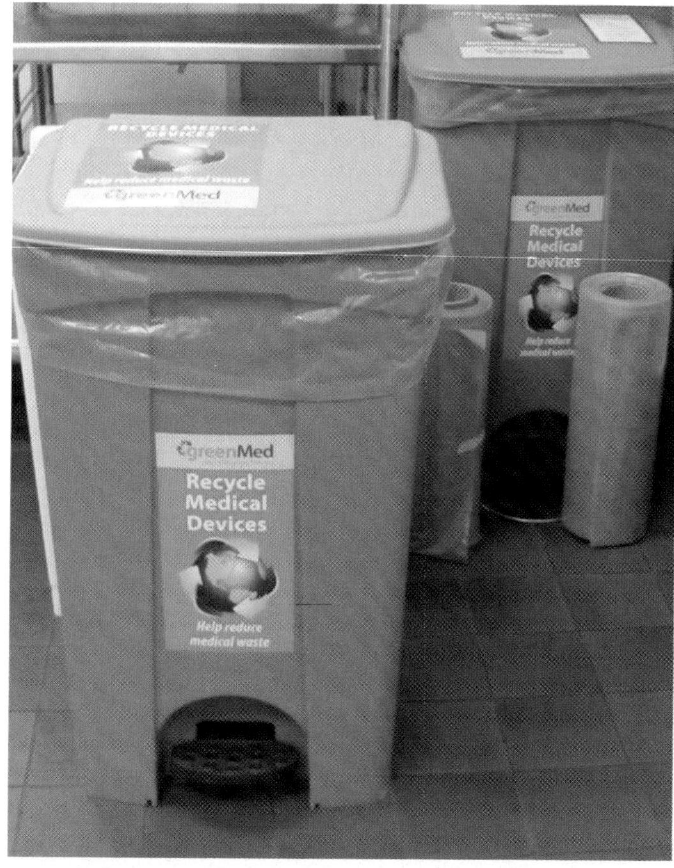

Figure 19.17

THE ROLE OF SP IN INVENTORY MANAGEMENT

Although the primary responsibilities of procurement, receiving, storage and distribution may be performed outside the SPD, SP technicians still play an important role in the healthcare facility's inventory management system. SP technicians are responsible for several key duties, including:

- Learning processes at their specific healthcare facility such as:
  - How orders are placed
  - How to identify items
  - How to locate items

  - How to properly dispense items
- Knowing how to stay informed of new products as they enter the system
- Understanding and following information contained on commercially sterilized packages
- Handling sterile products with care
- Reporting concerns such as:
  - Excessive, unexpected demand on specific products
  - Low quantities
  - Frequent outages
  - Storage issues

Each step in the life cycle of a sterile medical supply is an important one. Through keen observation and best work practices, SP technicians can protect the integrity of products until they reach their point of use.

INVENTORY REDUCTION

A key part of inventory management is the ability to reduce stock, instruments and sets where there is excess inventory. Standardization of instrument sets helps reduce the number of instruments needed in the facility. SP technicians can easily identify sets that have consistently unused instruments or sets that are infrequently used. Reducing the quantity of unused sets or the quantity of unused instruments in a set frees instruments that may be needed in other sets, or allows the department to create more sets that are used most frequently. This process also reduces the amount of replacement instruments needed in a facility.

Technicians can also identify stored items that are infrequently used or where too much of an item is available. Procedure and case carts need to be monitored to ensure all products placed on these carts are used.

Keeping excess inventory of any type causes a financial burden on the department budget and creates more work for technicians who need to clean, inventory and stock these supplies and instruments.

CONCLUSION

Inventory management is an important part of every healthcare facility. Managing inventory effectively and efficiently assists caregivers in providing quality care at lower costs. More importantly, it helps ensure that the items needed for patient care and treatment are available when needed.

When SP and SCM staff work together to manage and control inventory, they help create a safe environment for the patient, while increasing provider and patient satisfaction.

RESOURCES

Healthcare Sterile Processing Association. *Central Service Leadership Manual*, Chapters 7, 22, 23. 2020.

U.S. Food and Drug Administration. *UDI Basics.* https://www.fda.gov/medical-devices/unique-device-identification-system-udi-system/udi-basics.

STERILE PROCESSING TERMS

Operational supplies

Patient care supplies

Inventory

Reusable inventory

Consumable inventory

Distribution

Periodic automatic replenishment (PAR)

Automated supply replenishment system

Exchange cart system

Requisition system

Non-stock items

Sustainability

Chapter 20

The Role of Sterile Processing in Ancillary Department Support

Learning Objectives

As a result of successfully completing this chapter, the reader will be able to:

1. Discuss the role of the Sterile Processing department in supporting ancillary departments
2. Discuss strategies for managing patient care equipment
3. Explain the importance of communication and coordination as it relates to ancillary support

INTRODUCTION

While the Operating Room (OR) is the Sterile Processing department's (SPD's) largest customer, it is by no means its only customer. SPDs provide support for other areas of the healthcare facility by providing instruments, disposable supplies, and equipment. Providing service to diverse departments and ensuring they have all the proper items when needed can be challenging. This chapter focuses on common support services provided by SPDs.

IDENTIFYING THE SPD'S SCOPE OF SERVICE

The level of service provided by the SPD varies by healthcare facility. In some facilities, the services provided by the SPD are limited to fulfilling the needs of the OR and providing reprocessing and sterilization services for instruments used in other departments. In other facilities, the SPD may be responsible for providing sterile instruments, equipment and supplies to healthcare units throughout the facility [i.e., the Intensive Care Unit (ICU), Emergency Department (ED), Pediatric Intensive Care Unit (PICU) and Labor and Delivery (L&D)]. SPDs that provide services to areas outside of the OR must ensure that they develop a system that meets the needs of all patients and providers in the safest, most timely and cost-effective manner possible.

PATIENT CARE EQUIPMENT

Along with instruments and supplies, SPDs may manage a large portion of the healthcare facility's patient care equipment. Effective handling of this equipment is an important part of the SP technician's job. Managing it properly can have a significant impact on the facility and patient safety.

The importance of patient care equipment was identified as one of the Top 10 Health Technology Hazards for 2022. There have been many reports of damaged infusion pumps being used during patient care, which led to dangerous and possibly fatal errors. Damage included excessive wear and tear, mishandling and misuse, poor device design, or the use of improper cleaning agents or methods. **Patient care equipment** must be readily available when needed and be safe, functional, ready to use and free from soil and contaminants. SP technicians are responsible for ensuring that these requirements are met. They must also manage equipment in a manner that minimizes costs to the healthcare facility. An effective patient care equipment management program is essential for managing these costs.

> **Patient care equipment** Portable (mobile) equipment used to assist in the care and treatment of patients. Examples include suction units, temperature management units, infusion therapy devices, etc.

Specific policies and procedures should be developed for the cleaning, preparation and tracking of patient care equipment. Equipment that has not been properly cleaned poses an infection risk to patients and healthcare workers. That risk is magnified because the equipment may be handled by several workers during the course of preparation, storage and distribution. If it is not properly assembled and ready for use, there may be a delay in treatment if staff must obtain necessary components such as tubing, collection devices, and pads. Equipment that is not accurately tracked can become "lost" within the system. This lack of availability may cause treatment delays or add unnecessary expense for the healthcare organization.

There are numerous types of patient care equipment in healthcare today. Some general device categories include infusion therapy, temperature management, wound care, and suction. Examples of specialized categories include equipment used for maternal and infant care, bariatric care, patient monitoring, specialty surfaces, and beds. Many devices are cleaned, tracked and dispensed through the SPD. Specific types, models and brands will vary from facility to facility.

Basic Types of Patient Care Equipment

Understanding the purpose of basic types of patient care equipment can improve customer service. SP technicians must also understand requirements for cleaning, inspecting, preparing, storing, dispensing and tracking patient care equipment. Each step in the patient care equipment process is an important component of a comprehensive patient care equipment program.

A Closer Look at Responsibilities

SPDs maintain the flow of the patient equipment system. They also partner with the Biomedical/Clinical Engineering department (Biomed). Technicians in the Biomed/Clinical Engineering department perform safety inspections and function tests on medical equipment. They are specially trained to inspect, test and repair patient care equipment. SP technicians should not attempt to perform equipment testing and maintenance functions unless they have received specific training, complete competencies and approval to do so. Biomed technicians must also not clean used equipment unless they have been properly trained and have specific competencies geared toward cleaning medical devices.

When equipment enters a healthcare facility, it must be safety checked and tested by a Biomed technician before being cleared for patient use. These items must also receive periodic follow-up inspections, scheduled according to the equipment manufacturers' instructions for use (IFU) and the healthcare facility's policies. Biomedical professionals maintain complete records about routine checks and repairs and other important information for all patient care equipment in the facility.

The Joint Commission (TJC) requires that **preventive maintenance** (PM) standards be established for healthcare equipment. The following information should be recorded and maintained for each piece of patient care equipment:

Preventive maintenance (PM) Service provided to equipment to maintain its proper operating condition by providing planned inspection and detecting and correcting failures before they occur.

- Assigned equipment location
- Ownership status (rented, leased, owned, borrowed)
- Schedule for PM
- PM history
- Facility-defined PM standards
- Repair history

The SPD and Biomed department partner in several ways. Each time patient care equipment is returned to the SPD for cleaning, its PM sticker should be checked. Items due for a PM inspection should be routed to the Biomed department after cleaning instead of it being returned to service. **Figure 20.1** provides an example of a PM sticker. As part of their routine inspection process, SP technicians should also check for damaged (cracked, torn or frayed) electrical cords, cracked equipment casings, loose knobs and switches, and other signs of damage that should be corrected before the item is reused. All equipment that appears to need repair should be cleaned and sent to Biomed personnel for inspection. Equipment-related issues can be minimized when all staff remain alert to obvious signs of the need for equipment inspection or repair. This, in turn, increases the level of patient and employee safety. After any PM, inspection or repair made by Biomed personnel, the medical equipment should be cleaned according to the IFU prior to its return to service or storage.

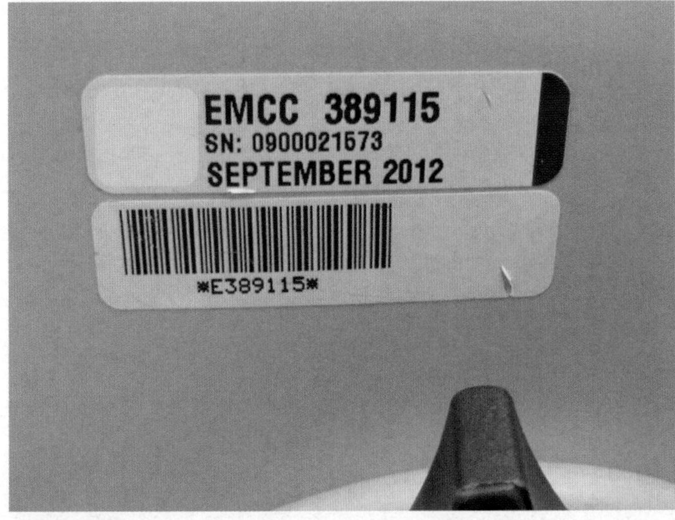

Figure 20.1

Handling Used (Soiled) Patient Care Equipment

All patient care equipment used must be considered contaminated and handled as such, regardless of its appearance. *Note: Patient care equipment may not be visibly soiled and may appear clean; however, it is likely to harbor microorganisms that could pose a threat to patients and staff.* In some facilities, SP technicians make routinely-scheduled rounds to pick up soiled equipment from user units (See **Figure 20.2**) and transport items to the decontamination area for cleaning. Sometimes, they may also make special trips to user departments to retrieve specific equipment. In either case, the equipment should be considered contaminated and transported according to soiled item transport guidelines. Consider the following when transporting soiled medical equipment:

- Using a closed cart to minimalize cross-contamination
- Choosing a route that minimizes contact with healthcare patrons (i.e., using staff hallways and elevators)
- Using personal protective equipment, such as gloves, when handling soiled equipment
- Performing hand hygiene procedures after removing gloves and when hands become soiled

Disposable components, such as pads, tubing and suction canisters, should be removed from each piece of equipment and discarded at the point of use. Only items that will be cleaned and reused should be transported to the decontamination area.

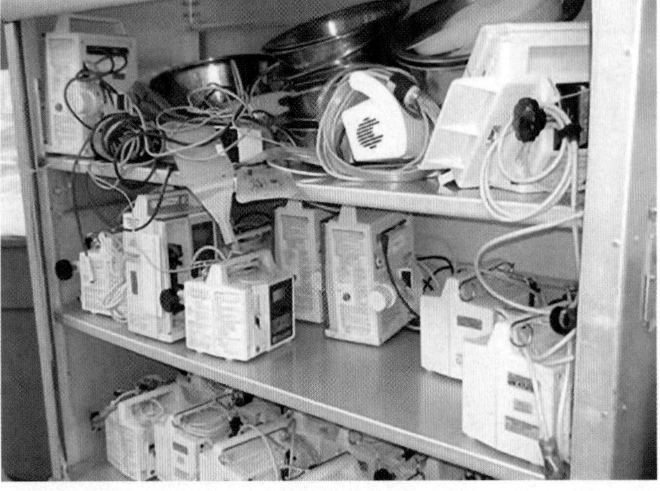

Figure 20.2

Cleaning Patient Care Equipment

Patient care equipment should be cleaned per the equipment manufacturer's instructions and the healthcare facility's infection prevention protocols. The manufacturer's cleaning instructions are typically found in the operator's manual that accompanies the equipment when it is purchased. Whenever a new item or patient care equipment is brought into the facility, SP technicians should receive written instructions about procedures for cleaning and handling. A review of the instructions should be performed to ensure the facility can process the item and that the facility has the required cleaning chemicals and necessary accessories. All surfaces, including cords, switches and crevices, must be thoroughly cleaned. (See **Figure 20.3**)

Managing Inoperative Equipment

Equipment that is nonfunctioning should be identified and tagged by the user. (See **Figure 20.4**) SP technicians must ensure that equipment tagged for repair is routed to the Biomed department after cleaning. If an equipment malfunction causes patient harm, it should not be disassembled or have its settings adjusted. It should be removed from service and returned immediately to the Biomed department for inspection and follow up.

Pay attention to detail

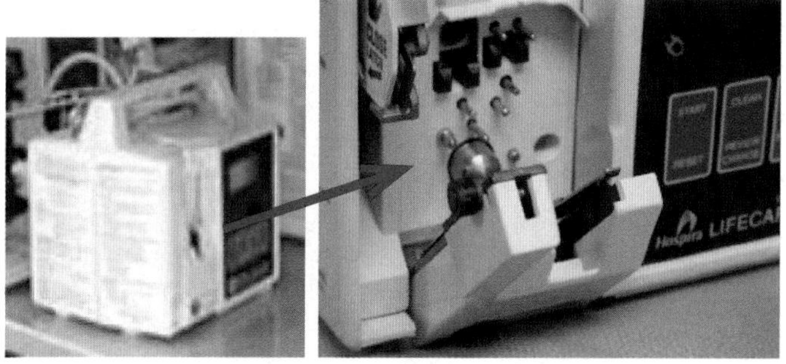

Figure 20.3 Follow manufacturers' instructions and clean all areas.

PREPARING EQUIPMENT FOR USE

Patient care equipment should be prepared for use and stored in a "ready to dispense" state. Preparation for use may include assembly, the addition of new disposable components, such as tubing and pads, and a check or replacement of batteries per the equipment manufacturer's assembly instructions. Clean items should be easily identifiable as "clean" with the use of bags, tags or labels.

Storage of Patient Care Equipment

After patient care equipment has been cleaned, inspected and assembled, it should be placed into storage until needed. In some cases, storage is confined to the SPD or a secure location nearby. Sometimes, however, patient care equipment may be stored in user units. This makes it more accessible for nursing and other patient care staff and reduces waiting time when the equipment is needed immediately. All equipment should be stored in a clean, secure location, away from high-traffic areas such as visitor hallways.

Some types of patient care equipment have battery back-up systems that must be recharged. An adequate number of electrical outlets is needed in all applicable storage areas to enable these items to be plugged in at all times for battery recharge. Critical items, such as defibrillators, may need to utilize "red outlets" or outlets connected to emergency back-up power. (See **Figure 20.5**) These outlets remain active in the event of a power failure. While this equipment is designed to run using electricity, there may be times when patients are moved while still connected to equipment—and during power disruptions, when the equipment must rely on pre-charged batteries to function.

Inoperative equipment should be tagged and routed to Biomedical/Clinical Engineering.

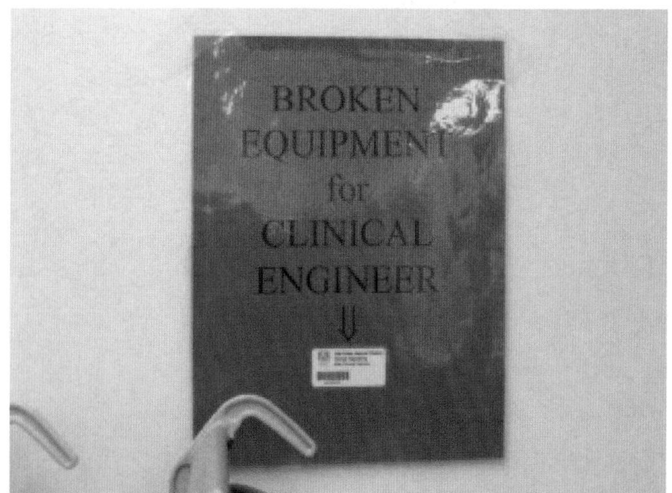

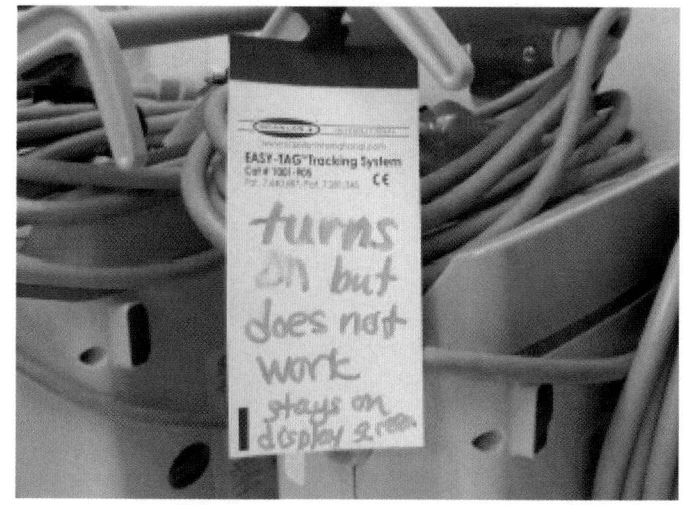

Figure 20.4

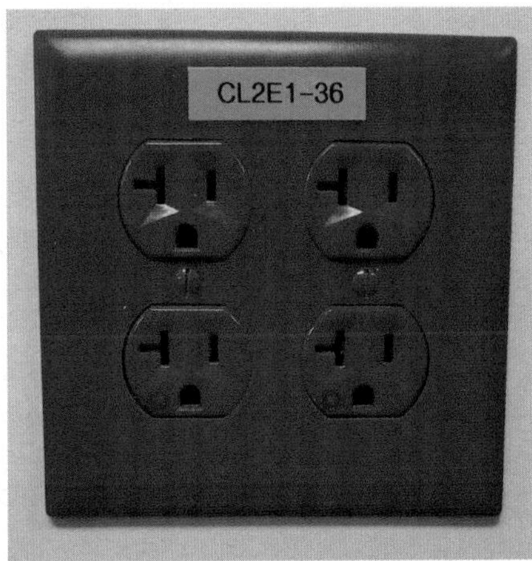

Figure 20.5

Tracking Patient Care Equipment

Tracking patient care equipment is a challenge for any SPD. The equipment is mobile and, in many cases, small. It can easily be placed in an incorrect location, set aside on a user unit or otherwise misplaced. Equipment that is difficult to locate can cause equipment shortages, which may delay treatment, necessitate short-term rental of replacement equipment, and increase the healthcare facility's operating costs.

There are several ways to track patient care equipment. It can be done manually or by using computerized programs that automate the tracking process with barcodes applied to the device. (See **Figure 20.6**) In some facilities, equipment is tracked with radio frequency identification (RFID) computer chips applied to each device that send signals to a locator system. Regardless of the type of tracking system used, the main goal is to provide information:

- About the current location of the equipment
- To charge patients for use of the equipment, if applicable
- On equipment usage and trends

Tracking patient care equipment allows SP professionals to monitor locations and ensure that equipment is available when needed. That information can also be used to justify additional equipment.

PROCURING NEW AND ADDITIONAL EQUIPMENT

New technologies and increased need (patient volume) often require healthcare facilities to procure additional patient care equipment. New equipment may be purchased, leased or rented, or it can even be loaned to the healthcare facility by a manufacturer. There are advantages and disadvantages to each approach, and the facility should make decisions based upon its specific needs.

Equipment Purchase

This method of equipment acquisition has been used by healthcare facilities for decades. Facility personnel identify the need for specific equipment, determine the type (model, style or brand) that is required, budget for its purchase and incorporate it into the system. The equipment is then owned by the healthcare facility.

Equipment Lease

As with purchasing, healthcare facility personnel must determine equipment needs. From there, they contract with a manufacturer

Equipment tracking using barcodes

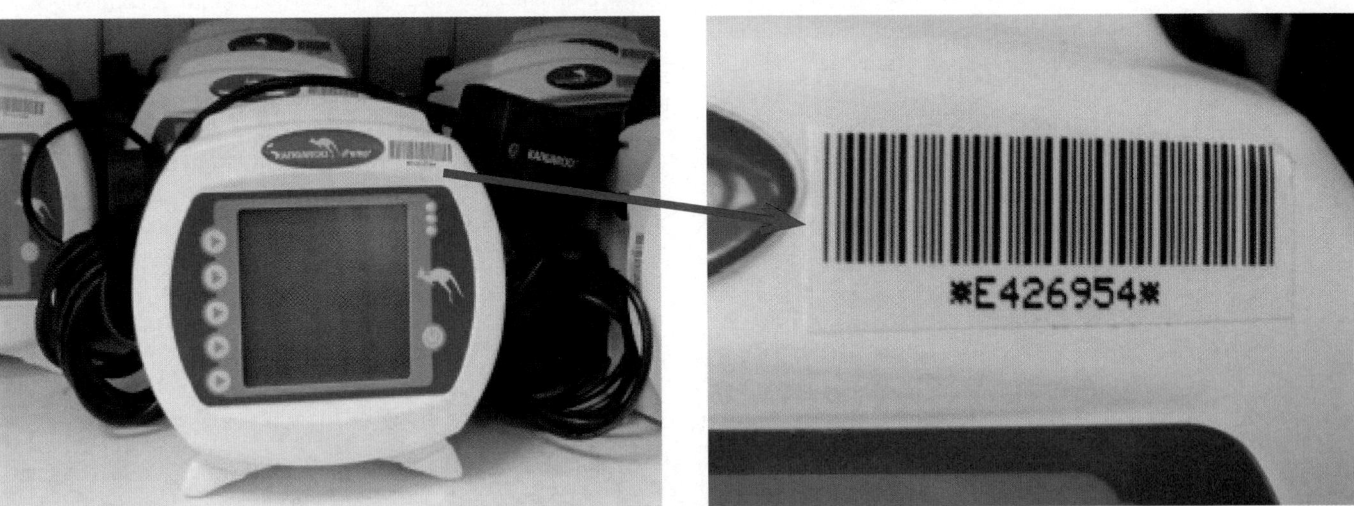

Figure 20.6

or leasing company to lease (use) the equipment for a specific time period. At the end of the contract, the healthcare facility can return the equipment (and acquire a newer technology) or purchase it.

Equipment Rental

Equipment rental differs from leasing because it is usually done on a short-term basis. For example, leasing contracts may be for months or years, but rental contracts may be as brief as a single day. When renting, the healthcare facility identifies an immediate need, usually because high patient volume has created a demand for existing equipment that has caused a shortage, or because of the unique needs of a specific patient. In either case, the healthcare facility then contracts for a short-term rental with an equipment rental company. It is important to return rental equipment as soon as the need ends to reduce rental costs associated with the equipment.

Manufacturer's Loan

Manufacturers occasionally provide equipment to healthcare facilities as part of an agreement in which the facility will use the manufacturer's disposable products such as pads, tubing and sleeves. Decisions about the type of equipment acquisition process that will be most beneficial to the healthcare facility should be made by facility administrators.

Whichever method is used to acquire equipment, the technician's responsibilities remain the same: to provide clean, safe and complete equipment and to maintain the availability of that equipment by coordinating workflow.

OTHER PATIENT CARE EQUIPMENT CONCERNS

Equipment Maintenance and Repair

All mechanical equipment must be properly maintained and will sometimes require **repair**. PM helps identify potential problems before they occur. PM is conducted on a routine, scheduled basis and is designed to ensure that equipment is in proper operating condition. Equipment repair is performed as needed when equipment fails to function properly, and when it appears to be damaged.

> **Repair (equipment)** Procedures used to return equipment to its proper operating condition after it has become inoperative.

Both PM and equipment repair should only be performed by trained Biomed equipment technicians or the equipment manufacturer.

PROCEDURAL SUPPORT

Procedure Trays and Kits

Procedures performed outside of the OR can be divided into two categories: those performed in a designated **procedure area** and those performed at the patient's bedside. In either case, safe and accurate instruments and supplies are critical to patient safety.

> **Procedure area** An area within the healthcare facility that performs invasive and minimally-invasive procedures that require instruments, supplies and equipment.

The SPD is the provider of sterile instrumentation and often provides trays and kits for procedural areas. Common procedure areas include the:

- Cardiac catheterization lab
- ED
- L&D
- Minor procedure rooms
- Radiology department
- Endoscopy department

Just as each procedure area provides a very different type of treatment, each area will also have different types of trays, instruments and supplies.

Disposable or Reusable?

When a facility determines whether to use disposable or reusable trays and kits, several factors are taken into account such as physician preference, logistics, storage and replenishment cost.

When reusable trays and kits are used, a process must be adopted to help ensure that instruments are returned to the SPD for reprocessing. When disposable instruments are used, SP staff must identify and remove disposable instruments that are inadvertently returned to the decontamination area so they are not reprocessed. Disposable instruments are not manufactured to withstand the harsh processes of repeated cleaning and sterilization.

Regardless of the type of tray used (disposable or reusable), the user department must identify the tray's contents.

Off-site clinic instruments

Packaging for sterilization

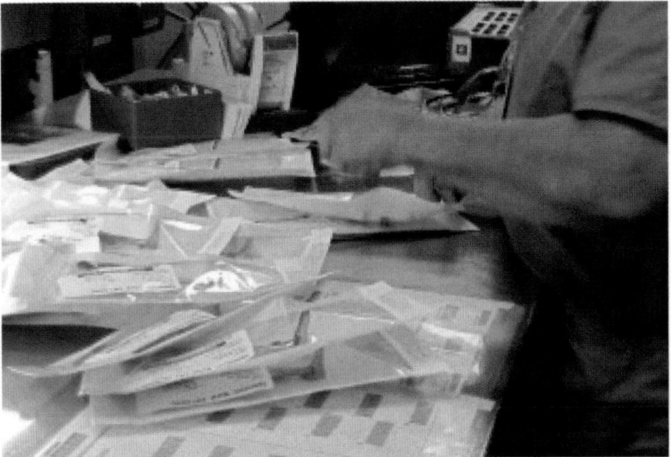

Sterile items ready for delivery

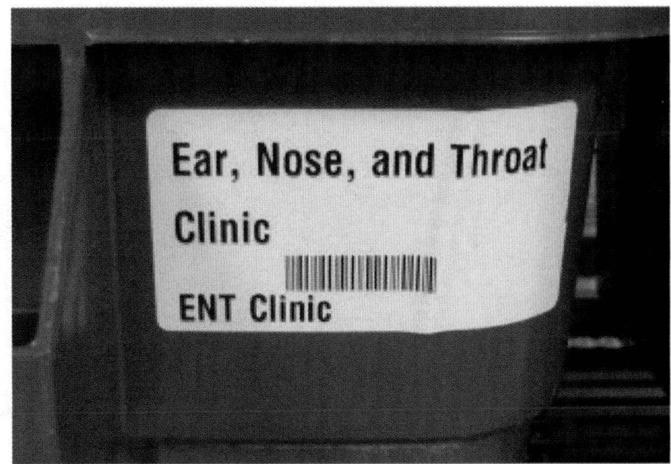

Figure 20.7

Managing Reusable Instruments

In addition to reprocessing instruments for ancillary departments, many SPDs also perform this function for offsite entities such as affiliated clinics. (See **Figure 20.7**) Care must be taken to help ensure that the process for transporting soiled instruments meets biohazard transport and infection prevention guidelines, and that the return of clean instruments follows specific protocols for sterile item transport.

If instruments are purchased and brought into the ancillary department through a channel other than the SPD, the user units must also provide the SPD with the manufacturer's written IFU. The instructions must be reviewed to ensure the item can be processed in the department.

As with the instruments used in the OR, the SPD should develop tray lists and written reprocessing protocols for all items processed for ancillary departments.

UTENSILS AND OTHER MEDICAL EQUIPMENT

SPDs may also be involved in handling utensils and other medical equipment. In many cases, the SPD is the only space in the building with the proper equipment and facilities to clean these devices. As with all items reprocessed through the SPD, manufacturers' reprocessing instructions should be obtained, made readily available to staff, and diligently followed.

COMMUNICATION AND COORDINATION ARE KEY

Any discussion of service to ancillary departments must address communication and coordination. Meeting the needs of many departments with various specialties can be challenging; therefore, careful planning and good communication are critical. For the system to run smoothly, everyone must understand and follow the appropriate process.

CONCLUSION

Modern healthcare facilities rely on equipment, instruments and supplies to provide patient care. Each healthcare department fills a specific need and requires specific items to fulfill its mission. The SPD provides valuable support to enable ancillary departments to provide quality patient care.

RESOURCES

U.S. Food and Drug Administration. *Medical Device Reporting 21 CFR 803.* 2014.

ECRI Top 10 Health Technology Hazards for 2022.

STERILE PROCESSING TERMS

Patient care equipment

Preventive maintenance (PM)

Repair (equipment)

Procedure area

Chapter 21

The Role of Information Technology in Sterile Processing

Learning Objectives

As a result of successfully completing this chapter, the reader will be able to:

1. Provide an overview of the use of information management systems in Sterile Processing departments
2. Discuss the use of computers and information systems to support activities within the healthcare facility and the Sterile Processing department
3. Review the advantages of instrument and equipment tracking systems

INTRODUCTION

Sterile Processing (SP) technicians must responsibly manage the equipment, instruments and supplies in their facilities. These items are in constant movement between departments as they are dispensed, used and replaced or processed. To maintain order and ensure the availability of items for patient care, SP staff must track each item to:

- Ensure that it can be quickly located
- Determine when consumable supplies should be replaced
- Monitor item usage
- Maintain accurate records of processes such as sterilization and distribution
- Assist with quality assurance processes and regulatory compliance
- Capture information for financial analysis

Historically, all recordkeeping (documentation) performed in the SP department (SPD) was done manually. Now, most departments use some form of automated information management system to track products and document processes. Some departments use a combination of manual and computerized tracking, while others employ a fully integrated information management model throughout the entire facility.

Some common types of computer-based information systems used in the SPD include those for instrument tracking, sterilization time and attendance information, case cart pick lists, patient care equipment tracking, inventory management, staffing analysis, and individual productivity data. (See **Figure 21.1**)

ROLE OF COMPUTER-BASED INFORMATION SYSTEMS

SP technicians must maintain and manage a significant amount of data as supplies, instruments and equipment are stocked and issued to the Operating Room (OR) and various other

Examples of computerization in Sterile Processing

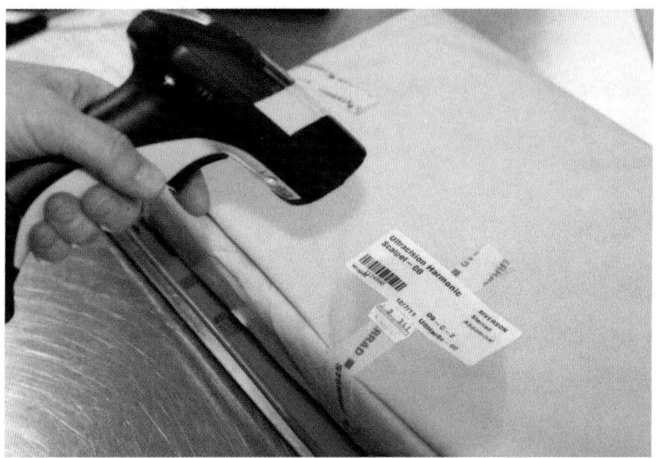

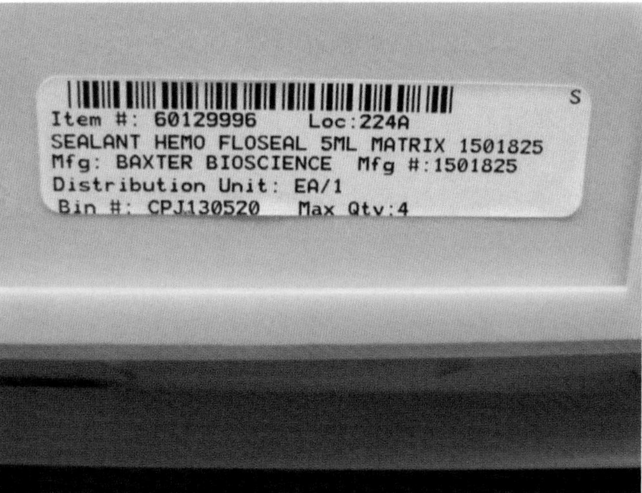

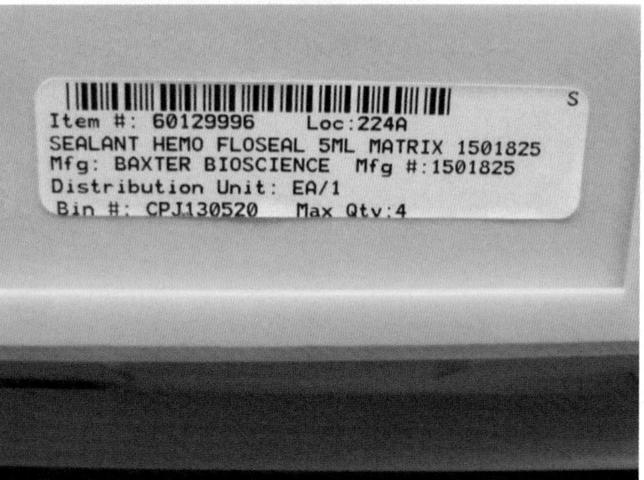

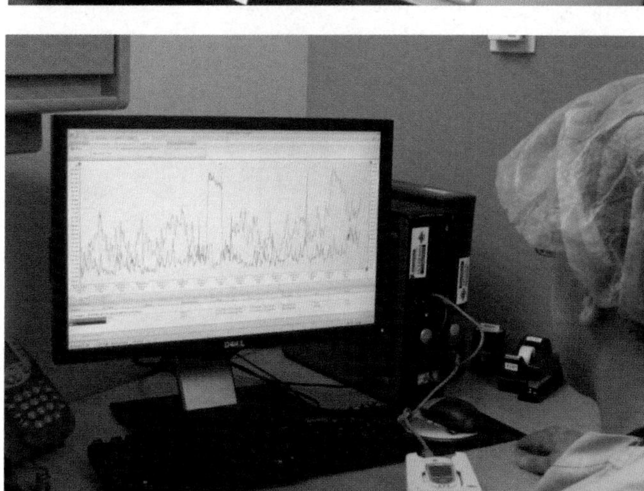

Figure 21.1

user departments. Computers can promote basic and advanced capabilities to support operational activities for healthcare Supply Chain Management (SCM) and SP. SP technicians require a solid understanding of how computers are currently used to serve the department's core mission and functions.

Computers and information systems continue to evolve rapidly. When SP personnel are involved in evaluating and/or selecting a new computer-based application or system, they must be aware of the latest trends and technological advancements that are relevant to their role in the healthcare setting.

Overview of Information Technology in the Healthcare Setting

The modern healthcare environment uses information technology to provide accurate and efficient management of a very complex set of business processes. Ideally, information technology and systems are used to ensure patient safety, demonstrate quality of care and provide efficient operational and financial management for the healthcare organization.

There are few, if any, aspects of healthcare where information technology or systems are not employed. While an organization may be currently using a mixture of computerized and/or manual processes, it is reasonable to assume that any of the manual processes in use are being routinely evaluated for conversion as resources and budgets allow.

To support the needs of the global patient population today and in the future, the healthcare industry is intensely focused on continual improvements to the environment of care and the ability to adopt and utilize all the tools available to provide high-quality healthcare at an optimal cost.

Increasingly, more emphasis is on point-of-care and point-of-use computing, with mobile solutions suitable for the bedside and use in SP work areas. (See **Figure 21.2**) This has become possible with the development of electronic recordkeeping systems and wireless network capabilities that provide real-time data communication. These systems can be supported with the use of laptop workstation-on-wheels (WOW) solutions, tablet-based computing, and even smartphones. Computer technology will continue to advance in this manner for the foreseeable future.

A clear understanding of the systems that can be utilized by SP management and staff is important for two critical reasons:

- The core mission is to support patient safety and quality patient care. Information systems can be used to ensure these objectives are accomplished.

- Using available systems appropriately will enhance the ability to provide efficient and cost-effective patient care.

It is also important to understand that many of the systems used in healthcare are integrated (interfaced), meaning they communicate with each other electronically. Integration is essential for eliminating redundant data entry, promoting efficiency and reducing the risk for inaccurate or conflicting data from being entered into the system.

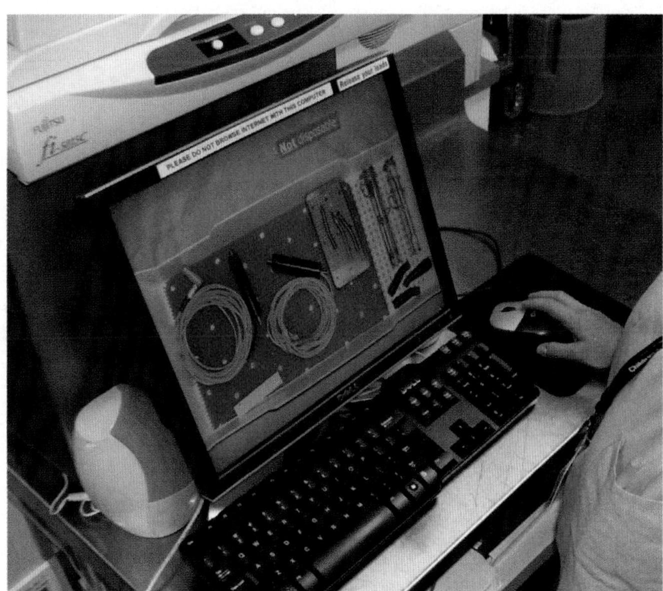

Figure 21.2

This is also important for the SPD because the department sometimes creates and manages information that feeds other systems. For example, if the department uses an electronic SP information system, information about inventory updates may be communicated to the OR scheduling system for use on physician preference cards.

The healthcare facility's information management system utilizes many components to meet a wide variety of needs. **Figure 21.3** provides an example of common components—clinical, operational, financial and public relations—that comprise that system.

Clinical information systems are at the heart of a healthcare provider's core mission because these systems capture data related to direct patient care.

- Admissions and registration, also known as admissions, discharge and transfer (ADT) systems, are used to manage inpatient and outpatient registration. This is important to SP technicians because patient census information is received from the ADT system.

- The electronic medical record (EMR) or electronic health record (EHR) is the library of data related to the care provided to a patient by the organization. Healthcare providers must comply with "meaningful use" requirements. This ensures the certified EHR technology is being used to improve quality, safety, efficiency and care coordination, while maintaining privacy of

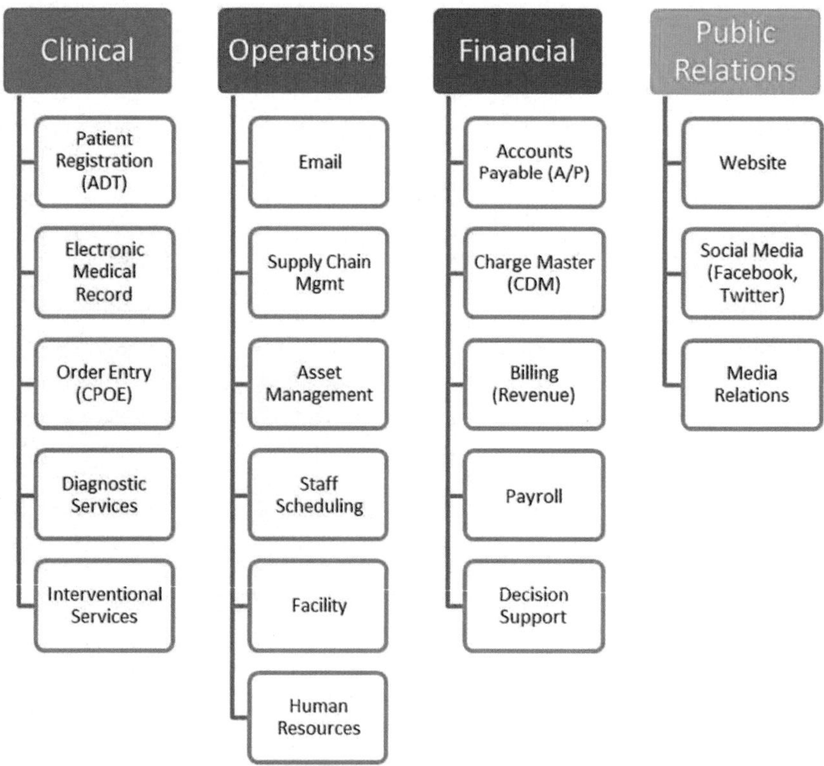

Figure 21.3 Example of healthcare information technology infrastructure

patient health information. *Note: The other clinical information systems will transmit relevant information to the EMR/EHR.*

- Centralized patient order entry (CPOE) systems are data portals used by physicians and other authorized caregivers to order tests, medications, supplies and equipment for patient use. The CPOE system also provides alerts when there are potentially conflicting orders created for a patient, such as allergies or medication incompatibility. This is important to SP technicians because automated requests for patient care items are generated by a CPOE system.

- Diagnostic and therapeutic services systems are used to manage the scheduling, procedures performed, and results reported for their respective departments, such as Radiology, Ultrasound, Vascular lab, EKG, Respiratory and Pulmonary Functions lab, Physical and Occupational Therapy, etc.

- Interventional services systems are used to manage scheduling, procedures performed, and results reported for their respective departments, such as the OR, Labor and Delivery (L&D) and the Cardiac Catheterization Lab. These systems are important to those in the SPD because information is received (schedules, pick lists, etc.) about the daily needs of the SPD's critical customers.

Operational systems are essential in managing the various functions within the organization that are not directly related to patient care.

- Email systems are a crucial platform for managing communication within any organization. Email reduces the need for voicemail and pagers.

- SCM or Materials Management Information Systems (MMIS) are used for managing the purchasing, receipt and inventory control functions within an organization. The supply chain system is essential to the SPD for many reasons, including inventory control and ordering of instruments and supplies.

Asset management systems (also known as tracking systems) are used to manage the use, processing and location of medical equipment (see **Figure 21.4**) and surgical instrumentation throughout an organization. These systems serve as tools for efficiently monitoring and controlling the utilization of surgical instruments and patient care equipment.

Figure 21.4 Barcode scanning systems are an example of computerized methods used to track assets such as equipment.

- Staff scheduling systems can be used to monitor compliance with the organization's timeclock policies, provide a mechanism to create work schedules, and analyze workforce needs and trends.

- Facility systems are used to manage the physical environment of the organization. Examples of commonly found facility systems are heating, ventilation and air conditioning (HVAC) for monitoring and managing temperature and humidity; fire control for managing fire alarms, sprinklers and magnetically controlled doors; public address for audible announcements; and access control for managing identification badge access to secure areas within the facility. These are important to SP technicians for managing the safety and quality of areas where items are processed and stored.

- Human Resources systems are used not only for recruiting and retaining staff, but also for managing employee benefits and monitoring compliance with regulatory requirements for staff.

Financial systems are essential for managing the organization's financial activities.

- Accounts payable (AP) systems – Used to manage payment to vendors providing products or services to the organization.

- Charge description master (CDM) systems – Used to manage a list of services and items that are chargeable to patients. The CDM system is designed to communicate (interface) with other software systems to support government-mandated standard billing requirements.

- Billing or patient accounting (revenue) systems – Used to manage the issuing of bills to patients/insurance payors and assist with collections of amounts due.

- Payroll systems – Used to track hours, calculate wages, taxes and deductions, and print and deliver checks.

- Decision support systems – Used to analyze operational and financial performance and provide key metrics to senior leadership. Decision support includes information related to the volume of procedures and services provided as well as the operational costs and revenue received. This is an essential tool used by leadership to evaluate the financial impact of services and programs offered by the organization.

Public relations systems are essential in managing the public perception of the organization.

- The facility's website is a significant portal for patients, employees and physicians to obtain information about the services and programs offered, including employment or volunteer opportunities; the facility's core mission and values; and other details such as phone directories, maps and directions. Patient portals also allow patients to view their medical records, receive and print lab results, retrieve consultation requests, and much more.

- Social media portals, such as Facebook and Twitter, are becoming increasingly important to hospitals because they are frequently used by patients to express their opinion about their experience with an organization (or learn about the opinions and viewpoints shared by others).

- Media relations resources include information that resides on other websites not directly controlled by the organization such as news articles on services provided.

TRACKING SYSTEMS FOR THE SPD

The processes and needs of the SPD have changed over the years. Advances in sterilization, instrument technologies, durable medical equipment, and supply inventory are ongoing, and costs for instrumentation purchase, repair and replacement have led to a greater need for improved asset tracking and management.

Overview

Tracking systems available for use in the SPD can forecast needs and identify processing costs and usage for trays and single instruments. These tracking systems can also help maximize equipment and inventory utilization to provide pertinent information as future budgets are developed.

Tracking Methods

There are several types of tracking systems and methods available. Examples include the use of barcodes to scan an item's last known location and radio-frequency identification (RFID) tags used for real-time tracking of patient care equipment.

System ease of use, cost and compatibility with other software systems in use are among the factors affecting purchasing decisions. Additionally, to ensure reliability, the tracking method must be compatible with the processing practices and technologies used by the facility.

A tracking system may typically be either a traditional installed software application with a database managed by facility information technology (IT) personnel or a web-based application with a database managed (hosted) by the software vendor and accessed through the internet. The latter, commonly referred to as **cloud computing**, may offer several advantages, including cost benefits and ease of installation.

Cloud computing The practice of storing regularly used data on multiple servers that can be accessed through the internet.

Integration capabilities are important when communicating critical information to and from the tracking system. OR scheduling system interfaces are typically desirable to both the SPD and the OR because they facilitate information about instruments, supplies and equipment needs based on the surgery schedule in real-time or near real-time forecasting.

Tracking Systems Meet Specific Needs

A tracking system must meet the specific needs of the facility that uses it. For example, in a multi-hospital health network, certain modules or special features in the system may be utilized by personnel at one site but not at other sites. This is generally due to differences in the complexity of processing or logistics between sites or departments. For example, a processing area that supports a small ambulatory surgery department may not have a need for the same tracking features that would benefit an SPD that supports a large inpatient OR.

In short, a well-developed tracking system has built-in flexibility and scalability that can allow SPDs to tailor the configuration to meet specific needs and allow for logical reconfiguration or changes as requested.

The continual need to update information is critical for the success of any tracking system, regardless of whether its primary use is for instrument processing, case cart pick lists, preference cards, inventory control or other purposes. (See **Figure 21.5**)

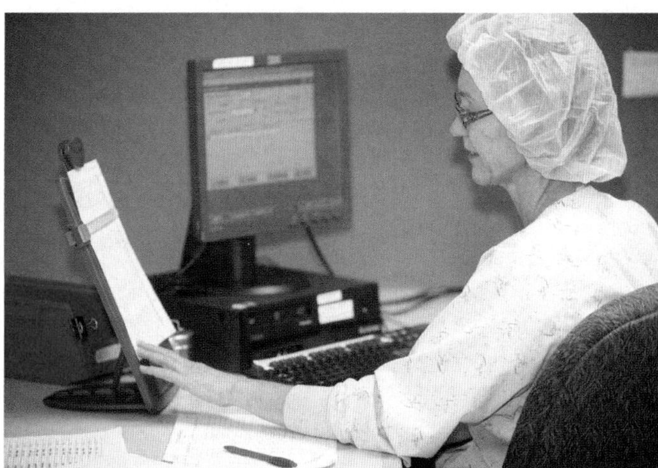

Figure 21.5 An SP technician updates information on preference cards.

Surgical instrument sets or single peel-packed items can be tracked (located) at the packaged and sterilized product level using one dimensional (1D) barcode labels. Small RFID tags, which can be used reliably within the sterilization process, can provide real-time location data when they are affixed to instruments or trays. It is likely that RFID technology will coexist with barcodes because use of a barcode promotes line-of-sight inspection by the user when scanning an item. This is an essential step in ensuring the sterile integrity of packaged products.

Individual instruments can be tracked (located) within a set or tray using two-dimensional (2D) data-matrix barcodes. These are marked directly on the instrument using a laser etching process or through the placement of a dot-type label. (See **Figure 21.6**) Individual instrument tracking ensures specific instruments are kept with a specific set. It can also locate specific high-cost, complex devices, such as powered, endoscopic or robotic instruments, for required preventative maintenance inspection. In facilities where the risk of exposure to emerging pathogens, such as Creutzfeldt-Jakob Disease (CJD), is high, individual instrument tracking is crucial for demonstrating the processing or dispensing actions taken in the investigation of a suspected or confirmed exposure.

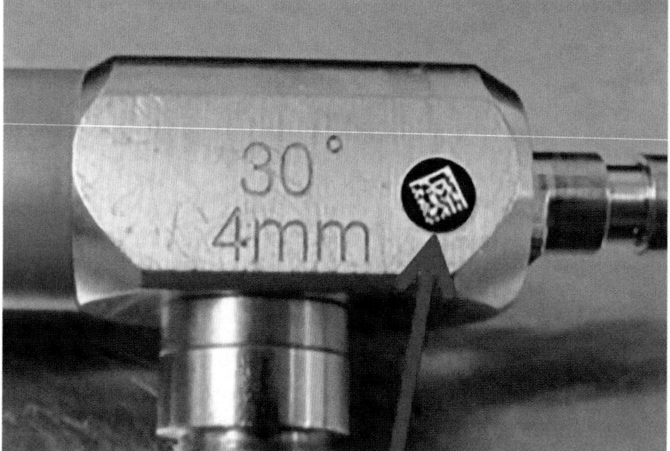

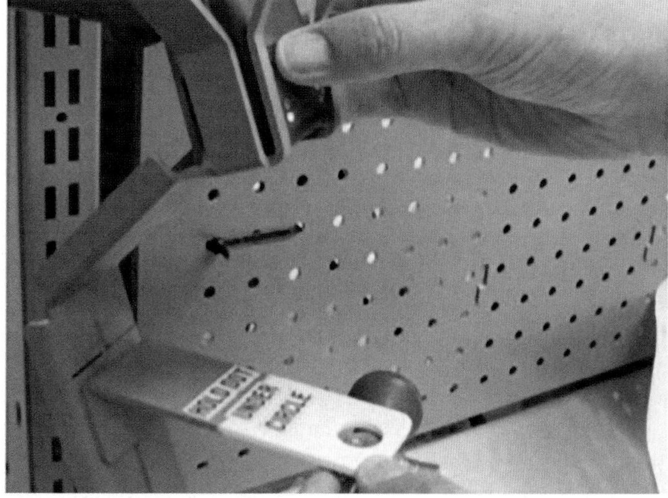

Figure 21.6 Dot matrix barcodes allow for individual instrument scanning and tracking.

System documentation and scanning can be done with many different types of devices. These include wireless mobile handheld devices (see **Figure 21.7**), systems wired directly to the computer terminal, fixed radio receivers that read RFID transponder signals throughout the facility, and manual entry of information into the computer.

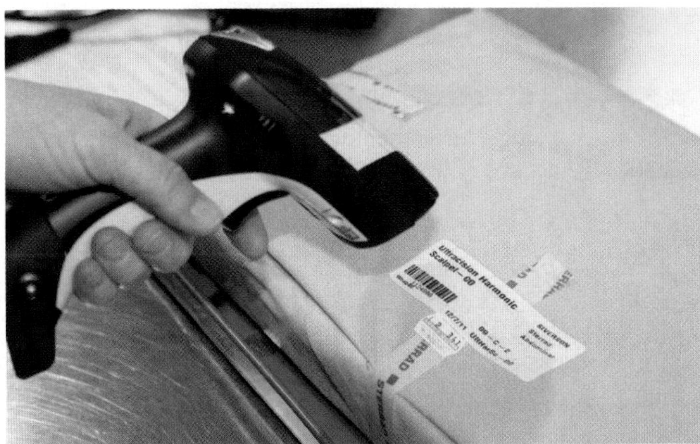

Figure 21.7 A handheld scanner is used to capture instrument information before an item is sterilized.

Decisions about system utilization should consider the specific environment to which the item(s) will be exposed. For example, the cleaning and sterilization processes for instruments and sets must be evaluated in detail during any implementation planning process to minimize the risk of any adverse effects on the tracking system. For example, chemical agents designed to be compatible for use with instruments (based on the materials used in their manufacturing) may negatively affects laser etchings, fade barcode labels, and make them unreadable to the scanner after repeated use. Heat generated during steam sterilization may damage RFID tags and impair their functionality. Water, chemicals, and drying temperatures used to clean case carts and other equipment may cause adhesives affix the RFID tags to dissolve. When this occurs, they can fall off or become damaged from water leakage. As these risks are recognized, manufacturers generally respond by making improvements to components or processes to ensure reliability.

FEATURES OF INSTRUMENT AND EQUIPMENT TRACKING SYSTEMS

Instrument and equipment tracking systems can provide many different features to assist SP professionals in the facility's OR, Finance, Nursing and Administrative departments. All tracking systems include some basic operating features; however, more advanced systems include additional features to enhance their usefulness.

Basic Systems

Basic instrument and equipment tracking systems typically can track (account for):

- Complete instrument sets and trays
- Specific equipment items
- The last known location of a specific instrument set, tray or equipment
- Cost and value of specific equipment and instruments, and the total cost of an instrument set/tray
- Number of complete processing and use cycles through which instruments and instrument sets have moved
- Usage of specific equipment
- Preventative maintenance (PM) schedules and repairs made to specific equipment and instrument sets/trays

Basic instrument and equipment tracking systems also provide other information, including:

- Complete tray lists for accurate tray assembly (see **Figure 21.8**) and equipment setup, such as:
  - › The name of the SP technician who assembled and inspected the set or equipment

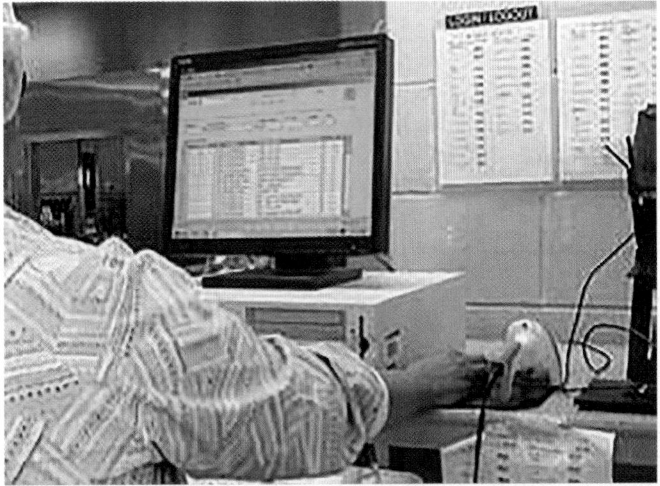

Figure 21.8

  - › The date the set or equipment was processed
  - › The sterilization and cleaning modality (process)
  - › The catalog number and manufacturer's name to identify instruments and associated equipment/supplies
  - › An image of the instrumentation
  - › Any acceptable substitutes for missing instrumentation
  - › Any special instructions required for assembly, such as tip protectors required for single skin hooks
  - › The quantity (individual and total) of instruments included in the set or tray

  - Identification of instruments missing from the set. *Note: These can be identified on the list and then be affixed to the outside of the set for identification and tracking.*

- Productivity reporting information:
  - Sets and instruments processed and completed during a specific work shift
  - Sets and instruments completed by specific employees *Note: This information is helpful for educational and training purposes.*
  - Equipment processed and distributed
- Quality assurance data for specific facility-based information such as:
  - Sterilization load quarantines or recalls
  - Biological monitoring standards and regulations
  - Educational and inservice documentation
- Financial data for documenting and managing:
  - Instrument replacement and repair
  - Equipment replacement and repair
  - PM notification
  - PM records
  - Utilization of instrument sets, trays and equipment
  - Productivity data and staffing requirements for peak operational workflow

Integrating/interfacing with clinical systems allows facilities to associate (link) instrument trays, sets and equipment to each patient's medical record. Today's tracking systems can also interface with sterilization and washer-decontamination equipment, automated endoscope reprocessors (AERs), and biological incubators.

Advanced Systems

Instrument and equipment tracking systems may also include some of the following advanced features that can be beneficial in certain healthcare facility applications:

- RFID that enables real-time location of an instrument or equipment item as it moves through the facility and the processing cycle. The real-time location of a complete instrument set or tray can also be assessed.
- Set-level tracking features to allow staff members to know the last scanned location of an instrument set or tray.
- Individual instrument level tracking features that allow staff to track a single instrument within a set or tray and identify the set into which a specific instrument was placed.

Tracking Loaned Instrumentation

Healthcare facilities often use loaned instrumentation. Loaned instrument tracking programs are available that can track loaned inventory in real time, provide communication to SP professionals regarding which instrument sets to expect, as well as provide instructions for use (IFU). Different types of systems are available that provide data to assist in the management of loaned instrumentation.

Tracking and Planning for SP Technicians

Commitment is required for any system to work, including tracking systems. Whether the system is computerized or manual, technicians need to be diligent in performing the scanning/location logging tasks. When SP technicians diligently perform the tracking processes, the system will provide information that allows technicians to locate devices and plan their shift. A few of the benefits include:

- Device location allows instruments, sets and equipment to be located quickly. If items are in transit to the user area, the customer can be informed of the device's location and how long until it will be delivered. On busy days when instrument sets are in full use, an accurate tracking system can let SP technicians know where each set is and allows SP staff to obtain and move items where they are needed.
- Video screens of the day's surgery schedule in the department allow for visualization of which phase each surgical case is in throughout the day. This information allows technicians to plan for turnaround items and allocate equipment and resources when they are most needed. Canceled or postponed case information allows SP technicians to retrieve and reallocate case carts, equipment and instruments to ORs that need them.
- Devices in need of PM can be identified so items are inspected in the timeframe that their manufacturers recommend.
- Damaged devices are noted in the system so that time is not wasted looking for these devices. Anticipated dates when items will be returned from repair can also be available. Systems can keep track of the number of times items that have been repaired or replaced, as well as the cumulative cost of these repairs.

Technology is a great resource with benefits that can be clearly recognized. Technology can be used to enhance processes, maximize time and improve patient safety. As with any automated, mechanical or digitized process, technology can fail, break or experience disruptions. It is important to have a clearly defined downtime process when interruptions occur. A computerized instrument tracking system used for instrument assembly is an example of an invaluable tool that the SPD can utilize. When tracking systems fail and instrument assembly cannot be completed digitally, the facility must have a back-up plan to keep instrument assembly moving. Manual copies of instrument count sheets should be regularly updated and available when experiencing down time. This is true for most processes in the healthcare facility. Patient care must continue even when technology is not cooperating. It is important to examine the processes in the SPD, identify processes and systems that rely on technology, and plan for the unexpected.

CONCLUSION

SP professionals must responsibly manage the equipment, instruments and supplies entrusted to them by their healthcare facility. An instrument and equipment tracking system helps facilitate this goal by capturing pertinent data, logging and documenting processes, practices and SP-related functions, and more.

As computer-based technology and information systems continue to evolve, additional capabilities will become available to help facilities better address operational activities and facilitate high-quality patient care. Even so, computers are only one part of a total information system. While computers and tracking systems provide numerous benefits, SP technicians are the key to providing efficient and effective services to help their department support the facility's core mission, which is to provide safe, high-quality patient care and customer service.

RESOURCE

Glandon GH, Slovensky DJ, Smaltz GL. *Austin & Boxerman's Information Systems for Healthcare Management,* 7th Ed. 2008.

STERILE PROCESSING TERM

Cloud computing

Chapter 22

Safety for Sterile Processing

Learning Objectives

As a result of successfully completing this chapter, the reader will be able to:

1. Explain the importance of safety and risk management in the Sterile Processing department
2. Review three common workplace hazards
3. Explain the importance of ergonomics and health awareness for Sterile Processing technicians
4. Identify strategies for accident prevention
5. Describe special safety precautions for handling ethylene oxide
6. Discuss the basics of a healthcare facility's internal and external disaster plans

INTRODUCTION

It has been said that "safety is no accident," and that statement couldn't be truer, especially for healthcare professionals who are responsible for keeping patients, employees and visitors free from injury.

Safety requires ongoing education, safeguards, proper planning and the combined implementation of safety systems to reduce risks, prevent injury and save lives. The Sterile Processing (SP) decontamination area is a perfect example of how safety systems and due diligence are essential for ensuring safety. The decontamination area operates in the presence of pathogenic microorganisms, which presents a real risk to those who enter. Engineering controls, such as managed air pressure, physical separation from clean areas, and personal protective equipment (PPE), are provided to minimize risk. Employees must be educated in biohazard safety and follow specific regulations, such as those established by the Occupational Safety and Health Administration (OSHA), to reduce the risk of injury. (See **Figure 22.1**) This chapter identifies common risks found in the Sterile Processing department's (SPD's) work areas and identifies ways to minimize the risk for injury.

RISK MANAGEMENT

Risk management is a method used to assess the risks of a specific activity and develop programs to reduce that risk. It also involves injury prevention and claims management (the settlement, defense and prevention of lawsuits).

> **Risk management** Methods used to assess the risks of a specific activity and develop a program to reduce losses from exposure to those risks.

Risk management originated in the insurance industry as the result of an increased number of medical malpractice lawsuits. Such lawsuits cost healthcare facilities billions of dollars. Healthcare facilities must effectively manage injury prevention for patients and employees as part of a risk management program. Various authorities, including The Joint Commission (TJC), require that healthcare facilities develop and implement procedures to ensure they meet minimum safety standards.

Risk management programs are designed to prevent accidents and injuries and ensure accurate reporting and follow up to help prevent similar incidents. After a situation is examined and hazards or unsafe practices have been discovered, risk management personnel ensure that corrective actions are taken to improve systems, behaviors and/or physical conditions to help prevent employee and patient accidents and injuries.

By following the protocols outlined in this textbook, as well as the manufacturer's instructions for use (IFU), standards and regulations, SP technicians can support patient safety.

COMMON WORKPLACE SAFETY HAZARDS

All jobs involve some risks. The key to working safely in any work environment is understanding those risks and taking appropriate steps to minimize them. SP technicians must understand potential hazards and pay close attention in work areas within and sometimes outside of their department. The assumption that "an accident or injury will never happen to me" creates a false sense of security that results in many injuries each year. Following safety protocols and incorporating them into all work practices is necessary for preventing injuries and accidents.

SPD Occupational Hazards

In the SPD, there are three different types of occupational hazards: physical, biological and chemical. (See **Figure 22.2**) Some of those occupational hazards can be present in all areas of the department. Physical hazards, such as heavy or awkward lifting, for example, can occur in any work area. Other hazards may be confined to a specific work area. For example, biohazard contamination will most likely occur in the decontamination area.

Examples of risk management in the decontamination area

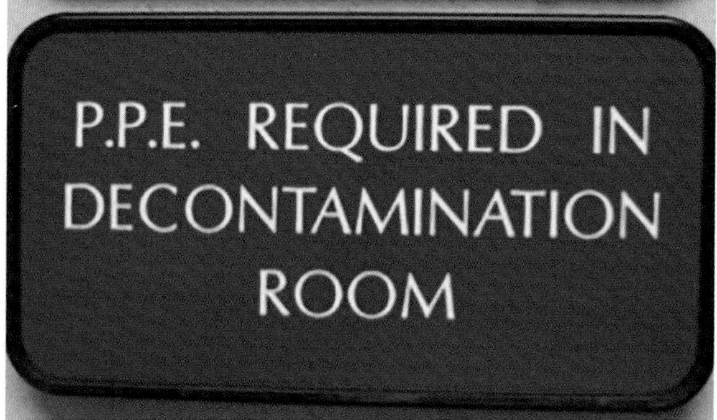

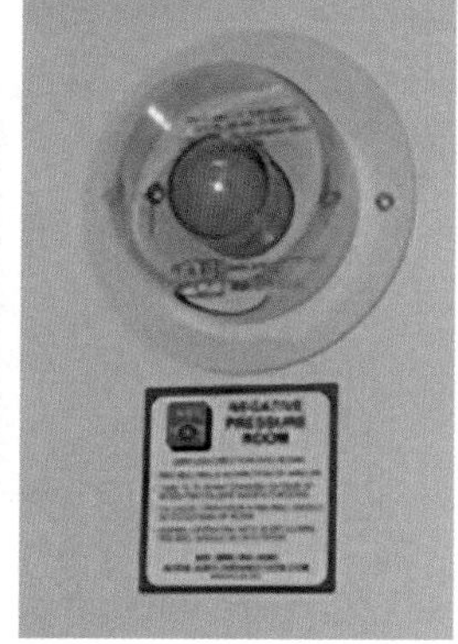

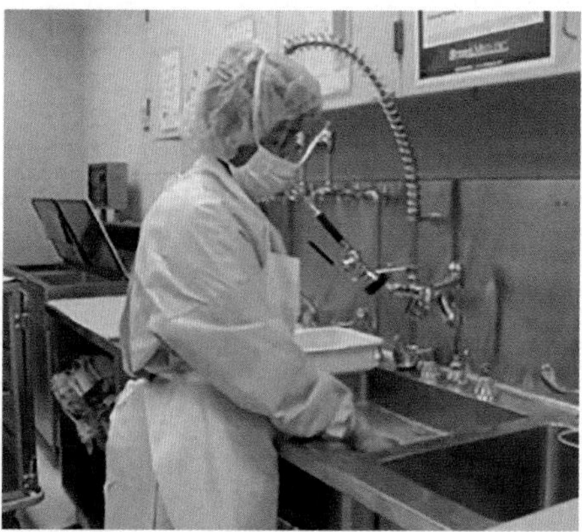

Figure 22.1

Physical safety hazards may be caused by the environment and the tasks performed within that environment. Due to the nature of the tasks performed, there are many potential physical hazards in the SPD. Physical hazards may include wet floors, cluttered walkways, heavy carts and sharp instruments. Fire is another physical safety concern.

Biological safety hazards (i.e., infectious waste and bloodborne pathogens) can potentially be found in any area of the department. Obviously, the decontamination area is the main area of concern for biological hazards.

Chemical safety hazards may be found throughout the SPD work areas. For example, solutions used in the decontamination area, sterilants used in the sterilization area, and some patient care products may pose chemical hazards within the department.

This chapter examines general safety hazards and outlines specific safety hazards by work area. The risk of injury from all of these hazards can be minimized by following safety protocols.

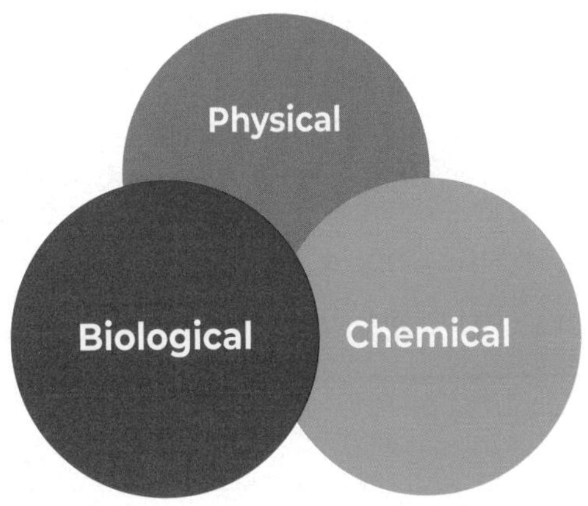

Figure 22.2 SP occupational hazards

GENERAL PHYSICAL HAZARDS

Ergonomic Concerns

General physical hazards include those related to **ergonomics**, slips, falls, electrical, and sharps. Ergonomics is the process of changing work or working conditions to reduce physical stress. SP technicians are exposed to many ergonomic stress factors such as repetitive motion, lifting and pushing.

> **Ergonomics** Process of changing work or working conditions to reduce employee stress.

Ergonomic stressors that employees may encounter include:

- Force – Heavy lifting or manipulating equipment or instrument sets.
- Repetition – Using the same motion, or series of motions, continually or frequently.
- Awkward positions – Assuming positions that place stress on the body such as reaching or twisting while lifting.
- Vibration – Rapid oscillation of the body or a body part.
- Contact stress – Continuous pressure between the body and a sharp edge.

Exposure to these stressors can cause numerous problems, including ligament sprains, joint and tendon inflammation, pinched nerves, herniated spinal discs and other injuries.

Problems, such as carpal tunnel syndrome from typing at a computer station, may develop gradually or from a single event such as from improperly lifting a heavy object. In either case, the injuries may cause pain, loss of work, and disability.

The number and severity of ergonomic injuries can be reduced if the work environment and work practices are adjusted effectively. To be effective, management commitment and employee participation are required. This forms the foundation for ergonomic improvements because a sustained effort, allocation of resources, and frequent follow up is needed. Staff member buy-in of equipment and work procedure changes is especially important.

Training can help employees to:

- Recognize the signs and symptoms of injuries, so they can respond to them
- Report potential problems
- Recognize jobs and tasks that present ergonomic stressors
- Understand how wasted movements can affect the body

Conducting a work site analysis can help identify conditions and aspects of work activities that increase injury risks to employees. A work site analysis also helps ensure that the corrective actions taken address the problems that create the hazard.

In an effort to reduce body stress, including fatigue, discomfort and pain, ergonomic solutions, such as ergonomic equipment, should be evaluated for use in the SPD. The following equipment can reduce factors that cause musculoskeletal disorders:

- Height-adjustable sinks – Move up and down depending on the height of the individual and can improve posture and reduce back strain and injury.
- Anti-fatigue mats – Provide a cushion between the user and hard floor and create micro movements within the leg muscles that aide blood circulation.

Lifts

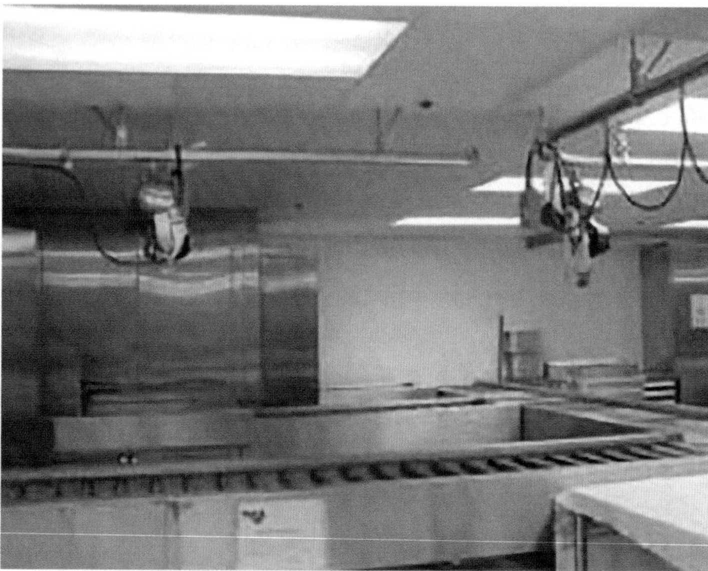

Transport carts

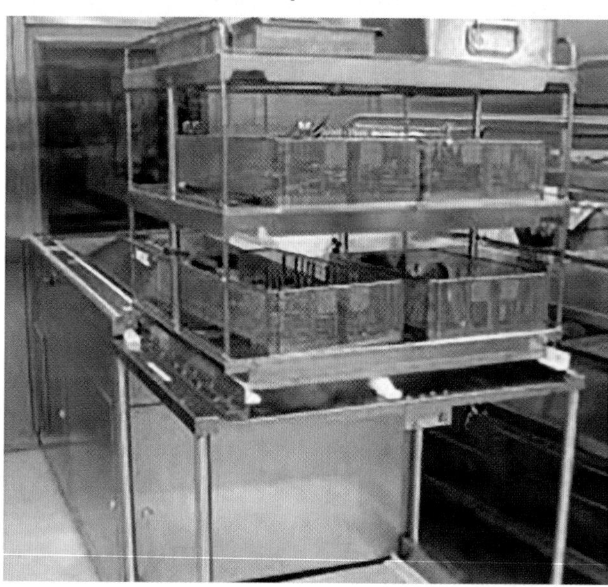

Figure 22.3 Ergonomic safeguards

- Auto-dosing dispensers – Reduce the amount of time and energy needed to move chemical and detergent bottles.
- Auto-loading washer-disinfector racks – Reduce back strain associated with pushing and pulling washer racks.
- Height-adjustable workstations – Move up and down depending on the height of the individual and can improve posture and reduce back strain and injury.
- Adjustable computer monitors – Move up and down or side to side depending on the individual to help improve posture and prevent awkward twisting or back strain.
- Printers and label makers – When located near workstations, these can reduce waste or repetitive movement.
- Utility carts – Can eliminate the need to carry instruments by hand to assembly areas and from the assembly area to the sterilizer cart. These carts can reduce back strain.
- Automated doors – Reduce pushing and pulling actions. Automated doors on cart washers and sterilizers can help reduce back strain associated with pushing and pulling.

*Note: **Figures 22.3** and **22.4** depict overhead lift systems, transport carts and height-adjustable worktables that can be used to reduce the risk for back injuries.*

Simple changes, such as stretching before work, shifting positions, learning and practicing good body mechanics, and breaking up repetitive activities, can help employees reduce the risks of ergonomic injuries. **Figure 22.5** shows proper lifting

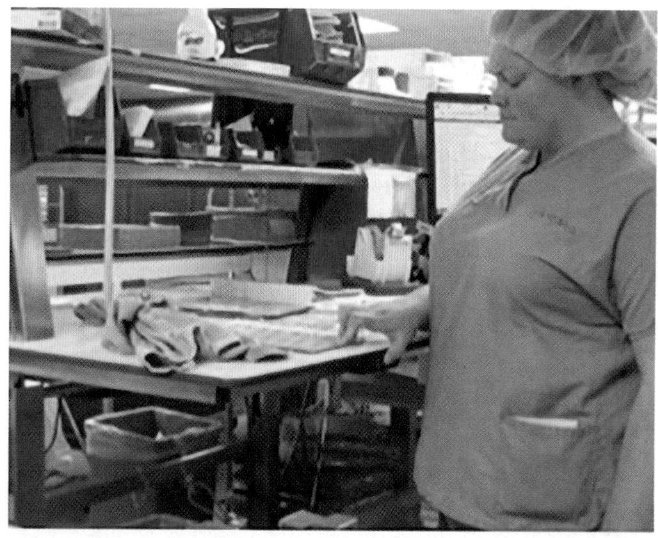

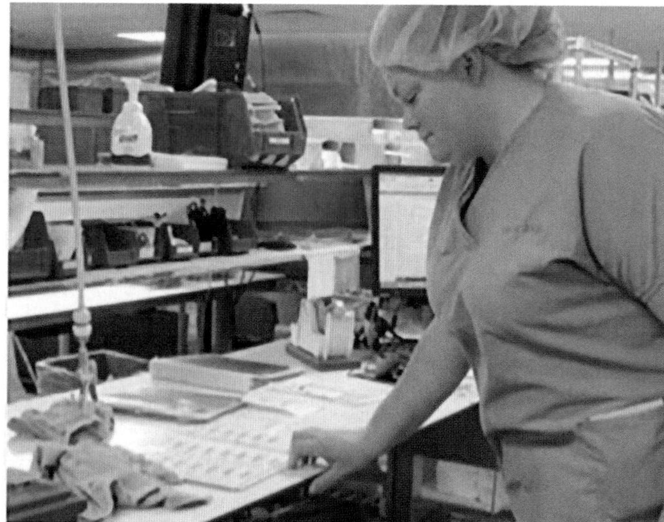

Figure 22.4 An SP technician demonstrates the range of a height-adjustable workstation.

techniques. **Figure 22.6** shows a technician practicing proper body mechanics while lifting a tray.

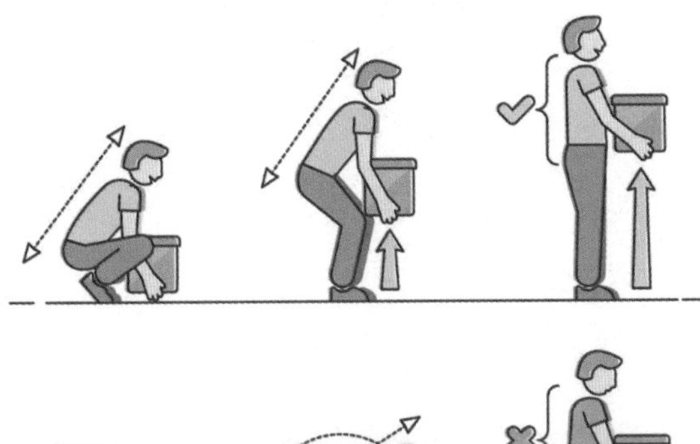

Figure 22.5

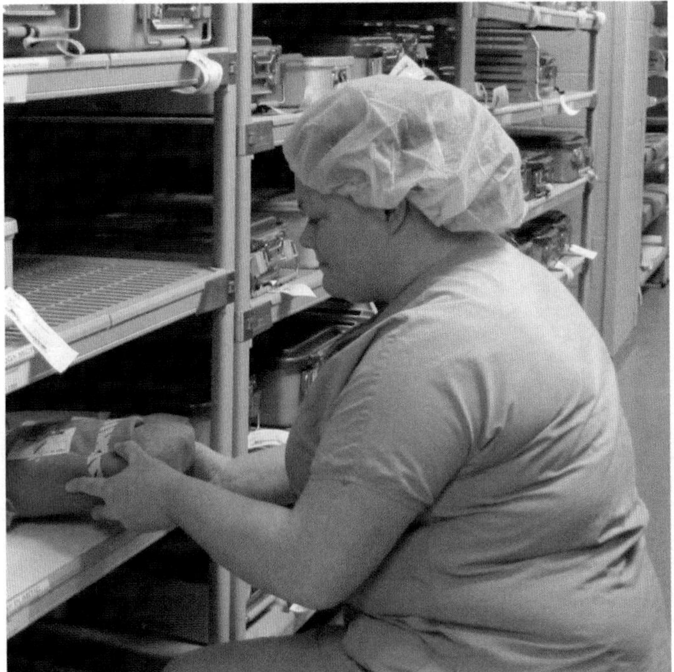

Figure 22.6

Proper lifting and pushing movements can prevent injuries. When loading and unloading carts from dumbwaiters or elevators, or receiving a cart into the department, it is essential to check the cart's weight before attempting to move it. **Figure 22.7** provides an example of a heavy cart that must be handled carefully. Ensuring that the wheels are straight and will roll over door spaces or uneven edges is important, as is unloading some items to lighten the cart if it is too heavy to move easily.

Other ergonomics improvements may include:

- Placing heavier instrumentation on the middle shelf within a storage rack
- Maintaining cart wheels or casters so they roll smoothly and without friction
- Positioning equipment, such as workstations, in a manner that reduces unnecessary movement
- Placing frequently used supplies near workstations

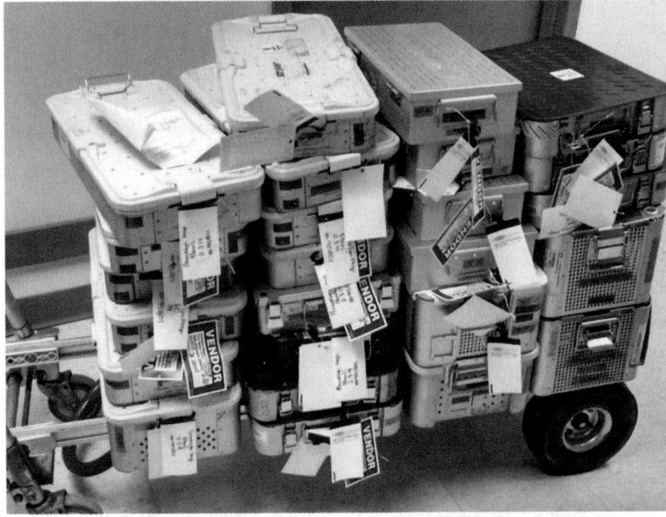

Figure 22.7 Example of a heavy loaned instrument cart

Slip and Fall Concerns

Slips and falls are always a concern in the SPD. Mobile equipment and wet floors increase fall risks. To reduce these risks, mobile equipment should be parked away from common traffic areas. Areas that often have wet floors, such as in the decontamination area, around the cart wash exits, and washer unload areas, must be kept as dry as possible, and spills should be wiped immediately. Non-slip footwear should be worn, and attention should be given to slippery floors. Signage, such as the wet floor sign pictured in **Figure 22.8**, alerts people to potential hazards.

Figure 22.8

Electrical Safety Concerns

Burns and shocks from electric equipment can result if safe handling precautions are not observed.

Technicians should carefully check all electrical cords to ensure they are intact, with no breaks in the insulation. Electrical cords on mobile equipment run a greater risk of being kinked or run over by a rolling cart, which can make the equipment unsafe. All plugs on electrical equipment must be three-pronged and grounded, and all electrical outlets must accommodate these plugs. Inspecting electrical cords for breaks and plugs for bent prongs is a responsibility of SP technicians. (See **Figure 22.9**) Identifying and reporting a potential hazard during cleaning or delivery can prevent injuries to patients and staff. Any new equipment brought into the facility should be tested for electrical safety, either by Facilities Engineering or the Biomedical (Biomed) Engineering department. Be sure to review the facility's policies and procedures for details.

Insulation leakage testing equipment, or voltmeters, are designed to use an electrical charge to identify nicks, tears or breaks in insulated instrumentation. Leakage or voltage testing devices are most commonly used on laparoscopic instrumentation. SP technicians can receive an electrical shock if the device is not properly grounded, or when contacting an active electrode. SP technicians should receive training followed by competencies prior to using these devices.

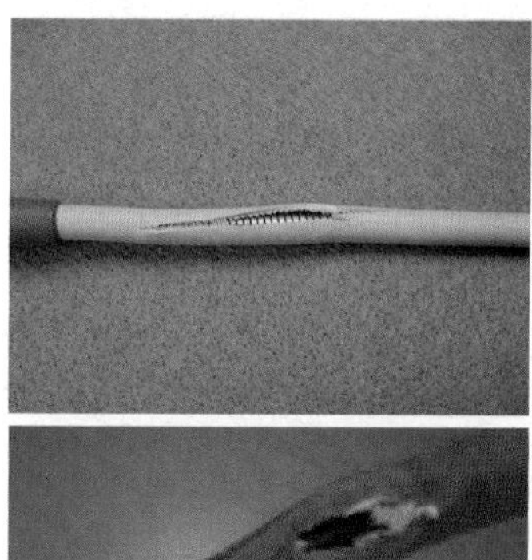

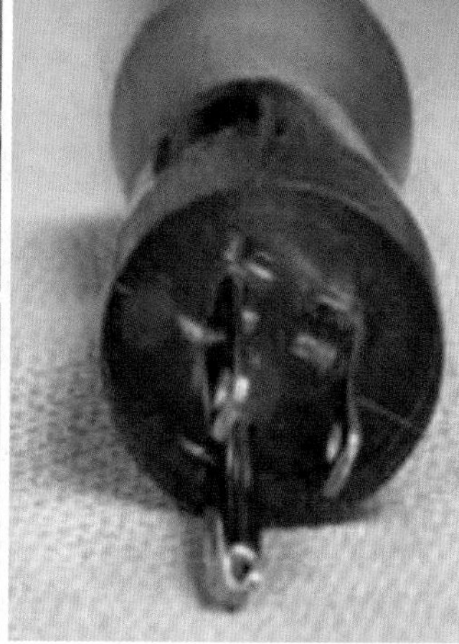

22.9 Check cords for damage.

Use Caution with Electrical Equipment

All electrical equipment can pose a hazard if it is used in an unsafe manner. For example, radios placed near water sources, such as sinks and ultrasonic cleaners, can lead to staff injury in that work area. Keep the work area safe from electrical hazards.

Sharps Concerns

Cuts and puncture injuries from sharps can happen in any area of the SPD. Sharp instruments can break the skin's surface and produce puncture wounds, lacerations and abrasions. If the injury occurs in the decontamination area, these injuries may result in exposure to disease.

Some general precautions to prevent sharps injuries include:

- Handling all sharps with care
- Not grasping several objects at once
- Ensuring that sharp ends point away from any part of one's body during transport
- Placing all disposable sharps, such as needles and blades, in the appropriate sharps container (see **Figure 22.10**)
- Not blindly reaching into an instrument tray. Sharps may be hidden and cause an injury

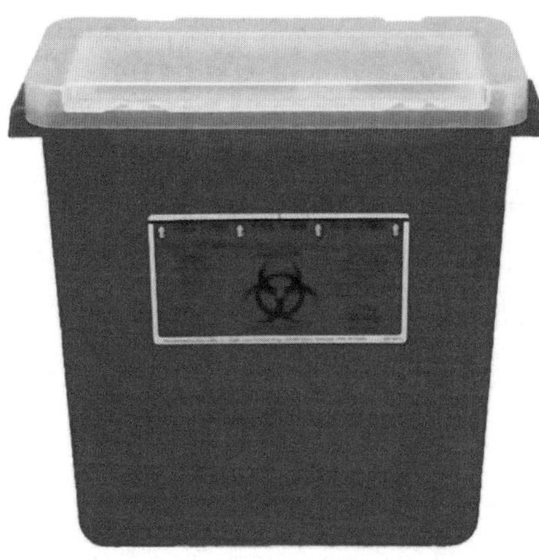

Figure 22.10 Sharps containers help prevent injury.

Sharps injuries can happen to anyone at any time. If a sharps injury occurs, it is important to promptly notify SP leadership and follow the healthcare facility's procedures, which may include following up with the facility's occupational health department.

General Chemical Hazards

Most chemicals used in the SPD are found in the decontamination area, although chemical hazards may be found in other areas of the department as well.

SP technicians must have basic training and an understanding of how and why each chemical is used in the SPD. They must understand how to handle the chemicals and any special precautions required such as PPE. Training should also include procedures for chemical removal and disposal. Not all chemicals

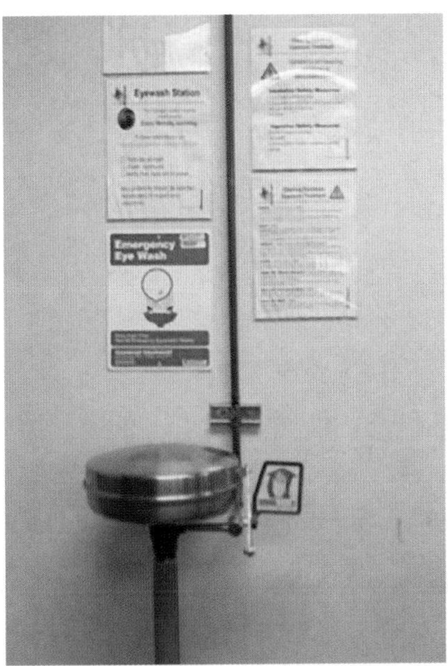

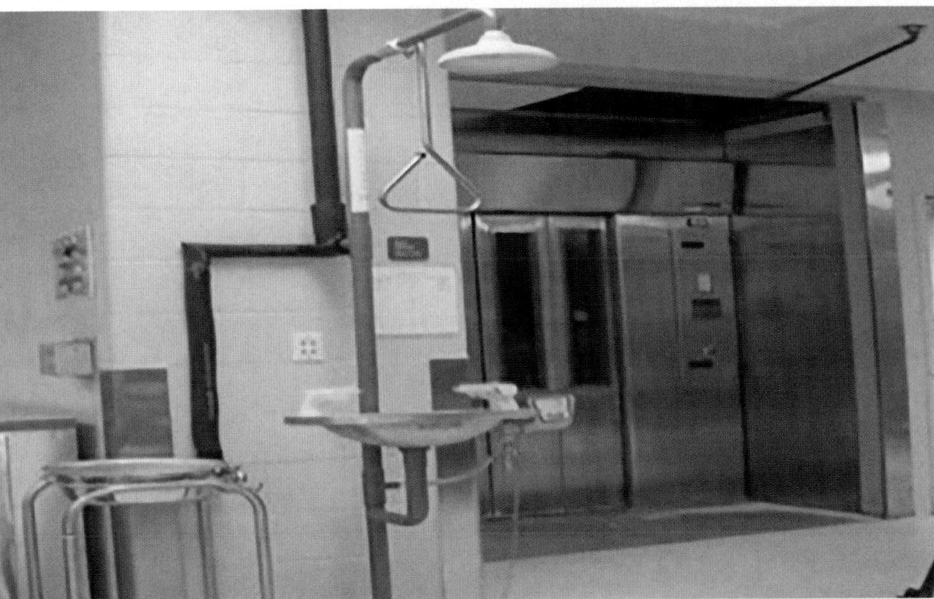

Figure 22.11 Emergency eyewash and shower stations

used in the SPD can be disposed of by simply pouring the chemical down the drain. Some chemicals require deactivation and dilution. Competencies should follow any training performed and should also incorporate procedures for addressing accidental spills. Spill kits assist with chemical cleanup and should be compatible with each chemical found in the department; they should cover worst-case scenarios and be readily available.

Chemical splashes are a common cause of eye injuries, so the use of eye protection is required. Eyewash stations are also required in areas where chemical injuries are a concern. (See **Figure 22.11**)

Hazardous Substance Concerns

Each state categorizes certain chemicals and substances as hazardous. Each SPD should have an easily accessible, understandable and current list of all hazardous substances with which employees could come in contact. This list should always be available to employees and not locked away or stored in an office. Most facilities today have a comprehensive computerized hazardous chemical list.

If employees are required to perform known hazardous tasks, it is important that they understand the safety procedures developed for that task. Prior to performing such tasks, employees must be given information about the hazards to which they may be exposed. This information should include identification of specific hazards, use of PPE, recommended safety measures, and emergency response procedures. Employers should take measures to minimize employee hazards. These could include increased area ventilation, respirators, the presence of other employees to assist, and the rehearsal of emergency procedures.

SP managers must develop a hazardous materials management program to help ensure the health and safety of employees, as required by state and federal regulations. Information about hazardous chemicals and substances must be available to all employees.

OSHA's "Employee Right to Know" regulations mandate that a comprehensive hazard communication program be in place to help ensure that employees know about the hazards around them. Components of an effective departmental hazardous substance management program include container labeling requirements, use of safety data sheets (SDS), employee information and training, procedures to manage and handle hazardous substances, employee monitoring, and **hazardous waste** management.

Hazardous waste Substances that cannot be disposed of in the facility's normal trash system.

Container Labeling

All containers with hazardous substances must be clearly labeled to specify contents and appropriate hazard warnings, and they must indicate the name and address of the manufacturer. All **secondary containers** must be labeled with an extra copy of the original manufacturer's label or with a generic label that identifies the chemical, hazard warnings, and directions.

Secondary container A generic container that is filled from a primary container or filled with a diluted solution. Secondary containers must be clearly labeled with content.

Safety Data Sheets

An SDS contains important information about product materials and properties that employees must know to work safely with any given product. SDS are developed and provided by the manufacturer of the product, and they are specific for each product. SDS contain at least 16 sections. The following is a list of the sections as they appear in the SDS:

- Section 1: Identification – Product name, manufacturer's name, address, telephone number, product item number (manufacturer's identification) and synonym names
- Section 2: Hazards(s) Identification – List of hazardous ingredients
- Section 3: Composition – Information about the ingredients contained in the product
- Section 4: First-Aid Measures – Emergency and first aid, including routes of exposure, symptoms and effects of exposure (See **Figure 22.12**)

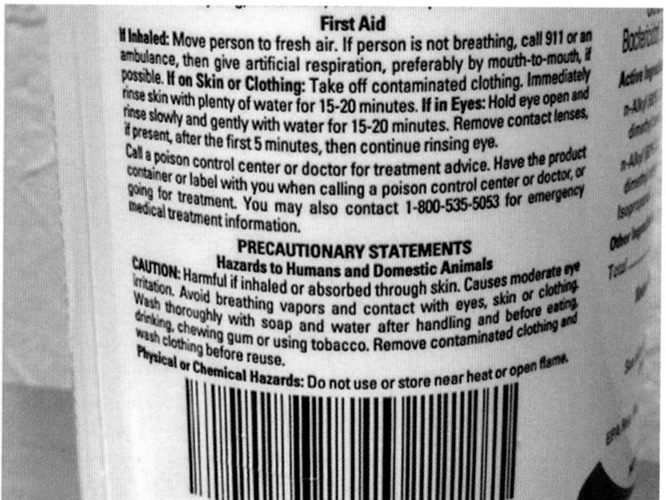

Figure 22.12 Container labels must include hazard warnings.

- Section 5: Fire-Fighting Measures – Fire and explosion information, flash point, flammable units, extinguishing media, special firefighting procedures, and unusual fire and explosion hazards
- Section 6: Accidental Release Measures – Spill or leak procedures, spill management and waste disposal methods
- Section 7: Handling and Storage – Storage recommendations, incompatible materials, and storage temperatures
- Section 8: Exposure Controls and Personal Protection Measures – Exposure limits, engineering controls and personal protective measures to minimize technician exposure
- Section 9: Physical and Chemical Properties – Data, vapor pressure, evaporation rate, water solubility, freezing and boiling points, specific gravity, acidity (pH), vapor density, appearance and odor
- Section 10: Stability and Reactivity – Reactivity data, stability, incompatibility, hazardous decomposition products, and conditions contributing to hazardous **polymerization**

> **Polymerization** A molecular reaction that creates an uncontrolled release of energy.

- Section 11: Toxicology Information – Health hazard data and effects of over exposure
- Section 12: Ecological Information – Provides information regarding environmental impact
- Section 13: Disposal Considerations – Provides guidance on proper disposal practices, including container use and disposal methods
- Section 14: Transportation Information – Information for shipping and transporting of the hazardous material.
- Section 15: Regulatory Information – Identifies safety, health and environmental regulations not found in other sections
- Section 16: Other Information – Indicates when the SDS was last prepared or when the known revision was made, along with other useful information

The employer is responsible for ensuring that SDS are readily available to employees who may work with or be in the vicinity of hazardous materials. (See **Figure 22.13**) In turn, employees are responsible for becoming familiar with the SDS information and consistently following the instructions given for the products they handle and use.

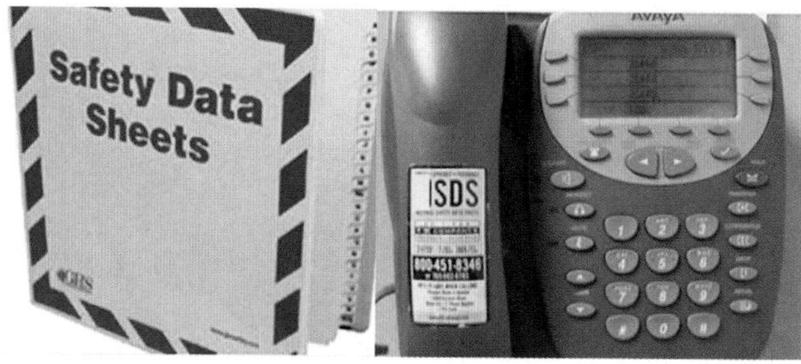

Figure 22.13 Safety data sheet information must be available to all employees.

Employee Monitoring

To prevent potential health hazards to workers, OSHA has established permissible exposure limits (PELs) for many chemicals used in sterilant and disinfectant formulations. These include ethylene oxide (EO), hydrogen peroxide (H_2O_2), and others.

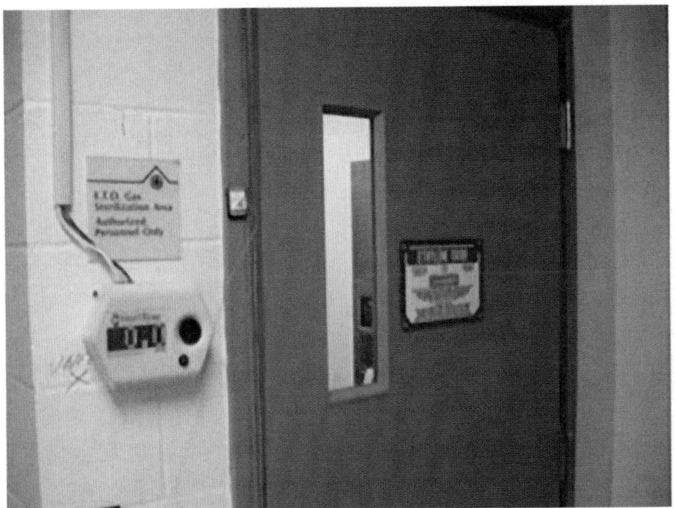

Figure 22.14 Example of a mechanical monitoring system

Glutaraldehyde is a chemical commonly used as a high-level disinfectant in the SPD. The National Institute for Occupational Safety and Health (NIOSH) recommends that exposure to glutaraldehyde be under 0.2 parts per million (ppm) time-weighted average (TWA) over an eight-hour work shift. The American Conference of Governmental Industrial Hygienists (ACGIH) recommends a ceiling value of 0.05 ppm, which should not be exceeded at any time.

Healthcare facilities are required by OSHA to:

- Provide adequate ventilation systems
- Establish safe work operating procedures
- Provide PPE
- Implement other methods to ensure that occupational exposure limits are not exceeded in the workplace

Mechanical monitoring systems can aid in the detection of chemicals present in the work area. These systems can detect the presence of chemicals at levels far below the level an employee would be able to detect by smell. (See **Figure 22.14**)

Personal monitors that measure individual exposure to chemical vapors by measuring the presence of specific chemicals in the employee's breathing zone are also available. (See **Figure 22.15**)

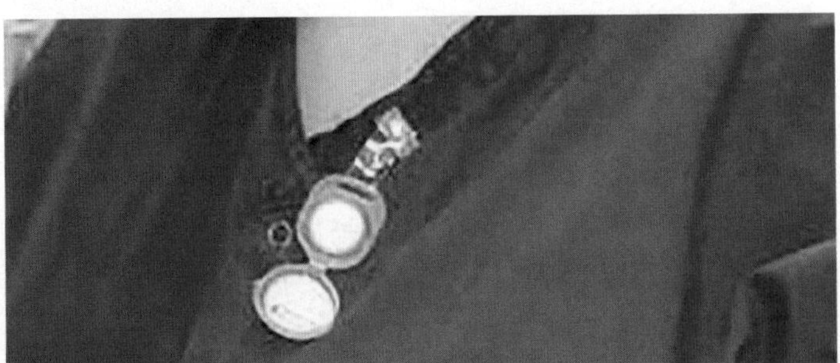

Figure 22.15

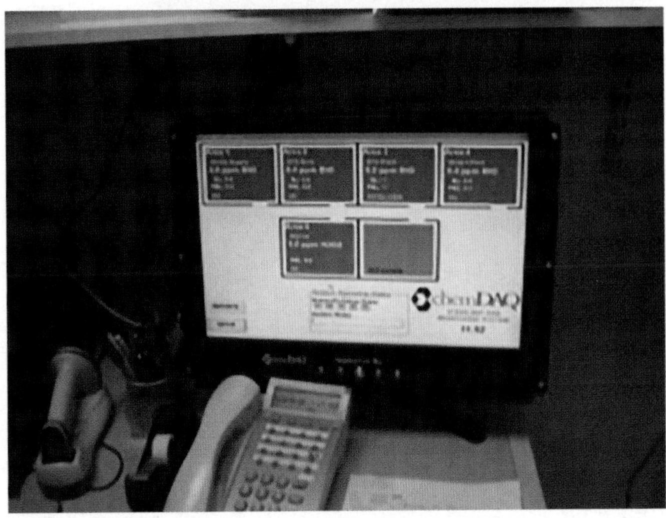

Fire Hazards

Fire requires three elements to be present at the same time; these elements make up what is known as the "fire triangle":

- A **combustible** or flammable substance
- A source of oxygen
- A source of ignition

To prevent fires, at least one of the elements in the triangle must be eliminated. (See **Figure 22.16**)

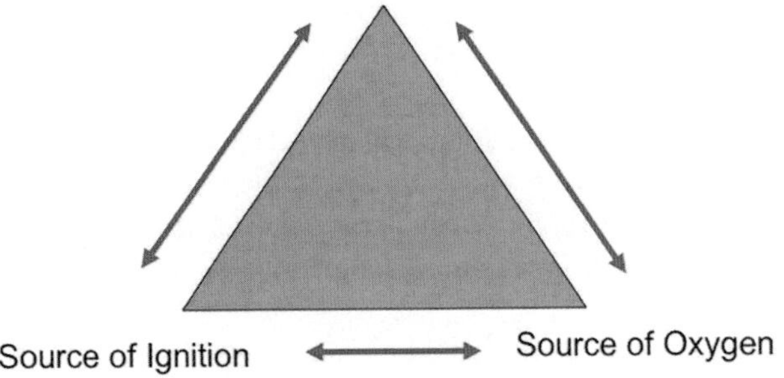

Figure 22.16 Fire triangle

Fire and Explosions

A fire occurs when the temperature of a flammable or combustible substance is raised high enough for the individual carbon and hydrogen atoms to combine with oxygen, and the resulting energy is released. If the material is a solid, it will burn only at its surface. In contrast, if the material is a volatile liquid, such as alcohol, which readily vaporizes, or a gas, such as EO, the flame front passes quickly through the substance. The result is an explosion accompanied by the instantaneous generation of large quantities of heated gases. Their rapid expansion creates a very loud pressure wave that can cause significant damage.

Combustible A substance that, if ignited, will react with oxygen and burn.

Combustible loading is the weight of combustible materials per square foot of area where the materials are located. The presence of large volumes of combustible materials and flammable substances poses unique risks. Large combustible loading created by single-use items and their wrappings in storage, and as trash, is especially dangerous. When these materials burn, large quantities of highly toxic smoke are produced. Even with hospital compartmentalization features that limit the spread of smoke and fire, a high-risk situation occurs; therefore, healthcare fire safety programs must include:

- Minimization of the combustible load
- Fire response plans
- Early detection
- Containment of the fire and combustible products
- Extinguishment
- Evacuation plans

Combustible Loads

It is important to minimize the volume of combustible substances because a prime rule of fire protection is: "Don't give fire a place to start."

Strategies to minimize combustible loads include:

- Ensuring that single-use items are safely stored by keeping them in areas with proper temperature and humidity.
- Minimizing trash buildup. Each facility must have an adequate trash handling program that includes covered trash containers of noncombustible construction and adequate volume at each site of trash generation.

Fire Response Plan

Every healthcare facility requires a comprehensive fire response plan, and all staff members in every department must know their specific role in these plans. The fire safety emphasis should begin at the time of new employee orientation and should continue with ongoing training.

Every healthcare facility is required to have and maintain sprinkler systems, smoke detectors, fire extinguishers, and audible alarms to warn and protect staff and patients. (See **Figure 22.17**) These devices must remain unobstructed.

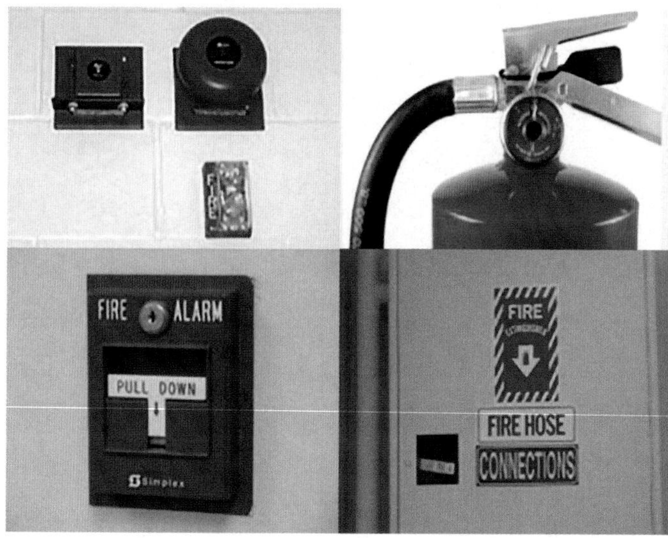

Figure 22.17 Examples of fire safety devices

Each SP technician must participate in their facility's fire training and become aware of the fire safety items within their work area. Carefully following the facility's fire plan is important for staff and patient safety. When a fire emergency occurs, everyone must understand their role and act quickly. Training may include:

- Location of nearby fire pull stations
- Location of nearby fire extinguishers
- All exit routes from the SPD to a safe designated location
- Fire emergency response (RACE)
  - › **R**escue or Remove – Any patients, guests or staff needing assistance must be evacuated per the facility's emergency evacuation plan.
  - › **A**lert or Alarm – Activate the fire pull station, call 911 and any internal emergency services.
  - › **C**onfine or Contain – Once everyone is removed from the area, close off or contain the fire as much as possible by closing doors.
  - › **E**xtinguish or Evacuate – Using the fire extinguisher, attempt to put out the fire (use the PASS method—Pull, Aim, Squeeze and Sweep) if comfortable performing the procedure. If the fire requires more than one fire extinguisher, evacuate to a safe designated location.

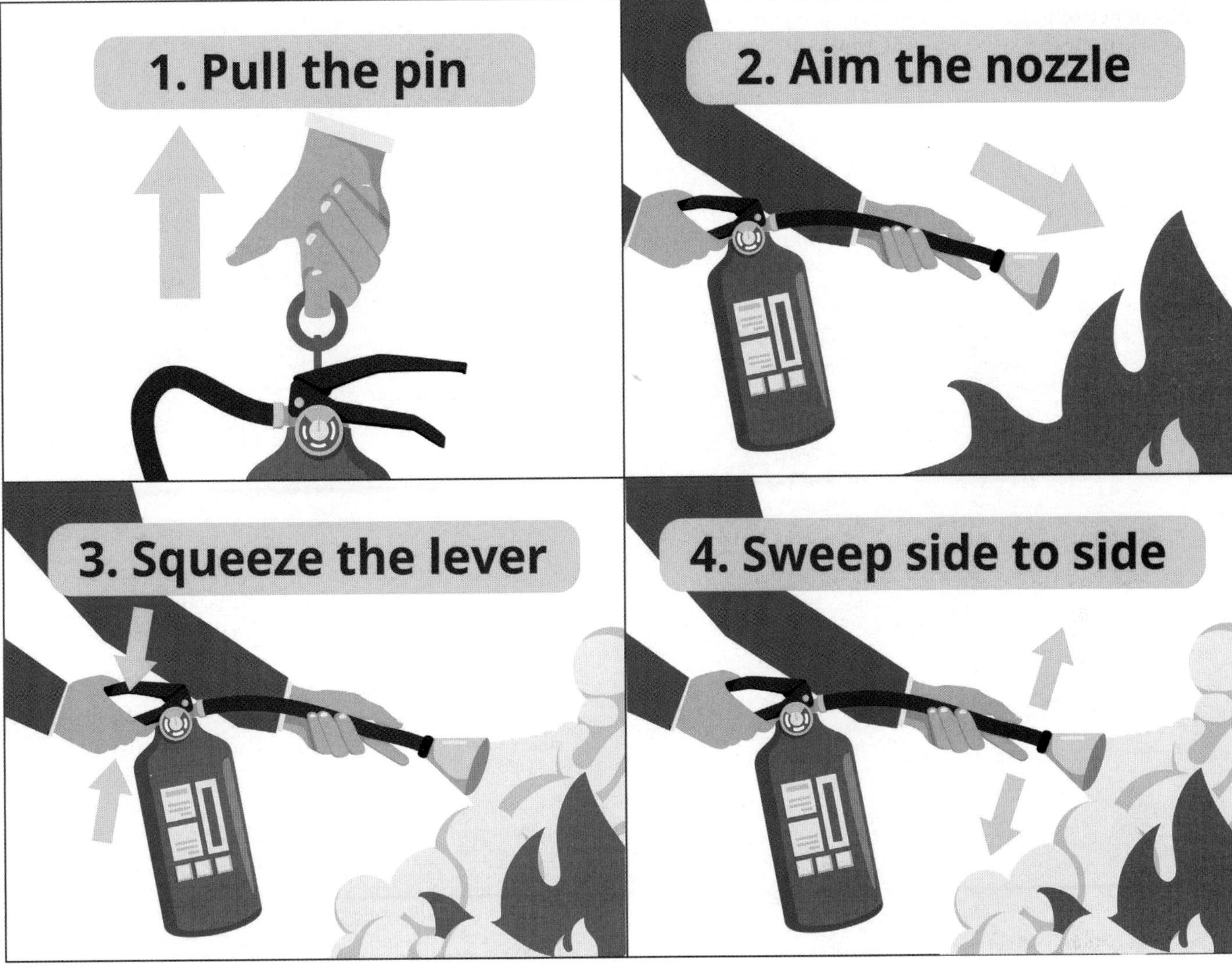

Figure 22.18

- How to use a fire extinguisher using the PASS method (see **Figure 22.18)**
  - **P**ull the pin of the extinguisher
  - **A**im the extinguisher at the base of the fire
  - **S**queeze the extinguisher to activate
  - **S**weep the extinguisher side to side at the base of the fire

Workplace Violence

According to OSHA, approximately two million people fall victim to **workplace violence** each year. All employees should pay attention to possible warning signs and they should:

> **Workplace violence** Any act or threat of physical violence, harassment, intimidation or other threatening or disruptive behavior that occurs at the work site.

- Immediately report to management any direct threats of violence or retaliation.
- Note behavior, statements or attitudes that are unusual, threatening or disconcerting.

Employees should be aware of their facility's specific policies on workplace violence and attend education programs that provide information on prevention and response (i.e., active shooter training). An active shooter is an individual actively engaged in killing or attempting to kill people in a confined and populated area; in most cases, active shooters use firearms(s) and there is no pattern or method to their selection of victims. Facility training should include how to respond when an active shooter is in the vicinity. These steps include:

1. Evacuate – If there is an accessible escape path, attempt to evacuate the premises.
2. Hide – If evacuation is not possible, employees should find a place to hide where the active shooter is less likely to find them.

3. Take action against the active shooter – As a last resort, and only when one's life is in imminent danger, attempt to disrupt and/or incapacitate the active shooter.

AREA-SPECIFIC SAFETY CONCERNS

Some safety concerns are common in specific work areas within the SPD, and it is important that all employees are made aware of those concerns and hazards. **Figure 22.19** shows a sign notifying personnel about the need for PPE in the decontamination area.

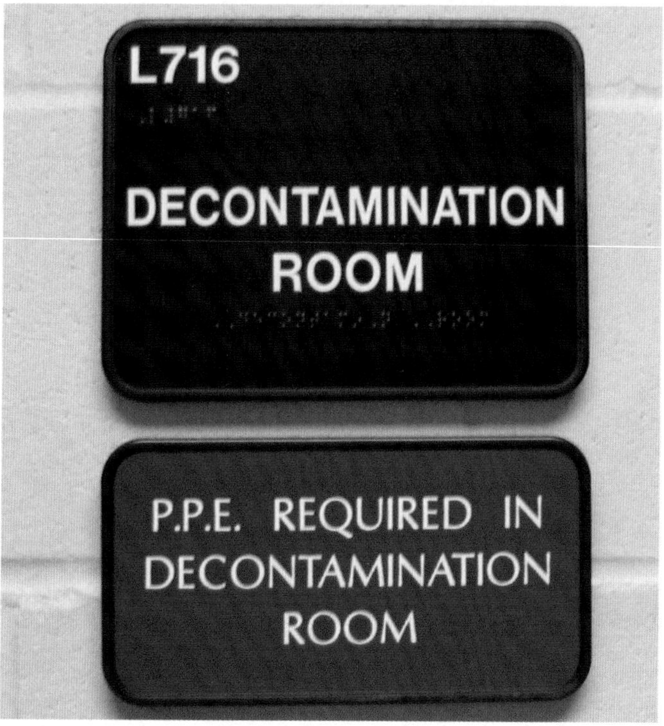

Figure 22.19

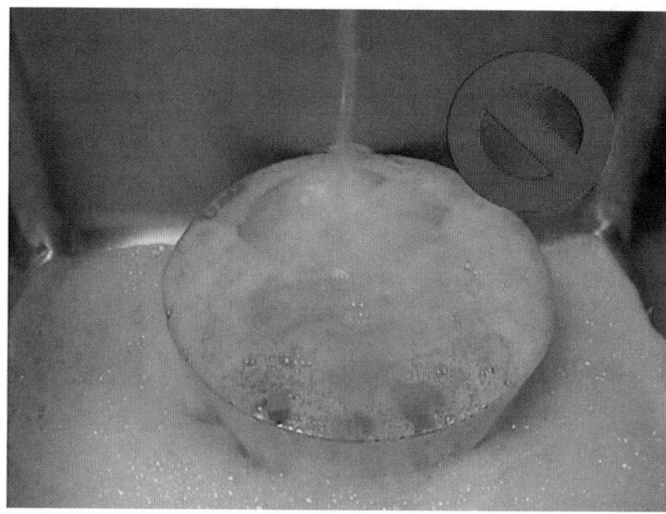

Figure 22.20 Foaming detergents can conceal sharp objects and increase the risk of injury.

Soiled Receiving and Decontamination Areas

Safety tips when working in soiled receiving and decontamination areas include:

- Never reaching into a basin or container that houses contaminated objects unless the objects in the basin are clearly visible. Instead, use a sponge forceps to grasp the object or pour out any solution that prohibits visual examination, and then remove objects from basins or containers one at a time. Never use foaming detergents when handling contaminated instruments in the decontamination sink, as the foam can prevent visualization of sharp objects. (See **Figure 22.20**)
- Never reaching into trash containers or sharp containers.
- Never removing scalpel blades in the SPD area. If a blade is found in the decontamination area, do not attempt to remove the blade without proper training.
- When processing reusable sharps technicians should separate them from other instruments and position them in a manner that protects anyone who may handle them.
- Following the manufacturer's recommendations for safe use of chemicals. Always wear recommended PPE to protect skin surfaces and mucous membranes from chemical burns.
- Following the manufacturer's recommendations for safe operation of cleaning and testing equipment.
- Using caution when walking and inspecting the floor for slippery surfaces. Utilize mats and non-skid footwear. (See **Figure 22.21**) If fluid is on the floor, it should be cleaned immediately.

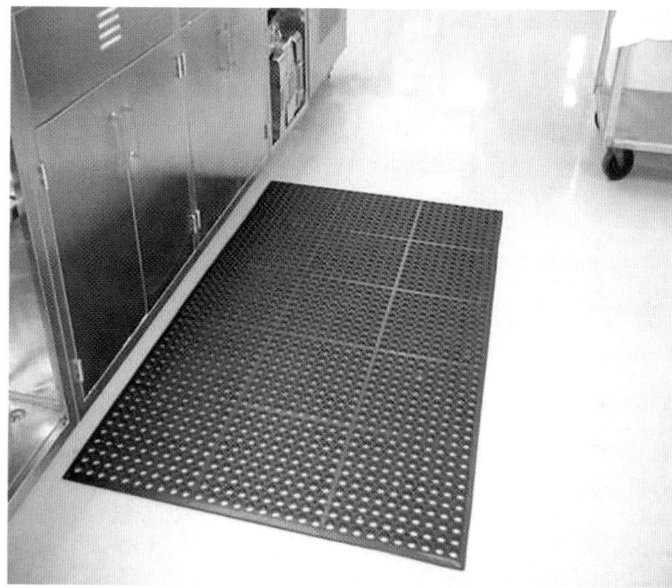

Figure 22.21

- When cleaning instruments in a sink, always scrub below the surface of the water to avoid the formation of **aerosols.** (See **Figure 22.22**)

Keeping sinks and other working surfaces at proper levels that provide easy access that reduces the risk for splashes and aerosolization as well as back and arm strain.

Aerosol A suspension of ultramicroscopic soiled or liquid particles in air or gas; a spray.

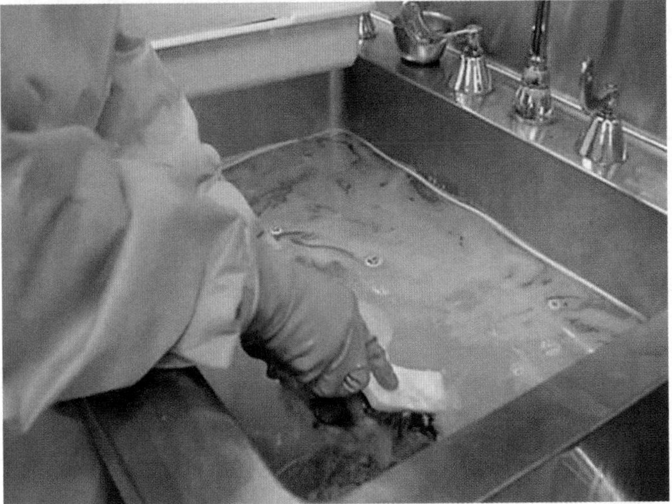

Figure 22.22

Preparation and Sterilization Areas

Safety tips when working in the SPD's preparation and sterilization areas include:

- Moving sterilizer carts to low- or no-traffic areas and other designated areas so that co-workers will be less likely to come in contact with hot carts (See **Figure 22.23**)

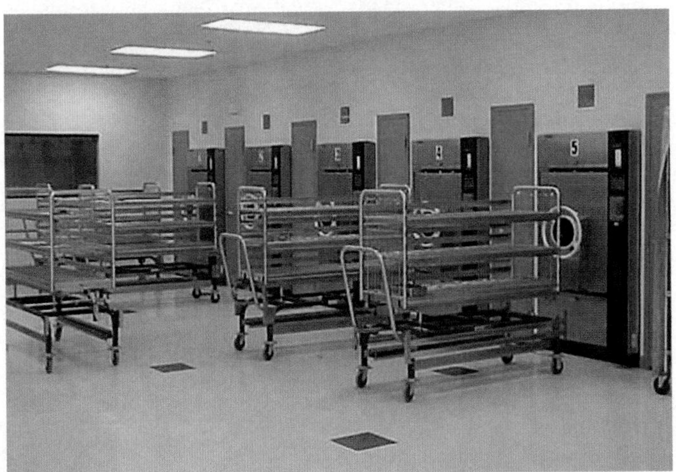

Figure 22.23

- Using thermal insulated gloves when handling steam sterilizer carts, washer baskets and other objects subjected to high temperatures. Hot sterilization carts, sterilizer doors and washer baskets can leave serious burns if not handled properly. (See **Figure 22.24**)

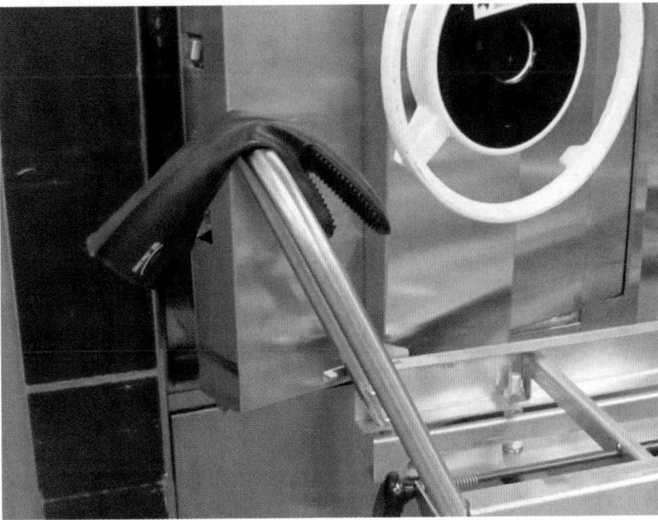

Figure 22.24

- Keeping sterilizer doors closed when not loading or unloading the chamber to protect co-workers from coming in contact with the hot inner door (See **Figure 22.25**)

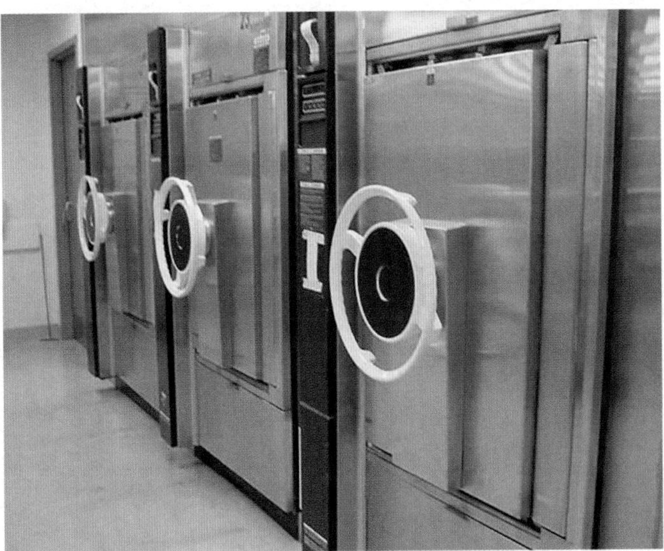

Figure 22.25

- Using caution when operating heat sealers. Keep away from heated components and be sure to follow the manufacturer's instructions.

- Being cautious when using a cutting edge to prepare paper/plastic peel packs

- Using caution when testing instruments for sharpness

- When lifting instrument sets, use the larger muscles in legs and arms. Hold the item as close to the body as possible, without touching the body.
- Following procedures for using and disposing of biological indicators
- Ensuring that proper signs and labels are posted to warn of hot surfaces or other hazards

Sterilization area

- Steam sterilizers – Use caution to avoid burns when working with steam sterilizers.
- H_2O_2 sterilizer safety – Use caution when handling H_2O_2 containers; damaged containers may release sterilant into the work area. Items in an aborted cycle may contain trace amount of H_2O_2 ,which can cause a chemical burn to unprotected hands and skin. Careful disposal of wrappers, peel packs and indicators should be performed with gloved hands.
- EO sterilizer safety – EO has been strongly regulated by the federal government for many years. In 1984, OSHA established a 1 ppm (in air) PEL, and a 0.5 ppm **action level (AL)** for EO. The PEL and AL limits are expressed as an eight-hour time weighted average (TWA). They represent the total allowable worker exposure during an eight-hour period and express it as an average exposure during the period.
- OSHA amended its rule on occupational exposure to EO by adding a 5 ppm **short-term exposure limit (STEL)** over a 15-minute period. The STEL is typically related to tasks such as performing sterilizer maintenance.

Action level (AL) Level of exposure to a harmful substance or other hazard at which an employer must take required precautions to protect the workers. It is typically one-half the permissible exposure limit (PEL).

Short-term exposure limit (STEL) Maximum concentration of a chemical to which workers may be exposed continuously for up to 15 minutes without danger to health or work efficiency and safety.

Sterilizer manufacturers now include many safety features on their EO sterilizers. These include negative-pressure airflow to help prevent exposures in the event the unit malfunctions during the cycle, and automatic mechanisms keep the sterilizer locked down until the aeration cycle is completed.

Safety precautions when working with EO equipment include:

- EO sterilization should be performed in a separate area, away from other department work areas.
- Healthcare facilities using EO must have an operational, dedicated ventilation system to remove fumes exhausted during the cycle. This exhaust system should be checked regularly to ensure that any fumes in the employees' breathing zone are captured. It is also necessary to have an audible and visual alarm that will sound in case of a malfunction.
- EO canisters should be stored in an approved containment locker. Check local regulations for the maximum amount of canisters allowed in the area. (See **Figure 22.26**)

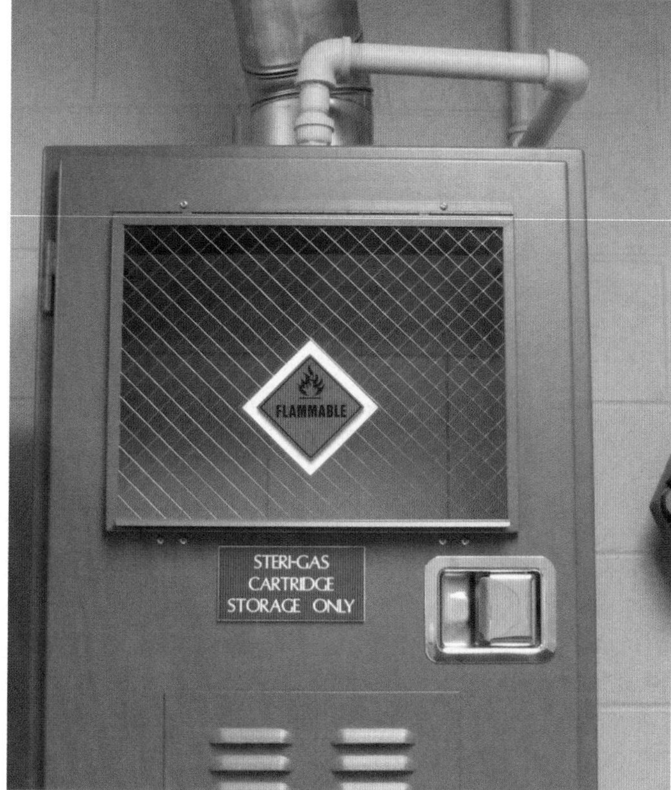

Figure 22.26

- Technicians must comply with all federal, state and local air quality and worker safety regulations relating to employee safety, discharge, air monitoring, and recordkeeping.
- The exposure of any person to EO must be reported immediately to the SP manager, employee health nurse or employee health service, and the Emergency Department. Employees must understand that several harmful effects can be contributed directly to EO. Exposure to EO can cause eye pain, sore throat, breathing difficulties, and blurred vision. Exposure can also cause, dizziness, nausea, vomiting, headache, convulsions, blisters and coughing. Both human and animal studies show that EO is a carcinogen that may cause leukemia and other cancers. EO is also linked to spontaneous abortion, genetic damage, nerve damage, peripheral paralysis, muscle weakness as well as impaired thinking and memory. In liquid form, EO can cause severe skin irritation upon prolonged or confined contact.

Supply Receiving, Break Out and Storage Areas

To ensure a safe and efficient supply receiving area, adequate storage space and traffic access must be available. Supply storage and shelving units must be secure and steady. Shelves should be arranged to facilitate maximum space efficiency and allow employees easy access to supplies. Heavy materials and items used most frequently should be placed on middle shelves to allow employees to easily and safely accessed them. Lighter, infrequently used items should be placed on higher shelves.

Employees should use appropriate equipment (e.g., steps, stands and ladders) to safely reach upper shelves. Climbing on shelves is not acceptable. Procedures for the safe operation of dollies, hand trucks or carts to handle bulk materials must be available, and employees must be trained to consistently comply with them. (See **Figure 22.27**)

Closed trash containers should be available to properly dispose of unwanted materials. Containers for the appropriate storage of hazardous or flammable materials must be readily available to avoid hazardous chemical exposure. Employees working in this area must also follow proper procedures when disposing of and removing hazardous materials. The SDS must be available for reference wherever these substances are used.

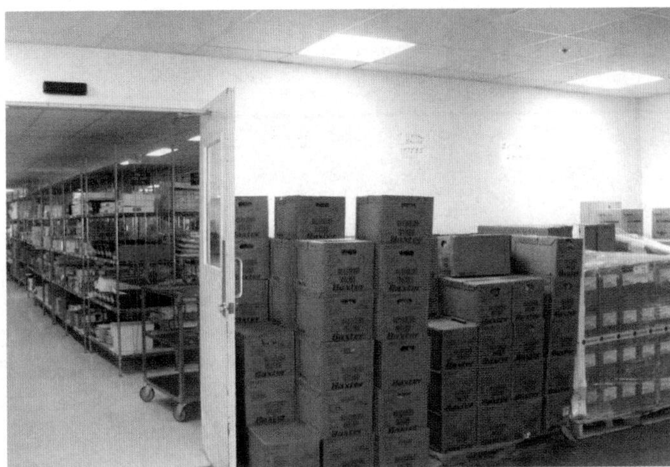

Figure 22.27

Safety tips for supply receiving, break out and storage include:

- Using caution when removing items from storage units or shelves. Allow time to perform the tasks and ensure adequate space is available to maneuver the items being received.
- Always cutting away from the body or to the side whenever a box-cutting tool is used. Retract the blade into the handle or cover the blade with a sheath when the device is not in use. Scalpels should not be used as a box-cutting tool.
- Avoiding twisting and jerking movements when picking up or removing objects from tight spaces.
- Inspecting work areas for objects left in pathways, or for equipment with parts that protrude into a traffic path. Aisles and doorways must always remain clear.
- Performing appropriate stretching exercises prior to work to avoid injuries to the back and other bodily areas affected by lifting, pushing and pulling.
- Using transport carts, when possible, to minimize lifting and carrying.

Equipment Storage and Transportation

Areas where supplies and equipment are stored while awaiting requests from patient care areas can also be dangerous. These areas can have substantial activity and often have limited space to move about freely. Many types of patient care equipment require electrical charging, so multiple electrical outlets must be available. (See **Figure 22.28**) All portable electrical equipment, including items used in the SPD and patient care areas, must comply with applicable electrical codes.

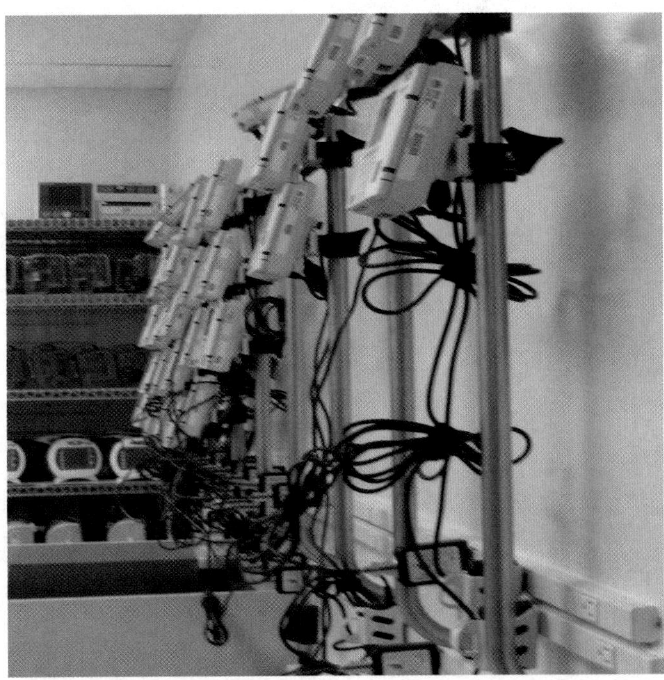

Figure 22.28

Adequate storage space should be provided, and shelving should be of adequate capacity and strength. Sturdy, easily controlled carts should be provided for transferring items.

Transporting supplies and equipment through the facility can pose several safety concerns. SP technicians must be aware of their surroundings and take extra care to help ensure they keep themselves and those around them safe as they perform their duties. Food service and patient transportation devices, such as gurneys and wheelchairs, may be in use in patient care areas. There may be corners and elevators that present hazards if proper techniques are not used by employees when transporting patients and other items.

Safety tips include:

- Avoiding excessive speed. Be prepared to stop quickly if a person steps into the hallway from a doorway. Always yield to patients.
- Using caution when approaching doorways, hallways, elevators and high-traffic areas.
- Not using a transport vehicle to push or prop open automatic doors.
- Not parking carts and mobile equipment in hallways where they may block traffic or door access. Always keep hallways clear for the free flow of traffic. (See **Figure 22.29**)

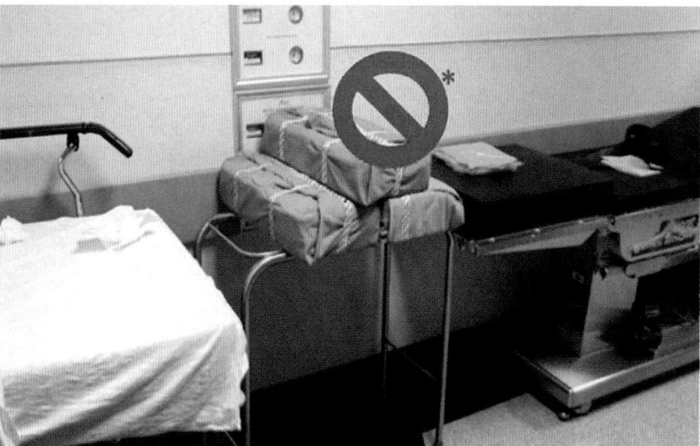

Figure 22.29 Never block hallways or access panels with carts. Never stack wrapped instrument trays.

- When transporting carts or equipment, ensuring that the path in front and on each side of the transport equipment is visible.
- Inspecting floors for uneven surfaces or defective tiles or edges to ensure that equipment being transported will not be thrown off balance.
- Using caution when approaching corners or intersections of hallways. Use safety mirrors whenever available.
- Using caution when pushing objects up or down hallway inclines. Push from behind when going up an incline (object goes before the person) and pull from in front of an object being transported down an incline (person goes before the object).
- Not riding or stepping on wheeled supply carts or other vehicles.
- Considering the use of powered carts, if available, for moving heavy or awkward loads. (See **Figure 22.30**)

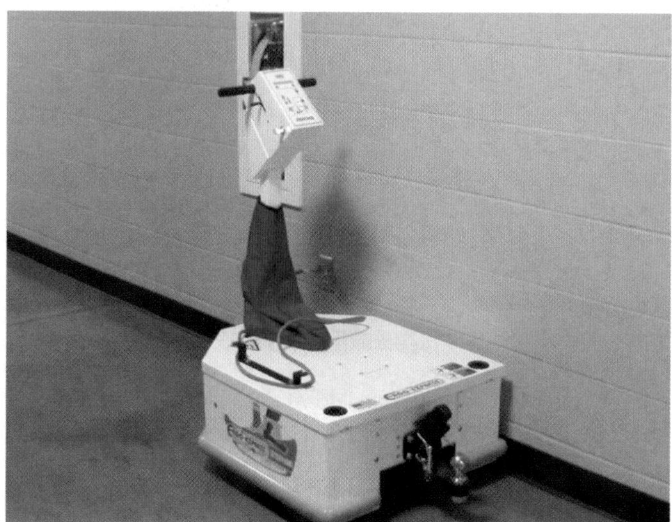

Figure 22.30

Clerical and Other Workstations

Poor workstation design can create issues for SP personnel. Repetitive activities, such as bending over sinks, sitting at a computer desk and standing while assembling instrument sets, should be evaluated in an effort to reduce unnecessary stress and strain. **Figure 22.31** shows an SP clerical workstation.

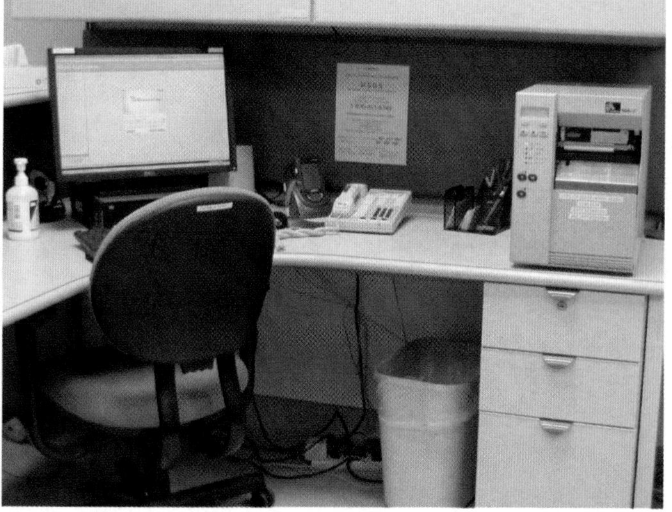

Figure 22.31

Safety tips in clerical and other workstations include:

- Ensuring the assembly work will be performed at levels that will lessen employee fatigue and strain.
- Ensuring that floors in work areas where employees must stand have fatigue mats to relieve leg strain.
- Providing appropriate chairs for computer and clerical workstations that properly support employees' backs.

- Ensuring that items are frequently used for routine tasks are stored within easy reach to avoid strain to the upper body from repetitive movements when retrieving the items.

- Exercising caution when using filing cabinets. When multiple drawers are open at the same time, the cabinet can tip over. Also, avoid leaving bottom drawers open when not in use because people can trip or fall if they open into a walkway. (See **Figure 22.32**)

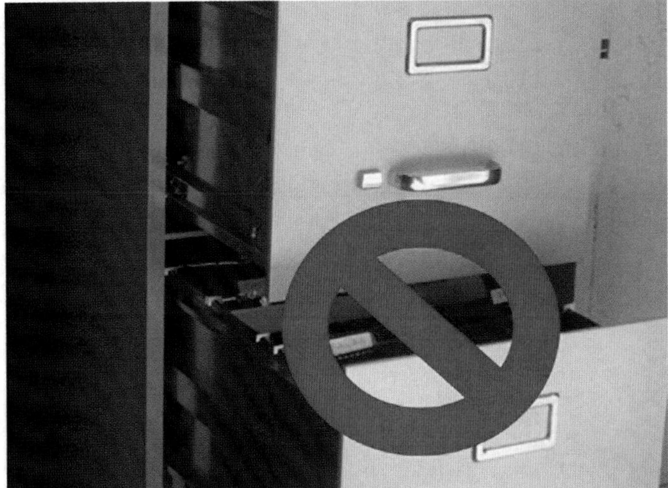

Figure 22.32 Open one file cabinet drawer at a time. Opening two drawers may cause the cabinet to tip.

Surgical Service Areas

SP technicians may have responsibilities that include services in surgery or other procedure areas. They should become familiar with possible hazards in all areas they visit and observe applicable safety policies and signage. These spaces have many of the same hazards found in other areas. Additionally, they may have hazards applicable to the use of lasers, X-ray equipment, and chemicals utilized during surgical procedures. Caution is required when entering areas when such equipment is in use. Specific safety precautions provided by the manufacturers should be reviewed and followed by employees.

Additional SP Safety Concerns

Equipment that is not functioning correctly may cause injury. A preventive maintenance (PM) program is required to ensure optimal operation and function of equipment used for SP activities. This equipment includes sterilizers, washer-disinfectors, heat sealers, and other processing equipment that should be routinely inspected and serviced by certified, experienced service personnel. Inspection records should be maintained, and copies should be readily available in the SPD. These records should be verified by the department's manager to ensure that the equipment used by SP employees is safe for use.

SP personnel should promptly report equipment in need of PM or repair.

Handling Compressed Gas Cylinders

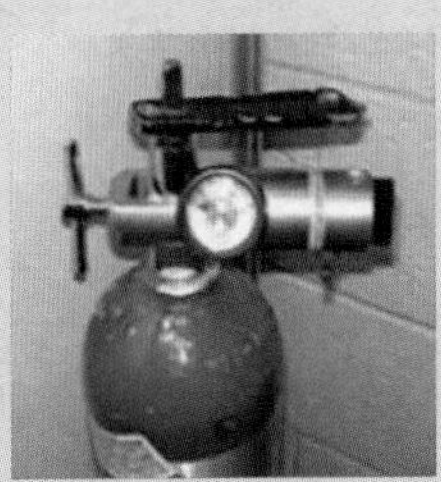

SP technicians are often involved in the handling, transport and storage of medical gas cylinders dispensed for direct patient care and treatment, or for use as equipment components.

These cylinders may contain oxygen, helium, nitrogen or other gases. Specific safety protocols should be used for each specific gas, and the protocols should be in compliance with the product's handling instructions in the applicable SDS. Medical gas cylinder safety precautions include:

- Never dispensing gas cylinders for use without a label.

- Securing gas cylinders at all times to prevent tipping. Place them in a secured holder for this purpose, or securely strap or chain them in an upright position.

- Handling cylinders carefully during transport. They should never be rolled, dragged or dropped.

- Using a cover cap to protect the cylinder's valve during transport.

- Using an appropriate regulator for the cylinder's contents. Cylinder regulators are gas-specific and not necessarily interchangeable.

- Inspecting threads on cylinder valves, regulators and other fittings for damage before connection.

- Clearly labeling all cylinders as "full," "in use" or "empty."

- Not storing empty cylinders with full ones.

- Ensuring gas cylinder regulators are equipped with either a hand wheel or stem valve. Stem valves require a key that should always remain with the regulator.

SP technicians should also be familiar with any emergency procedures that may be needed when using equipment. For example, SP technicians should be familiar with emergency shut-off procedures for any equipment in their work area. (See **Figure 22.33**)

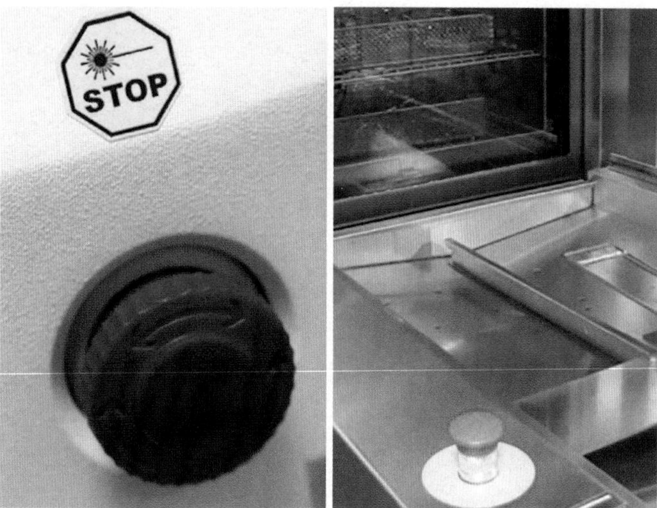

Figure 22.33 Know the location of emergency shut-offs.

DISASTER PREPAREDNESS

Disaster preparedness is an important component of the SP safety system. Each facility has developed a comprehensive response plan for internal and external disasters. An **internal disaster** is any situation with the potential to cause harm or injury to the healthcare facility employees or where the loss of utilities may drastically impact departmental operations. Examples of internal disasters include a hazardous chemical spill or leak, loss of power, or failure of a utility such as water, electricity or steam.

An **external disaster** is a situation where activities outside the facility impact departmental or facility operations. Examples that may necessitate activation of the external disaster plan include earthquakes, floods, hurricanes or other events that result in large numbers of seriously injured patients being sent to the facility. When an external disaster occurs, the entire facility is placed on alert, and personnel from each department are expected to perform tasks based on the situations present.

Disaster (internal) Situation with the potential to cause harm or injury to Sterile Processing or other employees, patients or visitors, or where the loss of utilities may drastically impact departmental operations.

Disaster (external) A situation in which activities external to the facility affects departmental or facility operations.

Disaster Plans

SPD disaster plans, like those of other departments, should be consistent with and support the facility's plans. Most facilities use an Incident Command System (ICS), a standardized approach to the command, control and coordination of emergency response. SP managers must ensure the SPD's disaster response activities and expectations are included in the overall ICS plan.

Elements of an SPD disaster plan typically include:

- An emergency call list outlining the lines of authority and the key individuals to be notified in the event of specific types of disasters. *Note: These may differ for each type of disaster.*
- Protocols for inventory replenishment and the delivery of emergency supplies. Usually, supply distribution department personnel are responsible for the maintenance of supplies and will deliver to an area for emergency patient care in times of disaster.
- Posted evacuation plans and practice drills for employees to ensure they know alternative ways to leave the department if their safety is at risk.
- SP technicians should actively participate in all disaster training and drills. It is important to understand roles and responsibilities during a disaster situation and be prepared to perform the assigned duties.

Biological Disasters

Many healthcare facilities have added biological incidents to their disaster plans. As with other types of disasters, SP technicians should know their role. Close communication with the Infection Prevention and Control department is critical in this type of disaster.

SPDs should utilize appropriate resources, such as the Centers for Disease Control and Prevention (CDC; www.cdc.gov) for up-to-date information regarding emerging biological threats. Other resources, such as the World Health Organization (WHO; www.who.org) can also provide guidance. In all instances, coordination between Infection Prevention and all areas impacted by the disaster is very important.

EMPLOYEE ACCIDENTS AND INJURIES

Even significant efforts to emphasize safety and accident prevention cannot eliminate all employee accidents, and SP technicians can still be injured on the job. If an injury occurs, it must be documented and reported to the appropriate administrative personnel, in compliance with OSHA regulations for healthcare facilities. An investigation is needed to provide information about the cause, the situation, and/or the behaviors that were involved to identify contributing factors, hazards or unsafe practices. Then, corrective actions must be implemented to revise the systems or physical conditions and address the behavior that caused the injury. This is necessary to help prevent future injuries or accidents.

Regardless of how insignificant an injury may seem, the appropriate manager should be informed immediately. Details regarding time, place, tasks performed and a description of exactly what happened must be recorded on the appropriate form. The form should then be submitted to the facility's safety officer, Human Resources (HR) department, Employee Health, or other entity, according to the facility's protocol.

A process should also be in place for SP technicians to report unsafe situations before an accident or injury happens. If an unsafe situation is identified, it should be reported immediately so the risk of injury can be minimized.

PATIENT ACCIDENTS AND INJURIES

SP professionals have a responsibility to help prevent patient and employee injuries, accidents and infections. They do so as they perform the important tasks of decontaminating, inspecting, testing, assembling, packaging, sterilizing, aseptically handling sterile items, and delivering items according to established procedures. When their job is done correctly, risk to the patient is greatly reduced.

When a patient incident occurs, it must be promptly investigated and documented. Any practices or physical conditions within the facility that can cause a patient injury must also be investigated and reported. All healthcare workers must report unsafe practices or hazards immediately to minimize accidents and prevent their recurrence.

EMPLOYEE INFORMATION AND TRAINING

No safety and risk management system can be successful without employee involvement. Each employee must understand their role and responsibilities in maintaining a safe environment. This requires education for staff at all levels of experience.

All new SP employees should attend a facility-provided health and safety orientation to become familiar with hazards and safety practices throughout the facility. They should also attend a department-specific orientation that focuses on (at minimum) the following:

- Notification of employees about any operations in their work area where hazardous substances are present
- Location and availability of written hazard communication program information
- Physical and health effects of any hazardous substances they may encounter
- Methods and observation techniques used to determine the presence or release of hazardous substances in the work area
- Strategies to lessen or prevent exposure to these hazardous substances through safe control and work practices and the use of PPE
- Steps the department has taken to lessen or prevent exposure to hazardous substances
- Instructions on how to read labels and review SDS to obtain appropriate hazard information
- Emergency spill procedures
- Disaster and fire plans, and the role of the SPD in their development and implementation

EMPLOYEE PREPAREDNESS

An important factor in safety and risk management is employee awareness and preparedness. Every employee should approach each shift and task with two questions in mind: "What can I do to ensure my safety and the safety of those in the facility?" and "What do I need to know to respond if I am faced with an emergency?" Some strategies to help ensure emergency preparedness include:

- Being familiar with safety policies. Ask questions if specific information is not understood.
- Being familiar with the chemicals used. Know how to handle them safely and what to do in the event of an emergency.
- Knowing how to work safely around equipment. Understand the hazards and know where emergency shut-offs are located.
- Being familiar with evacuation routes and the location of fire extinguishers and fire alarm boxes.
- Leaving each area safe. Wipe up spills, prevent trip hazards and do not cross-contaminate.
- Maintaining a safe environment at all times. Pay attention to detail and report anything that threatens the safety and well-being of those in the facility.

The success of any safety system depends on the individuals who work within that system. Creating and maintaining a culture of safety reduces risks for everyone.

CONCLUSION

SP technicians play an important role in every healthcare facility's safety program. It is important that all SP employees know the expectations and are able to perform efficiently and calmly during any type of situation that may arise. For the safety of patients, visitors, other employees and departmental staff, training and safety drills must be taken seriously, as should the adoption of safe work habits that help ensure preparedness for any unplanned emergency.

RESOURCES

U.S. Department of Homeland Security. "Active shooter - How to respond." https://www.dhs.gov/xlibrary/assets/active_shooter_booklet.pdf?t=149547415680.

ANSI/AAMI ST79:2017 & 2020 Amendments A1, A2, A3 and A4, *Comprehensive guide to steam sterilization and sterility assurance in health care facilities.*

Occupational Safety and Health Administration (OSHA). *Ergonomics for the Prevention of Musculoskeletal Disorders: Guidelines for Nursing Homes.* 2003.

OSHA. "Fact sheet: Ethylene oxide." https://www.osha.gov/sites/default/files/publications/ethylene-oxide-factsheet.pdf.

OSHA. "Fact Sheet: Workplace Violence." www.osha.gov/OshDoc/data_ General_Facts/factsheet-workplace-violence.pdf. 2002.

OSHA. "Hazard communication standard: Safety Data Sheets." Federal Register 56:64004. December 6, 1991. https://www.osha.gov/sites/default/files/publications/OSHA3514.pdf.

STERILE PROCESSING TERMS

Risk management

Ergonomics

Hazardous waste

Secondary container

Polymerization

Combustible

Workplace violence

Aerosol

Action level (AL)

Short-term exposure limit (STEL)

Disaster (internal)

Disaster (external)

Chapter 23

Success Through Effective Communication and Human Relations Skills

Learning Objectives

As a result of successfully completing this chapter, the reader will be able to:

1. Explain why Sterile Processing technicians must use effective communication and human relations skills
2. Define the term "professionalism" and list traits of quality-focused Sterile Processing professionals
3. Describe behaviors that can impact on-the-job success
4. Use basic tactics for effective communication in the workplace
5. Discuss approaches to improve teamwork
6. Define the term "diversity" and understand why it is important
7. Review common workplace communication issues

INTRODUCTION

The responsibilities of Sterile Processing (SP) technicians relate directly to patient health and well-being. SP technicians must have the knowledge and skills to address the sophisticated concepts addressed in this technical manual; however, they must also interact with other people in their department—and in other departments within the facility—as well as with vendors, suppliers and others. Doing so requires consistent use of communication and human relations skills. A Sterile Processing department (SPD) where all employees demonstrate professionalism and utilize effective communication skills is an ideal setting that can be accomplished when each SP technician adopts the behaviors and practices outlined in this chapter.

NEED FOR EFFECTIVE COMMUNICATION AND HUMAN RELATIONS SKILLS

SP technicians, like all other healthcare professionals, must have effective interpersonal skills. Effective communication is one facet of interpersonal skills because it allows a person to understand someone else's needs and interests. **Human relations** skills are also important because they allow people to use the information gained from communication to interact effectively with others.

Communication is the process of transmitting information from one person to another by use of words and non-verbal expressions such as body language. The concept of human relations involves the development and maintenance of effective interpersonal (between people) relationships that enhance teamwork and help ensure a positive work environment.

Human relations The development and maintenance of effective interpersonal (between people) relationships that enhance teamwork.

Communication The process of transmitting information and understanding from one person to another by use of words and non-verbal expressions such as body language.

Many communication and human relations principles are applicable on the job and most can be used off the job as well. While people are unique in many respects, they also share many commonalities, which may include specific needs, wants and desires—all of which help form a framework for human relations.

The use of appropriate communication and human relations skills is important whenever people interact. Today, much communication is done through the internet (computers, smart phones); however, technicians must also be comfortable with face-to-face verbal communication to effectively interact with their customers. Human interaction is critical in the SPD. The healthcare environment is very labor intensive, with many processes being equipment-dependent. Still, machines do not replace the need for human judgment and skills as SP technicians undertake their job responsibilities. SP technicians must work with their peers, departmental supervisors and managers. They also must represent their department as they interact formally and informally with staff members in other departments throughout the facility. SP technicians may also come in contact with patients, their families and visitors to the facility, including those conducting business with departmental managers. (See **Figure 23.1**) Regardless of the situation, effective communication and solid human relations skills are a must. It is also important to recognize that some SP professionals may understand details of inspecting and assembling complex surgical instruments and can apply specialized skills to operate sophisticated sterilization equipment, but they may have difficulty interacting with others. Proper use of communication and human relations skills is important for the success of all SP technicians in all healthcare facilities. Fortunately, these principles can be learned and are easy to apply on the job. The ability to do so is a characteristic of professional SP technicians.

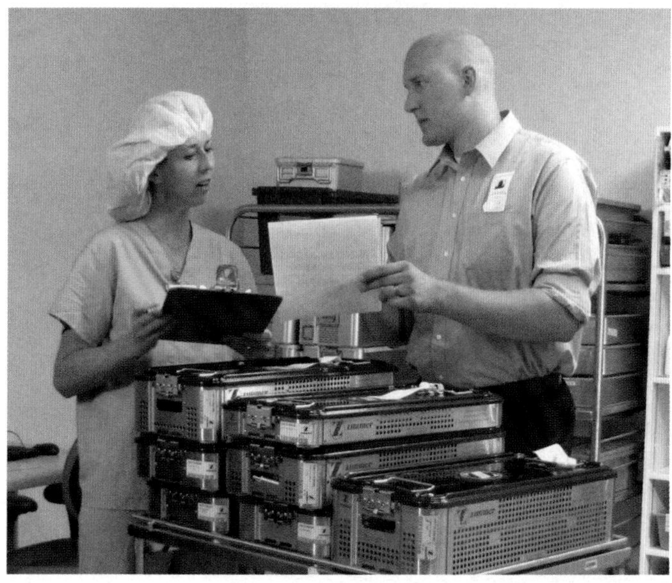

Figure 23.1

These days, when healthcare organizations face public scrutiny, the need for effective communication and the application of appropriate human relations skills continues, even when healthcare employees are off the clock. What one says (and does not say) and what one does (and does not do) reflects on the individual as well as their employer, regardless of where and how the communication occurs.

COMMON COMMUNICATION BARRIERS

Communication problems happen far too frequently. Even when everyone speaks the same language, common communication missteps can lead to errors, frustration and strained relationships. The following are some approaches that can lead to misunderstanding and prevent effective communication:

- Asking questions that can be interpreted differently, such as, "Can you come to work early?" (What time is "early"?)

- Relaying vague requests. Imagine a new technician answering a call to "Send up the old instrument that Dr. Smith used to use." (Which instrument?)

- Providing answers that do not give adequate or detailed information. Surgery, for example, may ask how long until a tray is ready, and the too-brief response could be, "It's in the sterilizer." (For how long? Is the cycle ending or just beginning?)

- Using **jargon** (slang or department-specific language) that may not be readily understood by others. An example could be stating to "Check the biological on the loaned trays and get them to eight. The TF has moved to first." Is this jargon or phrasing something a new employee would understand?

Jargon (slang) In the workplace, specialized words or phrases known only by people working in a certain position.

While adopting the communication principles discussed in this chapter will not resolve all communication problems, it will help address many of them.

SP TECHNICIANS ARE PROFESSIONALS

A professional is a person working in an occupation that requires extensive knowledge and skills to be successful in their role. A profession involves individuals with education and experience and who possess a specialized body of knowledge. Membership within a profession is usually controlled by licensing, registration and/or certification, and this certainly applies to SP professionals.

Professionals are proud of themselves and the work they do. They tackle their job effectively and efficiently and try to improve their profession in the process. A professional "goes the extra mile," is part of the team, tries to put forth the best possible effort to meet the facility's and department's goals and is truly interested in what is best for their fellow employees, customers and patients.

Professional SP technicians know what their manager expects of them and strive to consistently meet those expectations. They are effective communicators and are courteous and concerned about the problems encountered by other staff members.

A large part of job success is affected by how well employees get along with their supervisor. Ideally, both parties will demonstrate mutual respect and understanding. Still, friction can sometimes occur. When this happens, it becomes even more important to develop, maintain and improve the relationship. SP technicians should recognize that their boss may not be their friend or "buddy." A professional relationship will address job tasks and human relations concerns.

Those who obtain promotions and pay raises and most quickly attain career goals often enjoy the respect of their peers and supervisors. This respect is most likely experienced when an employee cooperates, is dependable and ambitious, and is willing to work hard to become successful.

MORAL, LEGAL AND ETHICAL CONSIDERATIONS

SP technicians must follow a professional code of conduct that includes moral, legal and ethical aspects of responsibility.

Moral conduct relates to basic principles about what is right and wrong. Patients who enter the hospital entrust their lives to the staff. SP technicians, like all healthcare employees, must honor this trust and carry out their duties in compliance with each detail and procedural step. They must accept responsibility to follow work schedules, maintain good attendance, and follow established policies and procedures in the best interest of patient care. Professional SP technicians also utilize resources wisely and do not question or ridicule others' beliefs or personal possessions.

SP professionals respect the rights of their co-workers. Additionally, they do not promote gossip or conduct that negatively impacts the best interests of their team, department or organization.

Legal behavior is determined by the authority of laws, and one must never overstep the limitations of these responsibilities. Laws protect staff as well as patients. Staff members are expected to perform job duties in the way they have been taught; therefore, technicians should not perform duties that have been designated for or assigned to a licensed or registered professional unless they meet those requirements. Technicians pay attention to details, follow each step in written procedures and instructions, and maintain thorough records and documentation.

Ethical behavior relates to what is right and wrong, relative to the standards of conduct for a profession. Ethical conduct is required of SP technicians at all times; however, the difference between what is "right" and "wrong" can be viewed from different perspectives.

How does one determine if a proposed action is ethical? Answering the following questions may be helpful:

- Is the proposed action fair?

- Does the proposed action hurt anyone (or could it)?

- Am I being honest as I undertake the proposed action?

- Can I live with myself if I do what I am considering?

- What if everyone did it?

- What are the consequences of my actions?

- Would I want my actions to become public knowledge?

Each day, SP technicians are faced with situations that require them to make moral, legal and ethical decisions. Understanding what is right (and the ramifications of doing what is wrong) can make those decisions easier.

COMMUNICATION BASICS

Some employees cannot effectively express their thoughts to co-workers; others may become distracted when someone speaks to them. A primary communication concern relates to speaking and another factor involves listening. Breakdowns with speaking or listening can interfere with the successful exchange of information between individuals.

SP technicians play an important role in their facility's communication process. They provide feedback, including ideas and suggestions to their supervisors who, in turn, communicate information up and down the chain of command. Each person's role in this communication process is vital to its success. (See **Figure 23.2**)

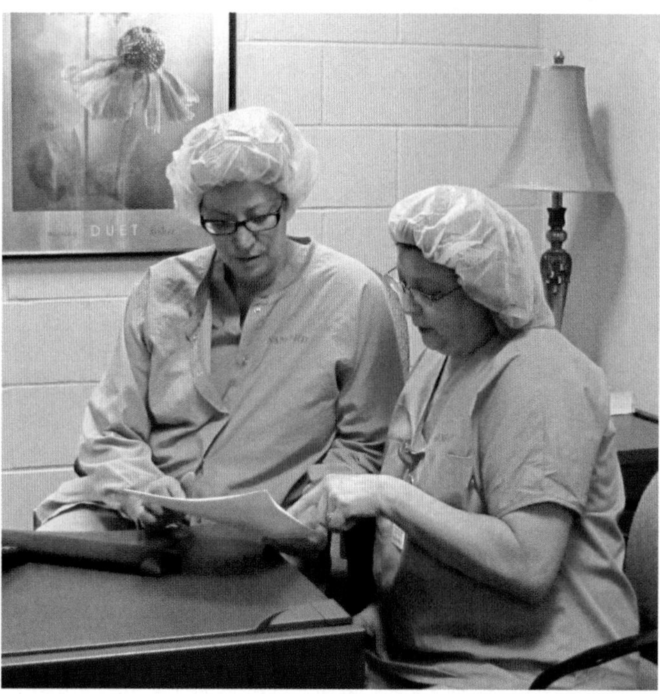

Figure 23.2

Some employees assume effective communication is easy (after all, people have been communicating their entire lives). In reality, the process is not difficult but it does require use of basic principles. Improving communication can be as simple as developing some basic speaking and listening skills.

Basic Speaking Skills

SP technicians speak to a diverse group of people on a daily basis. Consider using these principles when speaking with others:

- Unless carrying a facility-assigned phone, personal phones should be muted or turned off during the entire conversation. *Note: Due to the possibility of cross-contamination, personal electronics are not allowed in the SPD work areas.*

- Identify the main points in the message; organize what will be said and ensure that, while speaking, each main point is addressed.

- Stay focused. Do not ramble, digress or discuss points that are not critical to the message.

- Concentrate on the listener rather than on oneself. Remember that the main objective of speaking is to communicate.

- Use language that the listener will understand.

- Be professional. Use appropriate language, tone and volume.

- Answer questions or concerns honestly, even if the listener will not be happy with the answer. If one does not have an answer, let the listener know when they can expect to hear from you with the answer.

> **Infection Prevention and Technology**
>
> Phones and other personal technologies carried into the department from outside sources are highly contaminated with microorganisms, some potentially pathogenic. Most personal electronics cannot be properly cleaned and disinfected without causing permanent damage.
>
> Check with your department for specific policies regarding personal communication technologies.

Basic Listening Skills

A good portion of each day is spent speaking and listening. Some SP technicians spend more time speaking than listening. Skilled listening is a very important skill to acquire. Once people know they are being listened to, they will be more likely to communicate before their topic becomes a critical issue. Basic techniques to improve listening include:

- Focusing on what the speaker is saying and not becoming distracted. Don't let an uncomfortable physical environment cause a distraction. There may be few places within a busy SPD where the environment is ideal for effective communication, but it is important to try and make the best of it.

- Not being influenced by emotions. Avoid an immediate evaluation of the message and try to think about its content objectively.

- Staying engaged, even when the message seems familiar or unimportant, or when the speaker's opinion differs from one's own.

- Considering the speaker's perceptions as the message is heard. Understand the speaker's basic ideas before criticizing them.

- Avoiding simply listening for specific facts. There may be additional information that is an important part of the message.

- Not tuning out when listening to complicated information. Use feedback such as "I really don't understand what you are saying" or "Can you please say that in another way?" to inform the speaker that their message was not conveyed effectively.

- Allowing the speaker to finish and then reacting fairly to the message that was stated. Avoid formulating a response to the message while listening to the speaker.

- Taking notes, when appropriate, if the information is detailed or specific or if it will be helpful in the future.

Types of Communication

Communication flows through formal and informal channels within the SPD. Formal communication is structured and orderly, like classroom instruction, while informal communication has no structure and usually occurs during downtime, breaks, etc.

Examples of formal communication include:

- Instructions, advice and **coaching** by managers and supervisors (see **Figure 23.3**)

- Facility and departmental policies and procedures that help regulate behavior and work practices

- Discussions during departmental and other meetings

- Individual and group training presentations

- Facility and departmental bulletins, memos, newsletters, and related communication tools

- Performance evaluations

- Employee work schedules

- Conversations related to delegated project assignments

- Monitoring ongoing work activities

Coaching Positive reinforcement used to encourage SP technicians to follow proper work behaviors, and negative reinforcement to discourage inappropriate work behaviors.

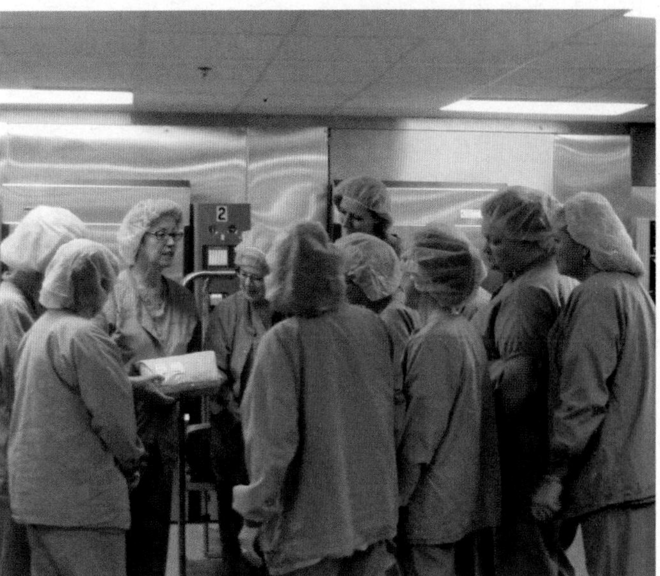

Figure 23.3

Informal methods of communication within SPDs include casual conversations between employees before, during and after work. Much of this communication is beneficial because it can improve working relationships of staff members. Unfortunately, informal communication can also be damaging. Consider, for example, rumors or other information circulated without knowledge of the source or concern about whether it is factual.

Rumors and "grapevine gossip" can negatively impact the team and the department. False information can cause anxiety and frustration and increase an already stressful work environment. In some cases, information may be factual but should not be shared with the team. For example, if a staff member learns of a fellow co-worker's personal problems, that information should not be shared unless the affected co-worker chooses to share it.

Gossip and rumors erode personal relationships and trust. They can waste time and shift the SP team's attention away from its real purpose.

Telephone and Technology Etiquette

The manner in which SP technicians answer and speak on the telephone reflects on their department, their facility and themselves. Each facility has policies and procedures to address professional expectations for telephone and technology etiquette. It is important to be aware of the facility's requirements and carefully follow them. (See **Figure 23.4**)

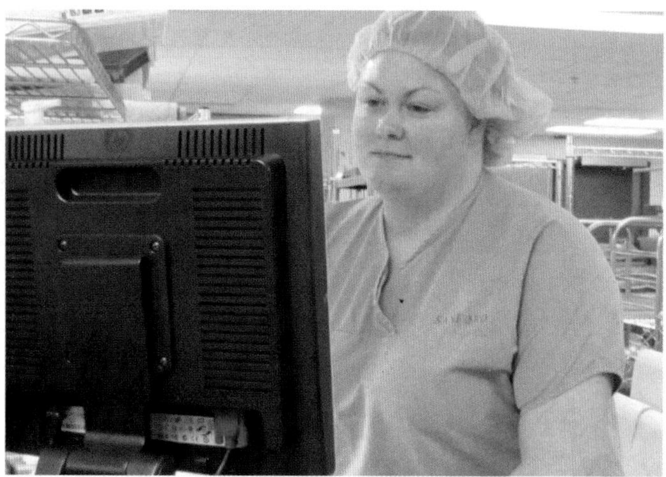

Figure 23.4

Whose Technology Is It?

Healthcare facilities and the Sterile Processing departments within them have invested significant financial resources in communications technology. It is increasingly difficult for many people to imagine how they could manage their professional and personal lives without seemingly constant access to computers, tablets, copiers, printers, smartphones and other telephones and other electronic communication equipment. With the convenience of technology, however, comes the opportunity for misuse when facility equipment is used for personal purposes (e.g., shopping on the internet, sending personal emails, and photocopying private or personal materials). Problems include time away from the job, increased facility expenses, and the blurring of the distinction between acceptable and unacceptable behaviors.

These concerns and other related issues are often addressed in facility policies and identified in employee handbooks and other documents. Professional SP technicians must know about these policies, understand their importance and consistently comply with them.

Music in the Workplace

Many SPDs allow music to be played in work areas. Music can promote a more comfortable atmosphere and may make the working experience more enjoyable. What follows are some guidelines for ensuring that music is enjoyed without creating distractions and jeopardizing the professionalism of the department.

The type or genre of music listened to at work reflects on the SPD and the healthcare facility. Do not listen to music that would be deemed unprofessional by the facility or its staff. When in doubt, don't play it. Lyrics should not be offensive to anyone in the department.

Music should be played at a low volume. Background music should allow staff to carry on a normal conversation without having to raise their voices. Music should not be heard in other areas of the department, public hallways, departmental offices, etc. If the telephone rings or a person needs to make a call, the music volume should not have to be turned down; it should barely be detected by the person on the other end of the call.

Time spent selecting, arranging and changing music must be kept to a minimum. Meeting the needs of patients and other customers is always the top priority.

Headsets or earphones should not be used because they can reduce the technician's ability to hear the telephone, machine cycle alarms, questions from co-workers, and other important sounds that are a part of the job.

Another concern created by advancing technology is the common availability of smartphones and other technologies that enable employees to text, speak, explore the internet, email and take photographs from almost anywhere. In addition to concerns regarding non-productive time, the Health Insurance Portability and Accountability Act (HIPAA), hospital policy and confidentiality concerns can become problematic if information captured in personal photographs or videos is shared outside the facility.

HUMAN RELATIONS

SP technicians may have the knowledge and skills required to do their job properly but they cannot be successful unless they know how to get along with their supervisors, peers and customers. Professional SP employees possess the following human relations skills:

- They recognize each of their fellow employees as individuals and, when possible, incorporate this understanding into how they interact with other staff members.
- They contribute effectively to their team because this benefits the department, facility, profession and the patient.
- They develop a genuine spirit of cooperation and teamwork amongst themselves, their peers and those at higher organizational levels.

It is relatively easy to talk about human relations skills' positive impact on the organization; however, it is much more difficult for SP technicians to consistently apply those skills. The workplace requires staff members to interact with many employees of different backgrounds, interests and job responsibilities. Such factors make it increasingly difficult to practice effective human relations.

There are numerous ways that SP technicians effectively apply their human relations skills on the job. For example, they:

- Take responsibility for maintaining positive working relationships with supervisors, peers and others in the healthcare facility.
- Set aside personal feelings for other SP employees on the shift, being sure to ask questions and assist challenging co-workers just as one would for co-workers with whom they are on friendlier terms.
- Act in a professional manner.
- Serve as a contributing member of the department and healthcare team.
- Accept the responsibility to continually learn and, when applicable, help their peers do the same.
- Promote cooperation among their peers. This is done by helping others, sharing knowledge and experience, and trying to understand others' perspective.
- Accept full responsibility for their own actions (or inaction) and not try to pass the blame to another person, shift or department.

Behaviors That Can Impede Success

Being successful in the workplace involves much more than having the technical skills to perform a job. The following are common behaviors that can impede success and, in some cases, lead to disciplinary action:

- Refusing to follow directions, orders, policies and procedures
- Being unwilling to adapt to change
- Talking too much and/or conducting personal business while at work
- Using personal electronics during assigned work time
- Demonstrating inconsistent and unreliable work behaviors
- Engaging in gossip and other behaviors that reduce group productivity
- Failing to get along with others
- Being dishonest and lacking in integrity on the job
- Failing to complete assignments in a timely manner
- Making or contributing to excessive errors
- Regularly missing work or being tardy
- Abusing substances

SP TECHNICIANS AND TEAMWORK

SP technicians must work as part of a team because the roles they perform relate directly to those being done by others. Consider, for example, that the main goal of every SP technician is to help patients. Teamwork is essential for ensuring that the patients are best served.

What one employee does (or does not do) affects the work of others and also impacts the success (or failure) of the SPD. For example, staff in the decontamination area may work intently to clean turnaround instruments as quickly and safely as possible, and the assembly technicians may assemble and package them as quickly as is feasible; however, if the instruments are not put into the sterilizer as soon as possible, a delay will occur that could impact the surgical staff and jeopardize patient care.

Teamwork is beneficial to the facility in other ways as well. For example, it can:

- Improve productivity through increased staff cooperation
- Increase employee job satisfaction
- Improve the work environment by creating a common purpose for staff members
- Decrease job-related stress

Factors Impacting Teamwork

Developing a culture where teamwork is valued and practiced requires the dedication and effort of each team member.

The following characteristics are vital for an effective team:

- Good **attitude** – A proper attitude is the most important factor driving effective teamwork. SP technicians' attitudes about their job, peers and patients impact their actions. An employee's attitude is often influenced by co-workers. If everyone on the team gets along, likes their jobs and the facility and wants to provide good service, each staff member will probably have a good attitude. By contrast, if a co-worker has a negative attitude about the job, supervisor or facility, and does not care about the quality of work, teamwork will suffer.

> **Attitude** Emotions that cause a person to react to people and/or situations in a predetermined way.

- Cooperation – To provide good service, one must be willing to assist and work with other employees.
- Promptness – When an employee is late to work or does not show up, the remaining members of the team must work harder. As a result, work quality and morale can suffer.
- Trust – An effective member of a team trusts co-workers and supervisors. Co-workers and supervisors also trust each team member.

Types of Groups

SP technicians belong to both formal groups and informal groups. Teamwork concerns are important for both types.

A healthcare facility is comprised of a formal group of employees who, at the highest organizational level, have the same boss: the Hospital Administrator and Board of Directors. As staffing plans are developed, smaller work groups are established. The SPD is an example of a formal group. Work in the SPD may be divided into other formal groups, including those relating to specific work areas and shifts.

Each formal work group has a formal leader who is responsible for coordinating and directing the group.

A task group is another example of a formal group. Members work together to perform essential non-routine activities. For example, a committee might address a specific concern, and a work team may develop a job breakdown for training purposes. After the task group's work is completed, the group is typically dissolved.

Informal groups develop for several reasons, including common interests of members; a desire to be "close" to others in a similar situation; economics; and a desire to satisfy specific but common personal needs. Informal groups may include employees who take lunch or other breaks together, work the same shift, participate in after-work activities, and carpool.

Informal work groups are not necessarily good or bad. Each can assist, harm or have no impact on the facility's efforts to attain goals. Informal groups can form cliques, exclusive groups of individuals who intentionally exclude others. These groups also frequently develop an informal communication system, called the "grapevine," which can spread rumors (a negative outcome) or provide helpful information.

Teamwork and Decision Making

In some healthcare facilities, SP technicians can participate in the decision-making process in their department by participating in cross-functional teams. A cross-functional team is a group of employees from different departments within the healthcare facility that works together to resolve operating problems. Consider, for example, a problem that involves instruments that are unavailable when needed in the Operating Room (OR). A cross-functional team comprised of OR, SP and staff from other departments may yield creative alternatives that would not be considered when a group with a narrower focus addressed the issue.

Relating Experience to Job Success

Experience should impact job success, but that is not always the case. The benefit that experience brings to the work situation is not equal to time spent on the job. In the fast-paced world of SP, ongoing professional development and continuing education are critical for one to make a full contribution. Unfortunately, experience can encourage some to develop an attitude of entitlement.

By contrast, experience can be invaluable because it provides insight about what has and has not been successful in the past. Experience can improve the knowledge and skills that help SP technicians become successful. This type of input is important when experienced staff members are encouraged to participate in the decision-making process or when individuals serve on cross-functional teams.

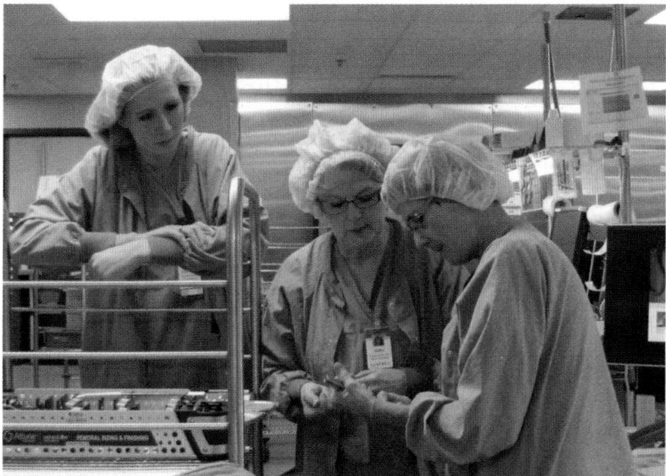

Figure 23.5

STERILE PROCESSING AND DIVERSITY

Diversity adds dimension to the SP work team. There are numerous aspects of diversity that shape values, expectations and experiences. These include education, family status, organizational role and level, religion, first language, income, geographical location, and more. Every person is unique and brings special qualities to the job.

Diversity The broad range of human characteristics and dimensions that impact the employees' values, opportunities and perceptions of themselves and others at work.

Developing a work environment where all co-workers are respected provides the following advantages:

- The creation of a welcoming and rewarding work environment improves job satisfaction.
- When people are valued, employee turnover and absenteeism are minimized and associated costs are reduced.
- A culture of understanding, respect and cooperation encourages teamwork.
- Diverse backgrounds create more creative alternatives as decisions are made and problems are resolved.

CUSTOMER SERVICE SKILLS FOR SP TECHNICIANS

Basics of Customer Service

Customer service refers to the relationship between the SP team and its customers. These customers include anyone who utilizes SP's services, including doctors, nurses, clinicians, patients and vendors. One brief positive or negative encounter with a customer can leave a lasting impression about the entire department. This impression can then be passed on to other customers.

Providing a service is not always easy. Some SP customers are the direct patient caregivers who, themselves, have customers (the patients). SP technicians must be committed to providing excellent support service, so their counterparts throughout the facility can also provide excellent service and care to the patient.

Providing exemplary service requires the consistent delivery of safe, high-quality products and services. Each employee must strive to do their part to support the facility's and department's goals. **Figure 23.6** provides an example of an SP technician working with a customer to solve a problem.

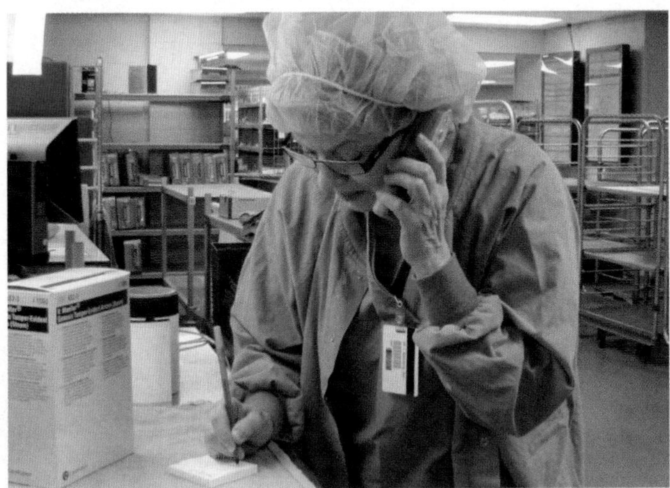

Figure 23.6

Each functional area and work shift in the SPD depends on others. The quality of each step in the processing cycle is affected by previous and subsequent steps. If decontamination and cleaning procedures are not done effectively or in a timely manner, the sterilization process may be ineffective and/or products may not be available when needed. SP technicians must function as a team to achieve quality customer service.

Self-discipline is very important, especially in difficult situations and encounters. SP team members must stay focused on real issues, maintain composure and not allow emotions or personalities to influence their performance. When it is necessary to say "no" to a customer request, it is important to explain the reasons and offer alternatives. If an error occurs, employees should be honest and work toward a resolution. Credibility and trust are essential, and customer trust must always be preserved.

Providing more personalized service is also beneficial. SP professionals should get to know their customers and, when possible, use their names when communicating needs and addressing special requests.

Cheerful, courteous and friendly behavior is also effective for promoting effective customer service. The provision of good service requires SP technicians to constantly assess the quality of their services, follow up on commitments, and solicit feedback. Quality service is a reflection of professionalism, and it requires maturity, self-esteem, competence, confidence and a positive attitude.

Emergencies and crisis situations are a reality in the healthcare environment; however, even during stressful times, a calm, professional attitude must prevail.

Cooperation with Operating Room Personnel

No two departments in a typical healthcare facility work more closely than the OR and SPD. The outcome of every patient procedure depends on effective communication and cooperation between personnel in these two fast-paced, ever-changing departments.

Much of the relationship between OR and SP staff is dependent upon mutual trust, communication and cooperation. To earn and maintain trust, each department must work hand in hand with the other and communicate effectively and often.

SP technicians should spend some time learning how each department and their respective procedures affect the SPD, and how the SP processes affect each department. This process makes it easier to see how less-than-optimal service can affect patient care and customers' opinions of the SPD. Spending time during orientation in different departments is an effective way of understanding how other departments operate.

Communication Is Critical

Differences in communication systems used by different departments can create challenges. Slang terms, jargon and nicknames used to describe medical instruments and supplies, for example, may not be familiar to all staff working in different departments. Also, instrument and supply needs change (often several times a day), and if information doesn't travel smoothly, frustration can increase and relationships may become strained.

Communication between OR and SP staff should be ongoing and not just occur when an incident occurs or after an issue has been identified. Also, simple actions, such as showing appreciation for the efforts and assistance of personnel in the other department, can help establish a stronger bond between both groups.

Handling Customer Complaints

Customer complaints can arise, even when the best procedures and protocols are in place (and even when staff diligently adhere to them). When facilities endorse the concept of empowerment, SP technicians can more easily resolve customer complaints by implementing a practice of **service recovery**.

> **Service recovery** The sequence of steps used to address customer complaints and problems in a manner that yields a win-win situation for the customer and the department.

SETTING PRIORITIES

There may be times when SP technicians face multiple tasks. How should priorities be established in these instances? The most important things should be done first. These might be identified by asking questions such as:

- What is the immediate need?
- What can I do to help my team?
- What task would I want done if I were the supervisor?
- What is the best use of my time right now?

It is not uncommon for priorities to change during a shift. For example, the addition of a trauma case will necessitate reprioritization of work tasks. SP technicians must be adaptable to changing needs and always put the patient first. **Figure 23.7** provides an example of instrument priorities being communicated through a communication board.

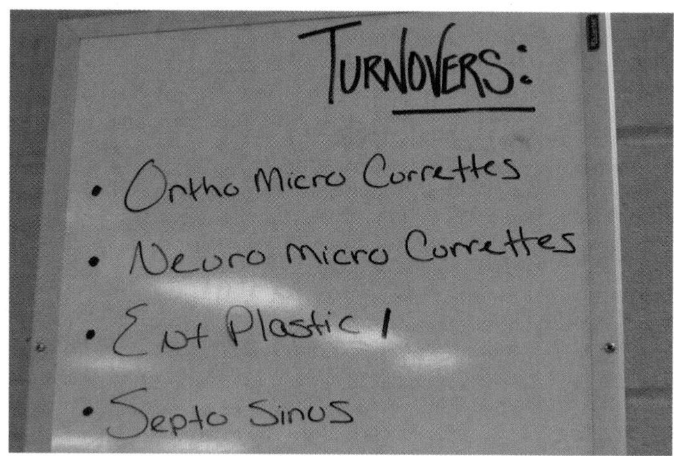

Figure 23.7

AVOIDING WORKGROUP COMPARISONS

Sometimes, SPDs fall into "shift wars," where some (or all) employees assigned to a specific shift begin to believe that the work they do is more important than others' work. For example, a day shift may wonder what the night shift does with their time.

In reality, not all shifts have exactly the same duties, and priorities do change throughout each 24-hour period. It is unrealistic to assume that all shifts work in exactly the same way and under exactly the same circumstances.

These types of comparisons can lead to misunderstandings between shifts and individual employees, which can then lead to communication breakdowns and negatively impact the ability to work as an effective team.

COMMITTING TO PATIENT CARE DURING DISASTERS

No one can predict when disasters will occur; however, each healthcare facility and SPD should anticipate the most likely crisis that may arise. From there, plans that incorporate the most appropriate responses to crises can be developed.

All SP technicians should be prepared to provide service during emergencies. To do so, they should:

- Study their department's/facility's disaster plans and ask questions, if necessary.
- Take disaster drills seriously.
- Keep the SPD informed of current contact information, so an accurate call-back roster will be available if it is needed.

- Make personal plans that will allow support of patient care. For example, SP professonals should have a back-up arrangement for childcare and family communications if remaining at the hospital is required for an extended time.

- Remember to remain calm and positive during a disaster. The stress level will be high, and making a conscious effort not to add to the stressful environment will benefit everyone.

- Focus on the job and what is needed to meet patient needs.

- Do not share patient information with anyone outside the hospital.

COMMUNICATING WITH THE MEDIA

Personnel from the news media will contact healthcare facilities for information. Each facility has trained personnel assigned to interact with the media. If approached or contacted by the media in any way, do not give out any information. Always refer them to the appropriately trained personnel. *Note: Information that may seem harmless, such as even saying a patient is in the facility, can be in violation of the patient's HIPAA rights; such an oversite can result in discipline, including termination.*

EMAIL

While everyone today uses email, it is important to project professionalism while using email at work. Composing a professional email makes it more likely that people will respond positively to your emails. It shows people that you are professional and polite, and makes it less likely to cause misunderstandings. Guidelines for writing professional emails include:

- Once something has been written, it becomes, in a sense, part of a "permanent business record." Unlike oral communication, there is no chance to retract an error or clarify a point that may offend or confuse the target audience.

- All emails should include an appropriate subject line. The subject line should be clear and as brief as possible. In today's busy facilities, emails with vague or cute subject lines are likely to be ignored, skipped or deleted.

- Only discuss public matters. The contents of emails should not be confidential or a topic that, if posted publicly or sent to someone unplanned, would embarrass the sender or the facility.

- Confidential information should never be sent over the internet. Even though many email systems are "secured," a recipient may forward the message to an unintended person who may not know to keep the information confidential. On occasion, email systems have also been compromised. Confidential information may be sent electronically only if using a facility-approved site such as an internal incident reporting and resolution program.

- Create a new email instead of continuing to "reply." At some point, including all of the previous replies becomes cumbersome and redundant. Include only the necessary information from the chain to support your message, such as the date and time of earlier pertinent responses, so the receiver does not have to hunt through an excessive number of emails.

- Do not use jargon, slang, generational terms or emojis. This practice is unprofessional and such messages are easily misinterpreted.

- Do not use humor, including funny sayings, comics or political cartoons. Not everyone has the same sense of humor, and some may be offended by the topic. Trying to be funny may also reduce the importance of your message.

- Keep the email brief. Supply only pertinent information and do not be redundant. People are too busy to read unnecessary information and may tend to ignore emails from those who send lengthy messages with too much or irrelevant information.

- Don't email when angry. When angry, it is easy to say something that could be regretted by the sender, recipient or both. It is always best to wait until some of the anger has passed and a clearer thought process can be used for communication. Remember, once sent, a message cannot be taken back.

- Be sure the punctuation is correct. Leaving out or using incorrect punctuation can be perceived as sloppy or not well thought out. It can also give the impression that the sender did not feel the message was important.

- Proofread the message before sending. Be sure the message is what was intended. Every email is a reflection of the sender. Misspelled words, poor grammar, punctuation errors and emotion (humor or anger) do not reflect favorably. These mistakes make the sender look careless.

Remember, once the message is in cyberspace, it no longer belongs to the sender. Others can edit, forward and share it, and the edited message may be sent to people for whom it was never intended.

SOCIAL MEDIA

Like email, social media is widely used today. Many of the rules for email are the same for social media. It is important to remember that social media is often shared, so a personal message may quickly travel around the world and be seen by hundreds of people. In addition to the rules stated for email, considerations for social media use include:

- Sharing any information about facility activities on social media may be infringing on a patient's HIPAA rights or go against facility policy.

- Sharing pictures that have not been approved may show something that is also an infringement on a patient's or staff members rights.

- Avoiding the mixing of work communication with personal communication. Discussing business information that has not been released to the general public can be detrimental to one's career. It is also inappropriate to discuss social gatherings and other non-business topics.

- Avoiding heated debates or conversations that may embarrass family, friends, co-workers or the healthcare facility. These conversations may be sent to others, including people who do not need or want the information.

- Using caution when posting and tagging pictures. Post only photographs that have been approved for social media sites and only to the approved sites. Posting unauthorized photos can be a violation of HIPAA requirements, the facility's confidentially policy, or both. Do not tag any person until a release to do so has been obtained.

- Being careful of the information shared. This also applies to personal accounts. It is common for organizations to look at personal social media accounts before scheduling an interview or making a job offer. Checking social media is also common during some disciplinary actions. Many times, evidence against the accused is retrieved from social media accounts. Misrepresenting personal information on social media, including being untruthful about job titles and employment information, can lead to termination of an existing position or the loss of a wanted position.

- Asking if the facility has a policy regarding the use of its name in online discussion boards, non-business accounts, and personal websites. Comply with the instructions as given.

CONCLUSION

SP technicians have challenging, critically important and ever-evolving responsibilities. Managing these duties effectively, consistently and efficiently requires good communication and human relation skills and an understanding that a well-operating department can only be had in the presence of a well-functioning team.

RESOURCES

Healthcare Sterile *Processing Association. Central Service Leadership Manual.* 2016.

Association of periOperative Registered Nurses. *Guidelines for PeriOperative Practice: Surgical Attire.* 2022.

STERILE PROCESSING TERMS

Human relations

Communication

Jargon (slang)

Coaching

Attitude

Diversity

Service recovery

Chapter 24

Personal and Professional Development for Sterile Processing

Learning Objectives

As a result of successfully completing this chapter, the reader will be able to:

1. Explain the meaning of personal development and how it can impact a career in Sterile Processing
2. List possible career paths available to Sterile Processing professionals
3. Review strategies for professional goal setting
4. Identify strategies to enhance professional skills and expertise
5. Understand the key aspects of resumé or curriculum vitae development
6. Understand the basic steps for the interviewing process
7. Identify opportunities for promotions and learn about positive personal behaviors and attributes that tend to get professionals noticed

INTRODUCTION

Learning is a lifelong endeavor, and change is inevitable. Never have these statements been truer than when applied to the field of Sterile Processing (SP). SP technicians must be prepared to encounter frequent growth in their positions. Whether SP technicians wish to stay in the Sterile Processing department (SPD) or seek advancement or promotion to other areas of the organization, **personal** and **professional development** will enable them to be proactive and more easily prepare for the change. This chapter highlights some of the resources and strategies available to help SP technicians grow and advance in their careers.

Personal development Activities that identify and develop talent and personal potential, improve your employability, and enhance quality of life.

Professional development Commitment to continuous learning and improvement; taking responsibility for your own development.

PERSONAL AND PROFESSIONAL DEVELOPMENT: WHAT IT IS AND WHY IT IS IMPORTANT

In some ways, personal development is the first step toward professional development. Personal development may be defined as any activity that identifies and develops talent and personal potential and improves employability and quality of life. Personal development can help individuals develop personally rewarding goals.

Professional development specifically refers to the skills and knowledge attained for both personal and career advancement. It provides the information and experience needed to progress in a career, stay competitive with other job seekers and, ultimately, become more employable.

Personal development is usually an individual endeavor—something a person does on their own time; however, more employers are recognizing the importance of investing in personal development. Employers may offer educational programs as part of the organization's employee benefits program to help staff learn more about time and stress management, teamwork, healthy lifestyles, and competency and career development. Ultimately, these programs are a win-win for both employees and the healthcare facility because personal development can create a workplace that is happier, healthier and more fulfilling. This environment can lead to greater productivity and quality in a department, which helps the healthcare facility meet its strategic goals.

Personal development should be a lifelong process, and it is more of a journey than a destination. Choose smaller goals that are attainable and build on those successes. For example, if a long-term goal is a college degree, set the first goal as successfully completing one college course. Upon successful completion of that goal, the individual can set their goal for the next class.

Strategies for Personal Development

Personal development involves four key steps:

Step 1: Identify the goal. What do you want to achieve?

Step 2: Identify the requirements for the goal. What will you need to achieve the goal?

Step 3: Identify personal strengths and areas that need improvement. What can you build on? What do you need to improve?

Step 4: Create an action plan with a timeline for meeting that goal. How do you plan to move forward?

Types of Professional Development

Professional development can be divided into two categories:

- Professional development to keep current in an existing job – Growth is inevitable in the SP field, and some professional development is mandatory, even for those who wish to remain in their current position. For example, changes in procedures, policies, instrumentation, products, and sterilization technologies, as well as changes in regulations and standards, must be adopted by every employee. Job growth in an effort to stay current is required of all SP technicians.

- Professional development to advance one's career – Some SP technicians have goals to advance their careers through position advancement and promotion. They participate in activities to improve their professional competency, enhance their existing skills and develop new ones. They move out of their comfort zone to take on new responsibilities and learn new things.

The job market, technology, regulations and practices are always evolving, and an employer may not provide staff with all the skills needed to keep up or move forward in the profession. Whether a person prefers to remain in a current position or dreams of advancement, it is essential to consider the benefits of taking ownership of one's career by continually improving knowledge and skills.

Learning opportunities through conferences, continuing education, and on-the-job training help SP technicians keep up with trends and changes in the SP field. (See **Figure 24.1**) This allows technicians to anticipate change more easily and helps them recognize professional opportunities.

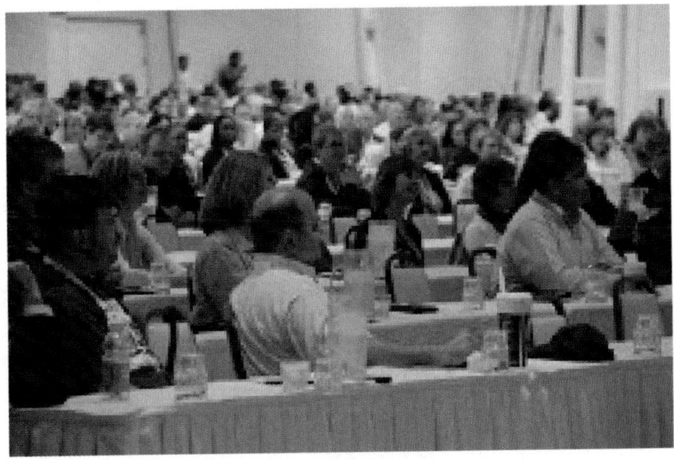

Conferences and workshops

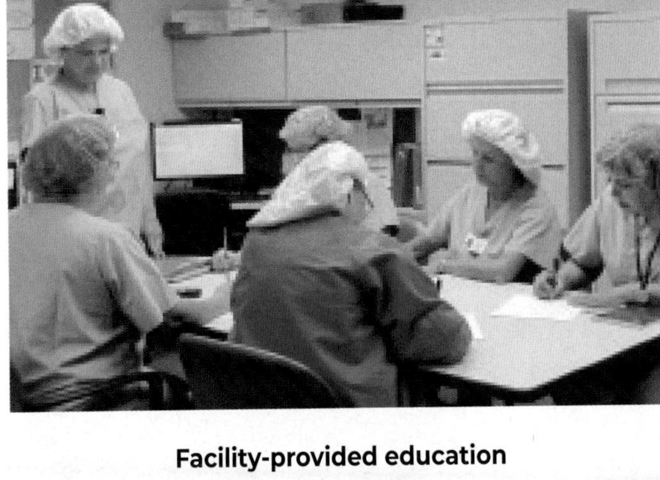

Facility-provided education

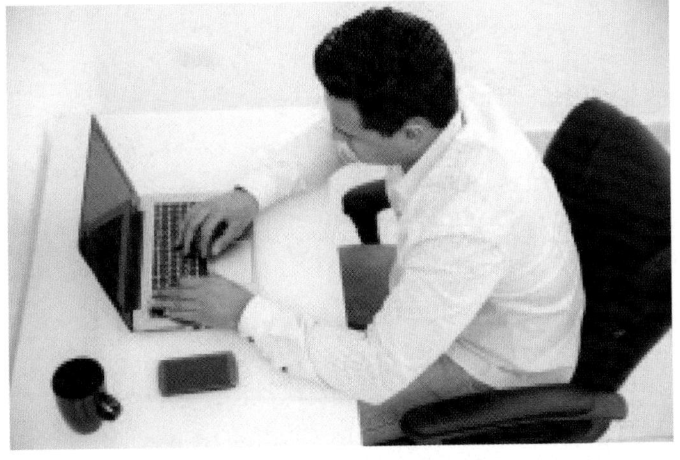

Independent study

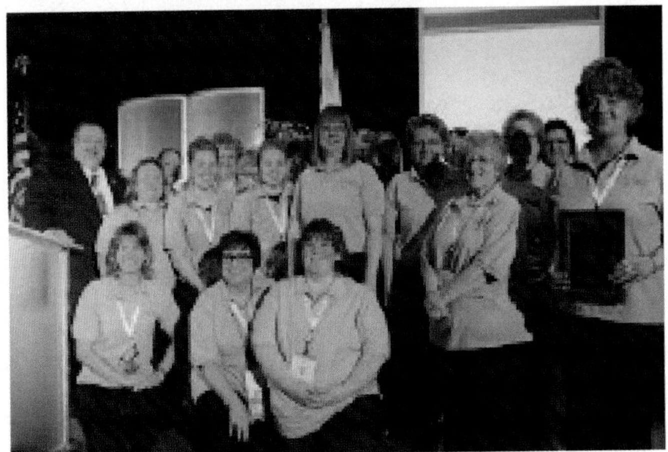

SP professional groups

Figure 24.1 Common learning opportunities

If an SP technician is a leader or would like to become one, professional development will provide the knowledge and confidence to influence and lead others by example.

Taking part in activities to improve professional competency will give SP technicians the skills they need to become more effective in their position. This will help demonstrate an ongoing commitment to the profession, improve employability with current and future employers, and lead to a more fulfilling and rewarding career.

An SP technician may be familiar with sterilization standards as a requirement of the job. If they are able to teach those standards to new employees, this will increase their understanding of the standards. Teaching an educational inservice or short course can sharpen one's technical skills and help develop training and public speaking skills. (See **Figure 24.2**)

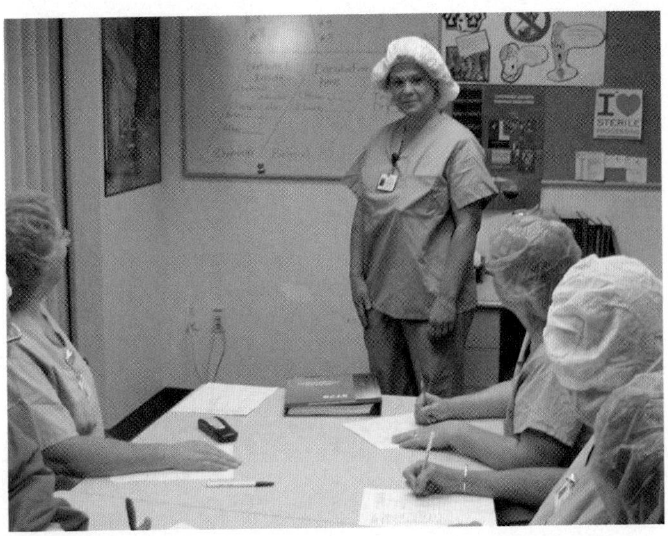

Figure 24.2

SP CAREER PATHS

While many SP technicians choose to remain employed in an SPD and become experts at their assigned duties, some seek different career paths. Common career opportunities for SP technicians include lead technician positions in the SPD, SP management positions, SP clinical educators, Operating Room (OR) core technicians, OR liaisons, faculty positions in local community and technical colleges, consultants, and vendor positions such as sales representatives and on-site product/service facilitators. (See **Figure 24.3**)

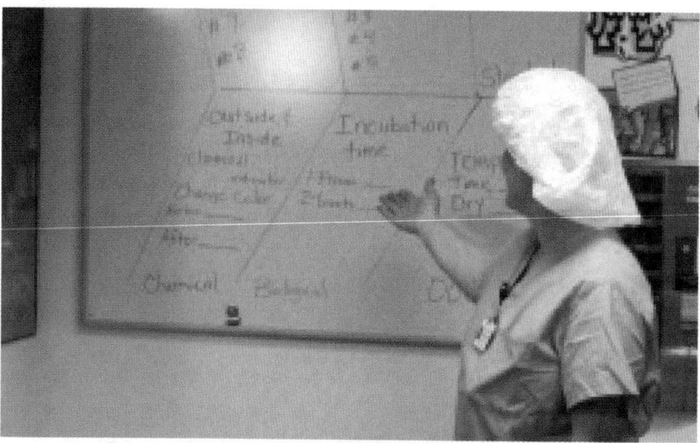

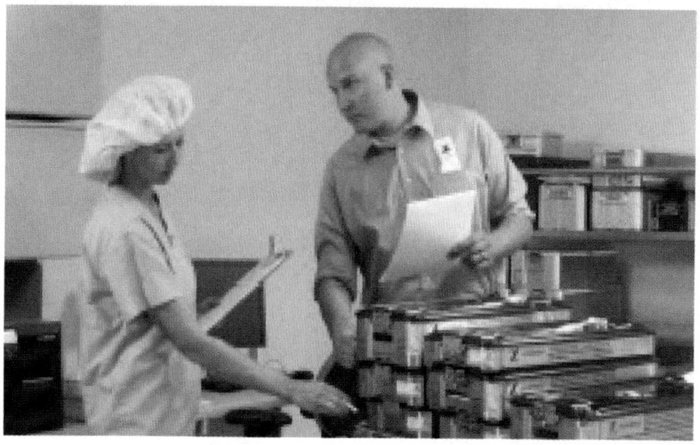

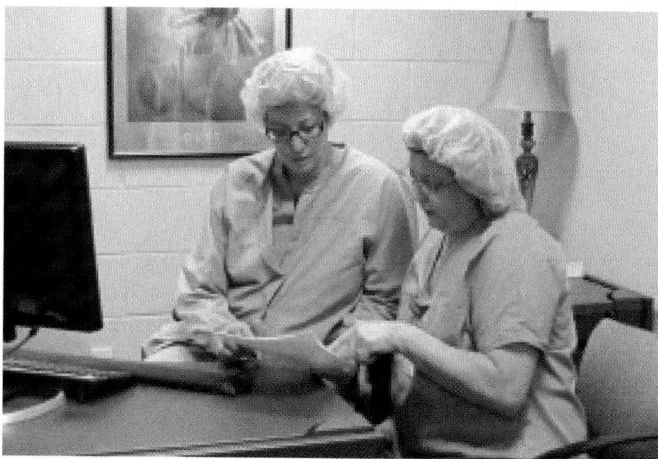

Figure 24.3 Examples of SP career paths

Each career path has specific requirements. It is prudent to research the needed requirements and develop personal and professional goals to move forward on a specific career path.

PLANNING CAREER GOALS

SP professionals looking to make their career more personally meaningful and rewarding should establish clear goals and periodically review them. This will identify activities and steps that will help meet those objectives.

As with personal development, professional development requires identifying areas in a present position in need of improvement and then moving forward with set goals. In many ways, the steps to take for professional development are similar to those one would take for personal development, with a specific emphasis on developing one's position and career advancement.

Strategies for Planning Career Goals

Step 1: Determine the goal for improving professional skills or employability.

Step 2: Identify the requirements for the goal. What will be needed to achieve it?

Step 3: Identify personal strengths and areas in need of improvement.

Step 4: Create an action plan with a timeline for meeting the goal.

Basic Technical Skills for SP Technicians

- Hand/eye dexterity
- Active listening and communication skills
- Problem solving
- Prioritization
- Ability to change tasks as needed
- Ability to evaluate job tasks for accuracy and completeness

ADVICE ABOUT CAREER GOALS

Personal development is a lifelong process, and professional development is a career-long process. Sometimes, employees get discouraged because they set lofty goals that do not materialize immediately. Most goals are achievable, but there may be many smaller goals to accomplish along the way before the larger goal(s) can be achieved. For example, if the goal is to become the SP Director, that will likely require meeting educational goals and attaining prior other leadership experience (i.e., as a lead technician or supervisor). When identifying what is necessary to achieve the final goal, be sure to identify individual steps that may be needed to prepare for that goal.

Those steps may include:

- Certification
- Attending educational conferences
- Becoming active in professional groups
- Engaging in on-the-job training in leadership, job and task-related skills
- Obtaining a degree
- Logging more time or developing more experience in a certain position

THE IMPORTANCE OF RESOURCES

One of the most important factors in attaining goals is finding the right resources to provide direction and support. Educational resources include publications, printed resources, courses, conferences, online information and other types of information designed to enhance knowledge about a specific process or topic.

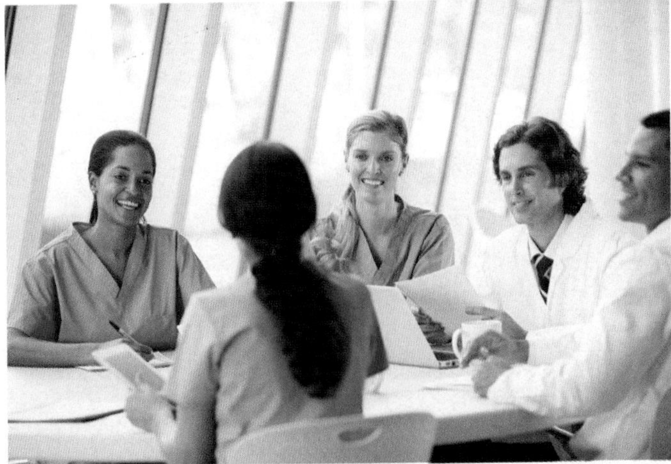

Figure 24.4

A Note About Online Resources

When using online resources, make sure the information and source are valid and current.

Developing professional resources within the SP field can provide a network with which to share information on issues pertinent to the department. SP peers may have already faced similar situations and may be able to share insights and information.

Do not underestimate the importance of developing a network beyond one's current specialty. OR professionals, infection preventionists, safety officers and biomedical engineers are a few of the healthcare specialists who can help SP technicians increase their knowledge about specific aspects of the field—and healthcare, in general.

There are several ways to build a network of resources. Becoming active in a local professional group or SP chapter is a great place to start. If there is no group in the area, contact local SPDs and explore the possibility of starting one. The first step can be as simple as gathering interested individuals at a local healthcare facility or business establishment.

PROFESSIONAL DEVELOPMENT ACTIVITIES

There are also ways to enhance existing skills and develop new ones to increase knowledge and professionalism and attain more expertise. **Figure 24.5** explores some ideas for professional development activities.

Social Media Information

Much information can be found on social media; however, it is important that whatever information one chooses to use is carefully vetted to ensure it is accurate.

DEVELOPING A RESUMÉ OR CURRICULUM VITAE

Every technician should develop and maintain a resumé or a curriculum vitae (CV); these documents are one of the keys to capturing the attention of hiring managers and obtaining a new role or position.

A resumé is a compilation of one's skills, education and accomplishments. It provides a prospective employer with information to help them determine if a job candidate has the necessary knowledge and skills to be successful in a specific role. A CV is an academic summary of the individual's experience, skills and accomplishments. CVs include personal teaching experience, awards, degrees and published works. There are key differences between the two documents. A resumé is usually used by professionals who are reasonably new to a job position or profession, and resumés are usually one to two pages in length. A CV is typically provided by professionals with extensive experience in the position being sought (or similar positions); this document is lengthier than a resumé and highlights accomplishments in the important areas of the new position.

Professional Development Skills-Building	
Desired Skill	**Skill Building Activities**
Public speaking: • Teaching • Presentations • Speaking in larger groups	• Start with smaller presentations such as reports and small inservices. Work up to larger presentations for larger groups. • Join a speaking development group. • Take a public speaking class.
Technical expertise	• Pursue additional knowledge through courses, certification, job shadowing and self-study. • Participate in committees through one's facility or local and national professional organizations. • Take steps to keep up with challenges in regulations, standards and technologies.
Team building skills	• Start by examining one's relationships with their current team. What can be improved? • Move outside one's comfort zone and work with different teams for short projects. • Read articles on team building.

Figure 24.5

One concept of professional development is building a resumé or CV through the advancement of skills. For example, if one aspires to become an SP staff educator, gaining experience presenting inservices, training new employees, or developing educational tools for the department can strengthen those skills.

Sometimes, obtaining a new position, either externally or through a promotion within the current healthcare facility, can be decided by a very small margin. For example, if an individual's resumé includes experience in staff education, that may offer an advantage in the selection process for an educator position.

Many templates exist to assist with writing a resumé or CV. Regardless of the chosen format, be sure to follow these simple rules:

- Be truthful.
- Research the duties of the job being sought and use personal experiences to help demonstrate to the employer or hiring manager that you are the best candidate for the job.
- Write the resumé or CV to the desired job position and include experiences that complement the job position.
- Include education and skills that complement the desired position.
- Organize information in a logical fashion and keep the information clear and concise.
- Spell out all acronyms to ensure clarity with the presented information.
- Use a resumé template. Numerous templates can be found at no charge on the internet.
- Carefully proofread the entire document to ensure there are no typographical or experience errors. Consider having another professional review the document as well.
- Ensure the resumé or CV is attention-getting for all the right reasons. Use a high-grade resumé paper and consider using a professional (yet slightly less-used) font. An off-white or pale-grey paper may also help differentiate one's resumé from others.
- Avoid injecting humor into the resumé or CV.
- Do not submit a personal photograph or video with the resumé or CV.
- Exclude sensitive information (age, marital status, religious affiliation, etc.).
- Keep the document updated so it is always ready when needed.

UNDERSTANDING THE INTERVIEW PROCESS

SP technicians are involved during the initial selection process, and they participate in performance evaluations that typically include an interview-like component. While much of process is controlled by the manager or another person conducting the interview, the interviewee (SP technician) can benefit from using basic speaking and listening techniques during these sessions. This is especially important because contemporary interviewing methods emphasize a participative approach whereby the person conducting the interview interacts with rather than "lectures to" the interviewee.

Interviewers may ask two types of questions: open-ended and closed-ended. Open-ended questions permit the interviewee to respond in an unstructured manner. Behavioral questioning is an open-ended approach that utilizes past behaviors to help predict future actions or behaviors. This type of questioning is used to help judge a candidate's problem-solving skills and focuses on how a candidate handled various work situations.

Examples of open-ended and behavioral questions may include:

- What do you think the role of a SP technician should be?
- Can you provide an example of a time when you communicated successfully with another person, even when that individual may not have agreed with your point of view?

Closed-ended questions call for a brief response. Examples may include:

- Do you like your job?
- Do you understand the correct way to do this task?

Many interviews include both open- and closed-ended questions. One important step in preparing for any interview is to carefully research the job and anticipate the types of questions likely to be asked, and then plan a response for them. A good response is one that answers the question and provides supporting details. This is an opportunity to display one's knowledge and understanding for the profession, not to provide "textbook answers. Along with well-thought-out responses, an interviewee should also prepare some questions for the interviewer. This demonstrates an interest for the position and allows the interviewee to participate in the interview process.

There are several different types of interviews. The most common is a face-to-face interview with either a Human Resources (HR) staff member or an SPD supervisor. (See **Figure 24.6**) In some instances, a candidate will meet with the HR person, followed by the SPD supervisor.

Some facilities use group interviews for many positions. These interviews include SP personnel and staff members from other departments like the OR. This type of interview may seem more stressful, however, if one researches the position and practices responses to anticipated questions, stress will be lessened.

Recently, online interviews have become more popular. This type of interview may be done for positions in another city or state but may be also done for any job opening, even when applying for a position in one's current facility.

Interviews should be approached thoughtfully and professionally. Dress professionally (even for online interviews), be punctual and take the interview seriously. Even if interviewing for a position at one's current place of employment, it is important to follow these general interview protocols to demonstrate professionalism and readiness for a change and added responsibilities.

Four Basic Steps for Any Type of Interview

Step 1: Ensure the exact purpose of the interview is known, along with the time, location and estimated duration.

Step 2: Be prepared for the opening conversation. Hopefully, there will be an initial discussion of mutual topics of interest to move the discussion away from ongoing work considerations to the specific topic. Professional SP technicians should have the confidence, pride, expertise, and positive attitude to allow them to be confident during the interview.

Step 3: Understand that questions will be asked. This is where the interviewee's anticipation of potential questions and ability to effectively speak and listen will be most useful. It is also where application of the speaking and listening tactics outlined previously will be most helpful.

Step 4: Recognize that the interview discussion can be reviewed. Ideally, the interviewer will provide a summary. The SP technician should provide reactions to this review so that both parties can agree on what was decided and which, if any, follow-up activities should be undertaken.

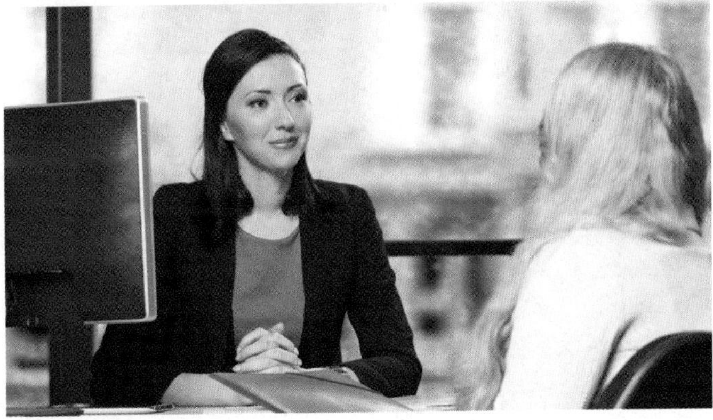

Figure 24.6

PROMOTIONS

Many SP technicians who perform their jobs well have opportunities for promotion to positions with additional responsibilities and, often, higher compensation. Those who accept these positions will likely find many differences in tasks, especially if they assume supervisory duties. Challenges arise when a staff member who has been a peer to other employees becomes their supervisor. Relationships change and must reflect the new supervisor/**subordinate** dynamic.

Subordinate An employee who is supervised by someone in a higher organizational position.

All management positions must consider the broader needs of the department and the healthcare facility before the specific needs of individual staff members.

SP technicians who are considering promotions should also recognize that some tasks will be different. Technicians with the knowledge and skills to perform cleaning, decontamination and related tasks, for example, may not be as comfortable performing supervisory activities, such as planning, coordinating, directing, controlling and evaluating.

Long-term planning that leads to promotion-related decisions should be an integral part of SP technicians' professional development process.

Positive Behaviors That Get Noticed

- Ability to work effectively on a team
- Practicing effective time management
- Being courteous, friendly and helpful
- Taking responsibility for actions, outcomes and personal and professional growth
- Collaborating with co-workers and outside departments
- Being respectful
- Demonstrating a "can-do" attitude
- Having good attendance
- Asking questions
- Mentoring others
- Working well with difficult co-workers
- Possessing critical-thinking skills

PERSONAL AND PROFESSIONAL DEVELOPMENT TIMELINES

Some personal and professional development goals are easier to attain than others. Promotions usually don't happen overnight, and preparing for promotions takes time as well. Personal and professional development timelines should be realistic and achievable. Goals require planning, commitment and an understanding that things don't always go as planned. When setbacks occur, and they sometimes do, it is essential to regroup and continue moving toward established goals.

Formal Education

Continuing formal education, either through a community college, technical college or four-year university, should be a consideration for anyone interested in career advancement. Many schools now have online classes and self-study programs that make it easier to continue formal education goals.

The first step is for the individual to decide where they want to be in the future and what the requirements of that position entail. Many management positions require some type of degree, for example. Depending on the position, a two-year Associate's or technical degree may be required, and other positions may require a four-year degree. If the ultimate goal is to remain in one's current position, obtaining some formal education may help maintain a position in an ever-growing field. Many technical schools have courses in communication, public speaking, planning, leadership, and time and project management, all of which are helpful skills for almost any vocation. While educational institutions typically encourage students to register for multiple courses during a quarter or semester, it is also possible to take only one course at a time. Starting with one course may be more manageable with many professionals' busy lifestyles. If it has been some time since the individual has left school, taking a course that is interesting and fun can help them re-acclimate to time requirements for school and study. Bear in mind that the course may have nothing to do with the workplace or specific position being sought; the important thing is that professionals seeking to advance their careers take steps to begin the learning and career advancement process.

CONCLUSION

The SP profession is dynamic and ever evolving and requires professional and dynamic individuals to help lead the way in education, systems development and departmental management. Through personal and professional development, SP technicians can not only enhance the skills necessary to improve within their current positions but they can also create new opportunities for career fulfillment and growth.

RESOURCES

Healthcare Sterile Processing Association. *Central Service Leadership Manual.* 2020.

Safani B. "Happy about My Resume. 50 Tips for Building a Better Document and Securing a Brighter Future." 2008.

McDaniel A. "The Young Professional's Guide to the Working World: Savvy Strategies to Get in, Get ahead, and Rise to the Top." 2013.

STERILE PROCESSING TERMS

Personal development

Professional development

Subordinate

In Appreciation

Developing any technical book relies heavily on researchers, authors, change to: photographers, content experts, reviewers and graphic designers. The Healthcare Sterile Processing Association would like to thank all who contributed to the development of the ninth edition of the *Sterile Processing Technical Manual.*

It is because of each contributor that this edition is sure to become a valuable and trusted educational resource for professional development and knowledge advancement.

Glossary

A

AAMI Abbreviation for the Association for the Advancement of Medical Instrumentation

ABC analysis Inventory management strategy that indicates storeroom controls should first address the relatively few items with the greatest value (A items) and should lastly consider the many items with the lowest value (C items)

Abdomen Part of the body between the chest and pelvis

Abduction Movement away from the midline; turning outward

Abort Failed or incomplete machine cycle caused by a malfunction

Abrasive Any of a wide variety of natural or manufactured gritty substances used to grind, wear down, rub away, smooth or scour

Abscess Area of tissue breakdown; a localized space in the body containing pus and liquified tissue

Absolute pressure (steam sterilizer) Gauge pressure (machine produced) plus (+) atmospheric pressure (14.7 pounds per square inch at sea level)

Absorbent towel All-cotton towel featuring a plain weave with only the warp yarns tightly twisted

Acceptance sampling Inspection of a sample from a larger lot to determine whether the lot should be accepted

ACGIH Abbreviation for the American Conference of Governmental Industrial Hygienists

Acid Compound with a pH less than 7.0 and with a sour, sharp or biting taste; compound with a water solution that contains positive hydrogen ions (e.g., HCl)

Acid detergent Organic, acid-based cleaning agent; best used for removing mineral deposits

Acid-fast bacteria Bacteria that do not decolorize when acid is added to the stained smear

Acidity Measurement of the amount of acid present

Acidosis Condition that results from a decrease in the pH of body fluids

Acid scrubber Type of ethylene oxide (EO) emission control device

Acquired immune deficiency syndrome (AIDS) Viral disease that attacks the immune system

Acquired immunity Immunity acquired by a person after birth

Action level Level of exposure to a harmful substance or other hazards at which an employer must take required precautions to protect workers; usually one half of the permissible exposure limit (PEL)

Activated (activation) Process by which a solution is combined with an activating chemical before use; glutaraldehyde, for example, must be mixed with an activating solution before use

Acute Short in time; relatively severe in degree

Acute disease Disease or disorder that lasts a brief time, comes on rapidly and is accompanied by distinct symptoms

Adhesion Holding together two surfaces or parts; band of connective tissue between parts that are normally separate; the molecular attraction between contacting bodies

Adipose Referring to fatty tissue

Adrenal Endocrine gland located above the kidney; suprarenal gland

Aerate To expose gas-sterilized items to warm, circulating air

Aeration Process in which sterilized packages are subjected to moving air to facilitate the removal of toxic residuals after exposure to a sterilizing agent, such as ethylene oxide (EO)

Aerator (ethylene oxide) Machine designed to speed up removal of ethylene oxide (EO) residuals from sterilized items by subjecting them to warm, circulating air

Aerobe Microorganism that requires the presence of air or oxygen for growth

Aerobic Requiring the presence of air or free oxygen

Aerosol Suspension of ultramicroscopic solid or liquid particles in air or gas; a spray

Affinity Attraction

Agar Extract of red seaweed used as a solidifying agent in culture media

AIDS Abbreviation for acquired immune deficiency syndrome, the advanced symptomatic and often fatal disease in the progression of an HIV infection

Airborne Suspended or carried in a gas or air stream

Air count Method of estimating the number of bacteria or microbes in a specific quantity of air

Albumin Protein in blood plasma and other body fluids that helps to maintain the osmotic pressure of the blood

Alimentary canal Pathway that food takes through the body's digestive system; also called digestive tract

Alkalis Chemicals that release an excess of hydroxyl ions (OH) in a solution to yield a pH greater than 7

Alkaline In solution; having a pH greater than 7

Alkalosis Condition that results from an increase in the pH of body fluids

Alkylation Chemical reaction where hydrogen is replaced with an alkyl group, rendering the cell unable to normally metabolize or reproduce (or both)

Allergen Substance that causes hypersensitivity; substance that induces allergy

Allergic Caused by allergy

Allergy Tendency to react unfavorably to a certain substance that is normally harmless to most people; hypersensitivity

Alveolus (pl. alveoli) One of millions of tiny air sacs in the lungs through which gases are exchanged between the outside air and blood; tooth socket

Ambient condition Environmental conditions, such as pressure, temperature and humidity, which are normal for a specific location

Amebiasis Infection with pathogenic amebas; acute amebiasis is called amebic dysentery

Amino acid Building block of protein; organic chemical compounds containing an amino group and a carboxyl group; forms the chief structure of proteins

Amitosis Directs the division of cells

Amniocentesis Removal of fluid and cells from the amniotic sac for prenatal diagnostic tests

Amniotic sac Fluid-filled sac that surrounds and cushions the developing fetus

Amoeba Protozoa that moves by extruding finger-like elements (pseudopods); also spelled ameba

Amoeboid movement Crawling movement of cells that occurs as the cell successively becomes longer and then retracts

Anaerobe Microorganism that grows only or best in the absence of oxygen

Anaerobic Bacteria that can live in the absence of atmospheric oxygen

Analgesic Relieving pain; a pain-relieving agent that does not cause loss of consciousness

Anaphylaxis State of hypersensitivity to a protein resulting from a previous introduction of the protein into the body; may result in death without treatment

Anastomosis Surgical or pathological formation of a passage between two normally distinct structures such as tubular organs

Anatomy Study of the structure and relationships between body parts

Anemia Reduction in the amount of red cells or hemoglobin in the blood, resulting in inadequate delivery of oxygen to the tissues

Anesthesia Loss of sensation (particularly of pain)

Aneurysm Bulging sac in the wall of a vessel

Angina Severe choking pain; disease or condition producing such pain

Angina pectoris Suffocating pain in the chest, usually caused by lack of oxygen supply to the heart

Animate Having life

Anion Negatively charged particle (ion)

Anionic Compounds with a negative electrical charge on the large organic portion of the molecule, which are relatively hydrophobic and lipophilic; used as synthetic detergents

Anorexia Loss of appetite

Anoxia Lack of oxygen

ANSI Abbreviation for the American National Standards Institute

Antagonist Muscle with an action opposite that of a given movement; substance that opposes the action of another substance

Anterior Toward the front or belly surface; ventral

Anthrax Infectious disease of cattle and sheep caused by a spore-forming bacterium (*Bacillus anthracis*), which may be transmitted to man through the handling of infected products

Antibacterial serum Antiserum that destroys or prevents the growth of bacteria

Antibiotic Substance produced by one microorganism that will kill or inhibit another microorganism

Antibody Protein produced in the body that reacts against a specific foreign molecule (antigen)

Antigen Substance that causes the body to produce antibodies

Antiseptic Solution that inhibits the growth of bacteria; usually used topically and only on animate (living) objects

Antiserum Serum containing antibodies given to provide passive immunity

Antitoxin Immune serum that neutralizes the action of a toxin

Anus Lower opening of the alimentary canal

Anvil One of the three middle ear bones; attaches to the hammer and stirrup

AORN Abbreviation for the Association of periOperative Registered Nurses

Aorta Largest blood vessel in the body

APIC Abbreviation for the Association for Professionals in Infection Control and Epidemiology

Aqueous humor Watery-like fluid between the cornea and the eye lens

Aqueous solution Liquid in which a chemical substance is dissolved in water

Arteriole Vessel between a small artery and capillary

Arrhythmia Abnormal rhythm of the heartbeat

Arteries Vessels that carry blood away from the heart

Arteriosclerosis Hardening of the arteries

Arthritis Inflammation of the joints

Asepsis Absence of microorganisms that cause disease

Asepsis (medical) Clean technique; procedures performed to reduce the number of microorganisms and minimize their spread

Asepsis (surgical) Surgical technique; procedures performed to eliminate the presence of all microorganisms and/or prevent the introduction of microorganisms to an area

Aseptic Free from pathogenic organisms; a means of preventing infection

Aseptic technique Any activity or procedure that prevents infection or breaks the chain of infection

Asphyxia Condition caused by lack of oxygen in inspired air

Aspirate To draw by suction. Example: When fluid is removed with a syringe and material is drawn into the lungs during inspiration

Assembly area A clean area of the Sterile Processing department where inspection, assembly and packaging functions are performed; sometimes called the preparation and packaging (prep and pack) area

Asset Something of value owned by an organization or person

Asset (current) Asset that is expected to be used within one year

Asymptomatic Shows no signs or symptoms of disease or infection

Atherosclerosis Hardening of the arteries caused by deposits of yellowish, fat-like material on blood vessel linings

Atom Fundamental unit of a chemical element

Atria Upper two chambers of the heart

Atrium One of the two upper chambers of the heart

Atrophy Wasting or decreasing in size of a part

Attitude Emotions that cause a person to react to people and/or situations in a predetermined way

Austenitic stainless steel Material also known as 300 stainless steel; it is nonmagnetic, cannot be heat hardened and is more corrosion-resistant than martensitic stainless steel

Autoclave Equipment that uses steam under pressure to sterilize, usually at temperatures of 250° or 270°F (121°C or 132°C)

Automated supply replenishment system Replenishment system in which items removed from inventory are automatically identified and tracked. When a reorder point is reached, item information is generated on a supply pick list in the central storeroom or by a contracted vendor. Items are then issued and transferred to the appropriate user area.

Automatic endoscope reprocessor (AER) Automated equipment designed to clean, disinfect and rinse flexible endoscopes

Autonomic nervous system Part of the nervous system that controls smooth muscle, cardiac muscle and glands; motor portion of the visceral or involuntary nervous system

Autopsy Examination of the internal organs of a dead body

Axilla Hollow beneath the arm where it joins the body; armpit

B

Bacillus (pl., bacilli) Rod-shaped bacteria; a genus of the family *Bacillaceae*

Bacillus *atrophaeus* Resistant microorganism used to challenge ethylene oxide (EO) sterilizers

Bacillus stearothermophilus See *Geobacillus stearo thermophilus*

Bacillus subtilis See Bacillus *atrophaeus*

Bacteremia Condition in which bacteria are in the bloodstream

Bacteria (sing. bacterium) Single-celled, plant-like microbes that reproduce by splitting; some cause diseases; also called germs

Bacterial count Method of estimating the number of bacteria in a sample unit

Bactericidal A substance that kills bacteria

Bactericide Substance that kills bacteria

Bacteriology Science of the study of bacteria

Bacteriostasis Condition in which bacterial growth is inhibited, but the organisms are not killed

Bacteriostat Substance that inhibits the growth of bacteria

Bacteriostatic Inhibition of bacterial growth, but without their destruction

Balance sheet Financial summary of what a healthcare facility owns (assets), owes (liabilities) and is worth (equity) at a specific point in time (e.g., the last day of every month)

Barcode Numerous machine-readable rectangular bars and spaces arranged in a specific way to represent letters, numbers and other symbols

Barrier cloth Fabrics made of blends or cotton/polyester

Barrier packaging Provides a barrier from microorganisms and allows aseptic presentation of the product at the point of use

Barrier properties Ability of a material to resist the penetration of liquids and/or microorganisms

Base Compound with a pH above 7.0 whose water solution yields negative hydroxyl ions (e.g., NaOH) and combines with an acid to form a salt and water; turns red litmus paper blue

Basophil Granular white blood cell that shows large, dark-blue cytoplasmic granules when stained with a basic stain

Benign Tumor that does not spread, is not recurrent or becoming worse; not malignant

Best practice Method or technique that has consistently shown results superior to those achieved by other means

Bevel Angle at which the point of a needle is ground

Bile Substance produced in the liver that emulsifies fat

Binary fission Typical method of bacterial reproduction in which a cell divides into two equal parts

Bioburden Number of microorganisms on an object; also called bioload or microbial load

Biocidal Process or ability to kill or control the growth of living organisms

Biocide Substance or microorganism that kills or controls the growth of living organisms

Biodegradable Readily decomposed by bacteria or enzymatic actions

Biofilm Collection of microorganisms that attaches to surfaces and each other and form a colony; the colony produces a protective gel that is difficult to penetrate with detergents and disinfectants

Biohazard signage Notices posted in easily seen locations that alert people in the area about the presence of harmful bacteria, viruses or other dangerous biohazardous agents or organisms

Biohazardous waste Waste containing infectious agents that presents a risk or potential risk to human health

Biological Relating to biology

Biological indicator (BI) Sterilization process monitoring device consisting of a standardized, viable population of microorganisms (usually bacterial spores) known to be resistant to the mode of sterilization being monitored

Biological transfer of infection Mode of transfer of infection from host to host by an animal or insect in which the disease-causing agent goes through a development cycle

Biology Science which studies living things, both animals and plants

Biomedical/Clinical Engineering department Healthcare department responsible for performing safety inspections and function tests on medical equipment; frequently abbreviated as Biomed department; Also known as Healthcare Technology Management department

Biopsy Removal of tissue or other material from the living body for examination, usually under the microscope

Blood Type of connective tissue fluid that transports many substances throughout the circulatory system

Body system Group of organs that work together to carry out a specific activity

Borosilicate Alkaline-free silicate glass with at least 5% boric oxide and used especially in heat-resistant glassware; a very hard glass (Pyrex)

Botulism Food poisoning caused by the toxin of an anaerobic, spore-forming bacterium (clostridium botulinum) in contaminated canned or smoked foods

Bowie-Dick test Test run daily to validate the vacuum function of the sterilizer; test should be run in an empty load and at the same time each day

Box locks Point where the two jaws or blades of an instrument connect and pivot

Bradycardia Heart rate of less than 60 beats per minute

Brain Main control unit of the central nervous system (CNS)

Brain stem Controls many automatic body functions such as heartbeat and breathing

Break out The process of removing commercially sterilized items from their outer shipping containers in an area adjacent to the storage area to prevent contamination that is present on the containers from being introduced into the storage area

Broad spectrum Term indicating that an antibiotic is effective against a large array of microorganisms

Bronchi Main passageway for air to travel from the trachea to the lungs

Bronchiole One of the small bronchial subdivisions that branches throughout the lungs

Buffer Substance that prevents sharp changes in the pH of a solution

Bursa Small, fluid-filled sac in an area subjected to stress around bones and joints

C

Calibration Comparison of a measurement system or device of unknown accuracy to a national standard of known accuracy to detect, correlate, report or adjust any variation from the required performance limits of the unverified measurement system or device

Cancer Uncontrolled growth of a tumor that spreads to other tissue; a malignant neoplasm

Cannulas Surgical instruments with a hollow barrel (or lumen) through their center; often inserted for drainage

Capillaries Vessels that serve as connections between veins and arteries

Capillary action Attraction or repulsion force caused by the surface tension of liquids in hair-like tubes

Capital equipment Item of major importance; usually defined by a set dollar amount and which is depreciated over the useful life of the equipment rather than being expensed at purchase

Capital (equipment) Assets that are relatively expensive, such as sterilizers or washers, that require significant advance planning for their purchase

Capsule Gelatinous, colorless envelope or slime layer surrounding the cell wall of certain microorganisms; a membrane or sack containing a body part

Carbohydrate Simple sugar or compound made from simple sugars linked together

Carbon dioxide (C02) Gaseous waste product of cellular metabolism

Carcinogen Cancer-causing substance

Carcinoma Malignant growth of epithelial cells; a form of cancer

Cardiopulmonary resuscitation (CPR) Method to restore heartbeat and breathing by mouth-to-mouth resuscitation and closed chest cardiac massage

Carditis Inflammation of the heart; myocarditis

Career ladder Plan projecting progressively more responsible professional positions that serves as a foundation for a professional development program

Caries Tooth decay

Carpals Wrist bones

Carrier Person who is infected with an infectious disease but displays no symptoms; although unaffected by the disease themselves, carriers may transmit the disease to others

Cartilage Type of flexible connective tissue

Case cart Prepared for an individual procedure; usually contains all instruments, supplies and utensils needed for a specific procedure

Case cart pull sheet (pick list) List of specific supplies, utensils and instruments for a specific procedure; used by Sterile Processing technicians to assemble the items needed for individual procedures

Case cart system Inventory control system for products/equipment typically used in an Operating Room that involves the use of an enclosed or covered cart; generally prepared for one surgical case and not used for general supply replenishment

CAT scan See Computed tomography

Catalyst Substance that influences the speed of a chemical reaction without being consumed

Catalytic converter Type of ethylene oxide (EO) emission control device

Cataract Opacity of the eye lens or lens capsule

Catheter Slender, flexible tube of rubber, plastic or metal used for draining a body cavity or injecting fluids through a body passage

Cation Positively charged particle (ion)

Cation resin tank Vessel into which untreated hard water flows, and in which sodium ions are exchanged for calcium and magnesium ions to produce soft water

Cationic Compounds containing a positive electrical charge on the large organic hydrophobic molecule and which exhibit germicidal properties

Causative agent (chain of infection) Microorganism that causes an infectious disease

Caustic Corrosive and burning; agent, particularly an alkali, that will destroy living tissue

Cautery Burner; means of destroying tissue by electricity, heat or corrosive chemicals. Thermocautery consists of a red– or white-hot object, usually a wire or pointed metallic instrument heated in a flame or with electricity.

Cavitation Process used by an ultrasonic cleaner in which low-pressure bubbles collapse (implode) and dislodge soil from instruments

CDC Abbreviation for the Centers for Disease Control and Prevention (part of the Department of Health and Human Services); investigates outbreaks and control various diseases

Cecum Small pouch at the beginning of the large intestine

Ceiling limit Maximum safe airborne concentration of a potentially toxic substance

Cell Basic unit of life; the smallest structural unit of living organisms capable of performing all basic functions of life

Cell membrane Outer covering of a cell that regulates what enters and leaves it

Cellulitis Diffuse inflammation of connective tissues

Centigrade Thermometer temperature scale with 100° between the melting point of ice at 0° and the boiling point of water at 100°

Central nervous system (CNS) Part of the nervous system that includes the brain and spinal cord

Centrifuge Device used to spin test tubes; used in the laboratory

Cerebellum Second largest part of the brain that controls muscle coordination, body balance and posture

Cerebrospinal fluid (CSF) Fluid that circulates in and around the brain and spinal cord

Cerebrovascular accident (CVA) Condition involving bleeding from the brain or obstruction of blood flow to brain tissue, usually resulting from hypertension or atherosclerosis; also called stroke

Cerebrum Largest part of the brain; controls mental activities and movement

Certification Association and industry recognition given to individuals with educational and/or work experience requirements who successfully complete an examination process that demonstrates their knowledge of subject-matter to be mastered for success in the position

Cervix Lower end (neck) of the uterus

Chlorofluorocarbon (CHC) Inert (inflammable) gas often mixed with a flammable gas to create an inflammable solution; has been used with ethylene oxide (EO) to create an inert gas

Chain of infection Six-step process of an infection spreading from one host to the next

Challenge test pack Used in qualification, installation and ongoing quality assurance testing of hospital sterilizers

Chamber Enclosed area that holds products to be sterilized

Chelating agents Chemicals that hold hard water minerals in solution and prevent soaps or detergents from reacting with the minerals

Chemical indicators (CIs) Devices used to monitor the presence or attainment of one or more of the parameters required for a satisfactory sterilization process

Chemical sterilization Process using a chemical agent to render a product free of viable microorganisms

Chemotherapy Treatment of disease without injury to patient with chemicals having a specific effect on microorganisms

Chickenpox Varicella; rather mild, highly contagious virus disease characterized by fever and the appearance of vesicles

Chisels Wedge-shaped instruments used to cut or shape bone

CHL Abbreviation for Certification in Healthcare Leadership, a certification offered by the Healthcare Sterile Processing Association

Chloride Compound commonly found in water created when chlorine is combined with another element or radical (e.g., salt and hydrochloric acid)

Chlorophyll Molecule in plants that absorbs sunlight and converts it to energy in a process called photosynthesis

Cholesterol Organic, fat-like compound found in animal fat, bile blood, myelin, liver and other parts of the body

Chromium Blue-white metallic element found naturally only in combination and used in alloys and electroplating

Chromogenic Producing a pigment

Chromosomes Rod-shaped structures responsible for inherited characteristics passed from parent to child

Chronic Referring to a disease (illness) that is not severe but is continuous, recurring, protracted and prolonged

Cilia (sing. cilium) Hair-like elements that spring from certain cells and, by their action, create currents in liquids. If cells are fixed, the liquid is made to flow; if cells are unicellular organisms suspended in the liquid, the cells move.

Circumduction Circular movement at a joint

Cirrhosis Chronic disease (usually of the liver) in which active cells are replaced by inactive scar tissue

CIS Abbreviation for Certified Instrument Specialist, a certification offered by the Healthcare Sterile Processing Association

CJD Abbreviation for Creutzfeldt-Jakob Disease, a debilitating, fatal brain disease; see Prions

Cleaning Removal of all visible and non-visible soil and any other foreign material from medical devices being processed

Clostridium Genus of cylindrical-shaped bacteria that are anaerobic, gram positive and spore forming

Cloud computing Practice of storing regularly used computer data on multiple servers that can be accessed through the internet

Coaching Positive reinforcement used to encourage Sterile Processing technicians to follow proper work behavior, and negative reinforcement to discourage inappropriate work behavior

Coagulase Enzyme that causes coagulation or clotting of blood serum

Coagulation Clotting (as in blood)

Coccus Round-shaped (spherical) bacterium

Coccyx Tailbone

Cochlea Coiled portion of the inner ear that contains the organs of hearing

Cold boil Cavitation that is not dependent upon heat for its bubbling action

Coliform bacteria Group of intestinal microorganisms of which Escherichia coli is a member

Collagen Flexible white protein that gives strength and resiliency to connective tissue, including bone and cartilage

Colon Main portion of the large intestine

Colonization Process that occurs when microorganisms live on or in a host organism but do not invade tissues or cause damage

Colony Visible growth of microorganisms seen in culture medium; usually obtained from a single organism

Colony count Determination of the number of visible clumps of bacteria derived from the multiplication of specific microorganisms on or in a culture medium

Combining vowel Letter (typically an "o") that is sometimes used to ease the pronunciation of a medical word

Combustible Substance that, if ignited, will react with oxygen and burn

Combustible Loading weight of combustible materials per square foot of area in which the materials are located

Combustion Chemical process accompanied by the rapid production of heat and light

Communicable Disease whose causative agent is easily transmitted from person to person by direct or indirect contact

Communication Process of transmitting information and understanding from one person to another by use of words and non-verbal expressions such as body language

Complication Secondary illness imposed upon a person with a primary illness

Compound Substance composed of two or more chemical elements

Computed tomography Imaging method in which multiple x-ray views taken from different angles are analyzed by computer to show a cross section of an area; used to detect tumors and other abnormalities; abbreviated CT or CAT (computed axial tomography)

Conditioning Treatment of products within the sterilization cycle but before sterilant admission to attain a predetermined temperature and relative humidity; may be carried out at atmospheric pressure or under vacuum

Conduction Heat transfer method in which heat is absorbed by an item's exterior surface and passed inward to the next layer

Conduction heating Process in which heat is transmitted in a solid substance from molecule to molecule by molecular impact or agitation

Conductivity (of water) Measurement of the ability of water to carry an electrical current

Congenital Present at birth

Conjunctiva Membrane that lines the eyelid and covers the anterior part of the sclera

Conjunctivitis Inflammation of the conjunctiva of the eye

Consignment inventory Inventory in the possession of the healthcare facility but still owned by the supplier

Consumable (inventory) Assets such as wrapping supplies, processing chemicals and other items that are consumed as healthcare services are provided to patients

Contagious Highly communicable; easily transmitted

Contaminate To render unfit for use through the introduction of a substance that is harmful or injurious

Contamination State of being soiled by contact with infectious organisms or other materials

Continuous quality improvement (CQI) Scientific approach that applies statistical methods to improve work processes

Contraception Prevention of fertilization of an ovum or implantation of a fertilized ovum; birth control

Convalescence Period during which recovery takes place following illness

Convection Process of heat transfer by the circulation of currents from one area to another

Convection heating Transfer of heat in a fluid or gas from one place to another by the motion of the fluid or gas

Copious Present in a large amount (such as large volume of rinsing water)

Cornea Clear portion of sclera that covers the front of the eye

Coronary Referring to the heart or arteries supplying blood to the heart

Corrosion Act of wearing away gradually by a chemical reaction

Corrosive Having the power to corrode or wear away

Cortex Outer layer of an organ such as the brain, kidney, or adrenal gland

Counterstain Second stain of a contrasting kind applied to a smear for the purpose of making the microorganisms treated with a primary stain more distinct

CPR Abbreviation for cardiopulmonary resuscitation

CPU Abbreviation for central processing unit

Craze Spiderweb cracking of plastics under chemical stress

CRCST Abbreviation for Certified Registered Central Service Technician, a certification offered by the Healthcare Sterile Processing Association

Crisis Change in a disease that indicates whether the result will be recovery or death

Critical devices Refers to the Spaulding medical device classification system; instruments or objects introduced directly into the bloodstream or other normally sterile body areas

Critical parameters Parameters that are essential to the sterilization process and require monitoring

Critical water Water treated extensively to ensure that microorganisms and organic and inorganic material are removed

Cross contamination Migration of contaminants from one person, object or work location to another

Cross-functional team Group of employees from different departments within the healthcare facility that work together to resolve operating problems

Cross infection Infection acquired from an animate or inanimate contaminated environment, usually accidentally

Culture Growth of microorganisms on a nutrient medium; to grow microorganisms on such medium

Culture medium Substance or preparation used for the growth and cultivation of microorganisms

Customer (internal) Physicians, nurses and other professional personnel served by Sterile Processing personnel

Cutaneous Referring to the skin

Cyanosis Bluish color of the skin and mucous membranes resulting from insufficient oxygen in the blood

Cycle buying Purchasing method in which an order is placed at a scheduled interval

Cycle (gravitation-displacement type; steam sterilization) Sterilization cycle in which incoming steam displaces residual air through a port or drain in or near the bottom of the sterilizer chamber

Cycle (sterilization) Defined sequence of operational steps designed to achieve sterilization; carried out in a sealed chamber

Cycle time Total elapsed time of a sterilization cycle from when the sterilizer door is closed and the cycle is activated until the cycle is completed and the door is opened

Cystitis Inflammation of the urinary bladder

Cytology Study of cells

Cytoplasm Clear, jelly-like substance of a cell between the cell membrane and nucleus

D

D-value Amount of time required to kill 90% of the microorganisms present

Debridement Surgical removal of dead or unhealthy tissue

Decontamination To make safe by removing or reducing contamination by infectious organisms or other harmful substances to an acceptable level

Decontamination area Location within a healthcare facility designated for the collection, retention and cleaning of soiled and/or contaminated items

Defecation Act of eliminating undigested waste from the digestive tract

Defect Variance from expected standards

Deflocculate To reduce or break up into very fine particles

Degeneration Breaking down (as from age, injury or disease)

Degerm To remove bacteria and other microbes by mechanical cleaning and applying antiseptics or disinfectants

Dehydration Excessive loss of body fluid

Deionization Process by which ions with an electrical charge are removed from water

Deionize To remove ions from a substance (such as water)

Deionized (DI) water Water that has had all minerals removed through an ion exchange process

Delayed processing Cleaning instructions for endoscopes that have not been processed within an hour after the completion of point-of-use treatment

Denatured alcohol Alcohol that has been rendered unfit for use as a beverage by the addition of substances that impart an unpleasant odor and taste (e.g., wood alcohol and benzene)

Density Degree of compactness; closely set; thickness

Deoxyribonucleic acid (DNA) One of two nucleic acids; essential for biological inheritance

Dermatitis Inflammation of the skin

Dermis True skin; deeper part of the skin

Detergent Cleaning agent composed of a surface wetting agent that reduces surface tension; a "builder" that is the principle cleaning agent, and a sequestering or chelating agent to suspend the soil; any chemical that causes oil or grease to dissolve in water and cleans the item on which it is used. Unlike soap, detergent does not contain fat or lye. Detergents may also have additional additives such as blood solvents or rust inhibitors.

Detergent/germicide Combination of a cleaning agent and disinfectant

Detergent/sanitizer Combination of chemicals that possess antibacterial and cleaning properties

Dextrose Glucose; simple sugar

Diabetes mellitus Disease in which glucose is not oxidized in body tissues for energy because of insufficient insulin

Diagnosis Identification of an illness

Dialysis Method to separate molecules in a solution based on differences in their rates of diffusion through a semi-permeable membrane; method for removing nitrogen waste products from the body by hemodialysis or peritoneal dialysis

Diaphragm Dome-shaped muscle under the lungs that flattens during inhalation; a separating membrane or structure

Diarrhea Loose and frequent bowel movements

Differential staining Staining technique to distinguish between different bacteria

Diffusion Movement of molecules from a region of higher concentration to a region of lower concentration

Digestion Process of breaking down food into absorbable particles

Dilation Widening of a part (e.g., pupil of the eye, blood vessel, or uterine cervix)

Diphtheria Acute, infectious disease of the mucous membranes of the upper respiratory tract; characterized by patches of *pseudomembrane* and caused by *Corynebacterium diphtheriae*

Diplococci Pairs of cocci

Direct contact Spread of disease from person to person

Disaster (external) Situation in which activities external to the facility affect departmental or facility operations

Disaster (internal) Situation with the potential to cause harm or injury to Sterile Processing or other employees, patients or visitors, or where the loss of utilities may drastically impact departmental operations

Disease State of illness characterized by marked symptoms caused by an infectious agent that produces a definite pathological pattern

Disinfectant Chemical that kills most pathogenic organisms but not all spores

Disinfectant/detergent Chemical compound that contains both a detergent and disinfectant. Usually, the action of both is compromised because of the combination.

Disinfection Destruction of nearly all pathogenic microorganisms on an inanimate (non-living) surface

Disinfestation Destruction of insects, rodents or other animals that transmit infections to other animals, humans or their surroundings

Displacement Process by which one element exchanges with another element through oxidation or reduction; chemical change in which one element, molecule or radical is removed by another

Dissection Process of cutting apart or separating tissue

Dissociation Physical breaking apart of a molecule

Distal End of an item that is farthest away from the point of origin (e.g., the distal end of the femur is closest to the knee); end of the instrument farthest away from the operator

Distill To vaporize by heat and then condense and collect the volatilized product

Distillation Changes from liquid to vapor to liquid; process for removing impurities from liquids

Distilled water Water that is heated to steam and then allowed to cool and condense

Distribution Movement of supplies

Diversity Broad range of human characteristics and dimensions that impact employees' values, opportunities and perceptions of themselves and others at work

DNA See Deoxyribonucleic acid

Doctor's (physician's) preference card Document that identifies a physician's needs (requests and preferences) for a specific medical procedure; usually contains information regarding the instruments, equipment, supplies and utensils used by a specific physician and may also include reminders for staff regarding the physician's preferences for patient draping, instruments and supplies

Dominant Referring to a gene that is always expressed if present

Dorsal Toward the back; posterior

Down time rate (equipment) Number of down days/ number of devices multiplied by 365

Droplet infection Infection transmitted by small drops (particles) of sputum or nasal discharges expelled into the air while talking, coughing or sneezing

Duct Tube or vessel

Duodenum First portion of the small intestine

Dust cover Protective plastic bag used to maintain the sterility of an item by protecting it from the environment; also known as a sterility maintenance cover or protective cover

Dye Material used for staining or coloring bacteria for microscopic examination

Dyspnea Difficult or labored breathing

E

Ebonize Exposure of an instrument to a chemical dip that blackens the metal

ECG Short for electrocardiogram; records electrical activity of the heart to determine if heart disease or other heart conditions are present

Economic order quantity (EOQ) Specific mathematical formula used to determine the most appropriate order quantity based upon usage and other variables

Ectoplasm Outer clear zone of the cytoplasm of a one-celled organism

Edema Presence of abnormally large amounts of fluid in intercellular tissue spaces of the body

EDI Abbreviation for electronic data interchange; process in which orders, invoices and other transactions are transferred electronically between the customer and vendor to create a paperless and more efficient system

EEG Abbreviation for electroencephalogram; records electrical activity of the brain

Effusion Escape of fluid into a space or part; the fluid itself

Ejaculation Expulsion of semen through the urethra

Ejaculatory duct Formed by joining the seminal vesicle with the vas deferens, through which semen moves during ejaculation

Electrocardiograph (ECG or EKG) Instrument to study the electrical activity of the heart; record made is an electrocardiogram

Electroencephalograph (EEG) Instrument used to study electrical activity of the brain; record made is an electroencephalogram

Electrolyte Compound that forms ions in a solution; substance that conducts an electrical current in solution

Electron Negatively charged particle that moves around the nucleus (central core) of an atom

Electroplating Process that uses electrical current in a solution to produce a metallic coating

Electrostatic Pertaining to the attractions and repulsions of electrical charges

Element One substance from which all matter is made; substance that cannot be decomposed into a simpler substance

Embolus Blood clot or other obstruction in the circulation system; the condition is an embolism

Embryo Developing offspring during the first two months of pregnancy

Emesis Vomiting

Emphysema Pulmonary disease characterized by dilation and alveoli destruction

Empowerment Act of granting authority (power) to employees so they may make decisions within their areas of responsibility

Empyema Accumulation of pus in a body cavity, especially the chest

Emulsification Dispersion of two mutually immiscible (unable to be mixed) liquids

Emulsifier Any ingredient used to bind together substances that typically do not combine, such as oil and water

Emulsify To break down large volumes of fat, oil and grease into small globules that are held in suspension

Encephalitis Inflammation of the brain

Encephalomyelitis Inflammation of the brain and spinal cord

Endemic disease One that occurs more or less continuously throughout a community

Endocarditis Inflammation of the endocardium (lining membrane) of the heart, including heart valves

Endocardium Membrane that lines the heart chambers and covers the valves

Endocrine Gland that secretes directly into the bloodstream

Endogenous Originating within the organism

Endometrium Lining of the uterus

Endoscope Instrument used to examine the interior of a hollow organ or body cavity

Endospores (spores) Microorganisms capable of forming a thick wall around themselves, enabling them to survive in adverse conditions

Endothelium Epithelium that lines the heart, blood vessels and lymphatic vessels

Engineering controls Controls (e.g., sharps disposal containers and self-sheathing needles) that isolate or remove bloodborne pathogen hazards from the workplace

Enteric Pertaining to the intestines

Enteric bacteria Bacteria living in or isolated from the intestinal tract

Entrained Process in which a liquid is suspended or carried in a vapor (e.g., water can become entrained in a stream of steam)

Environment Space that surrounds or encompasses a person or object

Enzymatic solution Contains special enzymes that dissolves proteinaceous materials

Enzyme Substance that initiates chemical changes, such as fermentation, without participating in them; a catalyst, usually protein, produced by a living cell with a specific action and optimum activity at a definite pH value

EPA Abbreviation for the U.S. Environmental Protection Agency

Epicardium Membrane that forms the outermost layer of the heart wall and is continuous with the lining of the pericardium; visceral pericardium

Epidemic Occurrence of a disease among many people in a given region at the same time

Epidemiology Study of the occurrence and distribution of disease; usually refers to epidemics

Epidermis Outermost layer of the skin

Epididymis Tube that carries sperm cells from the testes to the vas deferens

Epiglottis Leaf-shaped cartilage that covers the larynx during swallowing

Equipment (capital) Relatively expensive assets, such as sterilizers or washers, that require significant advance planning for their purchase

Equipment utilization rate Days used/number of devices multiplied by 365

Ergonomics Process of changing work or working conditions to reduce employee stress

Erythema Redness of the skin

Erythrocyte Red blood cell (corpuscle)

Esophagus Connects the throat to the stomach

Estrogen Group of female sex hormones that promotes development of the uterine lining and maintains secondary sex characteristics

Ethylene oxide (EO) Chemical (gas) used in low-temperature sterilization; performs as a very effective general purpose sterilant for heat or moisture-sensitive items

Etiology Study of the cause of a disease or the theory of its origin

Eustachian tube Tube that connects the middle ear cavity to the throat; auditory tube

Exacerbation Increase in the severity of a disease

Exchange cart system Inventory system where desired inventory items are placed on a cart assigned to a specific location. A duplicate cart is maintained in another location and exchanged on a scheduled basis to ensure sufficient supplies are available at all times

Excretion To eliminate or give off waste products (e.g., feces, perspiration, urine)

Exfoliate To remove dead cells from a surface using something like a brush or special substance

Exotoxin Soluble, poisonous substance excreted by a living microorganism; can be obtained in bacteria-free filtrates without death or disintegration of the microorganism

Expiration date Calculated by adding a specific period of time to the date of manufacture or sterilization of a medical device or component that defines its estimated useful life

Expiration statement Statement indicating that the contents of a package are sterile indefinitely unless the integrity of the package is compromised

Exposure time Time in which the sterilizer's chamber is maintained within the specified range for temperature, sterilant concentration, pressure and humidity

External solutions Solutions typically used for irrigating, topical application and surgical use (given orally or by inhalation)

Extracellular Outside the cell

Extraction Use of physical force (usually centrifugal or strike/impact) to remove excess water from a wash load prior to drying

Extraneous Outside the organism; not belonging to it

Extrinsic Coming or operating from outside

Exudate Accumulation of a fluid in a cavity or matter that penetrates through the vessel walls into adjoining tissue

F

Facultative Having the power to do something but not ordinarily doing it; capable of adapting to different conditions (e.g., a facultative anaerobe can live in the presence of oxygen but does not ordinarily do so)

Fahrenheit Thermometer scale in which the space between water's freezing point and boiling point is 180°; 32° is the freezing point and 212° is the boiling point. To convert from Fahrenheit to Centigrade scales, subtract 32 and multiply by .5556.

Failure mode and effect analysis (FMEA) Process to predict the adverse outcomes of various human and machine failures to prevent future adverse outcomes

Fallopian tubes Slender tubes that convey the ova (eggs) from the ovaries to the uterus

Families (chemicals) Groups of chemicals that have similar characteristics

Fascia Band or sheet of fibrous connective tissue

FCS Abbreviation for Fellowship in Central Service, a designation offered by the Healthcare Sterile Processing Association

FDA Abbreviation for the U.S. Food and Drug Administration

Febrile Characterized by or pertaining to fever

Feces Waste material discharged from the large intestine; excrement; stool

Feedback Step in communication that occurs when the listener asks a question, repeats information or otherwise helps the speaker know that the message has been correctly received; method to respectfully share ideas and information about a specific issue

Femur Upper leg bone

Fenestrated Having openings

Fermentation Decomposition of complex organic molecules under the influence of ferments or enzymes; usually associated with living microorganisms

Fertilization Union of an ovum and a spermatozoon

Fetus Developing offspring from the third month of pregnancy until birth

Fever Abnormally high body temperature

Fibrin Blood protein that forms a blood clot

Fibula Smaller bone of the lower leg

Filter Device secured to a rigid sterilization container's lid and/or bottom that allows the passage of air and sterilants; provides a microbial barrier

Filter retention system Mechanism on a rigid sterilization container that secures disposable filters in place

Filtrate Liquid that has passed through a filter

Fimbriae Finger-like projections extending from the fallopian tubes that draw ova (eggs) into the uterus

First in, first out (FIFO) A stock rotation system whereby the oldest product (that which has been in storage the longest) is used first

Fissure Deep groove

Fixative Substance used to keep things in position or stick them together; preserves or stabilizes biological material for examination

Flagella Long, hair-like structures extending from the cell wall of a microorganism that help an organism to move (especially in liquids)

Flammable Combustible substance that ignites very easily, burns intensely or has a rapid rate of flame spread

Flash sterilizer Sterilizer that uses higher temperatures for shorter exposure times (used for emergency sterilization of dropped instruments)

Flatus Gas in the digestive tract

Flexion Bending motion that decreases the angle between bones at a joint

Fluid invasion Damage to powered surgical instruments when water or solution enters the instrument's internal components

Focal infection Localized site of more or less chronic infection from which bacteria or their byproducts are spread to other parts of the body

Fomite An inanimate object that can transmit bacteria

Foot candle Amount of light equivalent to that produced by one standard candle at a distance of one foot

Forceps Instruments used for grasping, holding firmly, or exerting traction upon objects

Forging To form by heating and hammering

Formaldehyde Class of disinfectants most often used to disinfect hemodialysis equipment; also used as a preservative and fumigant. Should be used with caution because of its potential carcinogenic effect and irritating fumes.

Fractional sterilization Sterilization performed at separate intervals, usually for 15–minute periods over three to four days so spores will develop into bacteria that can then be destroyed

Fumigation Disinfection by exposure to a lethal gas/fumigant

Fumes Emanating from a gas or vapor (such as from a disinfectant)

Fungicide Substance that kills fungi

Fungus (pl. fungi) Type of plant-like microorganism; unicellular and multi-cellular vegetable organisms that feed on orgànic matter (e.g., molds, mushrooms and toadstools)

G

Gamma globulin Protein component of blood plasma that contains antibodies

Ganglion Collection of nerve cell bodies located outside the central nervous system

Gangrene Death of tissue due to loss of blood supply; accompanied by bacterial invasion and putrefaction (process of rotting or decay)

Gas State of matter in which molecules are unrestricted by cohesive forces; has neither shape nor volume and is neither liquid nor solid

Gas cylinder safety relief device Installed in a gas cylinder or container to prevent rupture of a cylinder by over pressures resulting from certain conditions of exposure; device may be a frangible (breakable) disc, fusible plug or relief valve

Gasket Pliable strip on sterilization containers that seals the lid and container to prevent entry of microorganisms

Gas pressure regulator Device that may be connected to the cylinder valve outlet to regulate gas pressure delivered to a system

Gastroenteritis Inflammation of the stomach and intestines with symptoms similar to enteritis and dysentery; often caused by an enteric group of bacteria (e.g., *Salmonella paratypih* and *Salmonella schottmuller*)

Gastrointestinal (GI) Pertaining to the stomach and intestine or the digestive tract as a whole

Gauge pressure (steam sterilizer) Pressure inside the sterilizer chamber above atmospheric pressure (14.7 psi at sea level)

Gene Biological unit of heredity; self-reproducing and located in a definite position (locus) on a specific chromosome

Generalized infection One involving the whole body

Genetic Pertaining to genes or heredity

Genus Group of one or more related species

Geobacillus stearothermophilus Highly resistant but relative harmless nonpathogenic microorganism used to challenge steam and dry heat sterilizers

Germ Microorganism that causes disease

Germicidal Related to the destruction of germs

Germicide Agent that kills germs

Glaucoma Disorder involving increased fluid pressure within the eye

Glucagon Hormone that can increase blood sugar level

Glucose Simple sugar; main energy source for cells; dextrose

Gonad Sex gland; ovary or testis

Gonorrhea Contagious venereal disease of the genital mucous membranes; caused by *Neisseria gonorrhoeae*

Gram Basic unit of weight in the metric system

Gram negative Losing the purple stain or decolorized by alcohol in Gram's method of staining; primary identification characteristic of certain microorganisms

Gram positive Retaining the purple stain or resisting decolorization by alcohol in Gram's method of staining

Gram stain Differential stain used to classify bacteria as gram positive or gram negative, depending on whether they retain or lose the primary stain (crystal violet) when subjected to a decolorizing agent

Gravity Pull toward the center of the earth

Greenhouse gases Any gases that absorb solar radiation and are responsible for the greenhouse effect, including carbon dioxide, methane, ozone and fluorocarbons

Gross soil Tissue, body fat, blood and other body substances

H

HAI See Healthcare-acquired infection

Halogen Any of the four very active, non-metallic chemical elements (chlorine, iodine, bromine and fluorine)

Hammer One of the three middle ear bones; attaches to the tympanic membrane

Hand bacterial count Method of estimating the number of bacteria present on one's hand

Hand hygiene Act of washing one's hands with soap and water or using an alcohol-based hand rub

Hardness Amount of dissolved minerals in water that alters the effectiveness of many disinfectants, detergents and soaps

Hazardous waste Substances that cannot be disposed of in the facility's normal trash system

HCFC Abbreviation for hydrochlorofluorocarbon gas; yields an inflammable gas when mixed with other gases

Health care products Medical devices, medicinal products (pharmaceuticals and biologics) and invitro diagnostics

Health Insurance Portability and Accountability Act (HIPAA) Act Privacy rule that provides federal protections for individually identifiable health information held by covered entities and their business associates and gives patients an array of rights with respect to that information

Healthcare-associated infection (HAI) Infection that is not present when a patient is admitted to a healthcare facility; refers to an infection that develops in a patient on or after day three of admission to the healthcare facility

Healthcare Information Management Systems Society (HIMSS) Global, cause-based, not-for-profit organization focused on improving health through the use of information technology

Heart Muscular organ that pumps blood throughout the body

Heat sink Heat-absorbent material; mass that readily absorbs heat

Heat-up time Time required for an entire load to reach a preselected sterilizing temperature after the chamber has reached that temperature

Hematocrit (Hct) Volume percentage of red blood cells in whole blood; packed cell volume

Hematoma Swelling filled with blood

Hemodialysis Removal of impurities from the blood by passage through a semipermeable membrane

Hemoglobin (Hb) Iron-containing protein in red blood cells that transports oxygen

Hemolytic Destruction of red blood cells with the liberation of hemoglobin

Hemorrhage Loss of blood

Hemostasis Stoppage of bleeding

Hemostatic forceps Surgical instrument used to control the flow of blood

Heparin Substance that prevents blood clotting; anticoagulant

Hepatitis Inflammation of the liver; usually caused by the hepatitis virus

Heredity Transmission of genetic characteristics from parent to offspring

Hernia Protrusion of an organ or tissue through the wall of the cavity in which it is normally enclosed

Herpes simplex Mild, acute, eruptive, vesicular virus; disease of the skin and mucous membrane

Herpes zoster Shingles; acute virus disease characterized by a vesicular dermatitis, which follows a nerve trunk

High efficiency particulate air filter (HEPA) Special filters with a minimum efficiency of 99.97%

High-level disinfection (HLD) Destruction of all vegetative microorganisms but not bacterial spores

HIPAA See Health Insurance Portability and Accountability Act

Histology Study of microscopic structure of tissues

HIV Abbreviation for human immunodeficiency virus; HIV infection is a chronic viral infection characterized by progressive destruction of the T-cell, which impairs the body's immune system; disease severity relates to the degree of immune suppression

HMO Abbreviation for health maintenance organization

Homeostasis State of balance within the body; maintenance of body conditions within set limits

Hormones Chemical messengers that travel through the blood and act on target organs

Host Animal, plant or human that supports the growth of microorganisms

HSPA Abbreviation for the Healthcare Sterile Processing Association

Huck towel All-cotton, low-linting surgical towel with a honeycomb-type weave

Human immunodeficiency virus Virus that causes AIDS

Human relations Development and maintenance of effective interpersonal (between people) relationships that enhance teamwork

Humerus Upper arm bone

Humidity Amount of water vapor in the atmosphere; expressed as a percentage of the total amount of vapor the atmosphere can hold without condensation

Hydration Act of combining with water

Hydrocarbon Chemically identifiable compound of carbon and hydrogen

Hydrogen ion concentration Degree of concentration of hydrogen ions in a solution used to indicate the reaction of that solution; expressed as pH (the logarithm of the reciprocal of the hydrogen ion concentration)

Hydrologic cycle Continual movement of water from the atmosphere to the earth and back to the atmosphere

Hydrolysis Splitting of large molecules by the addition of water (as in digestion)

Hydrophilic Refers to a substance that absorbs water; materials with an affinity for water

Hydrophobic Refers to a substance that repels/does not absorb water

Hyperglycemia Abnormal increase in the amount of glucose in the blood

Hypertension High blood pressure

Hypertonic Solution with a higher osmotic pressure than that of a reference solution

Hypoglycemia Abnormal decrease in the amount of glucose in the blood

Hypotension Low blood pressure

Hypothermia Abnormally low body temperature

Hypotonic Solution that is of less that isotonic concentration

Hypoxia Reduced oxygen supply to tissues

I

IAHCSMM Abbreviation for the International Association of Healthcare Central Service Materiel Management [now known as the Healthcare Sterile Processing Association (HSPA)]

Icteric Yellow pigmentation of tissues, membranes and secretions caused by the deposit of bile pigment; usually, a sign of liver or gall bladder disease

Idiopathic Of unknown cause

Idiosyncrasy Individual and peculiar susceptibility or sensitivity to a drug, protein or other matter

Ileum Last portion of the small intestine

Immediate-use container Use of a chemical that will be under the control of and used only by the person who transfers it from a labeled container to another container and only within the work shift in which it is transferred

Immediate use steam sterilization (IUSS) Process designed for cleaning, steam sterilization and immediate delivery of heat-resistant items for use in the procedure room

Immune Exempt from a given infection

Immunity Power of an individual to resist or overcome the effects of a particular disease or other harmful agent

Immunization Process of conferring immunity on an individual

Impact marker Tool that engraves with a forceful impact that indents and "breaks" the polished metal surface, leaving an inscribed marking

Impingement Spray-force action of pressurized water against instruments being processed to physically remove bioburden

Implosion Bursting inward; opposite of an explosion; occurs when cavitation in an energized solution collapses

Inactivation To stop or destroy activity

Inanimate Not endowed with life or spirit; not alive

Incipient Just beginning

Incompatible Not capable of being mixed without undergoing destructive chemical changes or antagonism

Incubate To maintain favorable for growth under optimum environmental conditions

Incubation period Period between when infection occurs and first symptoms appear

Incubator Apparatus for maintaining a constant and suitable temperature for the growth and cultivation of microorganisms

Indefinite Shelf life of hospital-sterilized items without a definite expiration date; based on the premise that shelf life is event related, not time related. Users must ensure that the integrity of the packaging is intact, clean and properly identified.

Indicator (quality) Measurable variable that relates to the outcome of patient care or employee safety

Indirect contact Transfer of infection from contaminated inanimate objects, fingers, water and food

Infarct Area of tissue damaged from lack of blood supply caused by blockage of a vessel

Infection Invasion of body tissue by microorganisms that multiply and produce a reaction

Infection control Control of active infectious disease; requires working knowledge of the usefulness and application of physical and chemical agents that suppress or kill microorganisms, and familiarity with the sources of potentially dangerous microorganisms, routes by which they spread, and their portals of entry into the body

Infectious Having the ability to transmit disease

Inferior Below or lower

Infestation Lodgment, development and reproduction of arthropods on a body or clothing

Inflammation Reaction of tissues to an injury; protective mechanism to an irritant on tissues

Inhibition Act of checking or restraining

Inoculate To implant or introduce causative agents of disease into an animal, plant or microbes onto culture media

Inoculated carrier Carrier on which a defined number of test organisms has been deposited

Inorganic Substance that does not contain carbon; material that has never been alive

Installation qualification (IQ) Obtaining and documenting evidence that equipment has been provided and installed in accordance with its specifications

Instructions for use (IFU) Information provided by a device manufacturer that provides detailed instructions on how to properly use and/or process the device

Instrument Utensil or implement

Instrument washer sterilizer (IWS) Combination unit that washes and sterilizes instruments to ensure the safety of processing personnel

Insulin Hormone that reduces the level of sugar in the blood

Integrated delivery network (IDN) System of healthcare providers and organizations that provides (or arranges to provide) a coordinated range of services to a specific population

Integrating indicator Chemical indicator (CI) designed to react to all critical parameters over a specified range of sterilization cycles and whose performance has been correlated to the performance of the relevant biological indicator (BI) under the labeled conditions of use

Intercellular Between cells

Interfaced Area or system through which one machine is connected to another machine in order to share information (for example, two computers may be interfaced, or a computer and a sterilizer may be interfaced)

Intermediate-level disinfection Process by which viruses, mycobacteria, fungi and vegetative bacteria are destroyed, but not bacterial spores

Intermittent (fractional) sterilization Destruction of microorganisms by moist heat for given periods of time on several successive days to allow spores during the rest periods to germinate into vegetative forms (which are most easily destroyed)

Interstitial Between; pertaining to spaces or structures in an organ between active tissues

Intracellular Within a cell or cells

Intravenous Within or into veins

In-use testing Evaluation of infection control chemicals, aseptic techniques, and sanitary and sterilization procedures under actual working conditions

Inventory Reusable equipment and consumable items used to provide healthcare services for patients

Inventory (consumable) Assets, such as wrapping supplies, processing chemicals, and other items, that are consumed as healthcare services are provided to patients

Inventory (official) Consumable products found in Sterile Processing departments and other storerooms, warehouses and satellite storage areas; included as an asset on a healthcare facility's balance sheet

Inventory (reusable) Assets, such as medical devices and sterilization containers, that can be reused as healthcare services are provided to patients

Inventory service level Percentage of items filled (available) when an order is placed

Inventory stock out rate Percentage of items that cannot be filled (are not available) when an order is placed

Inventory turnover rate Number of times per year (or other time period) that inventory is purchased, consumed and replaced

Inventory (unofficial) Consumable products found in user areas such as surgical locations and labs; unofficial inventory has usually been expensed to user units and is stored in various locations on the units

In vitro Referring to a process or reaction carried out in a culture test tube or petri dish

In vivo In the living body

Iodophor Disinfectant that is a combination of iodine and a solubilizing agent (or a carrier) and which slowly liberates or releases free iodine when diluted with water

Ion Electronically charged particle formed by the loss or gain of one or more electrons

Iris Circular, colored region of the eye around the pupil

Ischemia Lack of blood supply to an area

Islets Groups of cells in the pancreas that produce hormones; islets of Langerhans

ISO 9000 International standards used by participating organizations to help ensure that quality services and products are delivered consistently

Isolate To place by itself; to separate from others

Isotonic Solution having the same osmotic pressure as that of another solution taken as a standard reference

Isotope Form of an element with the same atomic number as another but with a different atomic weight

Issue Act of withdrawing supplies from storage for transfer to areas for use

IUSS See Immediate use steam sterilization

J

Jargon Specialized words or phrases known only by people working in a certain position

Jaundice Excess of bile pigments in blood, skin and mucous membranes, with a resulting yellow appearance of the individual

Jaw Two or more opposable parts that open and close for holding or crushing something between them

Jejunum Second portion of the small intestine

JIT Abbreviation for just in time; method of inventory distribution where a vendor holds inventory for an organization and on a regular basis delivers items that go directly to supply carts

Job description A Human Resources tool that identifies the major tasks performed by individuals in specific positions

Joint Any place where two bones meet

Julian date year Number of days that have elapsed since January 1 of a specific year; also known as Julian day number (JDN)

K

Kidneys Organs that remove excess water and waste substances from the blood in a process that yields urine

Killing power Ability of a chemical to kill bacteria under laboratory conditions and during in-use testing

L

Labeling Legend, work or mark attached to, included in, belonging to or accompanying any medical device

Lacrimal Referring to tears or tear glands

Lactation Secretion of milk

Lactic acid Organic acid that accumulates in muscle cells functioning without oxygen

Laminar airflow Filtered air moving along separate parallel flow planes to surgical suites, nurseries, bacteriology work areas and pharmacies; prevents collection of bacterial contamination or hazardous chemical fumes in work areas

Large intestine (colon) Digestive organ that dehydrates digestive residues (feces)

Larynx Voice box

Laser Device that produces a very intense beam of light

Latching mechanism Mechanical device that secures a rigid sterilization container's lid to the container's bottom

Latent heat Additional heat required to change the state of a substance from solid to liquid at its melting point, or from a liquid to gas at its boiling point after the temperature of the substance has reached either of those points

Lateral Farther from the midline; toward the side

Latex Common form of rubber used in the manufacturing of hospital and medical supplies

Latex sensitivity Sensitivity (allergic reaction) of some people to latex caused by exposure to latex that is improperly processed; symptoms range from skin rash, primarily on the hands, to an anaphylactic reaction

Leak test (endoscope) Endoscope processing procedure that ensures the device's flexible covering and internal channels are watertight

Lean Quality process that focuses on eliminating waste in the production of products

LED Abbreviation for light emitting diode

Lens Biconvex structure of the eye that changes in thickness to accommodate near and far vision; crystalline lens

Lesion Wound or local injury; specific change or morphological alteration by disease or injury

Lethal Pertaining to death

Leukemia Malignant blood disease characterized by the abnormal development of white blood cells

Leukocyte White blood cell

Ligament Band of connective tissue that connects a bone to another bone

Light-emitting diode (LED) Semiconductor diode that emits light when voltage is applied

Lipids Group of fats or fatty substances characterized by insolubility in water

Lipid virus Virus whose core is surrounded by a coat of lipoprotein. Viruses included in this structural category are generally easily inactivated by many types of disinfectants, including low-level disinfectants.

Liquid-proof Material that prevents the penetration of liquids and microorganisms

Liquid-resistant Material that inhibits the penetration of liquids

Liter Basic unit of volume in the metric system

Liver Organ that filters blood to remove amino acids and neutralize some harmful toxins

Load configuration All attributes defining the presentation of products to sterilization process, including: orientation of products within the primary package; quantity and orientation of primary packages(s) within secondary and tertiary packages; quantity, orientation and placement of tertiary packages on sterilizer pallets or within carriers; and quantity and placement of the pallets (or carriers) within the vessel or area

Load control number Label information on sterilization packages, trays or containers that identifies the sterilizer, cycle run, and date of sterilization

Loaned instrumentation Instruments or sets borrowed from a vendor for emergency or scheduled surgical procedures that will be returned to the vendor following use

Local exhaust hood System that captures contaminated air and conducts it into an exhaust duct; also called a venting hood

Local infection One confined to a restricted area

Logarithm Exponent indicating the power to which a fixed number (the base) must be raised to produce a given number

Lot (load) control number Numbers and/or letters by which a specific group of products can be traced to a particular manufacturing or sterilization operation

Low-level disinfection Destruction of some vegetative forms of bacteria

Lumen Interior path through a needle, tube or surgical instrument

Lungs Main organs of the respiratory system whose function is transporting oxygen into the blood and removing carbon dioxide from the blood

Lux Unit of illumination equal to one lumen per square meter

Lymph Fluid in the lymphatic system

Lymphatic system Series of tiny vessels throughout the body that carry lymph fluid to protect the body against disease

Lymphocyte White blood cell involved in antibody production

M

Macromolecules Large molecules (proteins, carbohydrates, lipids and nucleic acids) within a microorganism

Macroscopic Visible to the naked eye

Magnet status Award given by the American Nurses Credentialing Center to hospitals that satisfy factors measuring the strength and quality of nursing care

Magnetic resonance imaging (MRI) Method for studying tissue based on nuclear movement following exposure to radio waves in a powerful magnetic field

Maintenance insurance Equipment outsourcing alternative whereby a hospital retains control of its equipment but contracts with an insurance organization to manage and insure the costs involved in maintaining it

Malaise Indisposition; discomfort or feeling of ill health

Malignant Describing a tumor that spreads or a disorder that worsens and can lead to death

Malnutrition State resulting from lack of food or an essential component of the diet, or faulty use of food in the diet

Mandible Lower jawbone

Manufacturer's instructions for use (IFU) See IFU

Manufacturer Maker or producer of items or equipment

Martensic Metal, also known as 400 series stainless steel, that is magnetic and may be heat-hardened

Material Management department Healthcare department responsible for researching, ordering, receiving and managing inventory (consumable supplies); also referred to as Supply Chain Management

Mastectomy Removal of the breast; mammectomy

Mastication Act of chewing

Measles Rubeola; acute, infectious virus disease characterized by fever, catarrh, coryza, Koplik spots on buccal mucous membrane, and a papular rash

Medial Near the median plane of the body or the midline of an organ

Mediastinum Region between the lungs and organs and the vessels it contains

Medicaid Federal and state assistance program that pays covered medical expenses for low-income individuals; run by state and local governments within federal guidelines

Medical device Any instrument, apparatus, appliance, material or other article used alone or in combination, including software necessary for its proper application intended by the manufacturer. Such devices are used for the diagnosis, prevention, monitoring, treatment or alleviation of disease; diagnosis, monitoring, treatment, alleviation of or compensation for an injury or handicap; investigation, replacement or modification of the anatomy or of a physiological process; or control of conception.

Medicare Federal medical insurance program that primarily serves those older than 65 years (regardless of income), people under 65 with certain disabilities, and those of all ages with end-stage renal disease

MedWatch U.S. Food and Drug Administration's safety information and adverse event reporting system that serves healthcare professionals and the public by reporting serious problems suspected to be associated with the drugs and medical devices prescribed, dispensed or used

Meiosis Process of cell division that halves the chromosome number in the formation of their productive cells

Membrane Thin sheet of tissue

Memory Inherent ability of a substance to return to its original shape and contours

Meningitis Inflammation of the meninges

Menopause Time at which menstruation ceases

Menses Monthly flow of blood from the female reproductive tract

Mesentery Membranous peritoneal ligament that attaches the small intestine to the dorsal abdominal wall

Mesophiles (bacteria) Bacteria that grow best at moderate temperatures [68°F to 113°F (20°C to 45°C)]

Metabolic rate Rate at which energy is released from nutrients in the cells

Metabolism Total chemical changes by which the nutritional and functional activities of an organism are maintained

Metacarpals Hand bones

Metallurgy Science and technology of metals

Metastasis Spread of tumor cells

Metatarsals Bones of the foot

Meter Basic unit of length in the metric system

Methicillin-resistant Staphylococcus aureus (MRSA) Staphylococcus aureus bacteria that have developed a resistance to methicillin, the drug of choice; usually occurs with patients who have had antibiotic therapy for a lengthy period

Microaerophilic Microorganisms that require free oxygen for their growth but in an amount less than that of the oxygen in the atmosphere

Microbes Organisms of microscopic or submicroscopic size; includes viruses, rickettsiae, bacteria, algae, yeasts and molds

Microbiology Scientific study of the nature, life and action of microorganisms

Micron 1/25,000 of an inch or 1/1,000 of a millimeter

Microorganisms Forms of life that are too small to see with the naked eye (e.g., bacteria, viruses and fungi); also called germs and microbes

Midbrain Upper portion of the brain stem

Mil Unit of length or thickness equal to .001 of an inch

Mineral Inorganic substance; dietary element needed in small amounts for health

Min/max (minimum/maximum) System in which orders are placed to reach a predetermined maximum level when a predetermined minimum level is reached

Minimally invasive surgery (MIS) Surgical procedure associated with smaller incisions, less pain and bodily trauma, fewer complications, and a shorter length of stay; often performed through a cannula using lasers, endoscopes or laparoscopes

Minimum effective concentration (MEC) Percentage of the concentration of the active ingredient in a disinfectant or chemical sterilant that is the minimum concentration at which the chemical meets all label claims for activity against specific microorganisms

Mitosis Cell division that produces two daughter cells that are exactly like the parent cell

Mitral valve Located between the left atrium and left ventricle of the heart; bicuspid valve

Mixed culture Growth of two or more microorganisms in the same medium

Mixed infection Simultaneous process of two or more microorganisms causing an infection

Mixture Blend of two or more substances

Mode of transmission (chain of infection) Method of transfer of an infectious agent from the reservoir to a susceptible host

Molds See Fungus

Molecular attraction Adhesive forces exerted between the surface molecules of two bodies in contact

Molecule Smallest quantity of matter that can exist in a free state and retain all of its properties

Monel Trademark used for an alloy of nickel, copper, iron and manganese

Monitor To systematically check or test to control the concentration of a specific ingredient or the execution of a process; may include qualitative and/or quantitative measurements

Monitor To watch, observe, listen to or check (something) for a special purpose over a period of time

Mouth Opening through which air, food and beverages enter the body; beginning of the alimentary canal

MRC Abbreviation for minimum recommended concentration; minimum concentration at which the manufacturer tested the product and validated its performance

MRI See Magnetic resonance imaging

MRSA See Methicillin-resistant staphyloccus aureus

Mucosa Lining membrane that produces mucus; mucous membrane

Mucous Thick, protective fluid secreted by mucous membranes and glands

Mucous membrane Mucus-secreting membrane that lines all body cavities that open externally, including mouth, nose and intestines

Multi-parameter indicator Indicator designed for two or more critical parameters that indicates exposure to a sterilization cycle at stated values of the parameters

Murmur Abnormal heart sound

Musculoskeletal disorders Injuries or disorders of the muscles, nerves, tendons, joints, cartilage, and spinal discs

Muslin Broad term describing a wide variety of plain-weave cotton or cotton/polyester fabrics with approximately 140 threads per square inch

Mutation Change or alteration in the gradual evolution of a microorganism

Mycology Study of molds, yeasts and fungi

Myocardium Middle layer of the heart wall; heart muscle

N

Nasopharynx Portion of the pharynx above the palate

Natural immunity Immunity with which a person or animal is born

Necropsy Postmortem examination or autopsy

Necrosis Death of a mass of tissue while part of the living body

Needle holders Surgical instruments used to drive suture needles to close or rejoin a wound or surgical site; also known as needle drivers

Negative pressure Air pressure inside the room that is lower than the air pressure outside the room, causing the air to flow into the room with the lower (negative) air pressure

Neoplasm Abnormal growth of cells; tumor

Nephron Microscopic functional unit of the kidney

Nerve Bundle of fibers that receives and sends messages between the body and the brain; messages are sent by chemical and electrical changes in the cells that make up the nerves

Neuritis Inflammation of a nerve

Neuron Nerve cell

Neutral Neither acid nor base

Neutralizer Substance added to a medium that stops the action of an antimicrobial agent

NFPA Abbreviation for the National Fire Protection Association

Node Small mass of tissue, such as a lymph node; space between cells in the myelin sheath

Nomenclature System of names used to identify parts of a mechanism or device

Noncondensable gases Those that cannot be liquified by compression under the conditions of temperature and pressure used during the sterilization process

Noncritical device Refers to the Spaulding medical device classification system; device that come in contact with intact skin

Noncritical zone Area of a gown or drape where direct contact with blood, body fluids and other potentially infectious materials is unlikely to occur

Nonionic Atoms with no electrical charge; compounds containing a non-dissociated hydrophilic group, which forms a bond with water

Nonlipid virus Virus whose nucleic acid core is not surrounded by a lipid envelope; generally more resistant to inactivation by disinfectants

Nonpathogenic Not capable of producing disease

Nonpyrogenic Free from fever-causing substances

Nonstock items Items not kept in the central storeroom or Sterile Processing storage area but that are purchased from an outside vendor, as needed, and then delivered to the requesting department

Nontoxic Not poisonous; not capable of producing injury or disease

Nonwoven Fabric made by bonding (as opposed to weaving) fibers together

Normal flora Normal bacterial population of a given area

Nose Organ of smell; filters the air during breathing

Nosocomial Hospital-acquired infection (HAI); pertaining to a hospital; applied to a disease caused in the course of being treated in a hospital

Noxious Physically harmful or destructive to living beings

Nucleotide Building block of deoxyribonucleic acid (DNA) and ribonucleic acid (RNA)

Nucleus Functional center of a cell that governs activity and heredity

O

Occluded Closure of an opening

Ohm Unit of measurement that expresses the amount of resistance to the flow of an electrical current

Olfactory Pertaining to the sense of smell

Oncology Study of tumors

Operational supplies Supplies needed for Sterile Processing department (SPD) operations (e.g., detergents, sterilization wrap, sterilization testing products)

Ophthalmic Pertaining to the eye

Opportunists Microbes that produce infection only under especially favorable conditions

Optimum temperature Applied to bacterial growth, the temperature at which bacteria grow best

Order point (order quantity system) Method of reordering a predetermined quantity of products when a predetermined on-hand level is reached

Organ Part of the body containing two or more tissues that function together for a specific purpose

Organic Describing compounds containing oxygen, carbon and hydrogen; characteristic of, pertaining to or derived from living organisms

Organic materials Compounds containing oxygen, carbon and hydrogen; derived from living organisms; organic matter in the form of serum, blood, pus or feces that can interfere with the activity of disinfectants

Organism Living thing, plant or animal; may be unicellular or multicellular

Origin Source; beginning; end of a muscle attached to a non-moving part

OSHA Abbreviation for the Occupational Safety and Health Administration; concerned with promoting a safe work environment and employee safety

Osmosis Net movement of solvent molecules across a selectively permeable membrane from areas of higher to lower concentrations

Osmotic pressure Tendency of a solution to draw water into it; directly related to the concentration of the solution

Ossification Process by which cartilage is replaced by bone

Osteoblast Bone-forming cell

Osteomyelitis Inflammation of bone marrow

Osteoporosis Abnormal loss of bone tissue with the tendency to cause bone fractures

Osteotomes Chisel-like instruments used to cut or shave bone

Otitis media Inflammation of the middle ear

Outsourcing (equipment) Transfer of control of a hospital's equipment management system to an external entity

Ovaries Female reproductive organs

Ovulation Release of a mature ovum from a follicle in the ovary

Ovum Female sex cell (egg)

Oxidation Involves the act or process of oxidizing, which is the addition of oxygen to a compound with a loss of electrons

Oxidative chemistries Class of compounds containing an additional atom of oxygen bound to oxygen that uses oxidation to interrupt cell function

Oxidize To change by increasing the proportion of the electronegative part or change (an element or ion) from a lower to higher positive valence

Oxidizing agent Material that removes electrons from another substance

Oxygen Gas needed to completely break down nutrients for energy within the cell

Ozone A reactive and unstable oxygen molecule

P

Packaging Application or use of appropriate closures, wrappings, cushioning, containers, and complete identification up to but not including the shipping container and associated packing materials

Pandemic Very widespread epidemic (even of worldwide extent)

Paper (Kraft-type) Medical-grade paper packaging material used for numerous sterilization applications

Paracentesis Puncture through the wall of a cavity (usually to remove fluid or promote drainage)

Parametric release Declaring product to be sterile on the basis of physical and/or chemical process data rather than on the basis of sample testing or biological indicator results

Parasite Plant or animal that lives upon or within another living organism (host) from which it obtains nourishment and at whose expense it grows without giving anything in return

Par cart Distribution method in which a supply cart remains in a given location; is inventoried and is replenished on a regular basis

Parenteral Something that is put inside the body but not by swallowing (e.g., injection administered into a muscle)

Parietal Pertaining to the wall of a space or cavity

Par level (inventory) Desired amount of inventory that should be on hand

Particle Piece of matter with observable length, width and thickness; usually measured in microns

Particulate matter General term applied to matter of miniature size, with observable length, width and thickness (contrasted to nonparticulate matter without definite dimension)

Passivation Chemical process applied during instrument manufacture that provides a corrosion-resistant finish by forming a thin, transparent oxide film

Passive carrier Harbors the causative agent of a disease but without having had the disease

Passive immunity Immunity produced without the body of the person or animal that becomes immune, participating in its production (e.g., production of immunity to diphtheria by injection of diphtheria antitoxin)

Pasteurization Process of heating a fluid to a moderate temperature for a definite period of time to destroy undesirable bacteria without changing its chemical composition

Patella Knee cap

Pathogen Capable of causing disease

Patient care equipment Portable (mobile) equipment (e.g., suction units, temperature management units, infusion therapy devices) used to assist in the care and treatment of patients

Patient care supplies Items dispensed for patient treatment and care (e.g., catheters, implants and bandages)

Pathogenic Capable of producing disease

Pawl Pivoted tongue or sliding bolt on one part of an instrument; adapted to fall into notches or interdental space on another part to permit motion in only one direction

PEL Abbreviation for permissible exposure limit

Pelvis Basin-like structure; lower portion of the abdomen; large bone of the hip

Penicillin Antibiotic produced by the mold *Penicillium notatum*

Periodic automatic replenishment (often called PAR level or PAR system) Inventory replenishment system in which the desired amount of products that should be available is established, and inventory replenishment returns the quantity of products to this level

Penis Male organ of urination and intercourse

Peripheral nervous system (PNS) All nerve tissue outside the central nervous system (CNS)

Peristalsis Rippling motion of muscles in the digestive tract that mixes food with gastric juices to form a thin liquid

Peritonitis Inflammation of the peritoneum

Permissible exposure limit (PEL) Maximum amount or concentration of a chemical that a worker may be exposed to under Occupational Safety and Health Administration (OSHA) regulations

Perpetual inventory system Tracks all incoming and issued supplies to determine, on an ongoing basis, the quantity of supplies in storage

Personal development Activities that identify and develop talent and personal potential, improve one's employability and enhances quality of life

Personal protective equipment (PPE) Part of standard precautions for all healthcare workers to prevent skin and mucous membrane exposure when in contact with a patient's blood and body fluids; includes fluid-resistant protective clothing, disposable gloves, eye protection, face masks, and shoe covers

Pertussis Whooping cough

Petri dish Shallow, covered cylindrical glass or plastic dish used to culture bacteria and in which bacterial colonies may be observed without removing the cover

pH Measure of alkalinity or acidity on a scale of 0 to14; pH of 7 is neutral (neither acid nor alkaline), pH below 7 is acid, and pH above 7 is alkaline

Phagocyte Cell capable of ingesting bacteria or other foreign particles

Phagotization Process by which some cells can ingest bacteria or other foreign particles

Phalanges Bones that comprise the fingers and toes

Pharynx Throat

Phenol Carbolic acid (phenyl alcohol); colorless crystalline compound (C6H5OH) with strong disinfectant properties

Phlebitis Inflammation of a vein

Physiology Study of the functions of body parts and the body as a whole

PI Abbreviation for performance improvement; process to continually improve patient care that identifies performance functions and associated costs that affect patient outcomes and patient and family perception about the quality and value of services provided

Pick and pack Inventory control system for forms and office supplies; Items are shipped/charged to the customer as ordered in minimal quantities, and the customer is financially responsible for the vendor's agreed-upon inventory

Pick list Itemization of specific instruments and supplies needed for a surgical case or a medical procedure

Placenta Structure that nourishes and maintains the developing individual during pregnancy

Plague Acute, often fatal epidemic disease caused by *Pasteurella pestis* and transmitted to man by fleas from rats and other rodents

Plasma Largest component of blood; transports nutrients throughout the body and helps remove waste from the body

Plasmolysis Shrinkage of a cell or its contents due to withdrawal of water by osmosis

Plasmoptysis Escape of protoplasm from a cell due to rupture of the cell wall

Platelets Blood cells that help blood to clot

Pleura Serous membrane that lines the chest cavity and covers the lungs

Pneumonia Inflammatory consolidation or solidification of lung tissue due to presence of an exudate blotting out the air-containing spaces; see Exudate

Pneumothorax Accumulation of air in the pleural space

Point-of-use processing Process that occurs when a medical device is processed immediately before use

Poliomyelitis Viral disease in which there is inflammation of the gray substance of the spinal cord; commonly called infantile paralysis

Pollution State of rendering unclean or impure by adding harmful substances

Polycarbonate Type of plastic; group of thermoplastic polymers containing carbonate groups in their chemical structures

Polyethylene Thermoplastic polymer capable of being produced in thin sheets; exhibits good moisture-vapor barrier qualities but has a high sloughing tendency

Polymerization Molecular reaction that creates an uncontrolled release of energy

Polymerize Process of joining many simple molecules into long chains of more complex molecules whose molecular weight is a multiple of the original and whose physical properties are different

Polyp Protruding growth (often grape-like) from a mucous membrane

Polypropylene Thermoplastic polymer used in a wide variety of applications

Polystyrene Polymer made from the monomer styrene, a liquid hydrocarbon that is commercially manufactured from petroleum

Polyurethane Class of polymers composed of organic units joined by carbamate (urethane) links

Polyvinyl chloride (PVC) High-strength thermoplastic material widely used in applications; world's third-most widely produced synthetic plastic polymer

Porous Possessing or full of pores (minute openings)

Portability Not fixed; can be transported

Portal of entry (chain of infection) Path used by an infectious agent to enter a susceptible host

Portal of exit (chain of infection) Path by which an infectious agent leaves the reservoir

Positive air pressure Situation in which air flows out of a room or area because the pressure in the area is greater than that of surrounding areas

Posterior Toward the back; dorsal

Pounds per square inch gauge (psig) Measure of ambient air pressure; pressure that a gas would exert on the walls of a one cubic-foot container

ppm Abbreviation for parts per million

Preconditioning Treatment of product prior to the sterilization cycle in a room or chamber to attain specified limits for temperature and relative humidity; see Conditioning

Preconditioning area Chamber or room in which preconditioning occurs

Prefix (word element) Comes before the root word element

Premarket approval (PMA) U.S. Food and Drug Administration (FDA) process of scientific and regulatory review to evaluate the safety and effectiveness of Class III medical devices

Preparation and packaging Clean area of the Sterile Processing department where instrument inspection, assembly and packaging are performed; sometimes called the prep and pack or assembly area

Preservative Substance that prevents biologic decomposition of materials when added to them

Preventive maintenance (PM) Service provided to equipment to maintain its proper operating condition by providing planned inspection and detecting and correcting failures before they occur

Primary infection First of two or more infections

Prion Infectious protein particle that, unlike a virus, contains no nucleic acid, does not trigger an immune response and is not destroyed by extreme heat or cold

Procedural area Area within the healthcare facility that performs invasive and minimally-invasive procedures that require instruments, supplies and equipment

Process challenge device (PCD) Object that simulates a predetermined set of conditions when used to test sterilizing agent(s)

Process equivalency Documented evaluation that the same sterilization process can be delivered by two or more pieces of sterilization equipment

Process improvement Activity to identify and resolve task-related problems that yield poor quality; strategy for finding solutions to eliminate the root causes of process performance problems

Process indicators Devices used with individual units (e.g., packs or containers) to demonstrate that the unit has been exposed to the sterilization process and to distinguish between processed and unprocessed units

Processes (work) Series of work activities that produce a product or service

Processing area Where decontaminated, clean instruments and other medical and surgical supplies are inspected, assembled into sets and trays and wrapped, packaged or placed into container systems for sterilization; commonly called the preparation and packaging area if part of Sterile Processing, and "pack room" if textile packs are assembled there

Processing group Collection of products or product families that can be sterilized in the same ethylene oxide (EO) sterilization process; all products within the group have been determined to present an equal or lesser challenge to the sterilization process

Product family Collection of products determined to be similar or equivalent for validation purposes

Professional development Commitment to continuous learning and improvement; taking responsibility for one's own development

Progesterone Hormone produced by the corpus luteum and placenta; maintains the lining of the uterus for pregnancy

Prognosis Prediction of the probable outcome of a disease, based on the patient's condition

Prophylactic Agent used to prevent infection or disease

Prophylaxis Prevention of disease

Prostate gland Produces a fluid element in semen that stimulates the movement of sperm

Prosthesis Artificial replacement of a body part such as an arm or leg

Protective packaging Configuration of materials designed to prevent damage to the sterile barrier system and its contents from the time of their assembly until the point of use

Protein Complex combinations of amino acids containing hydrogen, nitrogen, carbon, oxygen and, usually, sulfur (and sometimes other elements); essential constituents of all living cells

Prothrombin Clotting factor; converted to thrombin during blood clotting

Proton Positively charged particle in the nucleus of an atom

Protoplasm Thick, mucous-like substance that is colorless and translucent and forms the biochemical basis of life found within the cell nucleus

Protozoan One-celled animal-like microorganism of the subkingdom, protozoa

Proximal End of an item that is closest to the point of origin (e.g., the proximal end of the femur is closest to the hip); end of the instrument closest to the operator

Prudent Marked by wisdom or judiciousness; wise

Pseudopodia False feet; temporary protrusions of ectoplasm to provide locomotion

psia Abbreviation for pounds per square inch absolute

Psychrophiles (bacteria) Cold-loving bacteria whose optimum temperature for growth is 59°F to 68°F (15°C to 20°C) or below

Pulse Wave of increased pressure in blood vessels produced by contraction of the heart

Pupil Opening in the center of the eye through which light enters

Pure culture Specific bacterial growth of only one species of microorganism

Purulent Containing pus

Pus Semifluid, creamy product of inflammation consisting of blood cells (mainly white), bacteria, dead tissue cells, and serum

Pyogenic Pus producing

Pyrex Type of hard glass made from borosilicate, which is alkaline free

Pyrexia Fever

Pyrogen Substance typically produced by a bacterium that produces fever when introduced/released into the blood

Pyrogenic Fever producing; byproducts of bacterial growth or metabolism

Q

Quadrant One part of four; to be divided into four equal parts

Qualified personnel Individuals who are prepared by training and experience to perform a specified task

Quality Consistent delivery of products and services according to established standards; integrates concerns for the customers (including patients and user department personnel) with those of the department and facility

Quality assurance Comprehensive and measured efforts to provide total quality; technical, statistical sampling method that measures production quality

Quality control Technical, statistical sampling method that measures production quality

Quarantine Isolation of infected people and contacts who have been exposed to communicable diseases for the time equal to the longest incubation period of the disease to which they have been exposed

Quaternary compound Group of disinfectants having derivatives of benzalkonium chloride as the active ingredient

R

Radiant heat Transmission of heat from one object to another without heating the space in between; process of emitting radiant energy in the form of waves or particles

Radical Group of atoms that behaves as a single atom in a chemical reaction

Radio frequency identification (RFID) Term used to describe a system in which the identity (serial number) of an item is wirelessly transmitted with radio waves

Radius One of the two bones in the forearm

Random numbers (table) Compilation of numbers generated in an unpredictable, haphazardous sequence used to create a random sample

Ratchet (or rachet) Part of a surgical instrument that "locks" the handles in place

Rationale Underlying reason; basis

Recessive Gene that is not expressed if a dominant gene for the same trait is present

Rectum Final several inches of the large intestine

Red blood cells Cells that carry oxygen throughout the body

Reflex Involuntary response to a stimulus

Refraction Bending of light rays as they pass from one medium to another of a different density

Regulation Rules issued by administrative agencies that have the force of law

Relative humidity (RH) Amount of water vapor in the atmosphere; expressed as a percentage of the total amount of vapor the atmosphere could hold without condensation

Remission Diminution or abatement of disease symptoms

Reorder point (ROP) Inventory level available when an order is placed to replenish inventory

Repair (equipment) Procedures used to return equipment to its proper operating condition after it has become inoperative

Requisition system Method of inventory distribution where items needed are requested (requisitioned) by user department personnel and removed from a central storage location for transport to the user department

Reservoir Carrier of an infectious microorganism; generally, refers to a human carrier

Reservoir of agent (chain of infection) Place where an infectious agent (microorganism) can survive

Resident bacteria Bacteria normally occurring at a given anatomical site

Residual (ethylene oxide/EO) Amount of EO that remains inside materials after they are sterilized

Residual property Capacity of an antiseptic or disinfectant to kill microorganisms over a long period of time after initial application

Resistance Ability of an individual to ward off infection

Resorption Loss of substance (such as bone)

Respiration Exchange of oxygen and carbon dioxide between outside air and body cells

Retina Innermost layer of the eye; contains light-sensitive cells (rods and cones)

Retractors Surgical instruments primarily used to move tissues and organs to keep the surgical site exposed throughout the procedure

Retroperitoneal Behind the peritoneum (kidneys, pancreas and abdominal aorta)

Reusable (inventory) Assets that are relatively inexpensive, such as medical devices and sterilization containers, that can be reused as healthcare services are provided to patients

Reusable medical device Intended for repeated use on different patients, with appropriate decontamination and other processing occurring between uses

Reusable surgical textile Drape, gown, towel or sterilization wrapper intended to be used during surgery or to assist in preparing for surgery; made from a fabric (usually woven or knitted), fabric/film laminate, or non-woven material intended for more than one use, with appropriate reprocessing between uses

Reverse osmosis (RO) Water purification process by which impurities are removed from water using a semipermeable membrane

Rhinitis Inflammation of the mucous membrane of the nose

Rib spreaders Retractor used to expose the chest

Ribonucleic acid (RNA) One of two types of nucleic acids; found in the nucleus and cytoplasm and involved in protein synthesis

Rigid container system Instrument container that holds medical devices during sterilization and protects devices from contamination during storage and transport

Risk management Methods used to assess the risks of a specific activity and develop a program to reduce losses from exposure to those risks

Rod Straight, slim mass of a substance related to microorganisms (e.g., rod-shaped bacteria)

Roentgenogram Film produced with of x-rays

Rongeur Surgical instrument used to cut or bite away at bone and tissue

Root cause analysis (RCA) Method of problem solving that "looks backward" to identify the root cause of a problem to help prevent its future occurrence

Root (word element) Tells the primary meaning of a word; also called base word element

S

Sacrum Lower portion of vertebral column

Safety data sheet (SDS) Written statement providing detailed information about a chemical or toxic substance, including potential hazards and appropriate handling methods; provided by the product manufacturer to the buyer and must be available in a place that is easily accessible to those who will use the product

Safety stock Minimum amount of inventory that must be on hand

Saline Containing or pertaining to salt; isotonic aqueous solution of sodium chloride for temporarily maintaining living cells

Saliva Secretion of salivary glands; moistens food and contains an enzyme that digests starch

Sanitary Relating to health; characterized by or readily kept in cleanness

Sanitize To reduce the microbial flora in materials or on articles, such as eating utensils, to levels judged safe by public health standards

Sarcoma Malignant tumor of connective tissue; form of cancer

Saturated steam Steam that contains the maximum amount of water vapor

Scapula Shoulder blade

Scissors Surgical instruments used to cut, incise and/or dissect tissue

Sclera Outermost layer of the eye; "white" of the eye

Scrotum Sac in which testes are suspended

SDS Abbreviation for safety data sheet

Seals (tamper-evident) Sealing method for sterile packaging that allows users to determine if packaging has been opened (contaminated) and helps them identify packages unsafe for patient use

Sebaceous Secreting or pertaining to sebum

Sebum Oily secretion of sebaceous gland that lubricates the skin

Secondary container Generic container that is filled from a primary container or filled with a diluted solution; secondary containers must be clearly labeled with contents

Secondary infection Superimposed infection occurring in a host that is already suffering from a previous infection

Selective action Ability to inhibit or kill one group of microbes and not another

Semen Mixture of sperm cells and secretions from several male reproductive glands

Semi-critical devices Refers to the Spaulding medical device classification system; devices that come in contact with nonintact skin or mucous membranes

Seminal vesicle Gland that produces semen

Sensitivity State of being susceptible

Sensitization Process of sensitizing or making susceptible

Sentinel event Unexpected occurrence involving death, serious physical or psychological injury, or the risk thereof

Sepsis Condition, usually with fever, that results from the presence of microorganisms or their poisons in the bloodstream or other tissues

Septic Relating to the presence of pathogens or their toxins

Septicemia Presence of pathogenic microorganisms or their toxins in the bloodstream; blood poisoning

Septum Dividing wall (e.g., between heart chambers or sides of the nose)

Sequestering agents Chemicals that remove or inactivate hard water minerals

Sequestration Removal or inactivation of water hardness elements by formation of a soluble complex or chelate

Serious injury Injury or illness that is life-threatening, resulting in permanent impairment of a bodily function or permanent damage to a body structure, or necessitates medical or surgical intervention to preclude permanent impairment of a body structure

Serology Science pertaining to serum

Serrations Parallel grooves in the jaws of surgical instruments

Serum Clear fluid exuded when blood coagulates

Service Activity that helps one or more people or groups of people

Service recovery Sequence of steps used to address customer complaints and problems in a manner that yields a win-win situation for the customer and the department

Shank Straight, narrow part of a tool that connects the part that does the work with the handle

Sharps Cutting instruments, including knives, scalpels, blades needles and scissors of all types. Other examples include chisels and osteotomes, some curettes, dissectors and elevators, rongeurs and cutting forceps, punches, saws and trocars.

Shelf carton Intermediate package used to protect the product; boxes intended to be stored in a clean or sterile environment

Shelf life Period of time during which product sterility is assumed to be maintained

Shelf life (disinfectants) Length of time a disinfectant can be properly stored after which it must be discarded

Shock Pertaining to circulation: inadequate output of blood by the heart

Short-term exposure limit (STEL) The maximum concentration of a chemical to which workers may be exposed continuously for up to 15 minutes without danger to health or work efficiency and safety

Sigmoid colon Last portion of large intestine

Sign Manifestation of a disease noted by an observer

Silicate Mineral commonly in water derived from silica in quartz and other components

Simple stain Staining technique using only one dye

Single-parameter indicator Designed for one critical parameter that indicates exposure to a sterilization cycle at a stated value of the chosen parameter

Six Sigma Quality process that focuses on developing and delivering near-perfect products and services

Skin This organ contains sweat glands that, through the process of perspiration, produces and eliminates sweat

Sloughing To cast off one's skin; to separate dead tissue from living tissue

Small intestine Organ in the digestive system where the greatest amount of digestion and absorption of nutrients into body cells occurs

Smear Thin layer of material spread on a glass slide for microscopic examination

SMS Abbreviation for spunbond-meltblown-spunbond; non-woven packaging material that is the most popular flat wrap

Soap Compound of one or more fatty acids, or their equivalent, with an alkaline substance

Softening (sequestering) Process of removing selected substances from hard water

Soft glass Made from alkaline materials that cannot be subjected to high temperatures without causing chemical reactions and possible shredding of the glass

Soluble Able to be dissolved

Solution Mixture with components evenly distributed

Solvent Liquid capable of dissolving another substance

Spaulding classification system Developed by Dr. E.H. Spaulding to divide medical devices into categories based on the risk of infection involved with their use

Species One kind of organism; subdivision of a genus

Sperm Male sex cell

Sphincter Muscular ring that regulates the size of an opening

Sphygmomanometer Device used to measure blood pressure

Spirillum Spiral-shaped bacterium of the genus spirillum; chief pathogens causing rat bite fever and Asiatic cholera

Spirochete Slender, corkscrew-like or spiral-shaped bacteria found on man, animals and plants, and in soil and water; moves in a waving and twisting motion; some cause disease

Spleen Lymphoid organ in the upper left region of the abdomen

Sporadic disease Disease that occurs in neither an endemic nor epidemic

Spore Microorganisms capable of forming a thick wall around themselves to enable survival in adverse conditions; a resistant form of bacterium

Spore strip Paper strip impregnated with a known population of microorganisms and that meets the definition of biological indicator

Sporicide Agent that destroys spores

Stain Substance used to color cells or tissues to differentiate them for microscopic examination and study; see Gram stain

Stainless steel Alloy of steel with chromium and sometimes another element, such as nickel or molybdenum, that is highly resistant to rusting and ordinary corrosion

Standard Uniform method of defining basic parameters for processes, products, services and measurements

Standard Precautions Method of using appropriate barriers to reduce the risk of transmission of bloodborne and other pathogens; applies to all patients, regardless of diagnosis or presumed infectious status

Standardization Being made uniform

Standards (AAMI) Voluntary guidelines representing a consensus of Association for the Advancement of Medical Instrumentation (AAMI) members that are intended for use by healthcare facilities and manufacturers to help ensure that medical instrumentation is safe for patient use

Standards (regulatory) Comparison benchmarks mandated by a governing agency; noncompliance may lead to citations and legal penalties

Standards (voluntary) Guidelines or recommendations for best practices to provide better patient care; developed by industry, non-profit organizations, trade associations and others

Staphylococci Gram-positive bacteria that grow in grape-like clusters

Stasis Stoppage in the normal flow of fluids such as blood, lymph, urine or contents of the digestive tract

Stat Abbreviation for the Latin term "statim," meaning immediately or at once

Statute Written and enforceable law enacted by a governing body

Steam Water vapor at 212°F (100°C) or above

Steam purity Degree to which steam is free of dissolved and suspended particles, water treatment chemicals and other contaminants

Steam quality Weight of dry steam present in a mixture of dry saturated steam and entrained water

STEL Abbreviation for short-term exposure limit

Stenosis Narrowing of a duct or canal

Stereotype Preconceived belief or opinion about a group of people applied to every person in that group

Sterilant/sterilization Physical or chemical entity, or combination of entities, that has sufficient microbicidal activity to achieve sterility under defined conditions

Sterile Completely devoid of all living microorganisms

Sterile field Immediate environment around a trauma site or surgical incision; includes all materials in contact with the wound, gowns worn by the surgical team (front panel from chest to the level of the operative field, and sleeve from the cut to two inches above the elbow), patient drapes (area adjacent to the wound) and table covers (top surface)

Sterile storage area Area of healthcare facility designed to store clean and sterile supplies and protect them from contamination

Sterility assurance level (SAL) The probability of a viable microorganism being present on a device after sterilization

Sterility (event-related) Items are considered sterile unless the integrity of the packaging is compromised (damaged) or suspected of being compromised, regardless of the sterilization date; sometimes referred to as ERS

Sterility (time-related) Package is considered sterile until a specific expiration date is reached

Sterilization Process by which all forms of microbial life, including bacteria, viruses, spores and fungi, are completely destroyed

Sterilization area Location of steam sterilizers, including the space for loading, queuing carts, cool down and unloading carts

Sterilization process monitor Physical/chemical device used to monitor one or more parameters to detect failures due to packaging, loading and/ or sterilizer functioning; cannot guarantee, assure or prove sterilization; measure physical conditions

Sterilization wrap Product intended to enclose another medical device to be sterilized by a healthcare provider and maintain sterility of the enclosed device until used

Sterilizer Equipment used to sterilize medical devices, equipment and supplies by direct exposure to sterilizing agent

Sterilizer (ethylene oxide) Sterilization equipment that utilizes ethylene oxide (EO) under defined conditions of gas concentration, temperature and percent relative humidity

Sterilizer (steam) Sterilization equipment that uses saturated steam under pressure as the sterilant

Sterilizer (steam, dynamic-air-removal type) Steam sterilizer in which air is removed from the chamber and the load by means of pressure and vacuum excursions, or by means of steam flushes and pressure pulses

Sternum Breastbone

Stethoscope Instrument that conveys sounds from the patient's body to the examiner's ears

Stilet (or stylet) Small, sharp, pointed instrument used to probe, stabilize needles or catheters for insertion, and remove obstructions from lumens of needles and tubes

Stockless inventory Distribution method in which supplies are stored by an outside vendor and delivered to the hospital on a regular basis in case lot quantities; minimum inventory is held and paid for by the facility, which is advantageous

Stock outs (inventory) Condition that occurs when reusable or consumable inventory items required to provide healthcare services to patients are not available

Stomach Pouch that serves as a reservoir for food that has been consumed

Strain Specific specimen or culture of a given species

Streptococci Bacteria which divide to form chains; members of the genus streptococcus which are gram-positive, chain-forming bacteria

Strikethrough Penetration of liquid or microorganism through a fabric

Subcutaneous Under the skin

Subordinate Employee supervised by someone in a higher organizational position

Suction devices Surgical instruments used to extract blood and other fluids from a surgical site

Suffix (word element) Comes after the root word element

Super-heated steam Occurs when dry steam becomes too hot compared to saturated steam; dry steam rises to a temperature higher than the boiling point of saturated steam (this commonly occurs when dehydrated linen is processed in a steam sterilizer). Due to the lack of moisture, dry steam is not an effective sterilant and will often char or burn items in the sterilizer.

Super heating Occurs when dry steam becomes too hot compared to saturated steam (dry steam rises to a temperature higher than the boiling point of saturated steam; commonly occurs when dehydrated linen is processed in a steam sterilizer); due to the lack of moisture, dry steam is not an effective sterilant and will often char or burn items in the sterilizer

Superior Above; in a higher position

Supply Chain Management Department that procures and distributes resources, manages supplies, goods and services to providers and patients; also known as Materials Management department

Surface tension Contractile surface force of a liquid that makes it tend to assume a spherical form (example: to form a meniscus); also exists at the junction of two liquids

Surfactant Substance that lowers the surface tension of the water and increases the solubility of organic compounds

Surgical drape Device made of natural or synthetic materials and used as a protective patient covering; isolates a site of surgical incision from microbial and other contamination

Surgical gown Devices worn by Operating Room (OR) personnel during surgical procedures to protect the patient and OR staff from transfer of microorganisms, body fluids and particulate matter

Surgical site infection Infection that occurs after surgery in the part of the body where the surgery took place

Surgical towel Absorbent product, typically made of cotton and intended to be used in a patient care procedure

Susceptible host (chain of infection) Person or animal that lacks the ability to resist an infection by an infectious agent

Suspension Mixture that will separate unless shaken

Sustainability Process(es) designed to reduce harm to the environment or deplete natural resources, thereby supporting long-term ecological balance

Suture Joint in which bone surfaces are closely united (e.g., skull); stitch used in surgery to bring parts together

Symbiosis Living together or close association of two dissimilar organisms with mutual benefit

Symptom Subjective disturbance due to disease

Synapse Junction between two neurons or between a neuron and an effecter

Syndrome Group of symptoms characteristic of a disorder

Synergism Action of an inactive material that improves or increases the action of an active material; case in which the sum of the actions of two or more active materials mixed together is greater than the sum of their individual actions

Synovial Pertaining to a thick, lubricating fluid found in joints, bursae and tendon sheaths; pertaining to freely movable (diarthrotic) joint

Synthetic Produced by chemical synthesis rather than of natural origin

Systole Contraction phase of the cardiac cycle

T

Tabletop sterilizer Compact steam sterilizer with a chamber volume of not more than two cubic feet that generates its own steam with distilled or deionized water added by the user

Tachycardia Heart rate greater than 100 beats per minute

Tamper-evident seals Sealing method that allow users to determine if sterile packages have been opened (contaminated) and help users identify packages that are unsafe for patient use

Tap water Treated water that is acceptable for drinking

Tarsals Ankle bones

T cell Lymphocyte active in immunity that matures in the thymus gland; destroys foreign cells directly

Technical information report (TIR) Developed by experts in the field and contains valuable information needed by the healthcare industry

Technical quality control indicators Process control measures utilized to assure that planned technical conditions within sterilizers and aerators are met

Tendinitis Inflammation of a tendon

Tendon Cord of fibrous tissue that attaches a muscle to a bone

Terminal disinfection Disinfection of a room after it has been vacated by a patient

Terminal infection Infection with streptococci or other pathogenic bacteria that occurs during the course of a chronic disease and causes death

Terminal sterilization Process by which surgical instruments and medical devices are sterilized in their final containers, allowing them to be stored until needed

Testes Male reproductive gland that forms and secretes sperm and several fluid elements in semen

Testosterone Male sex hormone produced in the testes; promotes the development of sperm cells and maintains secondary sex characteristics

Tetanus Constant contraction of a muscle; infectious disease caused by a bacterium (*Clostridium tetani*); lockjaw

Tetany Muscle spasms due to abnormal calcium metabolism as in parathyroid deficiency

Therapy Treatment of disease

Thermal disinfection Use of heat to reduce the amount of microorganisms (excluding spores) on a medical device

Thermal equilibrium Condition in which all parts of a system have reached the same temperature; in a steam autoclave or hot-air oven, when the temperature throughout the entire load is the same

Thermocouple Device composed of two lengths of wire, each of which is made of a different homogenous metal; used to measure temperature changes by connecting a potentiometer or pyrometer into the thermocouple circuit

Thermolabile Easily altered or decomposed by heat

Thermophiles (bacteria) Bacteria which grow best at a temperature of 122°F to 158°F (50°C to 70°C)

Thermostable Not easily affected by moderate heat

Thermostatic Controlled by temperature

Thorax Chest; thoracic

Threshold limit value (TLV) Refers to airborne concentrations of substances and represents conditions under which it is believed that nearly all workers may be repeatedly exposed day after day without adverse health effects

Thrombocyte Blood platelet; participates in clotting

Thrombus Blood clot within a vessel

Thumb forceps Tweezer-like instrument with smooth tip; used to grasp objects

Thyroid Endocrine gland in the neck

Tibia Large bone in lower leg

Time-weighted average (TWA) Amount of a substance employees can be exposed to over an eight-hour day

Tincture Liquid in which a chemical is dissolved in alcohol

Tissue Group of similar cells that performs a specialized function

Tissue culture Cultivation of tissue cells in vitro

Tissue forceps Tweezer-like instrument with teeth to grasp tissue

Titer Concentration of infective microbes in a medium; amount of one substance to correspond with given amount of another substance

Titration Volumetric determination against stand solutions of known strength

TLV-C Abbreviation for threshold limit value ceiling; concentration that should not be exceeded during any part of the working exposure; if instantaneous monitoring is not feasible, the TLV-C can be assessed by sampling over a 15-minute period, except for substances that may cause immediate irritation when exposures are brief

TLV-TWA Abbreviation for threshold limit value-time-weighted average; TWA concentration for a normal eight-hour workday and a 40-hour work week, to which nearly all workers may be repeatedly exposed, day after day, without adverse effect

TLV-STEL Abbreviation for threshold limit value-short-term exposure limit; supplements the TLV-TWA where there are recognized acute effects from a substance with toxic effects that result primarily from chronic exposures; STELS are the legal maximum average exposure for a 15-minute time period

Tolerance Ability to withstand or endure without ill effects

Tonsil Mass of lymphoid tissue in the pharynx region

Total acquisition costs All costs incurred by a facility to purchase a specific supply or equipment item from the point of authorization through its disposal

Total quality improvement (TQI) System that measures the current output of a process or procedure and then modifies it to increase the output, efficiency and/or effectiveness

Total quality management (TQM) Quality management approach based on participation of all members aimed at long-term success through customer satisfaction and benefits to all members of the organization and society

Toxemia General intoxication caused by absorption of bacterial products, usually toxins, formed at a local source of infection

Toxic Poisonous

Toxic anterior segment syndrome (TASS) Acute postoperative inflammatory reaction in which a noninfectious substance enters the anterior segment and induces toxic damage to the intraocular tissues

Toxin Poisonous substance produced by and during the growth of certain pathogenic bacteria

Toxoid Detoxified toxin that produces specific antibodies; neutralized specific toxins used to immunize against bacteria that produce specific toxins

TQM Abbreviation for total quality management

Trachea Windpipe

Tracheostomy Surgical opening into the trachea to introduce a tube through which the patient may breathe

Trait Characteristic

Transducer Device that converts energy from one form to another (e.g., an ultrasonic transducer changes high-frequency electrical energy into high-frequency sound waves)

Transmission Transfer of anything (such as a disease)

Transplant Portion of a bacterial culture that has been transferred from an old pure culture to a fresh new medium

Triage System designed to sort out or classify emergency room patients according to severity of injury or disease

Tricuspid valve Valve between the right atrium and right ventricle of the heart

Tuberculin Filterable substance produced in the growth of mycobacterium tuberculosis in culture media; when injected intracutaneously in people exposed to the tuberculosis bacillus or its products, a reaction is produced in 24 to 48 hours that consists of infiltration and hyperemia

Tuberculocidal Having the ability to kill tubercle bacilli

Tuberculosis Highly variable and communicable disease of man and some animals caused by the tubercle bacillus (Mycobacterium tuberculosis); characterized by the formation of tubercles in the lungs or elsewhere

Turbidity Occurs when water contains sediments or solids that, when stirred, make the water appear cloudy

Turnkey Of or involving the provision of a complete product or service that is ready for immediate use

Turnover/turnaround Describes instruments or equipment that must receive priority processing in order to be made available for another procedure

Tympanic membrane Membrane between the external and middle ear that transmits sound waves to the bones of the middle ear; eardrum

Type 5 (chemical integrators) Integrating indicators designed to react to all critical parameters over a specified range of sterilization cycles

U

Ubiquitous Present everywhere or in many places

Ulcer Area of the skin or mucous membrane in which the tissues are gradually destroyed

Ulna One of the two bones in the forearm

Ultrasonics Physical science of acoustic waves that oscillate in approximate range of 18 to 80 KHz.

Ultraviolet radiation (UV) Invisible component of sun's radiation; used infrequently to degerm air and inanimate objects

Umbilical cord Structure that connects the fetus with the placenta; contains vessels that carry blood between the fetus and placenta

Umbilicus Small scar on the abdomen that marks the former attachment of the umbilical cord to the fetus; navel

Unicellular Composed of a single cell

Universal precautions See Standard precautions

Unsanitary Deficient in sanitation; unclean to such a degree as to be injurious to health

UPC Abbreviation for universal product code

Ureters Tube-like structures extending from the kidneys to the urinary bladder that move urine between those organs

Urethra Tube that discharges urine

Urinary bladder Reservoir for urine

Urine Liquid waste excreted by kidneys

Use life (disinfectants) Length of time (or number of times) a disinfectant can be used after which the efficacy of a disinfectant is diminished

Utensil Instrument or container for domestic use; in hospitals, an item used for basic patient care (e.g., bed pan or wash basin)

Uterus Female organ within which the fetus develops during pregnancy

Utility water Water as it comes from the tap that may need further treatment to achieve the required specifications; primarily used for flushing, washing and rinsing

Uvula Soft, fleshy, V-shaped mass that hangs from the soft palate

V

Vaccination Introduction of a vaccine into the body

Vaccine Substance used to produce active immunity; usually a suspension of attenuated or killed pathogens given by inoculation to prevent a specific disease

Vagina Muscular canal in a female that extends from an external opening to the neck of the uterus

Validation Procedures used by device manufacturers to obtain, record and interpret test results required to establish that a process consistently produces a sterile product

Value analysis Study of the relationship of design, function and cost of a product, material or service

Valve Structure that prevents fluid from flowing backward (as in the heart, veins and lymphatic vessels)

Vancomycin-resistant enterococcus (VRE) Enterococcus bacteria that are no longer sensitive to vancomycin (transmission can occur either by direct contract or indirectly by hands)

Vapor Substance in the gaseous state that is usually a liquid or solid

Variance Difference between the amount of a supply that should be available (from records)and the amount that is available (from physical count) when a perpetual inventory system is used

Varicella Chickenpox

Varicose Pertaining to an unnatural swelling (e.g., varicose vein)

Variola Smallpox

Vas deferens Duct that transfers sperm from the epididymus to the seminal vesicle

Vasoconstriction Decrease in the diameter of a blood vessel

Vasodilation Increase in the diameter of a blood vessel

VD Abbreviation for venereal disease

Vector Carrier of pathogenic microorganisms from one host to another (e.g., flies, fleas and mosquitoes)

Vegetative bacteria Non-spore forming bacteria or spore-forming bacteria in a non-sporulating state

Vegetative stage Active growth of microorganisms (as opposed to resting or spore stages)

Veins Vessels that carry blood back to the heart

Vena cava One of two large veins that carry blood into the right atrium of the heart

Venereal disease (VD) Disease transmitted through sexual activity

Venous Relating to vein or veins

Ventilation Movement of air into and out of the lungs

Ventral Toward the front or belly surface; anterior

Ventricles Two lower chambers of the heart

Venule Very small vein that collects blood from the capillaries

Verification Procedures used by healthcare facilities to confirm that the validation undertaken by the equipment manufacturer is applicable to the specific setting

Vertebra One of the bones of the spinal column

Vesicle Small sac or blister filled with fluid

Viable Living having the ability to multiply

Virology Study of virus and viral diseases

Virucide Agent that destroys or inactivates viruses

Virulence Capacity of microorganisms to produce disease; power of an organism to overcome defenses of the host

Virus One of a group of minute infectious agents that grow only in living tissues or cells

Viscera Organs in the ventral body cavities (especially the abdominal organs)

Vital Characteristic of life; necessary for life; pertaining to life

Vitreous humor Fluid-filled compartment that gives shape to the eye

VRE Abbreviation for vancomycin resistant enterococcus; transmitted by direct contract or indirectly by hands. When enterococcus bacteria are no longer sensitive to vancomycin, treatment is a challenge.

W

Warranty Guarantee or assurance from a seller to the buyer that the goods or property is or shall be as represented

Washers Automated equipment used to clean, decontaminate or disinfect (low, intermediate, or low level) and dry medical devices

Wet pack Package or container that contains moisture after the sterilization process is completed

Wetting agent Substance that reduces the surface tension of a liquid and allows the liquid to penetrate or spread more easily across the surface of a solid

Wetting power Reduction of the water surface tension, which allows the water to run or spread evenly over the surface

White blood cells Cells that circulate in the blood and help defend the body against infection or foreign invaders

Wicking material Approved absorbent, non-linting material that allows for air removal and steam penetration and facilitates drying

Word elements Parts of a word

Workplace violence Any act or threat of physical violence, harassment, intimidation or other threatening or disruptive behavior that occurs at the work site

Work practice controls Controls that reduce the likelihood of exposure by altering the manner in which a task is performed (e.g., prohibiting recapping needles with a two-handed technique)

Work-related musculoskeletal disorder (WMSD) Injury to or disorder of the musculoskeletal system where exposure to workplace risk factors may have contributed to the disorder's development or aggravated a pre-existing condition

X

X-ray Radiation of extremely short wavelength that can penetrate opaque substances and affects photographic plates and fluorescent screens

Y

Yeasts Any of several unicellular fungi of the genus, Saccharomyces, which reproduce by budding

Z

Ziehl-Neelsen stain Method used to classify bacteria as gram positive or gram negative

Index

A

B

C

D

M

N

T